MEDITATION REVOLUTION

The Authors
(In order of their appearance in the text)

Douglas Renfrew Brooks, professor of religion and chairperson of the Committee on Asian Studies at the University of Rochester in Rochester, New York, has written *The Secret of the Three Cities: An Introduction to Hindu Śākta Tantrism*, published in 1990 by the University of Chicago Press, and *Auspicious Wisdom: The Texts and Traditions of Śrīvidyā Śākta Tantrism in South India*, published in 1992 by the State University of New York Press. His Ph.D. is from Harvard University.

Swami Durgananda, a member of the Sarasvatī Order of *daśanāmī sannyāsa*, took monastic vows in 1982 and has practiced Siddha Yoga since 1974. A former journalist, Swamiji was for many years the chief chronicler of events around Swami Muktananda. She also edited many of Muktananda's books, including *Play of Consciousness, Where Are You Going? A Guide to the Spiritual Journey*, and *I Have Become Alive.* She was the founding editor of *Darshan*, the Siddha Yoga magazine, and is one of the principal teachers of Siddha Yoga.

Paul E. Muller-Ortega is professor of religion at the University of Rochester in Rochester, New York. He is the author of *The Triadic Heart of Śiva: Kaula Tantricism of Abhinavagupta in the Non-Dual Shaivism of Kashmir*, published by the State University of New York Press in 1989 and a number of articles on Śaivism. His latest book, *Journey to Cidambaram: Meditations of Śiva, Hindu God of Ecstasy*, is forthcoming from SUNY Press. His Ph.D. is from the University of California at Santa Barbara.

William K. Mahony, professor of religion at Davidson College in Davidson, North Carolina, was the assistant editor of *The Encyclopedia of Religion*, a sixteen-volume edition published in 1987 by the Macmillan Publishing Company. He has written numerous publications, including *The Artful Universe: An Introduction to the Vedic Religious Imagination*, which is forthcoming from the State University of New York Press. He received his Ph.D. from the University of Chicago.

Constantina Rhodes Bailly is an assistant professor of religious studies at Eckerd College in St. Petersburg, Florida and the author of *Shaiva Devotional Songs of Kashmir: A Translation and Study of Utpaladeva's Shiva Stotravali*, which was published in 1987 by the State University of New York Press and reissued in 1994 as *Meditations on Shiva.* She received her Ph.D. from Columbia University.

S. P. Sabharathnam, on the faculty of the Muktabodha Indological Research Institute in Ganeshpuri, India, was for over twenty years a professor at the Vaishnav College in Madras and was also associated with the Department of Śaiva Siddhānta at the University of Madras. Among his published works are *Nādamenium Koyilile* (a treatise on Āgamic literature), *Atmopadeśa Śatakam* (Narayaṇa Guru's Malayalam work), and *Guruprakasam,* (a commentary on the *Kumarastavam*), all in Tamil.

MEDITATION REVOLUTION

A History and Theology of the Siddha Yoga Lineage

Douglas Renfrew Brooks
Swami Durgananda
Paul E. Muller-Ortega
William K. Mahony
Constantina Rhodes Bailly
S. P. Sabharathnam

AGAMA PRESS
Muktabodha Indological Research Institute

Published by Agama Press
South Fallsburg, New York, U.S.A.

Production by Dana Foote
Typesetting by Eastern School Press
Cover design by Chiquita Babb

First published 1997
Printed in the United States of America

Grateful acknowledgment is given for use of material from the following sources: Unless indicated otherwise, all passages noted from *Jñāneśvarī* are from *Jnaneshwar's Gita,* rendered by Swami Kripananda. Copyright © 1989 by State University of New York Press. Reprinted by permission of SUNY Press.

Quotations from *Daughters of the Goddess: The Woman Saints of India* by Linda Johnsen (1994, Yes International Publishers, St. Paul, MN 612–645–6808) are reprinted with permission of the publishers.

The cover illustration is a photograph of the sun; an artistic representation of the Blue Pearl, the light of God that the Siddha Yoga gurus teach is within every human being.

Library of Congress Catalog Card Number: 97-73501

ISBNs 0-9654096-1-9 (hc) 0-9654096-0-0 (pbk.)

The paper used in this publication meets the minimum requirements of the American National Standard for Information Sciences—Permanence of Paper for Printed Library Materials, ANSI Z39.48–1984.

Illustrations:
The cover photograph is by Arthur Nichols; the painting on p. 12 is by Shane Conroy; the photos on pp. 17, 21, 46, 522 are by Suvarna Shetty; p. 55, Dnyaneshwar Gadekar; pp. 87, 108, 120, 123, Gauri Hubert; pp. 142, 146, Susan Bransfield; pp. 157, 563, Melissa Markis; p. 160, Suzanne Gold; p. 536, Kanta Kraseski, p. 566, Elin Dickens.

Dedication

yatsatyena jagatsatyaṃ yatprakāśena bhāti tat /
yadānandena nandanti tasmai śrīgurave namaḥ //
Gurugītā 36

Contents

List of Illustrations / ix

A Note on the Translations and the Sanskrit / xi

Foreword / xiii
Gerald J. Larson

Acknowledgments / xvii

Introduction
The Experience of Perfected Yogis / xix
Douglas Renfrew Brooks

Part I
History

1 To See the World Full of Saints
The History of Siddha Yoga as a Contemporary Movement / 3
Swami Durgananda

Without Talking, He Gave Instructions:
Bhagawan Nityananda of Ganeshpuri / 7

'He Has Become Śiva':
Swami Muktananda and the Gift of Shaktipat / 25

When You Stand Next to a Fire, You Get Warm:
Swami Muktananda's Tours / 71

Everything Happens Through His Grace:
The Passage of Power / 115

Let Every Action Be an Offering:
The Mission of Gurumayi Chidvilasananda / 135

Part II
Theology

2 The Siddha
Paradoxical Exemplar of Indian Spirituality / 165
Paul E. Muller-Ortega

3 The Guru-Disciple Relationship
The Context for Transformation / 223
William K. Mahony

4 The Canons of Siddha Yoga
The Body of Scripture and the Form of the Guru / 277
Douglas Renfrew Brooks

5 The Self
A Vedāntic Foundation for the Revelation of the Absolute / 347
William K. Mahony

6 Shaktipat
The Initiatory Descent of Power / 407
Paul E. Muller-Ortega

7 Kuṇḍalinī
Awakening the Divinity Within / 445
Douglas Renfrew Brooks & Constantina Rhodes Bailly

8 Siddha Yoga as *Mahāyoga*
Encompassing All Other Yogas / 497
S. P. Sabharathnam

9 The Ashram
Life in the Abode of a Siddha / 521
William K. Mahony

Appendix 1: Siddha Yoga Publications / 569
Appendix 2: Swami Muktananda's Three World Tours / 575
Appendix 3: Siddha Yoga Courses and Intensives (1994) / 581

Notes / 589

Bibliography / 655

Index / 673

Author Index / 707

A Note on the Muktabodha Indological Research Institute / 711

ILLUSTRATIONS

1. Painting of the young Nityananda from a photograph taken September 24, 1926 / 12

2. Bhagawan Nityananda / 16

3. Nityananda in the village of Ganeshpuri, with his ashram, Kailas Bhavan, under construction in the background, ca. 1958 / 21

4. Swami Muktananda in Kasara, a sparsely populated region in western India, ca. 1953 / 30

5. Muktananda in front of his meditation hut in the village of Suki, 1955 / 37

6. The original rooms of Gurudev Siddha Peeth, then the Gavdevi Ashram, facing a rose garden, planted and tended by Muktananda, ca. 1958 / 43

7. Swami Muktananda with his guru, Bhagawan Nityananda, during darshan in Kailas Bhavan in 1959 / 46

8. After several years of growth, Shree Gurudev Ashram in the mid-1960s / 50

9. Swami Muktananda, in his meditation room at Shree Gurudev Ashram / 55

10. Malti, with her guru, Swami Muktananda, mid-1960s / 63

11. Swami Muktananda leading a chant, in the Bhagawan Nityananda Temple in Shree Gurudev Ashram, with Malti, playing a tamboura, a traditional stringed instrument / 68

12. Swami Muktananda on his first world tour, 1970 / 77

13. Swami Muktananda in the courtyard of the Oakland Ashram during his second world tour, 1974–76 / 87

14. Muktananda speaking on his third world tour / 108

15. Malti taking *brahmacarya dīkṣā* in preparation for *sannyāsa dīkṣā,* April 1982 / 120

16. Swami Muktananda bidding farewell to Swami Chidvilasananda, as she leaves Gurudev Siddha Peeth for her first meditation retreat as the guru, July 1982 / 123

17. A Caturmāsya Śrauta *yajña,* a 3,500-year-old Vedic ritual, held in Gurudev Siddha Peeth in 1990 / 137

18. Swami Chidvilasananda giving a talk in Mexico City in February 1996 / 142

19. Gurumayi visiting the Shrine of Our Lady of Montserrat in Spain, April 1996 / 146

20. Gurumayi giving a talk in Palm Springs, California, December 1995 / 157

21. Following a morning program in the Shakti Mandap, Gurumayi and some of her students on a walk on the grounds of Shree Muktananda Ashram; summer 1996 / 160

22. Zipruanna in the village of Nasirabad in northern Maharashtra / 171

23. Swami Muktananda with Hari Giri Baba in the village of Chalisgaon, 1953 / 173

24. Bhagawan Nityananda, in Kailas Bhavan, in Ganeshpuri village / 178

25. Sai Baba of Shirdi / 188

26. Gurudev Siddha Peeth, the Siddha Yoga ashram in Ganeshpuri, India, in the late 1970s / 522

27. Tansa Valley in Maharashtra, as seen from the gardens of Gurudev Siddha Peeth, 1981 / 527

28. The Swami Muktananda Samadhi Shrine at Gurudev Siddha Peeth, 1996 / 530

29. The Bhagawan Nityananda Temple at Shree Muktananda Ashram in South Fallsburg, New York, 1986 / 536

30. An aerial view of Anugraha, the oldest facility at Shree Muktananda Ashram, October 1996 / 563

31. The courtyard at Gurudev Siddha Peeth / 566

A Note on the Translations and the Sanskrit

Unless otherwise attributed, any translation and rendering of an original text is by the author of the chapter in which it appears.

For the reader's convenience, the Sanskrit and Hindi terms most frequently used in Siddha Yoga literature and courses appear throughout the text in roman type with simple transliteration. *Śaktipāta,* for instance, is shaktipat; *darśana* is darshan, and so on. Since the transliteration styles for Sanskrit words have varied considerably in Siddha Yoga publications over the years, quotes from the Siddha Yoga gurus reflect a variety of conventions. Also throughout the text, names of places and geographical features do not include diacriticals. Otherwise, the standard international transliteration scheme for South Asian languages has been used.

For those readers not familiar with Sanskrit, the following is a guide for pronunciation:

Vowels

Sanskrit vowels are categorized as either long or short. In English transliteration, long vowels are indicated with a macron, a horizontal line over the vowel, with the exception of the *e* and the *ai,* and the *o* and the *au,* which are always long.

Short	**Long**
a as in *cup*	*ā* as in *calm*
i as in *give*	*ī* as in *seen*
u as in *full*	*ū* as in *school*
ṛ as in *written*	*e* as in the Spanish *sera*
	o as in *know*
	ai as in *aisle*
	au as in *cow*

Consonants

The main differences between Sanskrit and English pronunciation of consonants are in the aspirated and retroflexive letters.

The aspirated letters have a definite h sound. The Sanskrit letter *kh* is pronounced as in *inkhorn;* the *th* as in *boathouse.*

The retroflexes are pronounced with the tip of the tongue touching the hard palate; *ṭ*, for instance, is pronounced as in *ant*; *ḍ* as in *end*.

The sibilants, which are often confused, are *ś*, *ṣ*, and *s*. The *ś* is pronounced as *sh* but with the tongue touching the soft palate; the *ṣ* as *sh* with the tongue touching the hard palate; the *s* as in *history*.

Other distinctive consonants are these:

c as in *church*	*ñ* as in *canyon*
ch as in *pitch-hook*	*ṃ* is a strong nasal
ph as in *loophole*	*ḥ* is a strong aspiration

Foreword

The term *yoga,* which is perhaps best rendered simply as any "disciplined meditation," refers to a wide variety of movements and practices that are especially characteristic of the spirituality of India. Yoga is as old or older than recorded history, its origins for the most part lost in the antiquity of Central, Western, and South Asia. It is possibly related to certain kinds of archaic shamanic traditions or other comparable techniques of physical and mental exertion (trances, auditory practices, fasting, and so forth) utilized from time immemorial for purposes of self-transformation, but there is not clear evidence for its specific beginnings. In India it is distinguished early on from two other modalities of spirituality characteristic of the religious life of South Asia, namely, *yajña* (sacrificial ritual) and *bhakti* (devotion to a particular deity), although it is also clearly related to ritual and devotion. One might well suggest that yoga as "disciplined meditation" represents a "ritual interiorization" as Mircea Eliade has suggested in his *Yoga: Immortality and Freedom,* an internal burning and cleansing that parallels the external burning of the sacrificial oblation. In this sense the practice of disciplined meditation is a form of sacrifice, the sacrifice of oneself.[1] Or again, one might well suggest that yoga represents a form of devotion insofar as disciplined meditation sometimes occurs in an environment of the apprehension of one kind of God or another. Certainly in the famous *Bhagavadgītā* of the early centuries of the Common Era, *bhaktiyoga* or the "disciplined meditation of devotion" is listed as an important, and even superior, form of yoga. Overall, however, it is fair enough to observe that there is usually a recognized distinction between the spirituality characteristic of ritual sacrifice, the spirituality characteristic of devotion to the gods, and the spirituality characteristic of the practice of disciplined meditation or yoga. Devotion and ritual may well serve as metaphors for certain modes of yoga, but for the most part yoga is understood as a unique form of spirituality in and of iself. To refer again briefly to Eliade, whereas shamanic practice, ritual observance, and devotion are largely "ecstatic" forms of spirituality (a moving outside of oneself, a "standing out") wherein the practitioner empties or loses ordinary awareness for the sake of being ecstatically "filled up" or, perhaps better, lifted up or lifted out for the sake of a new identity provided by the spirits or gods, in the practice of yoga there is much more of an "enstatic" focus, a going deeply within (a "standing within") for the sake of finding ultimate truth in one's innermost selfhood.[2]

In any case, while there are many kinds of yoga, and one can speculate endlessly about its modalities or varieties of manifestation, this particular book deals with one specific type and one specific tradition of yoga, namely, the Siddha Yoga of Gurumayi Chidvilasananda and her spiritual predecessors (gurus) in the tradition: the ascetic known as Nityananda, who lived in the early decades of the twentieth century in India and was a "born" Siddha or "perfected one" (and, hence, having no immediate predecessor); and his disciple to whom he passed on the lineage, Swami Muktananda, who began his work in the middle of the twentieth century. Today the movement in the United States is officially referred to as SYDA (the "Siddha Yoga Dham Associates") Foundation, or simply as Siddha Yoga, with primary headquarters or ashrams in Ganeshpuri (in the state of Maharashtra) in India and South Fallsburg (in the state of New York) in the U.S. There are also numerous other centers of the movement throughout the world.

The Siddha Yoga of Gurumayi is an unusual combination of Śaivite spirituality from ancient India, mainly of the Kashmir Śaiva variety, and what Agehananda Bharati has called the "yoga-oriented guru-disciple movements" of Hindu-based spirituality deriving from India that have become so popular in Europe and the United States (and elsewhere) since the middle of the twentieth century.

What makes this book particularly interesting, however, is that it is a serious historical and theological treatment of the movement by a group of sophisticated and critical scholars who are themselves followers of Gurumayi's Siddha Yoga. In other words, we are dealing here with critical scholars who do not shy away from advocacy. We are, of course, familiar with theological advocacy in Christian, Jewish, and Islamic scholarly circles and to some extent in some Buddhist scholarly circles (especially, for example, in the "theology" of a Bob Thurman or other advocates of contemporary Tibetan Buddhist ideology). With respect to Hindu-based groups, however, while there is a sizable sociological or "new religion" bibliography of a social scientific kind, there is very little sophisticated theological advocacy by serious historians of religion, and in this sense the present collection is a most welcome addition to our scholarly bibliographies.

Paul Muller-Ortega, Douglas Renfrew Brooks, William K. Mahony, Swami Durgananda, et al., offer herein a rich feast of historical and theological reflection that is sympathetic to the Siddha Yoga of Gurumayi but at the same time is fully faithful to the canons of critical inquiry characteristic of serious history of religions work. Whether, finally, one is persuaded of the merit of Siddha Yoga as a serious spiritual option is, of course, a matter of personal taste and inclination, but one very much hopes that this collection may be the first of many other collections that dare to move away from purely descriptive scholarship in order to address some of the great spiritual issues of our time.

GERALD JAMES LARSON
Rabindranath Tagore Professor
of Indian Cultures and Civilizations
and Director, India Studies Program,
Indiana University, Bloomington

Acknowledgments

This project would not have been possible without the help of Peggy Bendet, who served as manuscript editor and general project manager and who also contributed to the research, interviewing, and fact-checking. She was assisted by Louise Galland, whose aid in the research, the computer work, and the fact-checking process was also invaluable.

Many others contributed to the completion of the book. The authors would especially like to thank Hemananda, Swami Gitananda, Swami Shantananda, and Stratford Sherman for their continued interest and help at various stages, as well as our other readers, Frank G. Clarke of Macquarie University in Sydney, Australia; Stephan Fredman of the University of Notre Dame; Elizabeth Grimbergen of Allegheny College; David M. Katz of Case Western Reserve University; Gerald J. Larson of the University of Indiana at Bloomington, and, from the SYDA Foundation, Richard Gillett, Barbara Hamilton, David Kempton, Catherine Parrish, Venkappanna Shriyan, Lila Stewart, Melynda Winsor, and Pratap Yande. Any mistakes are, of course, the responsibility of the authors.

Thanks also to Amir Mohammadi, who helped to formulate the outline for the book; to William D. Eastman for support and advice; to Lissa Feldman for help in the research; to Tim Barnett for help in selecting the photographs; to Lise Vail, for copyediting; to Judith Levi of Northwestern University, who prepared the index; to Leesa Stanion, for proofreading; and to Julie Boland of the Siddha Yoga Documentation Archives for her patience in checking the accuracy of our quotations.

For the History section of the book, thanks to Frances Aitken, Sandra Hopson, Cynthia Kline, Swami Madhavananda, Pratibha Trimbake, and many other interviewers from the Siddha Yoga Historical Research project, who gave us material that would otherwise have been unavailable, and to Christopher Wallis, who helped in the preparation of the appendixes.

Introduction
The Experience of Perfected Yogis

Douglas Renfrew Brooks

THE EXTRAORDINARY MASTERS OF YOGA AND THE HISTORY OF UNDERSTANDING

At least from the time of the ancient Greeks, when Alexander the Great's general, Seleucus Nicator, sent the ambassador Megasthenes to the court of the Mauryan kingdom, the accomplishments of India's masters of yoga have been legendary in the West.[1] While too frequently yoga masters have been portrayed inaccurately, even at the superficial level there are examples among them that suggest the potential of human beings to accomplish the extraordinary or the seemingly impossible. From the rich textual history of yogic teachings, practices, and life stories we are struck immediately by the adepts' experiential claims and by accounts of their achievements as beyond the ordinary, whether physically, intellectually, or spiritually.

Before us is a record of experiences—however incomplete, unresearched, and even misinformed it may be—for which we have no simple explanations or categories for understanding. And while more than two thousand years have passed since our first accounts of the yogis (Sanskrit, *yogin*) appeared or since the sage Patañjali composed his *Yoga Sūtras*, we seem still to languish in analytically incomplete understandings and critically naive interpretations.

Only in very recent times have scholars begun more careful and serious studies of yoga and of the extraordinary masters, the "true gurus" (*sadgurus*) who practice and teach. While historical texts and traditional lore enable us to capture images of the *sadguru*, and to hear stories about the few who appear to have matched these ideals, we come at last to wonder if such persons still exist or if the romance of spiritual achievement is so much Shangri-la of a bygone era. Certainly, many in academic scholarship and the media seem bent on refusing the possibility of spiritual fulfillment even as they lionize the significance of the mundane. And yet the experiences of thousands of contemporary persons speak to their own startling life-transformations with just such great beings.

Swami Chidvilasananda has for more than a decade been a catalyst for spiritual awakening and an example for thousands who have met her, heard her teachings, and experienced transformation through their encounters with her. The disciple and spiritual heir of Swami Muktananda, who first brought his teachings of yoga and meditation to the West in the early 1970s, Swami Chidvilasananda has brought continuity, innovation, and expansion to the spiritual movement called Siddha Yoga that Muktananda set in motion.

It is Gurumayi Chidvilasananda's living example that has provided the impetus for this book, not to extol her virtues or to establish her as a model of the *sadguru* but rather as an inspiration to explore more deeply and with seriousness the phenomenon of the *sadguru* as an experiential reality. As authors we have chosen not to focus on our personal experiences as the basis of our understandings, though these experiences have not been excluded from our work. Rather we wish to take seriously the record of experiences of disciples for whom she is the *sadguru*. Simply put, Gurumayi Chidvilasananda has had just the sort of transformative influence that we as historians of religion understand to be at the very core of the *sadguru* traditions of mystical yoga. As a yoga master, her accomplishment is evident to even skeptical observers. But more significant is that as a living representation of the *sadguru* to her disciples, Chidvilasananda reveals the possibility that the ideals of the yoga tradition continue to be met even now at the end of the twentieth century, some twenty-two centuries since Megasthenes' reports and Patañjali's *Yoga Sūtras*.

The Western world has always been of two minds about the gurus it encounters. It has admired their displays of knowledge and tangible power and yet has found it difficult not to question their motives or to feel suspicious of their methods. The word *yoga*—like the term *guru*, which simply means "teacher"—may be familiar to Westerners but it is not one with which we are altogether comfortable. Unfortunately, there are still too few resources from credible scholarly sources that inform, correct, and enrich our understanding of the concepts and practices of yoga, resources that could lead us from impressions and hearsay to clearer interpretations and deeper appreciations. Moreover, some of the same uneasiness about yoga and gurus is present among those for whom these are not only familiar categories but native ones. In India, the yoga master is often loved and even worshiped but also feared and sometimes avoided—though perhaps not for the same reasons we in the West might imagine.[2] Traditional India has noticed as well that the yogis' experiences are as extraordinary as the tales of their deeds. In India, however, there is more credibility to these teachers and teachings, perhaps because there is more experience with the notion that the genuine masters of yoga have led others to similarly extraordinary self-understandings and personal transformations. Countless personal testimonies record that many who begin in disbelief and deny the possibility of spiritual breakthrough come to acknowledge it not as romantic hyperbole but as their own experience.

We as scholars have only recently begun to take these testimonies beyond the boundaries of our own academic skepticism.[3] Only very recently have we developed methods of study that insist on taking religious experiences seriously and not reducing them merely to social, cultural, or psychological phenomena. In other words, we begin now with the notion that what people say about themselves in good faith is "true," that sincere people are not attempting to mislead or deceive others with these reports about themselves. This initial affirmation of the integrity of those who report does not mean that these experiences or concepts cannot be subject to one or another type of analysis. Instead it is simply that, as scholars, we attempt to explain these persons and phenomena rather than explain them away.

At stake in recounting these tales of gurus and yoga is not a verification of events or even a credible account of different stories of self-transformation. Rather it is that the teachings and teachers of yoga speak consistently to levels of human experience for which there are no ready-made explanations either in nature or in science. The yogis are not only extraordinary themselves; they have led others to extraordinary experiences that cannot be dismissed because they have so often been replicated. In the modern West, William James's famous accounts in his *Varieties of Religious Experience* forever changed the way we deal with the spirituality of persons who have had life-transforming experiences. His work, which ushered in the study of religious experiences as both spiritual and psychological transformations, set the stage at the beginning of the twentieth century for the research we now see in the humanities and social and natural sciences. James's most basic lesson still remains our guiding principle of study: it is an error to dismiss or ignore the extraordinary accounts of otherwise ordinary human beings. Instead we must learn to take them as seriously as we take ourselves.

Clearly there are good reasons why the study of yoga and the examples of yoga masters have evoked strong reactions—both from those who have been deeply and positively affected and from those who deny any legitimacy to them whatsoever. Since yoga is at the heart of these claims to extraordinary insight and transformed experience, a basic understanding of its meaning is crucial before delving more deeply into the many levels of experience that result from its practice. There are important definitional principles with which we should begin.

THE DEFINITION OF YOGA

Though there are many different yoga traditions, *yoga* is not a term with "many meanings."[4] Rather, it is a concept used in different ways. In the most encompassing sense of the word, *yoga* means any concentrated effort directed toward accomplishing a goal. As the Sanskrit root *yuj-* suggests, one "yokes" oneself to a task; the originating image may be the comparison of the yoking of a horse to a chariot. Warriors before a battle were "called to the yoke," a ritual that prepared them physically, emotionally, and spiritually for the task ahead. The term suggests a heightened anticipation, a deliberate preparation, and a goal set upon with a commitment. Yoga then is a process, one through which a person makes a determined effort. It is twofold inasmuch as one both sheds the unnecessary or unwanted and reclaims or refocuses to achieve a goal through a well-understood process. Yoga sorts out and sets apart even as it joins together and unifies. In both of these senses it entails a singleness of purpose. As Swami Chidvilasananda puts it, "Yoga is the practice of concentrating the mind until it becomes one-pointed—that is, until it can focus on a single object without wavering."[5]

Yoga is always an endeavor of human accomplishment rather than a disembodied theory or theology. As one scholar has said, "*Yoga* is always of somebody, in something, with something, for some purpose. . . . *Yoga* then implies (1) the process of a difficult effort; (2) a person committed to it; (3) the instrument he uses; (4) the course of action chosen; and (5) the prospect of a goal."[6] Seen in this light, yoga is not as unfamiliar or foreign a concept as we assume. Instead, yoga is intrinsically human; the simplest and the greatest achievements of civilization require yoga. Without yoga what could ever be accomplished? Placed in the realm of spirituality, yoga is that by which we accomplish the fullest expression of our growth as human beings. To learn yoga is to advance one's own purpose for being human; to teach yoga is to have accomplished the goals that others recognize as most valued.

In all its varieties and forms in India, learning and practicing yoga begins with the prerequisite understanding that one must have a qualified teacher, a masterful guru under whose guidance every step on the path is sure and each accomplishment is given its appropriate value. One may have a guru for language study or the fine arts; one's parents are gurus; and there is, of course, the notion of the spiritual guru, the "one guru" (*ekaguru*) to whom the disciple offers her or his deepest spiritual yearnings. In certain traditions, the guru becomes far more than a teacher, mentor, and exemplary resource. The guru offers the grace-bestowing power (*anugraha-śakti*) of Self-awakening, which provides both the initial breakthrough and the continuing instruction for cultivating a life of spiritual discipline or sadhana (Sanskrit, *sādhana*). Such a *sadguru* not only kindles a latent spiritual fire but transforms the disciple's entire life into the pursuit of Self-realization. Yoga with the *sadguru*'s guidance becomes nothing less than the pursuit of divinity as one's own nature; as Swami Chidvilasananda says, "Yoga is that which unites the mind to the supreme Soul."[7] Disciples of the *sadguru* regard their master as having achieved this God-consciousness and as capable of leading them to that same realization within themselves.

Finding a genuine guru, one whose own experience leads and inspires the daily practice of diligent and committed students, has never been as easy as opening a phone book or asking for a doctor's referral. One must know how to distinguish the charlatan guru from the *sadguru*. The sources of Indian tradition are replete with instructions, admonitions, and criteria by which one makes this crucial distinction. Acutely aware of the kinds of power being vested in the *sadguru*, yoga tradition sources make clear that one does not relinquish his or her better judgment in choosing a guru. Further, one must know how to distinguish those gurus who may teach a skill or an art from the "one guru" (*ekaguru*) who can lead the student to a realization of the highest Truth.[8] Whatever arts or skills one acquires, the yoga traditions generally agree that the purpose of all such endeavors is to transform the entirety of one's life into a process or discipline of Self-realization under the guru's guidance.

But where does one look for the *sadguru*? How does one identify a genuine guru? How can one be sure that a guru's teachings are valid and that the path shown by a guru will lead to promised results? What makes a yogic discipline "authentic," that is, true to historical claims of being part of a tradition? These are all questions that naturally follow from a consideration of the definition of any "traditional" form of yoga and the accompanying notion of a necessary and supremely qualified yoga master. From the standpoint of the spiritual quest, worldly accomplishments necessarily follow from the rigors of spiritual discipline. For whatever other purposes to which yoga has been put, it has always been understood *first* as a spiritual discipline. Yoga implicates one's whole being and personality. It is not a mere addendum to improve the quality of one's life. From their traditional point of view, the masters of yoga are more than spiritual virtuosi, they are those human beings who have accomplished what all human beings ultimately aspire to attain.

RECLAIMING YOGA: A NEW STUDY OF AN ANCIENT PHENOMENON

In recent times, Westerners have acquired more examples and firsthand accounts of yogis, if not always better understandings or deeper insights. No longer romanticizing yogis as harmless eccentrics capable of sleeping on beds of nails, walking on hot coals, or contorting the body into pretzel shapes, we sometimes resort to more cynical views. From this "less naive" perspective, when the yoga master is called "guru" he is suspected of being a cult leader; he is condemned as a manipulative charlatan, feared to be a religious dictator who steals away reason from the sincere, and often reduced to a spiritual entrepreneur bent on profit and personal fame. These rather glib and superficial characterizations allow us to dismiss what we do not understand, and they commit a more serious error as well: they deny to Indian civilization, which has taken yoga and the masters of yoga seriously for more than twenty centuries, the same respect that is graciously offered to other, more familiar spiritual traditions. Further, such dismissals deny any validity to the human experiences that follow from the practice of yogic disciplines even though those experiences and practices bear tangible results. Before we deny or reject the results of these spiritual arts, we must ask ourselves if we are prepared to ignore as well the evidence they have produced.

Despite the remarkable transformations that have brought East to West and West to East and the twenty-two centuries that have passed since Alexander the Great's historians and chroniclers first introduced us to the great ascetics and practitioners of yoga, we seem to have acquired as many misunderstandings as we have insights when it comes to these mysterious arts and artisans. In the end, left with far too many negative images, we remain largely uninformed and even *mis*informed about those yoga traditions and yoga masters who have offered examples very different from these images.

This book seeks to correct some of these most basic misunderstandings as well as to foster deeper insights by focusing on one detailed example of yoga and its distinctive tradition of yoga masters.

SIDDHA YOGA: THE SPIRITUAL INTENTION OF THE LINEAGE GURUS

Our case study is Siddha Yoga, so named by Swami Muktananda to distinguish his own lineage and practice but more precisely to describe his deliberate spiritual intention (*saṅkalpa*) to transmit and so pass forward the continuance of his lineage according to his own will and command. As we shall see in the essays that follow, Siddha Yoga cannot be reduced to a canon of textual or oral resources, or a fixed set of teachings or practices, though it certainly makes use of texts, teachings, and practices. Siddha Yoga, like many other Hindu-inspired mystical yogas, understands its source to be the empowering intent (*saṅkalpa*) of the divinely aligned guru as its most distinctive trait.

Though in some traditional lineages of yogis the guru's *saṅkalpa* is vague or unformalized, even before Siddha Yoga became a worldwide movement, Swami Muktananda very carefully set forth the parameters of his lineage and described the requirements that must be upheld by its future leaders.[9] In other words, Muktananda left no doubt as to his intentions, including the creation of a spiritual lineage. He made explicit as well the necessary qualifications (*adhikāra*) of his successors for them to become empowered to carry out the guru's *saṅkalpa.* It is Gurumayi Chidvilasananda who today occupies the guru's "seat" (Sanskrit, *pīṭha;* Marathi, *gaddi*) as the inheritor of Swami Muktananda's Siddha Yoga. Before we consider Siddha Yoga's history and its teachings and practices, we should pause to reflect on this particular "yoga of perfected beings" (*siddhayoga*) and Swami Muktananda's "reinvention" of this term.

In historical sources the generic compound *siddhayoga* is, as Paul E. Muller-Ortega shows in his essay, "The Siddha: Paradoxical Exemplar of Indian Spirituality," rather obscure, rare, and unlike other generic compounds such as *rājayoga* or even *kriyāyoga.* In traditional textual sources and in popular nomenclature, *siddhayoga* has not been used to define a particular movement, a type of yoga, or a program of yogic studies. Rather, it only loosely refers to any yoga practiced or taught by perfected or "accomplished" (*siddha*) yogis. It was Swami Muktananda who transformed *siddhayoga* into a widely known proper noun and so made it the recognized designation of a specific spiritual movement.[10] This is noteworthy if only because other terms that compound with *yoga,* such as *kriyāyoga, mahāyoga,* or *rājayoga,* are not only more frequent in traditional literature but cannot be properly delimited as designative of a specific movement, school, or lineage. *Siddhayoga,* as a compound in the Sanskrit language and as a concept within the history of yogic literature, has had little history or textual use to suggest or confuse its meanings. While one might speak of the "yoga of siddhas" in a general sense, one of Swami Muktananda's contributions has been to reclaim this rare Sanskrit *compound* and to use it as a *single term,* as a name that aligns his own spiritual intentionality with teachings based on his particular understanding of the Siddhas and their lore.[11] In the West, as in contemporary India, "Siddha Yoga" has come to mean Swami Muktananda's designated lineage, his teachings, practices, and interpretations, and the institutions he founded—Gurudev Siddha Peeth in Ganeshpuri, India, and the Siddha Yoga Dham Associates (SYDA) Foundation in the West.[12] By the time of Swami Muktananda's third world tour in 1978, Siddha Yoga had become a worldwide movement with ashrams and meditation centers on every continent, and also had become the proper name associated with Swami Muktananda's lineage. At the same time, it was also Muktananda's clear intention to locate his lineage tradition within a much larger body of yoga traditions whose masters were called siddhas.

As this book makes clear, Siddha Yoga as Swami Muktananda conceived it was not an invention of his imagination nor is it what we would call today a New Age religion. Rather, "Siddha Yoga" is the name of Swami Muktananda's lineage and the very specific interpretive views it advances under the lineage guru's direction. Muktananda's teachings and interpretations are rooted in yoga traditions with predominantly Hindu sensibilities, most of which have ancient or medieval precedents or prototypes.[13] In the West, it is fair to say that "Siddha Yoga" has never meant anything else other than Swami Muktananda's lineage teachings, either in terms of "name recognition" or as a manner of identification.[14]

To put this matter more squarely within the realm of traditional understandings of theology (*siddhānta*) and systems of customary instruction (*sampradāya*), Siddha Yoga is the distinctive body of teachings, practices, and interpretations that follow from Swami Muktananda's spiritual intention to sustain his own lineage's transmissive power. While this book examines those teachings and attempts to refine our understanding of its canon, traditional resources, concepts, and values, we hope to make clear as well that Siddha Yoga should not be reduced merely to a body of teachings, texts, or practices. Rather, Siddha Yoga flows from Swami Muktananda's deep spiritual intentionality and discretion (*saṅkalpa*) and from his transmission of the power (*śakti*) that he bestowed on Swami Chidvilasananda.

When understood in this light, Siddha Yoga is not the "ancient" teachings of the lineage gurus per se, but the transmissive power of the awakened spiritual energy (*kuṇḍalinī*), which from the standpoint of Siddha Yoga has been passed down from one guru to the next in a clear succession (*paramparā*). As scholars we use the name "Siddha Yoga" then in two senses: first, to designate a particular succession of lineage gurus and second, to identify the experience of awakened spiritual energy that flows *through* this lineage. As swamis Muktananda and Chidvilasananda make clear, Siddha Yoga is an experience that properly speaking is conveyed and whose significance is explicated in *this* lineage in distinctive ways through the transmissive power of its gurus. This view ties the experiential dimensions of Siddha Yoga clearly to the particular teachings of this lineage's gurus.

Siddha Yoga continues to flourish today under Swami Chidvilasananda, at whose discretion alone these resources of teaching and practice are extended to other teachers. This important fact means that Siddha Yoga is not anything or anybody who claims to follow these teachings or who has the guru's blessing. But neither is it a stagnant or fixed body of teachings or dogmas. It is the guru who decides who and in what ways a person may speak in the name of Siddha Yoga.[15] This vitally important issue is discussed at some length in the essay entitled "The Canons of Siddha Yoga: The Body of Scripture and the Form of the Guru," where the notion of tradition formation is examined in light of the guru's role as the center of spiritual authority. Under Swami Chidvilasananda's direction Siddha Yoga is a living spiritual movement that continues to grow and to develop within the delineated boundaries and intentions that Swami Muktananda established.[16]

DEFINING SIDDHA YOGA IN TERMS FAMILIAR TO THE STUDY OF RELIGION

The Siddha Yoga gurus' claims to "an ancient spiritual tradition," as we will show, seem well grounded in historical and theological understandings and interpretations. Clearly, we can locate the vast majority of their views within the boundaries of Indian, and even more precisely, Hindu sensibilities and traditions of yogic mysticism.

As we have already noted, Swami Muktananda did not set out to create a "new religion," nor did he seek dissociation from his traditional contexts and inadvertently create a new type of "Hindu" religion. Siddha Yoga's origins are rather typical of the kind of lore surrounding siddhas. We see this clearly in the figure of Swami Muktananda's guru, Bhagawan Nityananda, who exemplifies the archetype of a certain type of siddha whose mysterious origins are part of traditional lore common to the history of siddha lineages.[17] In swamis Muktananda and Chidvilasananda we encounter gurus who envision themselves as thoroughgoing traditionalists. Yet both have sought to reform and to expand any narrow conceptions we might have of their Hindu-inspired spirituality so as not to mistake it with something it is not. While virtually all of the spirituality of Siddha Yoga can be understood as occurring under the large umbrella of Indian, Vedic, and Hindu religiosity, this does not prevent the Siddha Yoga gurus from using other sources, including texts, images, or tales from Christianity, Judaism, Islam, Buddhism, or Sikhism. Siddha Yoga's emphasis on attaining the experiential state of the siddha permits nearly any resource to be put to the use of teaching or practice directed toward this aim. It is also part of this study's larger objective to define precisely which aspects of these religious and spiritual traditions enter Siddha Yoga through the guru's choices and intentions.

Before considering our focus of study we should pause to take note of an important and potentially confusing feature of Swami Muktananda's understanding of Siddha Yoga.

As he began to introduce the teachings and practices of Siddha Yoga to Westerners, Swami Muktananda deliberately chose not to call them a "religion." In fact, he stated clearly that Siddha Yoga is not a religion.[18] And yet he also said that Siddha Yoga has for its purpose "to unfold the God-consciousness that lies hidden in all human beings."[19] Everything about this latter statement, along with other teachings about God, spiritual practice, ritual, mysticism, and scriptural truths suggests nothing other than a religion. From the most commonsense standpoint, Siddha Yoga has all the major features of a world religion. We must then ask what Swami Muktananda meant when he said that Siddha Yoga is *not* a religion.

From the perspective of the Siddha Yoga gurus, Siddha Yoga's foundational claim and most basic insight—that God dwells within each human being as his or her own truest Self—is common to many religions. This is a spiritual claim about the possibility of *experiencing* ultimate reality; it is not viewed as a dogmatic or doctrinal claim. As an experiential claim it is not meant to be defended argumentatively nor is it understood to be in conflict with other religions or religious concepts. Swami Muktananda's statement that Siddha Yoga is not a "religion" meant that Siddha Yoga does not exclude or vitiate the beliefs of other religions. Rather, he took what might best be termed a "standpoint of ultimacy" with regard to understanding the highest and most important sense of religious truth. The Siddha Yoga gurus teach that this "standpoint of ultimacy" is the highest truth. It is not merely a logical argument as such with assumptions, evidence, reasons, and a conclusion, though it is possible to argue for the truth of this statement. More importantly, the "standpoint of ultimacy" is the divine's own position, God's "place" within the realm of our deepest human experience. It is that final or ultimate reality, the conclusion of all spiritual quests, and it is that truth that must be experienced. In these ways, it is understood to be a truth that requires no argument. Put simply, the Siddha Yoga gurus teach that the highest truth is that point at which all differences between religions vanish and all religious positions converge in the singularity of the divine's own wish to unite humanity.

Undoubtedly, this standpoint of ultimacy is part of the Siddha Yoga guru's theology of nondualism, their belief that all of reality is ultimately one. For the Siddha Yoga gurus the cause of the divisiveness that poisons human relations is dualism, the notion that God is "other" than one's own deepest nature and that the perception of this "otherness" undermines our respect for the appearance of different forms. There is, from the Siddha Yoga point of view, but one reality that assumes different forms. In this assumption of many forms the divine singularity (*apūrvatā*) remains none other (*ananya*) than itself. It only makes sense then to believe that all religious truths converge into this divine oneness and that all religions will ultimately lead to this truth. Siddha Yoga teachings begin and conclude in this standpoint of ultimacy and so are seen by the gurus as not being in conflict with other religions. Significantly, this standpoint of ultimacy has done nothing to prevent the Siddha Yoga gurus from retaining their central beliefs, teachings, and practices in relatively unaltered and uncompromised forms, nor has it led them to require or commend others to compromise the integrity of their beliefs or practices.

From the scholarly standpoint, Swami Muktananda's statement that Siddha Yoga is not a religion becomes not a simple declarative statement to be taken at face value but *a matter of his theology*. The Siddha Yoga gurus have assumed theological positions we might call "inclusivism" (or "nonexclusivism") and "perennialism." Both of these positions we will need to examine more carefully. Following this line of interpretation we see the gurus' intentions to be that Siddha Yoga teachings are neither at odds with nor are they meant to supplant other religious teachings. To become a practitioner of Siddha Yoga is not to gain an *exclusivist* religious identity that will necessarily deny any other. Muktananda and Chidvilasananda maintain the view that one can plausibly remain, sustain, or even develop a Jewish, Christian, or other religious identity and still practice Siddha Yoga. These are, as far as they are concerned, noncompeting theologies and allegiances. From the gurus' perspective, not only does practicing Siddha Yoga not exclude having another religious identity, it is certainly possible to identify the basic Siddha Yoga teachings and practices within other religions. In this sense, other religious truths or traditions may be said to be "included" under the larger umbrella of Siddha Yoga without conflict or exclusion. Seen in more personal terms, disciples are not asked or encouraged to renounce religious, cultural, social, or spiritual connections to any other tradition or community to which they may belong or with whom they identify. The fact that Siddha Yoga disciples not infrequently *do* identify themselves as Christians, Jews, Hindus, and in other religious terms seems to bear out the Siddha Yoga gurus' contentions. It is similarly common for Siddha Yoga disciples to identify their own religious values, teachings, and practices with those taught in Siddha Yoga. This notion of noncompeting and nonexclusivist identity is precisely what we mean by saying that the Siddha Yoga gurus are religious *inclusivists.* Swami Muktananda summarizes the position this way:

> Siddha Yoga and meditation on the Self do not oppose any religion, sect, or code of ethics. . . . Siddha Yoga considers all castes, religions, and sects to be its own and loves everyone with an open heart. . . . Never hate any religion, for all religions are equal.[20]

To take the inclusivist position another step further, we need to consider the gurus' belief that Siddha Yoga's meaning is rooted in certain mystical experiences. At the core of *all* religious and spiritual traditions, they believe, are certain mystical insights and experiences. While the vocabulary, symbols, rituals, and other forms of religion might vary, the human situation and the goals of ultimacy originate in the same divine reality. Given this belief, it only makes sense to affirm that beneath our cultural, historical, and *religious* differences are common experiences of ourselves and of God. Identifying all religions with the same basic human issues and aspirations, swamis Muktananda and Chidvilasananda address these issues in the spirit of *perennialism.* Perennialism is that affirmation of the universal nature of the human spirit, accompanied by a religious boundary-crossing vision, in which problems and solutions are seen to be common to all people throughout time and in spite of location or culture.[21]

The perennialist vision does not trivialize historical differences or ignore the significance of situations that certain peoples or religions have experienced. Rather, the perennialist views these differences empathetically because they are common to all human beings, whether they entail suffering or joy. It is our common humanity and our common source in divinity that makes this respect for difference and a deeper empathy with all possible. At the source of our common humanity is a common divinity; that common divinity reveals itself through all religions rooted in basic human values. These simple principles provide the core of Siddha Yoga's perennialist vision. In Siddha Yoga's view we are all one humanity seeking a common goal: the deepest realization of the presence of God within ourselves. As Swami Muktananda writes, "The Supreme Being dwells in the space of the inner heart."[22]

It is when *religion* means the *ultimate* incompatibility of different spiritual teachings and practices that Swami Muktananda suggests that Siddha Yoga is not a religion. By this he means that religions cannot speak of having one God and not mean the same God. It is when (or if) *religion* comes to mean "my God as opposed to your God" that Muktananda dissociates Siddha Yoga from the concept. For the Siddha Yoga gurus, the ultimate unity of God and therefore of all religions is a mystical realization with worldly consequences such as respect, love for fellow human beings, and a willingness to accept differences in customs and forms. This mystical realization does not remove one from the world's religious, social, political, or cultural realities any more than it compels one to include them as part of Siddha Yoga's spiritual path. The Siddha Yoga gurus suggest that their spiritual understanding simply infuses these conventions and beliefs with deeper meanings. As Muktananda often said, Siddha Yoga's mysticism respects most social customs, especially those that uphold dharma, and insists on personal discipline.[23] For the Siddha Yoga gurus, the standpoint of ultimacy obviates duality's less-than-ultimate differences even as it permits (and supports) differences among traditions and in conventions of practice.

Siddha Yoga was not conceived as an "alternative lifestyle" meant to redefine the cultural or social conventions of a given time or place, though it is fair to say that it has created many of its own cultural and social realities. There are, for example, standards of modest dress within Siddha Yoga ashrams and the practice of some devotees assuming a spiritual name (after requesting one from the guru), though neither of these conventions need apply beyond the ashram. This is an important point since it is clear that

Siddha Yoga's purpose remains decidedly spiritual inasmuch as it seeks to be "nonintrusive" in matters of cultural, social, political, or religious life.

The standpoint of ultimacy has a common spiritual purpose quite apart from appearances or conventions: to unite people in their common quest to know God. Further, Siddha Yoga gurus actually endorse the religious, cultural, and social differences that extend from the greater common spiritual purpose of people who seek a deeper sense of happiness and human fulfillment. In other words, devotees are encouraged to sustain beliefs, practices, and customs that strengthen them in the pursuit of their highest spiritual aims. Perhaps this is one important reason it has been so successful in extending its message to peoples from around the world and of very different religious backgrounds. The forms or conventions of universal human values can vary because they are viewed as different possible means of supporting the search for ultimacy. To give one example, Swami Muktananda says that "Siddha Yoga respects marriage and does not condemn disciplined pleasure."[24] At the same time he notes that "Siddha Yoga highly respects the sacred vows of all monks . . . and other great souls who have renounced everything. It respects the fact that they perform actions in the world in a detached manner while seeing Shiva everywhere."[25] In both cases more is at stake than an endorsement of marriage and renunciation as supporting spiritual values; it is implied that Siddha Yoga does not consider particular *religious* differences to be based on conflicting human values. Muktananda's point is subtle: Shared human values require one who practices Siddha Yoga to respect and even to support those religious or cultural differences that do not undermine those values.

As for the purpose of religious disputes or debates, the Siddha Yoga gurus are equally unambiguous. Swami Muktananda states, "Siddha Yoga does not engage in arguments or debates about acceptance and rejection. When there is nothing different from Shiva [God], what can be accepted or rejected? Siddha Yoga upholds equality."[26] On this point he and Swami Chidvilasananda are both clear and uncompromising.

We might also see Muktananda's statement that Siddha Yoga is not a religion as particularly fitting in the context of the 1970s and early 1980s when *religion* was all too frequently a term used to divide, distinguish, and dissociate people from one another.[27] Saying that Siddha Yoga is not a religion is simply to say that it is not the only "real religion." In the spirit of inclusivism and with perennialist objectives, Muktananda sought less divisive ways to discuss human spirituality. He summarizes the Siddha Yoga gurus' position when he writes:

> This Siddha Yoga revolution is founded on high principles. It is an invitation to universal brotherhood. Because light, truth, and peace exist in all, we should love one another with respect for the Self in all. . . .

> Siddha Yoga takes no interest in differences. It does not argue about bigotry or cults. In Siddha Yoga, there is no room for cultism. . . . This field of knowledge is beyond human ambition, beyond the mind and imagination. . . .
>
> By respecting all, Siddha Yoga dispels the hatred that continually arises in the world.[28]

Swami Chidvilasananda continues in precisely the same vein. The Siddha Yoga gurus' inclusivist, perennialist vision seeks to affirm beyond cultural and historical differences the *human* condition and so affirm a common spiritual destiny. This is not to say that the gurus conceive teachings and practices that are "generic." Nor do they mean to dilute or reduce teachings to simplistic common denominators. Quite the contrary. The Siddha Yoga gurus affirm the integrity of each tradition's chosen path, its symbols, concepts, and practices. And like many other religious universalists, swamis Muktananda and Chidvilasananda have no particular stake in compromising their views. Simply put, affirming the integrity of Siddha Yoga views does not mean rejecting or even impinging on the views of others. This was, in fact, a *religious* principle of Muktananda's, one that he affirmed without argument and one he clearly believes to be true beyond argumentation. It is a vision rooted in his claim that all standpoints of duality, rooted as they must be in distinctions of difference, are not ultimate. It is a stance from within Siddha Yoga that continues today under Swami Chidvilasananda and one which we should assume to be a foundational principle. As Swami Muktananda has said:

> The task of Siddha Yoga is to put an end to the notion of duality—to distinctions of high and low, superior and inferior, rich and poor—to arguments and disputes, to the race-track competition among people, and to the futile rushing towards a dream of progress.[29]

The very existence of many religions only confirmed to Muktananda the notion that many paths lead to one goal. In fact, he held that genuine mystical experiences serve to *prove* the ultimate reality of the singular goal of all religions. Muktananda wrote, "Siddha Yoga affirms that the individual soul is nothing other than the Absolute. There is not the slightest difference between the individual and God."[30] While this is not a view with which everyone would agree, as far as Siddha Yoga is concerned, this claim is not meant as a rejection or a refutation of any other view. Further, this standpoint of ultimacy does not mean that others who do not share the notion are "wrong," "incorrect," or to be "condemned." In fact, this identification of the human soul with God means that no ultimate condemnation or rejection of others is possible since all human beings must be viewed as equals in the eyes of God. Again, it is important to point out that such "theological generosity" does not mean a compromise of position or a dilution of intellectual integrity. The Siddha Yoga gurus leave it to others to agree or disagree with their views.

Our aim as scholars has been to understand what Swami Muktananda meant when he said that Siddha Yoga is not a religion in light of his life as master practitioner of a mystical yoga, as a theologian, and as a prolific writer on spiritual subjects. Certainly by any scholarly criteria we might imagine, the teachings and practices of Siddha Yoga are most definitely religious and constitute a distinctive form of religion. This is not a claim at odds with Muktananda's own seemingly unambiguous statement. Rather it is a scholarly interpretation and an effort to *understand* Swami Muktananda's statement in the context of well-accepted definitions of religion.[31]

Cast in this light, Siddha Yoga is a religion that most closely resembles certain mystical traditions of yoga generally associated with Hinduism. As we shall see, particularly in the essay entitled "The Canons of Siddha Yoga: The Body of Scripture and the Form of the Guru," the primary textual and traditional resources favored by swamis Muktananda and Chidvilasananda belong to Hinduism. We should note, however, that this mystical Hinduism does *not* align itself with particular nationalist ambitions or political movements, be they Indian or otherwise. Swami Muktananda conceived of Siddha Yoga as entirely apolitical; Siddha Yoga does reject such cultural conventions as "Hindu" caste or discrimination based on race or ethnicity, and it has never supported any particular governmental party or political position. He wrote, "This meditation revolution does not violate the laws of any government. . . . It is not against any caste or social class. . . . It does not argue with either the good or bad qualities of any country."[32] This apolitical stance is similarly *not* anarchistic or opposed to government as such since, according to Muktananda, "it is people who constitute a nation, and spreading the teaching of the equality of all people makes a nation progress. The Siddha Path endeavors to spread this equality-awareness."[33] The Siddha Yoga gurus have as little interest in nationalism as they do in religion when claims of exclusive truth require rejecting others either on intellectual, theological, ethnic, racial, caste, class, or gender grounds.

While more will be said about Siddha Yoga's relationship to religion and other religions in the essays that follow, it is important to begin by noting that we encounter in Siddha Yoga a living, dynamic, and continuing tradition whose living master, Swami Chidvilasananda, not only presides over well-established precedents but continues to shape and guide the movement forward. It seems clear as well that future Siddha Yoga gurus may take the movement in directions as yet unknown. Our goal in this work is to suggest the contours and forms that have already appeared and the principles that will likely remain constant. Unlike other examples of mystical yoga we might choose to study, our case is not "a finished product" or "a bygone tradition," but rather one in which there is continuity with the past and expressions of innovative freedom as it moves into the future.

VIEWING SIDDHA YOGA FROM WITHIN THE CATEGORIES OF HINDU-INSPIRED MYSTICISM

To place Siddha Yoga in the historical context of Hindu-inspired mysticism it is important to make a crucial distinction from within this Indian context. Some yoga traditions have so encouraged secrecy or self-concealment in their teachings that they maintain the view that spiritual truths are beyond the comprehension of all except the guru. This empowers such gurus to teach without reliance on a common basis or foundation of understanding and to act without accountability to disciples or others.

In some cases, particularly in those mystical traditions classified generally as "Left-Current Paths" (*vāmācāra* or *vāmamārga*), this notion of truth creates a hierarchy of truths, a hierarchy of practices, and a strict hierarchy of disciples distinguished by their qualification for certain teachings and practices.[34] In such cases the principle of nonduality, which suggests a level of understanding entirely beyond the ordinary expectations of the world, becomes a means by which dramatically different measures of accountability are applied, distinguishing the guru from disciples. Placing the emphasis on the radical freedom that the guru enjoys in the state of perfection, the Left-Current Path guru lives and acts beyond any standard of conduct and may or may not exhibit the slightest concern for providing an example of discipleship. Because the siddha's realization is entirely beyond space and time, any rules, measures, or qualifications that might seem appropriate in the world simply do not apply.

Siddha Yoga aligns itself with a very different vision but one which does not forsake the notion of freedom (*svātantrya*) as the divine's most distinctive characteristic.[35] The key to understanding freedom as a spiritual quality and as the guru's own state is in the notion of the absolute autonomy of God. God is perfectly *free to choose*, which includes the choice to specify or to limit, to govern or to submit his own actions or intentions. The point is that every action or intention comes about in perfect recognition of this freedom rather than as an experience of being enslaved by past or present karma, habit, and custom, or by forms of any kind. Every action or intention is, in effect, a *choice* for freedom rather than a compulsion, a convenience, or a conscription. Like all siddha traditions, Siddha Yoga has not forsaken this ultimate freedom of the siddha guru to *choose* and so stand beyond predictability or limitation.

Siddha Yoga, however, is not a Left-Current Path in which the guru deliberately chooses to enact examples of this state of freedom by defiance or transgression of social, cultural, or religious norms. Left-Current gurus, in essence, make a point of asserting their freedom through countercultural or deliberately anti-mainstream values. Siddha Yoga is more correctly associated with the "Right-Current Paths" (*dakṣiṇācāra* or *dakṣiṇamārga*). In these traditions, the guru's achievements, like his teachings and practices, more frequently intend to exemplify the truths taught. The guru is no less free to act as a perfectly free being. However, Right-Current Paths seek no *deliberate or intentional forms* of countering social norms or values. According to the Right-Current, absolute freedom requires no demonstrations of countering norms and no boundary-defiance to create the notion of a boundless freedom.[36] Rather, by affirming the guru's prerogative to perfect spontaneity (*svecchā*), the Right-Current gurus may still baffle or amaze disciples and onlookers, but they do not intend to use concealment or defiance from social norms as a mode of teaching freedom. Furthermore, they are mindful of and sensitive to social norms.

The Siddha Yoga lineage of gurus, like all siddha traditions whether Left or Right, offers multiple examples of unconventional behavior and mysterious intentionality. There is, however, no rejection or self-conscious effort to abandon standards of truth from which disciples can gather a deeper understanding. In general in Right-Current traditions, such as Siddha Yoga, formal teachings, examples of discipline, and rules of conduct all speak to paradigms of truth that are deliberately less "anti-social" and so more intelligible to inexperienced disciples. While there still remain instances in which the gurus' teachings or actions are beyond the complete comprehension of disciples who are not yet fully realized siddhas, the gurus of the Right-Current choose freedom for its own sake rather than advocating freedom as a path in itself. Swami Chidvilasananda perhaps best exemplifies this point: Her teachings, practices, and behaviors provide the *model* of yoga for current Siddha Yoga devotees. This model practice, however, is not a limitation or a convention but a mode of teaching and a form freely chosen. The difference between Left and Right on this matter is quite straightforward: The gurus of the Right-Current uphold standards of truth that can lead one to understand that freedom requires no defiance of convention any more than it rejects willful self-limitation as a positive value.

This issue of the Siddha's perfect freedom is as subtle as it is important. Even disciples who have attained the goal of ultimate Self-realization and have achieved the guru's spiritual state continue to conduct themselves *as disciples.* And even those disciples who assume the guru's *role* do not have the license to forsake discipleship. We see this example clearly in Swami Muktananda's relationship to Bhagawan Nityananda and again in Swami Chidvilasananda's relationship to Swami Muktananda. In the case of Muktananda, he continued to conduct himself with complete deference and humility toward his guru even after his own enlightenment and after his guru had conferred on him the right to act as a guru.[37] Though he had been "made a guru," he never failed to act as a disciple. Similarly, Chidvilasananda sustains her own discipleship as a form of the siddha's achievement.

Moreover disciples who achieve Self-realization, and therefore the *state* of the guru, do not become gurus in the literal sense of starting their own lineages unless specifically empowered to do so by their own guru. In Siddha Yoga the line of succession as well as the conditions under which the lineage guru must conduct her or himself were spelled out explicitly by Swami Muktananda. While not all siddhas seek to create a single spiritual lineage, Muktananda clearly meant for his lineage to continue through one line of siddha gurus. This issue is treated separately from the Siddha Yoga gurus' wish that every Siddha Yoga student achieve the spiritual state of the guru. "Becoming the guru" as a spiritual state is not the same as having a claim to lineage leadership or to control of its teachings.

In Right-Current traditions, such as Siddha Yoga, the guru does not *deliberately* engage, personally or privately, in contradictory ideals, values, principles, concepts, or practices. Further, the guru is not diffident or disdainful of social conventions. As we noted, this does not mean that the siddha is in any way "restricted," since to be in the state of the siddha is to be perfectly free. Rather, it means that disciples are given clear instructions or have among themselves very explicit understandings of the limitations that apply to one who is not yet a siddha. Right-Current traditions have as one of their important features the notion that the guru will not abuse or overstep certain ethical or personal boundaries in the guru-disciple relationship. This is precisely because, as we have said, certain standards by which the truth is made known to all are made part of the guru-disciple relationship. William K. Mahony's essay on the guru-disciple relationship addresses this extremely subtle understanding of the guru's behavior versus the disciple's own recognition of the siddha's achievement of transcendence. At the heart of the issue is the question: What is a siddha guru, according to Siddha Yoga, and how are we to understand the experience of spiritual awakening that empowers the guru to act as he or she does? Suffice to say for now that Siddha Yoga is not a convention-defying path that eschews the ethical standards of the world nor is it one that *relies on* a double standard for guru and disciple. Again, this is not to say that the *same* standards apply to guru and disciple, but only that there is no deliberate effort to abuse the notion of having standards in order to assert the siddha's perfect freedom.

As Swami Muktananda says, "A Siddha lives in total freedom."[38] And yet the example of the Right Current is similarly invoked when he states, "The behavior of a great being is the greatest example for others, and they follow it. Become true, sublime, perfect, and pure. Never lead people in the wrong direction."[39] It is in this context that we must endeavor to understand the Siddha Yoga gurus within the larger vision of mystical yoga traditions. Swami Chidvilasananda makes the point that the siddhas themselves not only teach disciplined freedom but create it. She writes, ". . . [W]hen you hear the words of the sages and Siddhas, your entire being is purified."[40]

TO STUDY THE ESSENTIAL TEACHINGS OF SIDDHA YOGA

Among the many teachings with which we might begin a study of Siddha Yoga as Swami Muktananda originally conceived it, none better captures its essence than his deceptively simple statement:

> Honor your Self, worship your Self, meditate on your Self.
> God dwells within you as you.

Here we find the very core of Siddha Yoga's teachings. It is the message of the siddhas who, having achieved this experience for themselves, assume the form of the guru to lead spiritual seekers to this same experience. The guru's most remarkable gift is the power of Self-awakening or shaktipat (Sanskrit, *śaktipāta, śaktinipāta*) which begins the grace-filled process of yogic purification and inner transformation. No concept is more crucial to understanding Siddha Yoga as a path of the guru's grace (sometimes called *gurukṛpāyoga*) than this mystical notion of shaktipat and the shaktipat guru. While Paul E. Muller-Ortega's article on shaktipat has this subject as its focus, virtually every other essay makes an important point about it. Crucial to the Siddha Yoga view is the notion that shaktipat *begins* the process of yogic purification and leads one ever deeper into the process of self-purification and awakening. In many other yogic traditions such a breakthrough initiation is only offered at the conclusion of years of preparation and selfless-service (*sevā*). Shaktipat is conceived as the *conclusion* of the process. In Siddha Yoga, however, as in certain other mystical lineages, shaktipat *begins* spiritual discipline and can occur whether or not one becomes a devotee or seeks to immerse oneself ever deeper in the processes of Self-awareness. Like an earthquake, the tremors of shaktipat are felt throughout one's being and across the span of an entire lifetime. As the Siddha Yoga gurus teach, however, this initial experience of shaktipat is enriched and fostered by further encounters with the guru who continues to infuse the grace-bestowing power (*anugraha-śakti*).

The shaktipat experience is undoubtedly at the very heart of Siddha Yoga and warrants a thorough examination from many different perspectives. While a matter of deep significance within the traditions of Kashmiri Śaivism and in other mystical yogas, shaktipat has been given perhaps the most prolific explication of its meaning and implications by the Siddha Yoga gurus.

As they understand it, shaktipat is rooted in traditions as ancient and as mysterious as life itself. It is shaktipat that represents the guru's most divine gift and embodies the guru's grace. The energy unleashed by the guru's shaktipat is the latent divinity within, Kuṇḍalinī Śakti, pictured as the serpentine power who stirs from sleep to begin a journey extending throughout the subtle body to arrive ultimately at the state of her own intrinsic perfection when the yogi achieves Self-realization. As the guru all the while directs Kuṇḍalinī's progress with loving care and full awareness of the disciple's needs, the seeker is aided by the rigors of spiritual discipline and enriched by scriptural study, faith in God, and deepening self-understanding. At last, by the disciple's self-effort *and* the guru's grace, Kuṇḍalinī Śakti, who is the form of empowered consciousness (*citi-śakti*), reaches her true destination and is reunited with the eternal Lord, Śiva, who is the absolute consciousness in the form of one's own direct experience of the realized Self. Siddha Yoga, drawing freely from the images of mystical Hindu-inspired yoga, adopts a vision that places God within the embodied form of the person and offers a process of transformation through which all aspects of the personality are brought to a subtle, inner awareness of the divine's residence in the body. Put in terms familiar to mystical yoga, the fully awakened goddess Kuṇḍalinī brings the yogi to the state of *jīvanmukti*, "liberation while yet embodied." This ultimate freedom is precisely what Siddha Yoga sees as the constant, inner state of the siddha guru. However, it is *not* a state reserved *only* for the siddha guru. Rather, it is the hope of every disciple on the path of yogic self-effort and divine grace.

Siddha Yoga is nothing less than the path of the guru's grace by which the seeker comes to revel in the blissful reality that everything is God, and God is none other than the deepest experience of one's very own Self. This too is a deceptively simple statement that gives us pause to reflect on certain values and assumptions that are part of the Siddha Yoga worldview.

For Siddha Yoga, neither is God wholly "other," distant from creation or apart from human nature, nor is the Self different from the God who dwells in the heart of every human being. The Siddha Yoga gurus teach that this basic truth is present in all the world's religions; God is beyond any disputes or boundaries that divide or confound us. As difficult as it may seem to fathom in the face of so many examples in history to the contrary, the siddhas teach that every person can achieve this realization of the inner perfection of Self when they become completely identified with the ubiquitous divinity of God. This realization was, according to Swami Muktananda, the experience of his own guru, Bhagawan Nityananda, who led him to this supreme truth, and then commanded him to bring it to the world. It is said to be a universal truth, capable of being affirmed in every time or place and not dependent on the ways of the world or limited to one spiritual path. As Gurumayi Chidvilasananda says, "This is the message of all the saints from all cultures and traditions." However, in order to see God in oneself, in others, and indeed in all things, Swami Chidvilasananda further makes clear that "you have to turn within." The key practice by which this "turning within" brings Self-realization is meditation. Meditation, then, is both process and the state of Self-discovery.[41]

Siddha Yoga does not assume a state of "original sin" nor does it view human nature as ultimately separate from or other than its divine source. We may bring misery to ourselves as human beings, but this is not because we lack the power to achieve ultimate joy in this life. Chidvilasananda makes clear that this is a matter of yogic practice rather than a doctrine. She writes:

> [I]f you want to realize the purpose of human birth and enter the abode of supreme bliss, then you have to change your view of life. . . . Much of your life has been created from your unlimited supply of negative concepts. Purify them. . . .
>
> The yoga of discipline is not about confining yourself to an unknown world filled with strange phenomena. Nor is it about doing penance for your sins. I want to clarify this: you are not following discipline to get rid of your sins. You are following discipline because you want to drink this nectar, this ambrosia.[42]

While the seeker's task requires living a life committed in every moment to this arduous path of unremitting self-effort, founded in practices leading to the purification of thought, intention, and action, the goal is viewed as neither remote nor unrealistic.

Arguably almost the entire history of Western civilization and spirituality has sustained a rather different view of human nature, namely, that humans are sinful or limited in a way that precludes human perfection. Perfection is a state reserved for God alone; to claim human perfection as a potential is either heresy or delusion. This is not only a religious or spiritual value in the West; it is also a psychological one. As Freud might have it, we are at best a little neurotic. Similar assessments of our negative potential for health and ultimate fulfillment abound. Siddha Yoga, in line with other mystical paths, begins from another place: Human beings are divine intrinsically and have only to re-cover and un-cover this nature. Once the process is completed, the divinity within takes the form of every action, thought, intention, and deed. No longer separated from God, the yogi experiences the great *so 'ham,* the mantra that reveals the mystery of "I am that" divine reality. This realization breaks down once and for all the dualism that ignorance, desire, and deep latent impressions (*saṃskāras*) impose on body, speech, and mind. Reveling in the ecstatic bliss of the perfectly realized Self, the yogi attains the consciousness that reunites him or her with God.

Dualistic theologies in which God must be "other" to be ultimate may not agree with either the assumptions or conclusions of this worldview. However, from the standpoint of nondualism or, to put it differently, from the realization of the unity of the One and the many, even these disagreements and distinctions vanish.

It is similarly important to note that Siddha Yoga, like other mystical yogas and nondualist theologies, affirms that the *process* of Self-realization and mergence with the divine occurs with austerity, endurance, and ultimate commitment to the goal. Swami Chidvilasananda writes:

> Austerity develops endurance, which is the backbone of yoga. In yoga, you need that power of endurance. Constantly enduring whatever happens, never falling apart. You should never give yourself a chance to fall apart because when you do it becomes a tendency, and it happens over and over. . . . You have many obstacles to overcome, so you must gain strength as you walk the path.[43]

From the Siddha Yoga standpoint it is possible then to become truly contented and fulfilled in this life and to achieve a discipline, a yoga, that eliminates negativity of every sort. Swami Chidvilasananda writes:

> When you behold the Truth with your eyes, when you behold God . . . then all that is negative, all that is destructive and evil, will walk away from your life. Only glory and auspiciousness will dwell in your house.[44]

Siddha Yoga maintains that the committed seeker has before him the example of the guru's own perfection and the inspiration born of his or her own glimpses of the cherished ultimate goal, gained from the guru's most precious gift, the grace-bestowing power of shaktipat.

Eventually, whether in this birth or in others to follow, the disciple comes to realize that God, Self, and guru are ultimately one and that the multiplicities of the world are but the play of the divine's own intelligent and mysterious consciousness. The key to realization, however, is this relationship between guru and disciple and the notion that what is passed between them is ultimately an inner transmission of enlightenment in which the sense of humanity is not diminished or set aside but rather is enriched, enlivened, and fulfilled. Perfection does not appear the same in all siddhas any more than the intrinsic unity of being (*sat*) and consciousness (*cit*), or its blissful nature (*ānanda*), is compromised by achieving different forms.

In fact, Siddha Yoga has no difficulty in using or adopting different forms as a manner of inspiring yogic discipline and of leading the disciple to the highest nondual (*advaya*) awareness. While it may seem ironic that forms and images are used to direct human consciousness to the realization of formlessness, this is not a strategy that is uncommon to mystical yoga, especially those traditions inspired by the nondual Śaivism of Kashmir.[45] Pictures of the gurus, along with images from the pantheon of Hindu deities and saints, are especially important to this process of remembrance (*smaraṇa*) of the truth and recognition (*pratyabhijñā*) of one's deepest nature.

To iconoclasts and those unfamiliar with images and idols this notion can be disturbing, not simply foreign. Siddha Yoga has not shied away from this Hindu-inspired notion, and its ashrams and centers are filled with the pictures of the gurus and divine images. Again, unfamiliarity can be quite misleading. Swami Chidvilasananda makes their purpose unambiguously clear:

> In the ashram when people come for the first time, they ask why we have so many photos of the Guru and so many statues in the garden. There is a purpose: it is so we will always remember, so we will see with discipline. Once the eyes see the form of the Guru, then everything the Guru upholds, everything the Guru stands for is invoked. When you see the statue of a deity, everything the deity stands for, that the deity contains is invoked. And then that is what you see, that great energy.[46]

From this perspective, forms represent the dynamic flow of the divine's own consciousness as it takes on manifestation. The yogi learns, in effect, through forms to see the divine in everything and everything as a form of the divine. Coming to appreciate this vision is in Siddha Yoga, as in other mystical yoga traditions, an important feature of a highly disciplined spiritual practice and a process meant to advance self-transformation.

The perfection of the siddhas is not a static or inert reality but rather a living, dynamic, and fluid expression of consciousness taking on the guise of time, space, and the universe as we know it. What marks the siddha as a being different from those not yet enlightened is that the siddha remains forever *brahmaniṣṭha,* "in the state of residing (permanently) in the absolute." This too takes the form of its own divine will, for God is perfectly free (*svātantrya*) even as he remains ever the same (*nitya*), blissful (*ānanda*), and perfectly self-aware (*svasaṃvid*). Thus, according to Siddha Yoga, the yoga of the siddhas will remain a living knowledge embodied in preceptors and teachings and ultimately in siddha gurus who will pass it down from master to student for time immemorial, as they always have.

While the siddha's way is traditionally also deemed a secret path for which few are yet prepared, with the life and teaching of Swami Muktananda we witness a revolution among siddhas: the successful creation of a tradition that has introduced these esoteric teachings to thousands of people from all over the world.

REACHING SCHOLARLY UNDERSTANDING

As scholars we do not take issue here with any of the spiritual affirmations and beliefs of the Siddha Yoga gurus. It is not our task to confirm or deny their statements. We should also make clear that our methods of study are not rooted in suspicion or hidden agendas. We have no desire to undermine Siddha Yoga's beliefs or practices. Rather, we seek deeper understanding and to that end we use the traditional tools of historical, critical scholarship as it has been developed in the West at least since the time of the Enlightenment. However, we should also make clear that, from our point of view, there is no such thing as a purely "objective" scholarly opinion, utterly detached from judgments and without its *own* standpoint. Having a personal stance, even one that arises from within the tradition about which we speak, is no liability and not something for which we feel the need to apologize or which we care to defend. As one among us put it, if we were studying the taste of mangoes, offering our honest observations about them, we would not believe that one who has never tasted mangoes has any advantage over one who has. At stake is credible, honest, and well-researched scholarship, not a pretense to objectivity that does nothing to advance those goals.

Too often scholarship on religious and spiritual subjects assumes extreme positions, posturing either to endorse and advocate without saying so openly, or to offer explanations that rationalize for the sake of "explaining away." Certainly advocacy can be rooted in honest scholarly interests and scholarly explanations can be without subversive agendas. In this work we seek historical, critical, and analytical honesty in understanding even as we take the experiences of the Siddha Yoga gurus, the teachings, and the accounts of followers with utmost seriousness. The goal is a deeper understanding of the origins, sources, teachings, and practices of Siddha Yoga, one that is grounded in the history of this tradition.

In this book, the aim is to take seriously Siddha Yoga's dramatic development and self-conscious transformation as a spiritual movement over its first thirty-five years, first as its seeds were planted by Bhagawan Nityananda, then under Swami Muktananda's initial formulation, and now as it is guided by Swami Chidvilasananda. The goal is to describe and explain the origins and development of Siddha Yoga from the standpoint of historians of religion. This is not a book of Siddha Yoga teachings or experiences, though both of these subjects are of interest. It is a book *about* Siddha Yoga and not a handbook of Siddha Yoga practice.

Our strategy is to trace the origins and sources of this now worldwide movement from its humble beginnings as a local manifestation of Hindu-based spirituality, beginning with Swami Muktananda's own guru, Bhagawan Nityananda, in the obscure Tansa Valley of Maharashtra in western India. We examine historical and theological developments up to their current formulations under Swami Chidvilasananda and begin the process of studying Siddha Yoga as an inclusivist world religion, a distinctive form of mysticism, and a type of human experience that neither denies others' experiences nor compromises its own worldview. Our primary concern is to describe and explain Siddha Yoga within the contexts of its historical, intellectual, and doctrinal sources; we see Siddha Yoga as a religious phenomenon and a spiritual movement rooted in Indian spiritual traditions and emerging out of them to create its own distinctive interpretive visions.

INTRODUCING THE ESSAYS

Each of the essays of this book takes up an aspect of Siddha Yoga that is crucial for understanding its origins, development, teachings, and practices. We do not pretend to cover every subject of importance and have restricted ourselves to limit the extent of coverage brought to bear on the topics we have selected. Difficult decisions were made about the book's content simply to bring it to some manageable size and scope. As our research progressed, we realized just how vast was the subject of Siddha Yoga when we considered all of its related sources and connections within the Indian tradition.

The decisions we reached about content, scope, and presentation were, like the essays themselves, done in very close collaboration and consultation. While individual (or collaborating) authors took responsibility for conceptualizing and composing each essay, "finished" pieces underwent a rather remarkable process of collective consultation and critical examination. Reconsiderations, clarifications, and input from the collective authorship were then incorporated into individual revisions. Put simply, this is less a "collection" of works than a single work with multiple contributors who spent nearly as many hours working together as apart.

Interestingly, the result of this collective and collaborative effort is a series of lengthy and focused essays, each of which can be read independently of the others. However, it is also the case that each essay was constructed with the others in mind and in light of the contents, methods, and aims that appear in the work as a whole. What a reader finds in one essay may appear (and often does) in others—especially when the subject is important and our understanding deepens with shifting or multiple perspectives. Even as each essay was designed to stand on its own to permit the reader to follow its line of presentation as a coherent work, it is also the case that a discerning reader can move from essay to essay, studying a concept or idea thematically by using the index as a guide. A reader may wish to cross-reference ideas or topics, gain multiple views of a single concept, or engage a single concept from a number of vantage points. We leave the readers to decide how the book might prove most engaging and useful to them. Our primary strategy has been to offer multiple vantage points from which to consider our larger subject, Siddha Yoga, and to address the issues, themes, concepts, and values that define its scope and direction. However one goes about reading the book, we aim to provide as much depth and insight as possible without making the reading presumptive of prior knowledge or other scholarly literature. Certainly this work does not mean to be "the final word" on any of these issues or subjects, and we look forward to future expansions and reevaluations.

The only tools one needs to read this book are a genuine curiosity and a willingness to consider with seriousness the complexity of the subject. Our hope is to achieve a balance between thoroughly credible scholarship and genuine accessibility. Though this might disappoint some scholars who will find portions of the work to be elementary or reiterative of well-understood materials, our aim has been a kind of intellectual self-sufficiency in presentation. Our presentation of foundational materials reiterates well-received scholarly opinion rather than idiosyncratic views. In addition, there is much in this book that is thoroughly original and highly innovative both in content and method. Again, our aim has been to create honest, credible, and well-researched scholarship that remains open to revision based on new data or understandings.

Our work begins with Swami Durgananda's "To See the World Full of Saints: The History of Siddha Yoga as a Contemporary Movement." This essay sets the stage for the entire work by offering the first comprehensive narrative history of Siddha Yoga, beginning from the time of Swami Muktananda's guru, Bhagawan Nityananda. In order to appreciate more fully the essays that describe key concepts, practices, or situations, one should consider Siddha Yoga's unfolding history as the setting in which they take shape and gain their meanings. It is here that these theological ideas and practices find their living counterparts in the gurus' histories and in the history of the movement.

This opening essay also stands apart from the rest in a few important ways. We should take note both of its extraordinary content and its methodology. It is the only essay not written by a professional historian of religion, though such a qualification would hardly suffice to accomplish its important task. In fact, Swami Durgananda's position from within Siddha Yoga offers the reader insights and perspectives that no amount of archival study could possibly have accomplished. Much of the *content* of this essay—its detailed and thorough accounts of events and lore—could not have been recreated by anyone other than an eyewitness. Its most compelling feature, however, is that it is far more than a simple recounting of events. Rather, it brings the reader directly into the extraordinary story of this lineage and its growth; it relies as much on fact and documented evidence as it does on the power of its narrative voice. From the scholarly perspective, Swami Durgananda's essay is a form of cultural and social anthropology of religion. What this means is that she offers us a well-researched historical view from the vantage point of an observer who has also been a deeply involved participant.

Anthropologists, like other social and natural scientists, now widely accept the premise that every observer of an event is also *part* of the event itself. There is no "standing apart from" a phenomenon when one is standing in the midst of it, observing it. To observe is, in one way or another, to participate. The *degree* to which an observer can report with accuracy and honesty even as he or she participates has always been a matter of anthropology's methodological discussion, particularly during the last twenty years.[47] The well-known anthropologist Clifford Geertz offers a helpful and healthy perspective on how firsthand study and the "insider's report" stands the tests of credibility. He links the importance of framing history and the community's different voices in the context of the anthropologist's quest for credibility:

> The ability of anthropologists to get us to take what they say seriously has less to do with either a factual look or an air of conceptual elegance than it has with their capacity to convince us that what they say is a result of their having actually penetrated (or, if you prefer, been penetrated by) another form of life, of having, one way or another, truly "been there." And that, persuading us that this offstage miracle has occurred, is where the writing comes in.[48]

Undoubtedly Swami Durgananda has both penetrated and been penetrated by the Siddha Yoga she describes. Her strategy as a researcher of the facts, of legend, and of events, as well as her privileged position as an oral historian-participant, is precisely what permits the penetration and the insight that lends this essay its distinctive voice. We are not only persuaded that Swami Durgananda has truly "been there" but that her words can and do transport the reader to those times, places, and events. No less than such a "privileged insider" could have offered such depth or understanding of this history. No other sort of "observer" could possibly have taken us as deeply into the heart of the persons, events, images, and concepts that make up Siddha Yoga's history. Her single voice takes on the character of many different voices—historian, journalist, devotee—each of which brings with it its own perspective and insight. An astute reader will notice the subtle shifts in tone to this single voice, each of which lends this historical account its narrative power and insight.

The issues or events that cannot be verified by others who might undertake similar research must be left to meet Geertz's tests of measured conviction. We leave it to readers to decide how far Swami Durgananda has come in meeting Geertz's criteria of conveying seriousness and credibility to the account. What is clear, however, is that Swami Durgananda's account of this history will be recognizable to those who shared in some of it and that her effort will enrich and enliven the understanding of those for whom this narrative begins the study of Siddha Yoga and the larger phenomenon of the guru.

Paul E. Muller-Ortega's essay on the concept and phenomenon of "The Siddha: Paradoxical Exemplar of Indian Spirituality" is the natural extension of the history of Siddha Yoga. The siddha is the spiritual ideal, the paradigm, the goal of spiritual practice, and the force behind the creation of mystical yoga lineages. This essay begins the project of examining the key subjects, teachings, and practices of Siddha Yoga and, in the larger sense, sets the stage for our focusing on the primary concepts that define siddha traditions. Muller-Ortega centers on the Siddha Yoga gurus' and particularly on Swami Muktananda's understanding of the siddha as the "perfected being." His goal is to place the Siddha Yoga gurus' understanding in the context of India's mystical and esoteric literature and history. Muller-Ortega is careful not to overextend the scope of his project since the term *siddha* and the yogic tradition of siddhas is far too vast for any single essay (or even any one book) to exhaust.

What we have before us in "The Siddha: Paradoxical Exemplar of Indian Spirituality" is a remarkable piece of scholarship that probes the Siddha Yoga conception seen in light of the esoteric resources of the Tantras and of Kashmiri Śaivism, particularly the work of the great philosopher Abhinavagupta. We are offered not only a careful study of Swami Muktananda's concept but a typology of meanings whereby we can gain a deeper appreciation of how this term has been and can be used in the context of mystical Indian yoga. This typology then extends further to the notion of a siddha lineage and Swami Muktananda's interpretations of the siddha's transmissional powers. The siddha is treated both as an embodied being and as a state of consciousness, thus taking us even further into the notion of *siddhi*s, "spiritual accomplishments," which culminate in enlightenment or liberation (*mokṣa*). This essay might well be read in conjunction with several others that describe the Siddha's path, particularly those that describe the practices that lead to becoming a siddha ("Siddha Yoga as *Mahāyoga*: Encompassing All Other Yogas" and "Kuṇḍalinī: Awakening the Goddess Within"), the Siddha's grace-bestowing power ("Shaktipat: The Initiatory Descent of Power"), and the context in which these practices and accomplishments take place ("The Guru-Disciple Relationship: The Context for Transformation").

William K. Mahony's "The Guru-Disciple Relationship: The Context for Transformation" places the accomplishment of the siddha and the notion of the siddha guru in the context of the fundamental relationship that defines tradition and lineage learning. The subjects of guru, discipleship, and the transmission of lineage power are essential aspects of Siddha Yoga, both as a spiritual tradition and as a developing movement and institution. In siddha traditions, the emphasis placed on the guru and the sorts of relationships the guru has with disciples involves issues of the most sensitive and mystical kind. As a *guruvāda*, a "way of the guru," Siddha Yoga vests an enormous power and responsibility in this figure. No subject has, in fact, been more controversial or sensitive, either in Indian traditions or in Western understandings of the guru phenomenon. In the latter case of the West, we have no directly comparable figure: the guru is far more than simply one's teacher and mentor. And because we have no such directly comparable concept, that of the guru is particularly difficult and even troublesome. From the time of Plato's critique of the Sophists and Christianity's notion that only Jesus of Nazareth holds the two-natures of humanity and divinity within him, we in the West have either been suspicious or exclusive in our understandings of the human as divine and the divinely human figure. Mahony's thorough and serious treatment of the relationship of guru and disciple offers us fresh insight and a powerful tool for understanding the issues and the stakes involved. A reader might well profit from reading this essay in conjunction with those on the siddha, shaktipat, and "The Canons of Siddha Yoga."

Having considered the history of Siddha Yoga, the spiritual goal of siddhahood, and the relationship of guru and disciple, our study moves forward to consider the body of teachings and practices that define Siddha Yoga as a form of Hindu-inspired mystical yoga. "The Canons of Siddha Yoga: The Body of Scripture and the Form of the Guru" is an effort to describe and explain the body of scriptural resources that the Siddha Yoga gurus have selected as the basis of their teaching and practice. It investigates the choices that determine which teachings and practices are regarded as sacred and authoritative, and provides a basic understanding of the different strands of literature and tradition that are brought together by the Siddha Yoga gurus. What are the sacred texts of Siddha Yoga and where did they come from? These texts form the "canon" of Siddha Yoga.

Though the term *canon* may seem unfamiliar to many, beyond its formal meaning is a rather simple idea. Every community, be it religious, cultural, or political, seeks to understand its beliefs and values. In this process of self-definition and self-understanding, the community creates a "tradition," literally, that which it "carries forward." Canons are forms of tradition; they are the collections of ideas, values, and practices that present the community's authoritative vision. Put more formally, a canon is an enumeration or register of resources *and* it is that ideal norm, that standard by which persons, places, or things are adjudged to be within the boundaries of tradition. While a canon is most often understood as a collection of enduring scriptural resources, whether written or oral, this definition may prove to be too narrow or even incorrect. In the case of Siddha Yoga, the canon constitutes not only the texts chosen by the guru, but the guru *is* the canon—that is, the guru is that authoritative resource by which and through whom teachings and practices *become* sacred. While this may seem a novel idea or one that goes beyond our usual associations of "canon" with "authoritative texts," scholars in other religious traditions have recently created similar paradigms of understanding.[49]

To understand a canon, like the canon of Siddha Yoga, we must ask questions about the sources of authority in regard to the teachings, practices, and forms that tradition takes. But more than this, our study of the "canon" of Siddha Yoga creates a theoretical foundation for understanding *how* choices are made, what principles of choice are invoked, and how that decision-making process has been developed. In other words, we are interested not only in the selections made and in the selection process, we are interested in what forms the canon might take apart from texts or other fixed forms of authority. The key to understanding Siddha Yoga's notion of the sacred scripture is the role of the guru and the way the guru infuses into texts, teachings, or practices the intentionality (*saṅkalpa*) that creates the authority we call "canonical." This study of canon-making is an important undertaking if we are to gain a deeper understanding of how a *guruvāda,* or "guru's teaching," actually *becomes* a tradition, both scripturally rooted and organically transforming in the process of lineage transmission. The essay offers a model of interpretation that probes the relationship between scriptures and historical precedents and the absolute freedom and the authority the Siddha guru has in defining and perpetuating tradition.

With a deeper appreciation of the resources and structures by which to understand Siddha Yoga as a guru-centered mystical yoga, we move on to a series of pieces that describe and explain key concepts that inform essential practices.

William K. Mahony's essay entitled "The Self: A Vedāntic Foundation for the Revelation of the Absolute" addresses the central issue of Siddha Yoga mysticism: Self-realization. Here the issue is interpreted through the lens of the tradition known as Vedānta. We are introduced to the concepts, sources, and interpretations that define the crucial experiential issues concerning spiritual enlightenment. Focusing on the concept of the "Self," Mahony pays special attention to the resources of the nondualist or Advaita Vedānta traditions, tracing them back to their original scriptural sources and detailing their history. This agenda not only permits him to define the scope of Vedānta teachings but to place Siddha Yoga in the context of their histories, theologies, and interpretations. Mahony takes the reader to a new level of understanding Vedānta by placing the Self in the context of Siddha Yoga's teachings on the guru's grace-bestowing power. And from studying Siddha Yoga, we gain important insights into the practice of Advaita Vedānta philosophy. Self-realization becomes, as we see here, not only a goal but a systematic process of spiritual discipline empowered by the siddha guru's gifts of wisdom and of love.

The process of Self-realization in Siddha Yoga begins with the truly mystical process known as shaktipat. Shaktipat begins the unfolding of spiritual awareness that leads to the siddha's perfection. Paul E. Muller-Ortega's essay, "Shaktipat: The Initiatory Descent of Power," presents genuinely original scholarship on a subject that is almost entirely unknown and unexplored. While shaktipat is a centerpiece of Siddha Yoga teaching, Muller-Ortega shows through careful historical study how scriptural resources treat this deeply secret and mystical notion of spiritual awakening. Tracing the development of this concept from the work of the eleventh-century mystic Abhinavagupta, Muller-Ortega offers remarkable insights into Siddha Yoga's notion of shaktipat and creates through his study of Siddha Yoga a deeper appreciation of shaktipat as a mystical experience. The agenda of this essay, like that of the others in this book, is twofold: first, to contextualize the topic within the broader scope of the Indian traditions of mystical yoga, and second, to consider it within the more specific realm of Siddha Yoga's understandings and interpretations. To historians of religion as well as to those interested in Siddha Yoga, this essay presents a level of understanding about mystical yogic traditions that has been hitherto unavailable in any previous scholarly work. No topic is more important for understanding the distinctive contribution of the Siddha Yoga gurus to the practice of mystical yoga nor is any more genuinely mysterious and powerful to the yoga itself. One might best read this essay in conjunction with "The Siddha: Paradoxical Exemplar of Indian Spirituality" and "To See the World Full of Saints: The History of Siddha Yoga as a Contemporary Movement" to gain a better grasp of how this mysterious power of shaktipat manifests in persons and in events. One might also consider it in light of the two following essays on Kuṇḍalinī and *mahāyoga,* which offer a context for understanding the source of this particular manifestation of the guru's grace-bestowing power (*anugraha-śakti*).

Having received shaktipat, the Siddha Yoga practitioner embarks on a spiritual journey. While outwardly the effects of shaktipat are held to transform a disciple's life, Siddha Yoga focuses primarily on the transformations that occur as the practitioner turns within and engages in meditation and Self-reflection. This inner journey of Self-realization is nothing other than the awakening of the goddess Kuṇḍalinī through the process of *kuṇḍalinīyoga.* "Kuṇḍalinī: Awakening the Divinity Within," coauthored with Constantina Rhodes Bailly, offers a description of the basic elements of this mystical theory and practice and proceeds to examine the interpretations of the Siddha Yoga gurus. The essay's focus is on the particular facets of the Kuṇḍalinī phenomenon to which Siddha Yoga attaches importance and on precisely how Kuṇḍalinī factors into Siddha Yoga's understanding of the inherently abiding divinity that exists within the yogi's subtle body. We are treated here as well to a discussion of the nature of the divine as an inner presence, the role of mantra in spiritual practice, and the effects of Kuṇḍalinī's awakening on the consciousness of the yogi.

To complement *kuṇḍalinīyoga*'s more descriptive theological agenda, the essay "Siddha Yoga as *Mahāyoga*: Encompassing All Other Yogas" by S. P. Sabharathnam establishes the theoretical and practical relationships between Siddha Yoga and other schools, traditions, practices, and forms of yoga. Its primary aim is to show how Siddha Yoga incorporates and adapts these various and complex phenomena into its own distinctive formulas and formulations.

While other topics and subjects might well have received as exhaustive treatment as those we selected for this volume, we believe these few provide the vital core of teachings and practices. However, crucial to understanding them is the context in which they appear. The ashram (Sanskrit, *āśrama*) is the abode of the siddha, the place where the siddha takes residence and offers the opportunity for disciples to concentrate their spiritual practices.

The concluding essay entitled "The Ashram: Life in the Abode of a Siddha," by William K. Mahony, describes the context within which Siddha Yoga teachings and practices have been formulated and continue to flourish. The ashram as a spiritual retreat center, as an ideal community, and as the guru's extended form of teaching and practice are all subjects Mahony treats in detail. The aim of this work is to give a historical context as well as a conceptual understanding of certain opposing concepts—such as sacred and profane, and spiritual exertion and supreme rest—as connected with ashrams and their broader influence, particularly viewed in light of the example offered by Siddha Yoga. As Mahony shows, the ashram is the center of Siddha Yoga's spiritual life and its reality as a religious institution. More importantly, Mahony demonstrates that the ashram is an extension of the guru's body of teachings and practices. In this way the ashram becomes both a practical instrument of the guru's yoga and a mystical extension of the guru's grace, leading disciples to Self-realization.

This work has been an ambitious undertaking for all involved, from its initial conception to its final editing and refinement. Rarely do scholars have the opportunity to work as closely or in such close collaboration on a single project and rarer still is the chance to learn as much from one another over such an extended time. We hope our readers experience at least some of the joy it has been for us to create this work and that their insight grows as much as has ours.

Sadgurunāth mahārāj kī jay!

Part I
History

Chapter One

To See the World Full of Saints

The History of Siddha Yoga as a Contemporary Movement

Swami Durgananda

> *My work in this world is to start a meditation revolution. . . . I want to see the whole world full of saints. I want to see everyone happy.*[1]
>
> Swami Muktananda, 1982

Swami Muktananda, who gave the Siddha Yoga meditation movement its name and established its contemporary identity, always linked his path to the ancient tradition of the Indian sages—a tradition drawn from the mists of prehistory and, as he often said, kept alive through lineages of enlightened beings. At the same time, the contemporary history of Siddha Yoga as a movement is essentially the story of three spiritual masters and their disciples. Bhagawan Nityananda, a silent and entirely unconventional holy man who dressed only in a loincloth and gained fame for the miracles that occurred around him, laid the foundation of the present Siddha Yoga transmission. His disciple Swami Muktananda, whose roots in the yogic culture of India combined with his modern outlook to make him a far more accessible figure, formulated Siddha Yoga's teachings, created its institutions, and brought its mysteries to public view. Swami Chidvilasananda, Swami Muktananda's disciple, is equally at home in both Eastern and Western cultural contexts. She has brought Siddha Yoga to maturity as a global spiritual movement. Connected by the bond of discipleship, heirs to the same stream of spiritual power, these three masters nonetheless present very different personalities and teaching styles. The development of Siddha Yoga reflects their varied temperaments and experiences as well as the underlying identity common to all three.

Nonetheless, this is not merely the story of three spiritual personalities. It is also the history of how an esoteric spiritual path, based on the intensely personal and private relationship between guru and disciple, has expanded to become a worldwide movement, its pathways through consciousness made available to many people who know nothing of its origins or traditions. In the early 1970s, following an instruction from his guru, Swami Muktananda set out to create what he later called a "meditation revolution." His stated goal was to awaken as many people as possible to the vast potential for power and joy that lies within the human heart. As he put it in a sort of mission statement that appeared in his book *Secret of the Siddhas*: "The main task of Siddha Yoga is to unfold fully the God-consciousness that lies hidden in all human beings."[2] The means he taught for achieving this unfoldment was meditation, but with a special ingredient. Swami Muktananda, by the evidence of thousands of his students, had inherited from his guru the power to pass on his own spiritual force, shakti (Sanskrit, *śakti*), in a special transmission called shaktipat (Sanskrit, *śaktipāta*: "descent of power"). This little-known and mysterious initiation, described most fully in certain scriptures of the Śaiva tradition,[3] historically had been given only by rare gurus to highly prepared disciples.

In shaktipat, a Self-realized—siddha—guru awakens the *kuṇḍalinī*, the evolutionary energy that yogic tradition holds lies dormant in every human being. Once awakened, says a modern text, "It [*kuṇḍalinī*] makes a person both spiritual and talented, and [makes him] acquire the capacity to work in any sphere of life with competency. He is, as it were, permanently infused with an elixir of life, elevating him morally, intellectually, and spiritually."[4] "In Siddha Yoga," Swami Muktananda said in a 1975 interview, "when you get the grace of a Siddha Guru who has received that grace from his Master, the inner divinity, or divine power—called Kundalini Shakti—is awakened. This is called Shaktipat initiation. Once this power is awakened through grace, it automatically takes you to higher and higher levels of [inner] experience until you reach a state of equanimity."[5] Several generations of Siddha Yoga students have attested to the powerful effect shaktipat has had on their inner and outer lives. Many say that it has opened them to a vision of the divine unity behind the material world, and that this shift of vision has radically and positively reordered their relationships, their attitudes toward work and love, and their moral and ethical behavior. As Swami Chidvilasananda said in 1993, "Putting this divine act [of shaktipat] into words makes it sound so simple and easy, but what actually happens within, hidden from the senses, is something marvelous. It can only be deciphered by the deepest part of you, yet your whole being is rejuvenated by its light."[6]

In later years, Swami Muktananda wrote that ordinarily a guru can give shaktipat only to a few people at a time, and then only after those people have prepared themselves through a long process of self-purification that usually includes years of service and study. However, all three

Siddha Yoga gurus have been able to give shaktipat at will and without requiring lengthy preparation from those who receive it.[7] Swami Muktananda set out to offer this powerful form of spiritual initiation on a wide scale, ultimately even developing a program, the Intensive, that allowed shaktipat to be offered in a weekend.

This profoundly innovative act of open-handed shaktipat has been the basis of the Siddha Yoga movement. Equally important has been its teaching of radical nonduality, summed up in the simple phrase from Swami Muktananda's autobiography, *Play of Consciousness*: "Everything is God."[8] Swamis Muktananda and Chidvilasananda have provided their students with a body of doctrines and practices, distilled from the vast reservoir of Indian tradition, designed to lead them by a path combining both personal effort and guru's grace to the point where they can experience this world and themselves as divine.

Most importantly, Swami Muktananda and, to an even greater extent, Swami Chidvilasananda have offered the guru-disciple relationship as the source of grace and guidance not just to a few but to anyone who sincerely follows their teachings. Offering their own lives as the model, they have promised that any seeker willing to give him or herself fully to the path of Siddha Yoga can achieve the state that the Indian scriptures hold out as the ultimate goal of human life—*mokṣa*, "freedom from the cycle of birth and death."[9] Siddha Yoga thus rests on an implicit premise that dedication to its practice can lead to the most powerful shift in awareness possible for a human being.

Over the years since Swami Muktananda inaugurated his "meditation revolution," the style in which shaktipat is transmitted and the forms that students adopt in following the path have been refined and vastly expanded as its adherents have grown in number from a small intimate circle to a worldwide movement in which many students receive initiation before physically meeting their master. So, on the surface, the culture surrounding Gurumayi Chidvilasananda, the contemporary head of the lineage, contrasts strongly with the lifestyle that presented itself to a devotee of Bhagawan Nityananda.

For example, a newcomer arriving in the 1990s at Gurumayi Chidvilasananda's ashram in South Fallsburg, New York, would find a culture in which distinctly Hindu elements—Sanskrit chanting; traditional methods of relating to the teacher; the invocation of deities like Śiva, Lakṣmī, and Sarasvatī—exist side by side with a Western organizational style, a sophisticated use of video technology, and a distinctly contemporary flavor in the articulation of its teachings. Whereas Bhagawan Nityananda rarely spoke, Gurumayi Chidvilasananda is a notable lecturer whose writings demonstrate equal familiarity with the teachings of the Indian scriptures and the complexities of life in modern society. Her teachings are often delivered to several thousand people at a time, and she regularly gives shaktipat initiation via satellite television to students in as many as ninety Siddha Yoga centers worldwide. Whereas Nityananda's followers, according to contemporary evidence, tended to be villagers, workers, religious mendicants, businessmen, and the occasional dignitary from southern and western India, Gurumayi's come from a wide range of professions and cultures. There are centers of Siddha Yoga meditation in twenty-nine countries besides India, including South Africa, Poland, and Russia. Bhagawan Nityananda received devotees in a stone hut whose assembly room felt cramped when twenty-five people were present. Nowadays the main Western Siddha Yoga ashram occupies a former hotel, and more than a thousand people can be seated in its spacious and comfortable meditation halls. The organization of these modern ashrams has little in common with the casual arrangements that prevailed in Bhagawan Nityananda's environs.

Yet though its exterior culture has evolved, those who enter deeply into the teachings and the practice of Siddha Yoga maintain that the essence of the path, and the fundamental experience of its participants, remains unchanged. From Bhagawan Nityananda's time to the present, students of Siddha Yoga have reported the same life-changing experiences of spiritual awakening, expressed the same devotion to and confidence in their guru, and followed the same fundamental teaching, summed up in Swami Muktananda's aphoristic phrase, "Meditate on your inner Self; God dwells within you as you." All three Siddha Yoga gurus have made the same implicit promise of grace and guidance on the spiritual journey to the students who take refuge in them.

This section of the present book—Part I—will trace the contemporary development of the Siddha Yoga movement, from its beginnings in the village of Ganeshpuri in western Maharashtra, India, to its present-day international expansion. We will look at how the teaching methods and institutions of Siddha Yoga have evolved to meet the changing needs of its students, and how the essential elements of the tradition—the guru-disciple relationship, shaktipat, and meditation—have been translated into the idioms of different cultures as the Siddha Yoga masters widened the context of practice.

Without Talking, He Gave Instructions: Bhagawan Nityananda of Ganeshpuri

Siddha Yoga's contemporary history begins in the 1930s in the Tansa River Valley of the western Indian state of Maharashtra. In 1932, this region, just ninety kilometers from Bombay, was still mostly jungle, sprinkled with rice fields and a few small hamlets, and known for the natural hot baths (*kuṇḍ*) that laced the riverbed and bubbled up from underground. The local market town, Vajreshwari, held a temple sacred to a goddess (*devī*) of the same name, and the whole valley was believed by the inhabitants to be under the protection of the Vajreśvarī *devī.** The original primitive images in the temple had been restored in the eighteenth century by a Peshwa ruler, Chimaji Appa, to celebrate a victory over the Portuguese. The temple was an important and popular pilgrimage site, visited by yogis as well as seekers of religious blessings. However, most of the inhabitants of the surrounding area were profoundly poor—members of the casteless aboriginal (*ādivāsī*) tribes, who struggled for bare survival, occupying leaf huts and making their living by hunting and gathering or by working, for pitifully low pay, for the local *patils* (Marathi: "landed farmers"), of the region.

Legends abounded about the valley, which like many rural regions in India claimed a connection to bygone spiritual glories. One persistent piece of local lore associates the region with the Dandaka Forest described in the epic *Rāmāyaṇa*; Lord Rāma and his brother Lakṣmaṇa were said to have passed through the area in their search for Rāma's abducted wife Sītā. Another legend describes how the ancient sage Vasiṣṭha performed a fire ritual (*yajña*) in the area; the hot springs were supposed to have been created by him for the convenience of the sages who were his guests. Mandagni Mountain, which shadows the area north of Vajreshwari, was said to have been named for Agni, the fire god invoked in Vasiṣṭha's sacri-

---

*The legend holds that in ancient times, a sacrifice was held in Tansa Valley by a sage, Vasiṣṭha. Indra, the chief of the gods, felt threatened by the spiritual power unleashed in the sacrifice and sent his thunderbolt (*vajra*) to destroy it. Vasiṣṭha prayed to the goddess Pārvatī, consort to Śiva, who immediately appeared to catch the thunderbolt and save the sacrifice from destruction. Hence the name Vajreśvarī, "goddess of the thunderbolt."

fices; in the 1930s, according to local reports, yogis still lived in hidden caves on its slopes.

Two miles from Vajreshwari in a tiny hamlet named Ganeshpuri stood an obscure Śiva temple, walled in rock and housing a rough natural stone *liṅga,* the pillar-shaped form symbolic of Śiva's creative power. The temple had an interesting natural feature: From its rock roof dripped a perpetual trickle of water that fell on the *liṅga.* Local people considered this a sign of special blessedness, since the stream performed a constant *abhiṣeka,* or ritual bath, of the *liṅga* beneath it. Though the temple was little used, one of the local families had taken care of it since the eighteenth century, living on a small government pension, and as is often the case with small temples in India, had assumed virtual ownership of the site.

Sometime in 1923, a tall, loincloth-clad yogi known as Nityananda (which literally means "eternal bliss") walked into Tansa Valley. He came from South India, where he had a reputation as a wonder worker, and though initially little was known of him in this region, it was not long before the villagers of Vajreshwari and nearby Akloli began to pay him their respects.

One morning in 1936, two devotees from Akloli accompanied Nityananda to the Śiva temple in Ganeshpuri. Gangubai Bhopi, the wife of the caretaker, happened to be sweeping the temple when they approached. As she told the story in an interview in 1989, her immediate thought on seeing this tall, shaven-headed figure standing outside the narrow doorway was that Nityananda was a Muslim. "You can't come in," she shrieked, frightened that the touch of a non-Hindu would desecrate the temple. At that, one of his companions explained, "He's not a man; he's a god."*

Gangubai, a devout and simple person, said that these words electrified her. "I came out and caught hold of his feet," she reported fifty years later. "[I said] 'Baba, forgive me, I said the wrong things. I didn't recognize you.'" The yogi laughed and asked to whom the temple belonged. On being told that it belonged to the government, he asked if he could stay there. Gangubai agreed. She helped him build a wooden hut with a cow-dung floor, and Nityananda took up residence.

From the beginning, say witnesses, Nityananda manifested marvels. Gangubai later recalled how a few weeks after his arrival the saint announced that he would give a feast for the local *ādivāsīs,* who lived habitually in a state near starvation. That same day, a truck arrived filled with sacks

*In the Indian tradition, God-realized persons are said to have become one with the ultimate reality. For this reason they are often referred to as being divine themselves. Such saints as Shirdi Sai Baba and Ramakrishna Paramahamsa were often addressed as "Deva" (literally, "shining one" or "god") by their devotees. Nityananda himself came to be called Bhagawan, meaning "beloved one," a term often applied to deities.

of rice and *dal*. Several days later, according to Gangubai, another truck lumbered through the jungle, this one loaded with cooking utensils. None of the villagers knew where these windfalls had come from, whether they had been sent by a devotee or arranged for by Nityananda. They simply assumed that Nityananda somehow manifested them by his *vibhūtis*, his "supernormal powers." After that, truckloads of vegetables would show up at regular intervals, and Nityananda's feasts became an important source of nourishment for the local residents. He fed everyone who came without regard for numbers, and according to Gangubai and other local eyewitnesses, there was always enough.[10]

Hagiographies of Indian saints typically include tales of feasts where a single pot of rice serves hundreds without running dry, and the devotees' reminiscences of Nityananda in Ganeshpuri are filled with such incidents. He reportedly exhibited other extraordinary powers as well. First, his detachment from the body was remarkable. He went without clothes in all weather, often sitting for days on end on a rock or on the bare ground, and ate only what was given to him. His favorite expression for material wealth as well as for the worldly concerns of his devotees was *miṭṭi*—"dust!" He would sometimes lie for hours without moving, in a state of *samādhi* (absorption in God), radiating an atmosphere that devotees have described as intoxicatingly blissful. In fact, his devotees used to watch him in fascination, sometimes for hours. "His skin was like a dark shining jewel filled with divine radiance," wrote Swami Muktananda in his biography of his guru, *Bhagawan Nityananda of Ganeshpuri*. "His forehead was high and arched, and his face completely captivating. . . . A river of love poured forth from his glance. . . . Now and then he would laugh out loud, and the sound of that laughter still rings in the ears of those lucky enough to have heard it."[11]

Nityananda was considered to be an *avadhūta*, a saint absorbed in a transcendental state, beyond body-consciousness and beyond the ordinary conventions of human life.[12] He spoke little and his words and actions were notoriously cryptic. At the same time, he would often reveal information about the lives of his devotees that later proved true, and his psychic powers were said to include mind reading. Many devotees say that when they went to see him with a family problem or a sickness, he would sometimes tell them what to do about their problem before they had a chance to voice it. He was also known for bilocation. Swami Muktananda described how a government official once put Nityananda in jail as a vagrant, only to release him when passersby noticed Nityananda on the road outside the jail at the same time that the jailers knew him to be inside his cell. Then there was his habit of producing objects out of thin air: many South Indian devotees claim to have seen him, when asked for a ticket on a train, pull out a fistful of tickets from his loincloth.[13] "Local people saw him walking on the waters of the Pavanja River," wrote Swami Muktananda in *Bhagawan Nityananda of*

Ganeshpuri. "Many times he fed thousands of people with sweets, and no one knows where the sweets came from."*

BHAGAWAN NITYANANDA'S EARLY LIFE

As in the case of Sai Baba of Shirdi and Swami Samarth of Akalkot, two modern-day siddhas[14] renowned for their supernatural powers and much sought after for blessings, the known facts of Nityananda's life history are sketchy and difficult to separate from the hagiography. Most of the available reports on his early life come from uneducated villagers and include incidents recalled after fifty years, undoubtedly colored by time and by the tendency of the devotees of charismatic yogis to mythologize the object of their devotion. The most commonly accepted version holds that Nityananda's parents lived in the town of Qualandi in Kerala State and worked as servants in the house of a lawyer named Ishwara Iyer. One story declares that Nityananda's mother found him in the forest while she wandered in search of food and simply adopted him as her son, but the truth of this account is not known. His childhood name was Ram. All who knew him in those years agree that from an early age he manifested an unusual yogic state.[15]

Nityananda's patron, Ishwara Iyer, was known in Qualandi as a devout brahmin (Sanskrit, *brāhmaṇa*) with a high degree of proficiency in yoga; it was accepted by many in his circle that he acted as a guru to the young Nityananda. Krishna Nair, an Indian high court judge who lived next door to the Iyers as a boy, said that Nityananda always showed Ishwara Iyer the respect due to a teacher. Swami Muktananda also acknowledged that a guru-disciple relationship existed between the two.[16] At the same time, Swami Muktananda and most of Nityananda's other devotees maintained that though Nityananda honored Ishwara Iyer as his guru, the saint belonged to the class of accomplished yogis referred to in Abhinavagupta's *Tantrāloka* as *saṃsiddhika-gurus* or *janma* ("born") *siddhas*. Such yogis are said to come into the world in the Self-realized state, rather than having to achieve it through yogic practice or by service to a teacher—the methods by which an ordinary yogic practitioner attains mastery. Such a being,

---

**Bhagawan Nityananda of Ganeshpuri*, p. 7. Swami Muktananda always pointed out that Nityananda's unusual powers were never deliberate attempts to astonish or impress, but rather arose naturally as a result of his inner state. In *Play of Consciousness* (p. 20), he writes, "He [Bhagawan Nityananda] did not attach any importance to *siddhis*, miraculous powers; he believed that compared to God's miracle of Self-manifestation, all other miracles are insignificant. . . . [I]t is quite natural for *siddhis* to live in Siddhas. They become active in such beings without being invoked and keep dancing around them unbidden."

Muktananda once said, accepts a guru out of respect for the tradition of gurus, rather than because he really needs a mentor.*

Even the name "Nityananda" was not an official monastic title, but simply a description of the saint's blissful inner state. "Because he loved to smile," wrote Swami Muktananda, "people came to address him as Nityananda, one who is always in bliss."[17] Nityananda's South Indian devotees say that he was given his name by Ishwara Iyer. The story goes that after some years in the Himalayas, Nityananda returned to Qualandi because his benefactor was very sick and had been praying for his return. When Ishwara Iyer saw him, he circumambulated the young yogi, saying, "Ah, my Nityananda has come, my Nityananda has come." From then on, he was known as Nityananda.[18]

Nityananda's "Miraculous" Powers

Nityananda was still an adolescent when his yogic powers began manifesting publicly, and he took to the roads before he was twenty. According to his own statements, he spent time doing yogic practices in the Himalayas (devotees say he spoke familiarly of most of the famous holy places in India), but in the 1920s he began to be seen again in towns and villages in the South Indian states of Kerala and Karnataka. He usually traveled on foot, eating whatever was given to him, often wearing nothing at all. (Later, devotees persuaded him to dress in a loincloth.) It was at this time that the stories began to circulate. His touch was said to be healing, and village folk throughout the countryside told of his miraculous cures. Someone's wife was cured of a tumor after Bhagawan Nityananda blessed her; someone else's cousin recovered miraculously from typhoid. Soon, people began to lie in wait for him and even run after him, begging for a healing for themselves or a sick relative. Sushila Shenoy, a resident of Vajreshwari who met Nityananda when she was a bride of thirteen in the village of Mulki, near Mangalore, described how he would pick leaves from a tree and throw them down on the visitors:

> Bade Baba** [Nityananda] would climb up the tree and sit on it. Then villagers would gather around the tree and keep calling him, "O Baba, O Baba, O

---

*Swami Muktananda said, "Even though [Nityananda] was a self-born Siddha, still he had to have a Guru. Even Lord Krishna had a Guru called Sandipani. It is the spiritual law—one has to have a Guru. And Lord Rama, who was also an incarnation of God, had a Guru called Vasishtha." (*Bhagawan Nityananda of Ganeshpuri*, p. 76).

**Both Nityananda and Muktananda were called Baba, an affectionate term meaning "father," by devotees. In later years, devotees came to refer to Bhagawan Nityananda as Bade Baba (literally "big" or "senior" father) to distinguish him from Muktananda, who was known to Nityananda's devotees as Chhota (literally "little" or "junior") Baba.

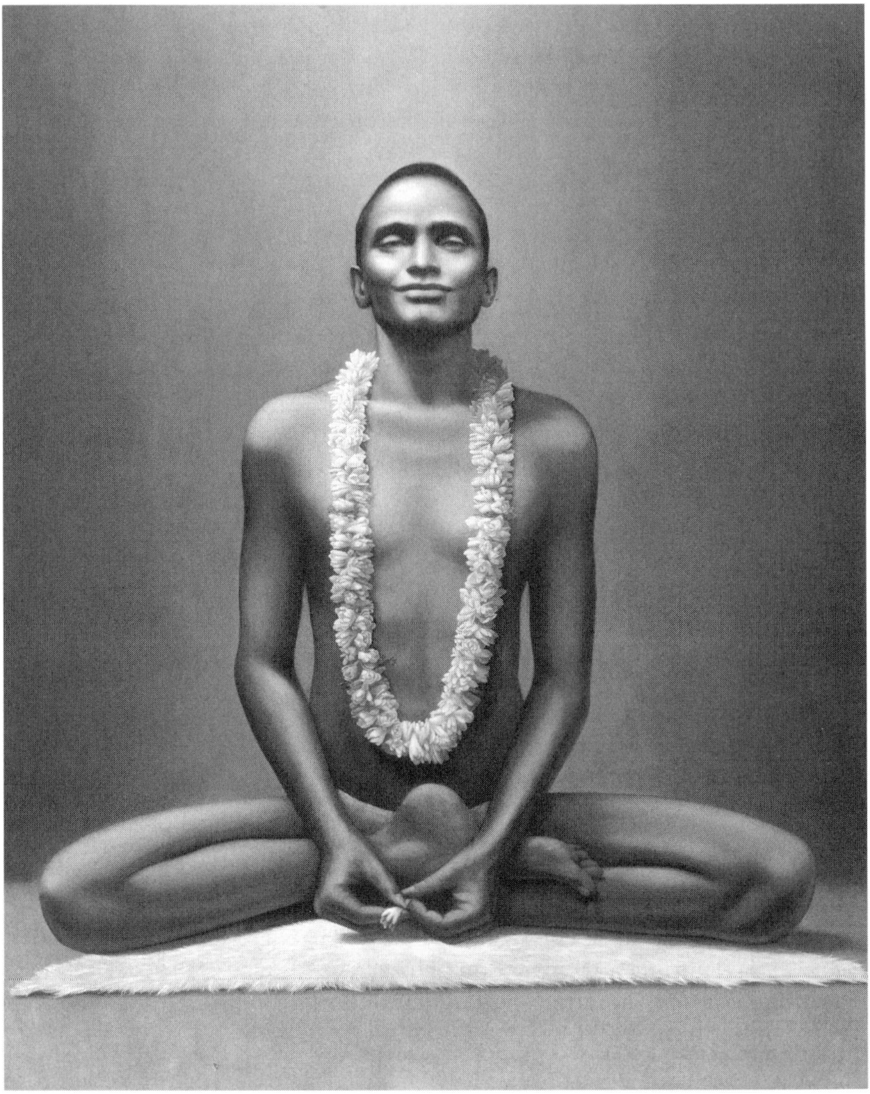

Fig. 1. Painting of the young Nityananda from a photograph taken September 24, 1926

> Baba." . . . He would never talk to the villagers or even look at them. Sometimes he would pick some leaves and throw them at people. . . . So the villagers would follow him on the road, and they would say, "O Baba, I'm feeling sick, I have got a headache, my tummy is aching." Then after a couple of days we would find out that Bade Baba gave this plant and someone extracted juice from it, and the [person] was cured.[19]

Sushila Shenoy added, "The poor people knew he was a saint, but we didn't." Even those who went to him for cures did not necessarily know him as a guru. However, there were families in the Mangalore area who followed him as a spiritual teacher and, according to Sushila Shenoy, he would sit in their house and give spiritual discourses. "Otherwise, he would walk around and then suddenly go to someone's house. He was very pure. If he found or sensed purity in your house, he would go there."

One of his first devotees was a woman named Tulsi Amma, a devout widow who had a small following as a spiritual teacher. Said Shenoy, "Tulsi Amma was staying in a small place. Bade Baba would go and sit there, and he started training her. He was very strict. Then he told her to build a *maṭha* [monastery], and he would sit there in the state of an *avadhūta.* One had to feed and bathe him at times." Tulsi Amma collected some of Nityananda's remarks, and later published them in a small book called *Chidakash Gita,* written in Kannada and later published in English.*

Because Bhagawan Nityananda so often went naked, owned nothing, and had no visible means of support, he often aroused the suspicion of the police. In *Bhagawan Nityananda of Ganeshpuri,* Swami Muktananda recounted one charming tale of how the police tried to arrest him for forgery. Swami Muktananda said that in the 1920s Nityananda had decided to build an ashram in some jungle caves (originally built as a fortified encampment) near the town of Kanhangad in Kerala state.** Architecture was an avocation of his: He would design buildings by drawing with a stick in the dust, and the workers would build according to his rudimentary plans. For this project, he hired local workers to cut a road and dig wells. On pay day, he would tell them to look under various rocks and stones for their money—which always turned up as promised. When word got around that this naked *avadhūta* was running a construction project, the local police suspected him of printing counterfeit money and demanded that he show them his mint. Bhagawan Nityananda led them deep into a jungle, dove into a crocodile-infested pool and came out with fistfuls of money, shouting, "Here's my mint. Come and see!" From then on the local police left him alone.[20]

---

*This book is highly edited and may represent Tulsi Amma's own interpolations of Nityananda's cryptic words; Swami Muktananda never recommended the book to his students and seems not to have recognized its authenticity within the Siddha Yoga canon.

**The Kanhangad ashram still exists, maintained by devotees of Bhagawan Nityananda.

Others, however did not. Sometimes village toughs harassed him by throwing stones. Evidently, it was the physical harassment Bhagawan Nityananda suffered in his native South India that eventually drove him out of the region and led him to settle in the state of Maharashtra, and eventually in Ganeshpuri.[21]

Bhagawan Nityananda and the Ādivāsīs

Nityananda had not been long in Ganeshpuri when his reputation as a miracle worker began to attract devotees from nearby Bombay, many of them transplanted South Indians who had known of him in their native place. Gradually a small hamlet, with restaurants, rest houses, flower stalls, and the other accoutrements of a traditional Indian pilgrimage site sprang up around him; to this day, the economy of Ganeshpuri village rests largely on the services it provides for pilgrims to the shrine where Bhagawan Nityananda's body is buried. Nityananda himself often went out of his way to provide material help for devotees; several of the flower sellers and restaurant owners in the neighboring area were originally set up in business by the saint.

More significantly, he began not only to feed but to provide means to clothe and educate the local *ādivāsīs*, who had been regarded by most local people as little better than animals. Vasu Shetty, an old devotee, recalled:

> All the land in the area was in the hands of landlords. The landlords paid these *ādivāsīs* for the work they did by way of grains. These people didn't get enough food—they starved. To fill their stomachs, they hunted in the forests, they ate leaves. They made a skirt-type of dress out of leaves. These people didn't even know how to milk a cow. Bade Baba came here and taught them how to milk the cows. He gave two pairs of clothes to all the poor men and a sari to all the women. He gave away clothes and food to whoever came.[22]

Bhagawan Nityananda also set up a school for the local children, as well as a center that fed them daily. The Balbhojan ("children's food") Center he created exists in Ganeshpuri village to this day.

In fact, several devotees of that time maintain to this day that one of Nityananda's motives for settling in Ganeshpuri was to look after the *ādivāsīs*. Ani, an *ādivāsī* devotee from the hamlet of Gavdevi, adjacent to the present Gurudev Siddha Peeth ashram, said in 1976:

> Nityananda Baba did so much for us. . . . He fed our children, and he clothed us. He built a medical center for us. He hired us all to work on the roads, he built all the roads. . . . Where all the money came from no one knew. He used to sit under the *adhumbhar* [a tree of the *Ficus* variety] tree to pay all the people who were working on the road. Where did the money come from? He used to pull it right up from under where he was sitting, paper notes and all.[23]

Bhagawan Nityananda regularly enlisted the visiting devotees, albeit casually, in giving employment to the *ādivāsīs*, and he could be creative in the means he devised for teaching the *ādivāsīs* elementary life-skills. Gopal Karkera, an officer of the Shree Bhimeshwar Sadguru Nityananda Trust,* recalled:

> The *ādivāsīs* were in the habit of begging money from visitors; Nityananda told them, "Don't give money like alms. Ask them to carry your bag and then you pay them something. Like that, teach them: 'Do work and then you will get money.'"[24]

BHAGAWAN NITYANANDA AS A TEACHER

Few devotees experienced Bhagawan Nityananda as a conventional guru or teacher of yoga. Most seekers sought him out not so much for his instruction as for his deeds—his protection and blessings—and their effect on their daily lives.

There is no doubt, however, that Nityananda gave teachings. To householders, he might give simple instructions that allowed them to integrate their spiritual and worldly lives. "He would say, 'Do your duty first, look after your parents, have faith. Remaining in the family, keep remembering the Lord,'" recalled Gopal Karkera.[25] To his more spiritually advanced disciples, he was likely to give instructions that pointed to a radical nondualism. Once, walking by a river near the village of Ganeshpuri, he looked at a boulder and said to Swami Muktananda: "Do you see this rock? See the miracle? See the doing of universal Consciousness? Here it has become a rock, here it has become a tree, and here it has become a human being."[26] The teaching that Swami Muktananda was later to take around the world—"Meditate on your inner Self, God dwells within you as you"—was based on Bhagawan Nityananda's instructions to his devotees. So was another of his essential teachings, "See God in each other." "Why do you worship Śiva outside," he once asked Muktananda, who had just returned from performing a ritual at the Śiva temple. "Śiva is within. Worship him there."[27] Swami Muktananda also used to quote a remark his guru made to him when Muktananda turned up with an Upaniṣad under his arm. Nityananda tapped his head and said, "Do you know how this book was made? It was made by a brain. The brain may make any number of books, but a book cannot make a brain. You had better let go of the book and meditate."[28] Nityananda was not denigrating scholarly knowledge as such—in later years he often praised Swami Muktananda's learning. Instead, he seems to have been pointing out that Muktananda should tap the source of direct, experi-

*This trust administers the shrine that has grown up around Nityananda's tomb.

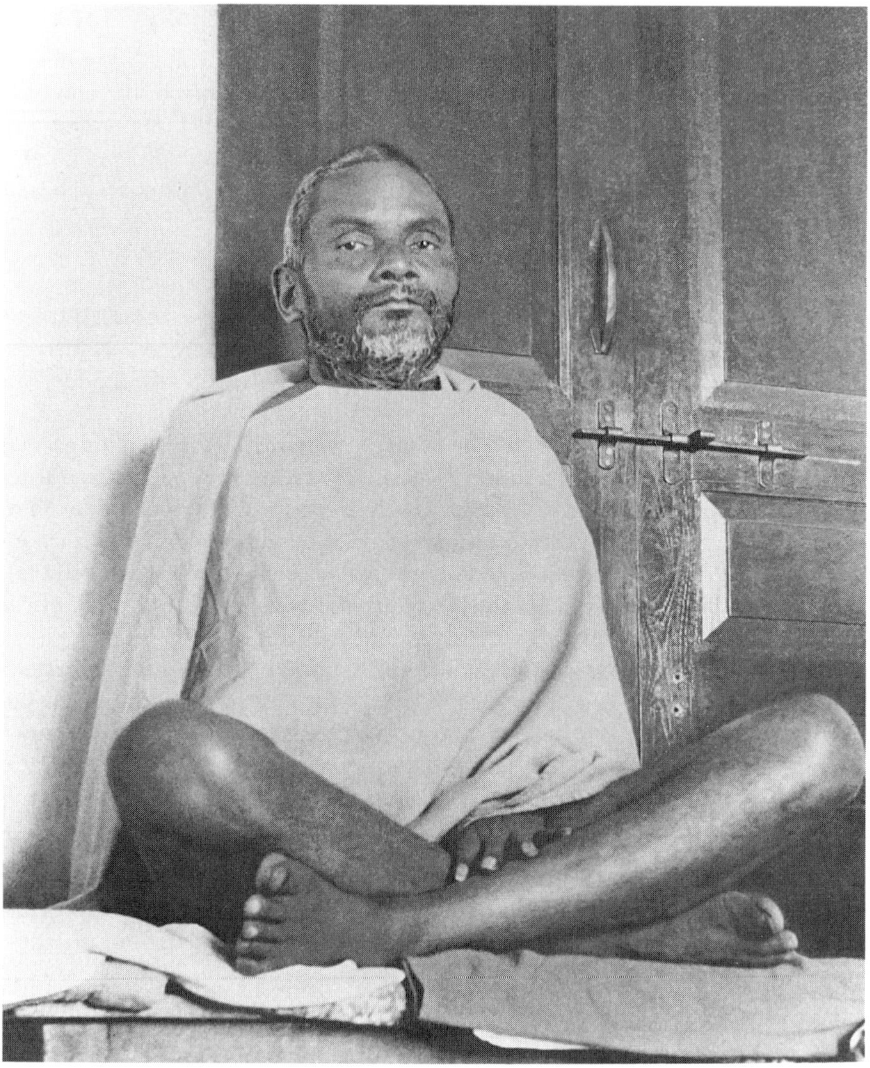

Fig. 2. Bhagawan Nityananda

ential knowledge that only meditation inspires. And in fact, Swami Muktananda went on to say, from that moment he stopped relying on books for knowledge and began to look for the truth in meditation.

Normally, Bhagawan Nityananda's teachings were delivered in such cryptic language that not everyone could understand what he really meant. As Swami Muktananda said of the atmosphere around Nityananda:

> If he ever spoke, he might say two or three words, and those three words were enough for a person's entire life. . . .
>
> [He] didn't write any books. He used to speak a little and people have collected his words and put together some books. He spoke in aphorisms and mixed different languages together. He might say just three words, "Give this there." Give it where? There were so many places, so many people!
>
> He used strange words. Sometimes he would say, "Hmm"—that's all. The people who had been with him for a long time could understand his words, so they interpreted them to others. For instance, they would say, "Baba said you should leave."
>
> There were times when he would speak very straightforwardly and simply. Somebody might go to him and say, "Baba, I came for your darshan."
>
> Sometimes he answered, "Hey, you dimwit! Don't I live in you? Why do you have to come here for my darshan? Have your own darshan. I am in you. Why do you have to have my darshan. Don't I live within you?"
>
> That was his state. He was a Siddha. He was beyond your rules, beyond your customs, beyond your disciplines. Siddhas live a strange life.
>
> . . . As people kept watching him, they would feel him inside themselves; they would feel knowledge arising within them. . . . Without talking, he gave instructions. Without giving the touch, he awakened the inner shakti. He did not have to hold question-and-answer sessions. Without speaking, he answered people's questions.[29]

Many devotees' reminiscences of Bhagawan Nityananda agree on the uncanny effect of his silent presence on a person's inner state. Swami Muktananda wrote: "Sitting in his presence, everyone meditated spontaneously."[30] Said Vasu Shetty: "Bade Baba would just look at all the people. He would hardly talk. He might at times give very short instructions so the queue would move. No one would dare to talk. Just by hearing his voice, people would get affected and remain at peace. If you just glanced at him, peace would come and settle in your heart."[31]

Witnesses testify to the great power in Bhagawan Nityananda's glance. Vasu Shetty recalled: "We people could not look at him, there was so much radiance. If Bade Baba looked at you with both his eyes, you simply would have to close your eyes. It was like when you look at the sun, your eyes water. Similarly, we could not withstand the gaze of Bade Baba. We would have to look down, at our feet."[32]

A significant distinction between Bhagawan Nityananda and more conventional teachers was his method of giving spiritual initiation. Since Indian tradition holds that there can be no progress in spiritual life without initiation, a seeker who enters into relationship with a guru usually receives a formal, often ceremonial initiation. Bhagawan Nityananda, as Swami Muktananda later said, had no need for such ceremonies. Instead, he would usually give his blessings through a piece of fruit or a casual look.* Swami Muktananda often said that the uniqueness of his guru lay in this capacity to transmit spiritual knowledge and spiritual awakening spontaneously, without any apparent effort or even, necessarily, any conscious intent. Moreover, in significant contrast to less powerful gurus, who might give initiation to one or two people at a time, usually through a ritual and only after requiring their disciples to purify themselves for a long time by mantra repetition or service, Bhagawan Nityananda was able to initiate seekers without demanding any special austerities of them. He could do this, Swami Muktananda later explained, because Nityananda was in a state of such complete oneness with God that he could purify a seeker's consciousness for him. Indian tradition holds that the impressions of past thoughts and actions stay with a human soul, creating both his present character and future destiny, causing that soul to be reborn again and again in order to live out the consequences of past deeds. In order to escape the cycle, a seeker must live out or dissolve all these accumulated karmas; certain yogic practices have as their goal the dissolution of an individual's karmic traces. According to Śaiva Siddhānta, one of the traditions that describes shaktipat, shaktipat initiation takes place when the accumulated effects of one's positive and negative actions are evenly balanced; seekers undergo purification in order to burn off the negative past impressions that create imbalance. A siddha guru has the capacity to take on the negative karmas and, as Swami Muktananda often said, burn them through the power generated in meditation.[33]**

---

*Swami Muktananda said, "When people used to watch my Baba, they would receive shaktipat just like that. They didn't have to receive the mantra from him. Just by watching him, changes would occur in them. If he threw an object at a person, say a banana, and if that person ate that, then he would receive shaktipat. He didn't need to have initiation, or any ritual, or any ceremonies. This is the characteristic of a Siddha." (From an unpublished transcript, February 11, 1977)

**The *Kulārṇava Tantra* (13.133) also cites the ability to take away karmas as one of the defining characteristics of genuine guru:

> As in the vicinity of fire all butter gets melted, so in the proximity of the holy Guru, all sins dissolve.

Translation by Ram Kumar Rai (Varanasi, India: Prachya Prakashan, 1983), p. 258.

A devotee recalled watching Bhagawan Nityananda transmitting spiritual energy to a friend of his:

> Nityananda was standing there, and this other man was standing in front of him. . . . I saw a blue light coming [from Bade Baba's eyes], like the light that comes when you hold a flashlight in the darkness, a blue light going in and entering his forehead like this. It was going from Nityananda's eyes to this man's forehead, like a continuous light entering. The man shouted "*Om*" and then fell down. He was shaking on the ground like a bird. I saw all this. I wept like a child, because [I thought], "I have brought one man and he dies here." Then Bhagawan left him and came to me. He was breathing [into] my nose, and he said, in Hindi, "Be strong. Be strong." It took about half a dozen times to make me stronger; otherwise I was weeping loudly like a child. Later, I made inquiries with other friends, narrated this story to them. They said, "That is what is known as shaktipat."[34]

As this account makes clear, Bhagawan Nityananda's disciples knew that he conveyed a special kind of initiation. Yet until Swami Muktananda explained it many years later, few devotees understood exactly what the term *shaktipat* meant, or understood the significance of the yogic movements (*kriyās*) sometimes including falling or shaking that might occur as a result. Devotees who received Nityananda's favor would experience spontaneous states of meditation, and people reported that their minds became still and joyful in his presence. However, not many had the courage to question the master about what he was doing.

Bhagawan Nityananda's "Yogic Fire"

In fact, during his early years in Ganeshpuri, most people besides the children kept a respectful distance from Nityananda. He showed great fondness for children; the Ganeshpuri youngsters played freely around him at all hours, and he would sometimes bathe and feed them with his own hands. With adults, however, he could be fierce. Vasu Shetty recalled:

> He was very hot. He would get hot with people. He would begin reciting that person's living habits; his past bad habits; his mistreatment of his mother, sisters, and other women. He would even throw stones. People with bad habits and vocations were afraid to come to Bade Baba. But in his later years he became peaceful and silent, and then all types of people would come for darshan. . . . Anyone could come and go."[35]

Nityananda's "hot" behavior was highly characteristic of traditional yogic culture, which abounds with legends of yogis like the ancient sage Durvāsas, whose propensity for hurling imprecations at those who broke the rules of dharma is described in numerous tales from the *Purāṇas*, the books of ancient legends and lore that provide most of the religious stories cherished in Indian culture. The fiery behavior of great yogis is a means by which they purify their disciples, teach them control of their inner tendencies, and free them from attachment to praise and fear of criticism. The yogic tradition promotes inner control and the transformation of physical and subtle impurities, a process that is compared to the purification of gold in fire. So, in the *Śiva Saṃhitā,* one reads of the yogic fire that burns away inner impurities and is reflected in the outer behavior of yogic masters, whose words and gestures are said to contain a fire that can burn away the impurities and incorrect understanding of the disciples. Part of the guru's function, according to the tradition, is to correct his disciples' understanding and to turn them away from materiality, egocentricity, and selfish preoccupations. One of the customary means the guru employed was known as *daṇḍa*—literally, "rod"—an exchange in which the master would signal disapproval or get the disciple's attention by shouting or, occasionally, striking him. The Sufi, Sikh, and Zen traditions are rife with accounts of how a disciple's awakening or spiritual transformation resulted directly from the master's blows. A couplet (*doha*) by the poet-saint Kabīr gives some insight into the disciple's experience:

> Master is the potter,
> Disciple the pot:
> The Master puts him on the wheel
> And removes his rough corners—
> He raps the pot on the outside
> But inside keeps
> His hand of support.[36]

In fact, this sort of behavior seemed quite normal in the Indian culture of those days, where nearly every schoolteacher enforced classroom discipline with a stick.

Devotees say that Bhagawan Nityananda's demonstrations of fierceness served three other basic functions. First, they kept unsavory people away—a significant benefit, since Nityananda used to be approached by gamblers wanting tips on the horses as well as by criminals wanting blessings for nefarious schemes, and his ferocity was the only means of defense against their importunities. (According to one eyewitness, some intrepid souls used to attempt to turn even his displeasure to their advantage by betting on the numbers according to how many rocks Nityananda threw at them![37])

Second, the aloof, stern, or apparently fiery demeanor of the saint served as a screening method for separating the serious seekers from the merely curious.

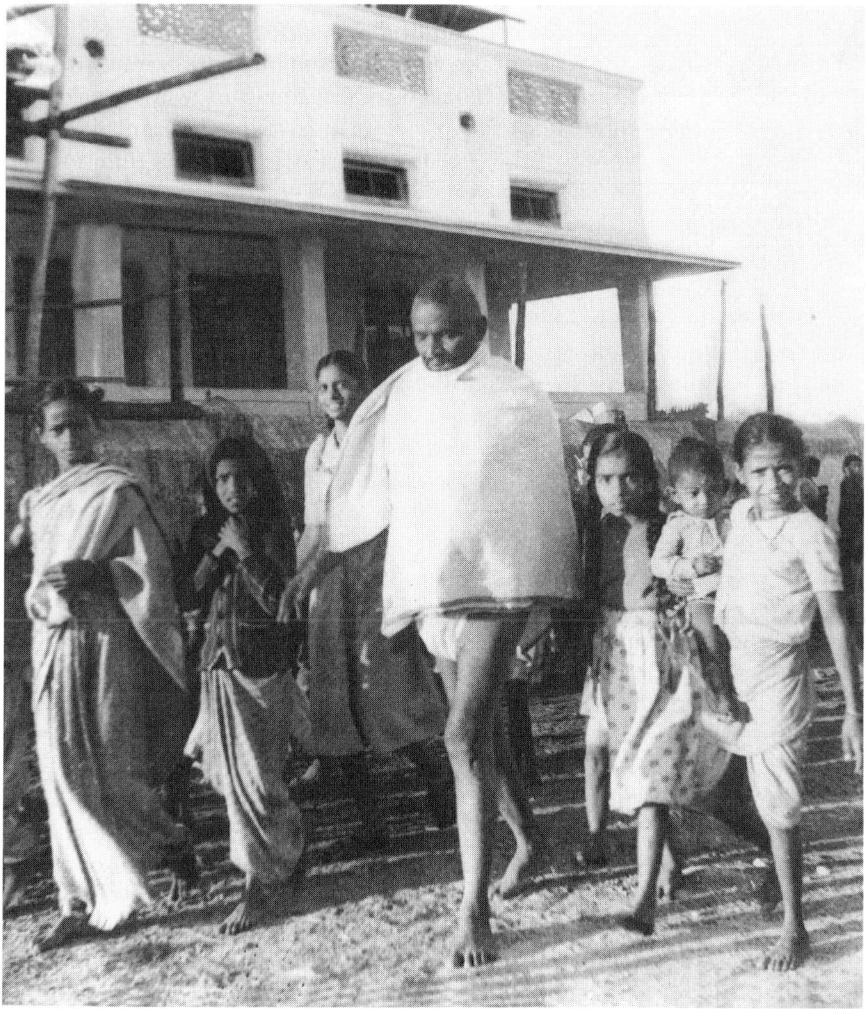

Fig. 3. Nityananda in the village of Ganeshpuri, with his ashram, Kailas Bhavan, under construction in the background, ca. 1958

There was also an esoteric function served by Bhagawan Nityananda's strong words. As the *Avadhūtagītā* and the *Śrīmadbhāgavatam* relate, the ways of *avadhūtas* are the reverse of those of ordinary people.[38] Specifically, Nityananda's brusque words were a vehicle by which he gave blessings. It used to be said that every insulting term carried boons, and people with worldly difficulties or problems would find that if they were strong enough to bear Nityananda's ferocity and kept visiting him, their troubles would go away. Said Swami Muktananda, "There was shaktipat in his abusive terms; there was shaktipat in his sticks."[39]

The Development of Ganeshpuri

As Bhagawan Nityananda's fame grew, the social base of his circle also broadened. Beginning in the early forties, a steadily growing number of middle-class and wealthy devotees came regularly from Bombay, until in the final days of Bhagawan Nityananda's life, thousands of people were willing to brave the rough roads and primitive domestic arrangements of Ganeshpuri for the sake of having a glimpse of him.

Accommodations were minimal. By 1940, the simple shack built by Gangubai and her husband had become a small ashram known as Vaikunth. Built of black stone with a thatch and tile roof, the structure contained a small, dark room where Bhagawan Nityananda stayed and a larger room where recitations of scriptural texts were sometimes held and where devotees gathered. However, except for the rare devotee who might be invited to pass the night in the hall of Bhagawan Nityananda's ashram, no one visited longer than a day, for there was simply no place to stay.

As time went on, Nityananda began to make arrangements for visitors. He renovated a small temple called Anasuya Mandir, and would direct sadhus (Sanskrit, *sādhu*: "mendicant") to stay there for a tenure of no more than the traditional three days. The village headman would provide rice and dried beans, which the sadhu could cook in water from the hot springs. Eventually, devotees opened restaurants and built dwellings in the neighborhood.

Organization of Bhagawan Nityananda's Circle

The culture around Bhagawan Nityananda, according to all reports, was marked by a certain carefree anarchy. Devotees, religious pilgrims, and seekers of blessings mingled with opportunists wishing to benefit from his popularity. Swami Muktananda sometimes spoke of how members of the so-called inner circle vied to prove their closeness to the master, jockeying for position and boasting of the blessings they had received. The penchant for intrigue that has characterized humankind since the beginning of recorded history also exists in Indian culture, and memoirs of the life around many Indian saints reveal that even devotees of God are not immune from greed, jealousy, and status-seeking. Swami Venkatesananda, a disciple of the well-known saint Swami Sivananda of Rishikesh, wrote in *Sivananda Yoga,* his biography of his guru, of how Swami Sivananda used to give refuge to virtually anyone who asked for help, including many whose motives were obviously unspiritual. Once, when Sivananda was asked why he allowed one such character—described as a "raw candidate"—in his ashram, he said, "Never mind. . . . [B]y bringing him here . . . I've ensured that there is one rogue less in Delhi!"[40] The memoirs of devotees of other Indian saints, including Ramakrishna Paramahamsa and Akalkot Swami, remark on this same fact: it appears that the compassion of the saints makes them willing to let certain devotees work out worldly tendencies in their ashram setting, perhaps in the hope that prolonged exposure to the ashram atmosphere will eventually bring about reform. The presence of such characters also tests other devotees, challenging them to develop inner strength and confidence in their own convictions.

Through it all, Bhagawan Nityananda remained serene, absorbed in his own state of constant, open-eyed meditation. His darshan (Sanskrit, *darśana:* "sight"), the experience of seeing him and receiving the blessing emanating from his silent presence, was the focus of all activity. However, by the mid-1950s, when hundreds of people began coming each Sunday for his darshan, it was not always easy to catch a glimpse of him. On holidays, devotees sometimes stood in line for hours and never knew whether they would see him sitting up and speaking or lying with his back turned, apparently asleep. Many didn't care; they said that even the sight of his back could fill the mind with peace and contentment.

Once the governor of Maharashtra announced his intention of visiting the saint. When he arrived with his entourage, entering the modest ashram with a government official's usual pomp, Nityananda refused to see him. After waiting for several hours, the governor sent his entourage away and said humbly that his wish was not to pay a state visit, but to seek Nityananda's blessings as a simple seeker. The change in the official's attitude had an immediate effect. Even before the message had been taken, Nityananda sent for the governor and began giving him spiritual instruction.[41]

Bhagawan Nityananda made few attempts to organize the life around him or to order the lives of his devotees. As Vasu Shetty described it:

> He never gave instructions, do this or do that. He used to give hints. He would say, "Such and such a place was so dirty, now it is so clean and tidy and looks good." So indirectly he would indicate, and listeners would get encouraged and start doing similar seva [service].[42]

Later chroniclers of Siddha Yoga would note this administrative laissez-faire as a major difference between Bhagawan Nityananda and his successor, Swami Muktananda, whose organizational acumen allowed him to lay the groundwork for the world movement that Siddha Yoga would become.

'He Has Become Śiva': Swami Muktananda and the Gift of Shaktipat

When Swami Muktananda arrived on the scene in Ganeshpuri, sometime in the mid-1940s, no one in Bhagawan Nityananda's circle had any idea that this modest *sannyāsī* would be Nityananda's successor. As Swami Muktananda himself wrote in later years, he made no attempt to become part of the hierarchy of Nityananda's ashram. Instead he sat silently in the back of the hall—so unobtrusive that for years many of the devotees regarded him as inconsequential. Yet at the time he met Bhagawan Nityananda, Swami Muktananda was already a yogi of great accomplishment.

SWAMI MUKTANANDA'S EARLY LIFE

Unlike Nityananda, Swami Muktananda came from a wealthy family; his father owned a large tract of land near the town of Mangalore, in the coastal region of Karnataka State.* He had several siblings, but the formative figure of his early life was his strong-willed and deeply religious mother.[43]

Swami Muktananda's earliest biographer, Swami Prajnananda (Pratibha Trivedi) began her account of his life with a remarkable story, one that resembles the legends surrounding the births of many Indian spiritual masters, from Buddha to Ramakrishna Paramahamsa.[44] Her source appears to have been Muktananda's sister, who was not herself a devotee, so we can assume that it must have been an accepted part of their family history. The story goes that after having been without a son for many years,

*Although Muktananda always kept his birthplace and family name a secret, as is customary with traditional *daśanāmi sannyāsīs*, he did once point out his house to some close devotees, and several of them, including Swami Prajnananda, later visited the place and met his sister and brother. Muktananda's village was between Dharmasthala and Mangalore, on the banks of the Netravati River. Venkappanna Shriyan and others have described it as being a very large one-story dwelling, built in the characteristic style of the region, with big verandas and a family cremation ground on the property.

Swami Muktananda's parents went on pilgrimage to the nearby Dharmasthala temple of Mañjunāth Mahādev, a form of Lord Śiva. There they prayed for the birth of an heir. Several days later, a holy man visited the wife, gave her the mantra *Oṃ Namaḥ Śivāya,* and told her that if she repeated it, God would soon bless her with a son. The mantra seemed to work; the boy, born on the full moon of the month of Vaiśakh, was named Krishna. May 16, 1908, is commonly accepted as his date of birth.*

Swami Muktananda used to say that his mother had such faith in the mantra *Oṃ Namaḥ Śivāya* that at mealtimes she would hold his hand and refuse to allow him to take a bite until he repeated the mantra the traditional eleven times. Years later, he would receive the same mantra in initiation from his guru.

Krishna's earliest ambition was to grow up to be a sage: "I had great love . . . for holy men," he later said. "Even then there was only one thing on my mind, and that was the miracles performed by these holy men, how to receive their grace, what would happen if a holy man cursed someone, and so on."[45] His father, like many wealthy men in his part of India, held readings of religious stories in his house and even sponsored festivals where tales from the lives of gods and sages were acted out. Krishna loved the stories of saints. When he and his friends acted out these tales among themselves, he would always insist on taking the part of the sage.

When young Krishna was somewhere between twelve and fifteen, an apparently casual meeting altered the course of his life.** He was at school, playing with a group of boys, when Nityananda entered the schoolyard. Many of the children knew Nityananda, since during his periodic visits to the area, he often used to come to the schoolyard to play with them. "Gurudev loved children," Swami Muktananda later said.

> . . . [S]o whenever he came to our school all of us would leave our classes and follow him. The moment we followed him, he would start running and shout-

---

*Birth records in rural India were not always kept carefully during the early years of this century, and to this day one meets village-born Indians who are not sure of their exact age or the precise date of their birth. Traditionally birthdays are marked according to the phase of the moon rather than by date. Moreover, as a *sannyāsī,* a renunciant monk, who had "died" to his conventional identity, Swami Muktananda was not forthcoming about details of his early life. *Sannyāsīs,* having renounced their name and family, generally do not disclose former identities, and though Muktananda did speak occasionally of his early life, he always did so without mentioning names or dates. This date was established by Swami Prajnananda, based on a notation she found in one of Swami Muktananda's notebooks.

**Swami Muktananda sometimes said that he was fifteen years old at this time, so, given his generally accepted birth date, it would appear that the year was 1923. However, since Athani Shiva Yogi, a holy man whom Muktananda met shortly after leaving home, died in 1921, Muktananda must have left home before that time. This argues that either he was twelve or thirteen when he had this encounter with Nityananda, or that he was born earlier than 1908.

> ing. We would run after him, and then he would climb up a tree and sit on a branch. . . .
>
> He would go into a candy store, reach into the containers, throw candy to the children, and then take off once again. Still, the shopkeepers never complained, because whenever he gave away candy, their sales went up.[46]

On this day, Nityananda walked up to the young Krishna, embraced him, and stroked his cheek. Muktananda, speaking of this incident in later life, said:

> I had this feeling that I wanted to become like him, that that would be much better than anything else.[47]

Years later, Muktananda was to identify this crucial moment with his guru as the first turning point of his life. Young Krishna's longing for God now intensified so dramatically that six months after this incident, he quietly slipped out the gate of the family compound, tossed his clothes back over the wall after him, and took off down the road in his loincloth. He went without saying a word to his parents—not, as he later made clear, because he was unhappy at home, but because he was afraid that his wealthy and influential parents would find a way to bring him back if he let them know his plans. In leaving home to search for God, the boy was following a course of action that was not unusual in the India of his day. What made Muktananda remarkable was not that he took this road but that, once having made his choice, he never abandoned it. Throughout Muktananda's life, his ability to make a decision and pursue it with wholehearted, single-minded perseverance was noticed by everyone who knew him. Decisiveness in action was one of the most striking qualities of his character.

With Siddharudha Swami

Early in the boy's wanderings, he came to Hubli, in northern Karnataka, the famous *maṭha* of Siddharudha Swami, a Śaiva yogi and reputed siddha. Very tall, with hands that hung almost to his knees, Siddharudha was at that time one of the most well-loved of the Śaiva saints of Karnataka. His ashram fed hundreds of people a day. This *maṭha* still stands in its original form, and is still the center of a community of devotees. Siddharudha's ashram was in many ways a traditional *gurukula*, a "master's clan," where disciples came to live with their guru, imbibing spiritual principles through practice, service, and study. It contained features that would later turn up in Swami Muktananda's own ashrams. For example, the mantra *Oṃ Namaḥ Śivāya* was continually chanted there, and a program of scriptural study was conducted by some of the resident monks. Muktananda would later set up similar study programs for his students.

Swami Muktananda studied Vedānta at Hubli and may have also received instruction in Śaivism from a saint named Mallikarjuna Swami. He used to tell the story of how Kabirdas, his teacher of Vedānta, taught him an important spiritual concept by the age-old method of demonstration:

> He gave me a candy and said, "Eat it." I ate it. He asked, "How did you like it?
>
> I said, "It was very sweet."
>
> "Who knows it was sweet?" the teacher asked.
>
> "Somebody," said the boy.
>
> "That somebody is the Knower," said Kabirdas. "And the Knower is the Self."[48]

As he pondered this, Muktananda had a revelation of the phenomenon of the witness-consciousness, the detached inner observer, or witnessing "I" that Advaita philosophy identifies as the true inner Self.

Swami Muktananda later said that he was able to imbibe the teachings given at Siddharudha Swami's ashram (and later at the ashram of Siddharudha's disciple Muppinarya Swami, where he went to live for a time after Siddharudha's death in 1929) because he offered *gurusevā*, "service to the guru."[49] The *Bhagavadgītā* describes the tradition that governs spiritual learning by saying that a seeker obtains knowledge from the guru through humility, enquiry, and service,[50] and in the *Chāndogya Upaniṣad* can be found several stories about seekers who were able to receive mystical knowledge by serving one who possessed it.* This would become a cornerstone of later Siddha Yoga practice—indeed, the main practice of many Siddha Yoga students.

The Upaniṣadic knowledge taught by these early teachers proved formative in Muktananda's education. In later years, when Swami Muktananda spoke of the Self, of the spiritual journey, of the purpose of human life, he usually spoke in Upaniṣadic language and imagery, and often quoted the writings of Śaṅkara and his disciples.[51] Moreover, the ways and customs of traditional *sannyāsīs*, which form a significant subculture in the spiritual life of India, became deeply embedded in Swami Muktananda's character.

By his own account, young Krishna received initiation into the Sārasvatī Order of the traditional *daśanāmi sannyāsa* in the mid-1920s in Hubli.** It is traditional for monks to be given religious names that correspond to their character and interests, so the name he received—

---

*Satyakāma Jābāla tended the cattle and Upakosala the ceremonial fires of their respective gurus and were in this way prepared to receive the highest teachings. *Chāndogya Upaniṣad* 4.4.1–5.2.8.

***Daśanāmi* means "ten names"; the *sannyāsīs* are so called because Śaṅkarācārya, the founder of the formal orders of renunciant monks, created *maṭhas*, monasteries, which became the homes of ten monastic orders. Swamis Muktananda and Chidvilasananda belong to the Sārasvatī Order.

Muktananda means "bliss of spiritual liberation"—indicates the degree of his focus on this goal.

The Years of Wandering

In 1930, Muktananda began a period of wandering. He would say later that for twenty-five years he crisscrossed the whole of India. He traveled in the Himalayas and visited most of the famous pilgrimage sites in central and South India. However, his main interest was in visiting saints. He had been convinced by his reading and by his mentors that the path to God could only be discovered, as he once put it, in the company of the friends of God. In other words, he was looking for a guru. So whenever he heard of a saint rumored to be possessed of special knowledge, he sought him out; he often used to say that he had met over sixty great saints in his life, including Anandamayi Ma and Ramana Maharshi.[52]

Swami Muktananda stayed at the *maṭha* of Shivananda Swami in Davangere, reading texts on Vedānta like the *Vicārasāgara, Pañcadaśī, Yogavāsiṣṭha,* and *Pañcakaraṇa*; in later years, he would demonstrate familiarity with much of the Indian scriptural canon, from the Upaniṣads and the Vaiṣṇava Bhakti texts to the epics and Purāṇas and the Śaiva and Śākta Tantras. He studied the Rāmāyaṇa with a swami in his hermitage in the Vindhya hills—located in northern Maharashtra and southern Madhya Pradesh—where he served by picking up cow dung for the fires. Moving farther north and east, he lived in the ashrams of Śaiva teachers in Varanasi, including a saint named Lingananda Swami, who once sent Muktananda to stay for twenty days in one of the city's famous cremation grounds. Along the way, he studied Āyurvedic medicine until he was sufficiently proficient to be in demand as a *vaidya*, an Āyurvedic physician. He became an adept at *haṭhayoga*; throughout most of his life his body had the supple strength characteristic of prolonged *haṭhayoga* practice. Over the years, he also picked up various minor arts, including sword-fighting, gardening, and music, so that along with his scriptural knowledge he demonstrated skill as a musician, singer, and cook and a knowledge of architecture (he later helped design some of the buildings at his Indian ashram).

Swami Muktananda traveled mostly on foot, carrying only a water-bowl and a staff. Often he went for days without eating—he had taken a vow not to beg for food or shelter—and slept under bridges or in the open through monsoon storms and piercing Himalayan cold. Once, after days of starvation, he ate mud mixed with water filtered through a cloth. In Haridwar, in the foothills of the Himalayas, he slept through cold winter nights by covering himself with the sheet from the burial shrine of a saint. In Varanasi, he ate *chapatis* (flat bread) smeared with clarified butter left over from the funeral pyres. He suffered from recurrent malaria and dysen-

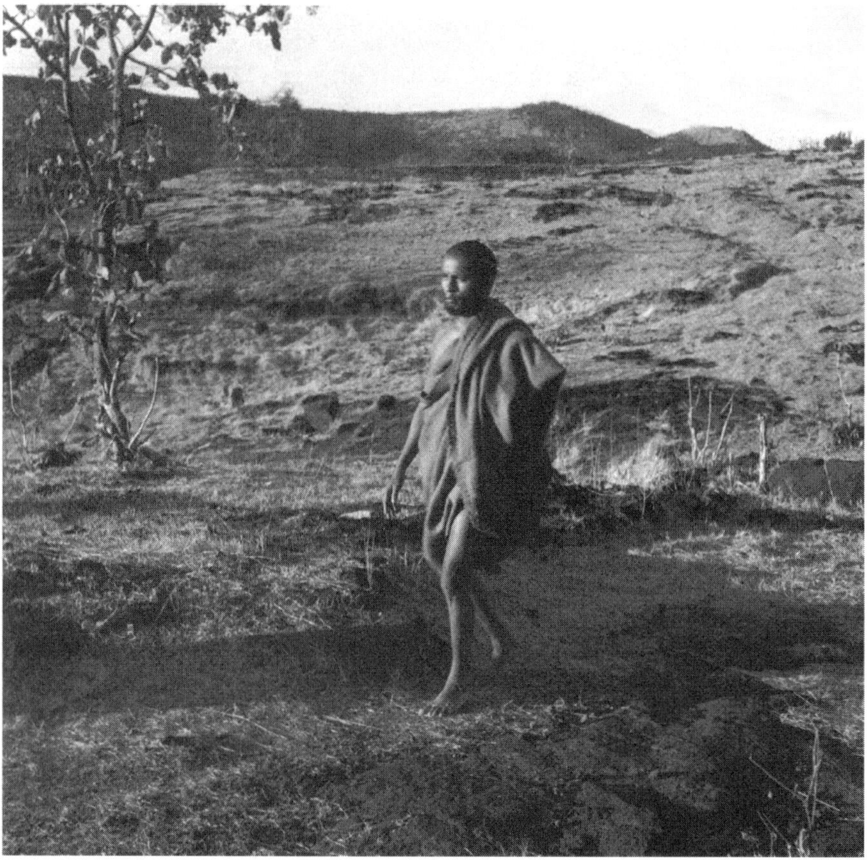

Fig. 4. Swami Muktananda in Kasara, a sparsely populated region in western India, ca. 1953

tery.[53] Yet Swami Muktananda often spoke of this period as one of the happiest times of his life. When a student asked him how he had been able to endure such hardships, he replied:

> [H]ardship did not feel like hardship. There was only one thing that filled my mind: How will I find God? Who will show God to me?
>
> There was nothing else I was concerned about. I didn't care whether I lived or died or how I would get food or drink. I would keep walking throughout the day, and wherever I was when the sun set, I would lie down and sleep. If anybody invited me for tea or some food, I would accept and then resume my walking."[54]

Swami Muktananda in Maharashtra

Muktananda was in his early twenties when he first came to the state of Maharashtra. The weaving town of Yeola, in Nashik District, became his home base, from which he would come and go for the next twenty years. In Yeola, he learned to speak Marathi and began to memorize and sing the *abhaṅgas*, the devotional songs of Maharashtrian poet-saints like Eknāth, Jñāneśvar, Nāmdev, and Tukārām.

The Maharashtrian countryside is poor and rugged, known for dramatic vistas, deep jungles, and vast stretches of desert-like hills. The spirit of the Maratha people matches the land, their temperament being both warlike and profoundly religious. In the seventeenth century, Maratha warrior-kings were among the few Hindu rulers in India to stand against the Moguls. Having given birth to one of the most enduring popular religious traditions in India—the Vārkari movement, spearheaded by the thirteenth-century saints Jñāneśvar and Nāmdev and the sixteenth-century saints Eknāth and Tukārām—Maharashtrian spirituality kept alive the egalitarian spirit as well as the popular devotional forms of the medieval *bhaktas*, whose devotion was their primary path to God. Most of the Maharashtrian poet-saints had been householders, many of low caste. Swami Muktananda (who used to say that his was one of the few ashrams in India where members of the brahmin caste, who usually eat apart, were asked to take their meals in the same room as everyone else) was deeply influenced by this egalitarian religious tradition, which combined intense devotional love for the form of God (*saguṇabhakti*) with a monistic vision that emphasized the formless unity of God and the devotee (*nirguṇabhakti*). He especially loved the practice of chanting, which he always extolled for its power to purify the mind and kindle inner bliss. "The divine Name has enormous importance," he once said. "I started chanting the divine Name from a very young age. Right from my early life I have been fond of holding week-long chants and singing the divine Name. As a result my ferry reached the other shore, while I saw the boats of many great Vedantins getting sunk midway."[55]

In several of the towns he visited frequently, Muktananda organized groups of young men to chant devotional songs, a practice that he would later introduce in his ashrams. Devotees of those days have shared numerous reminiscences of the power generated at these sessions of chanting. Once, during a chant of *Hare Rāma, Hare Kṛṣṇa* in Yeola, a local brahmin named Panduranga Shastri saw a figure dancing before the altar. He felt sure that he was seeing Lord Kṛṣṇa in his form as a child; later, according to the accounts of several witnesses, the devotees saw tiny footprints in the dust.[56]

Babu Rao Pahelvan was a young weaver who met Muktananda soon after the swami arrived in Yeola, and became a lifelong disciple. He recalled in an interview that from the first, Muktananda attracted devotees. Even the brahmin scholars (Sanskrit, *paṇḍitas*) of the town came to him for advice and respected his knowledge:

> Even then Baba showed his special luster. He had more light than others. His faith was something you could not shake; he had faith in God and in himself too. Watching him over the years was like watching a person climb a ladder. He went higher, but it was the same person who began the climb who finished.[57]

Meeting the Master

In the mid-1940s, events began to lead Swami Muktananda to his guru. In his wanderings, he had actually visited Nityananda on occasion. "I would go and stay with him for a few days. Then he would tell me to go and travel some more. So I would leave. . . . But then I would miss him and go back to see him again."[58] Then, in the mid-1940s, Muktananda became close to a siddha named Zipruanna. Zipruanna was a naked renunciant who lived like a vagrant in Nasirabad, a village near Jalgaon, yet exhibited the omniscience and blissful equanimity that Swami Muktananda said he had learned to recognize as evidence of the enlightened state.[59] It was Zipruanna who told him that Bhagawan Nityananda was his guru. Swami Muktananda later described the incident:

> He said, "O you crazy one, God is within! Why do you seek Him outside?"
> I said, "Instruct me."
> "That is not for me to do," he replied. "Go . . . to Ganeshpuri and stay there. Your treasure lies there. Go and claim it."[60]

In this way, after years of wandering, Swami Muktananda began his time of discipleship to the siddha who had first set him off on his journey many years before. He said later:

I was overjoyed. No—I was fulfilled. After a bath in the hot springs, I went for his darshan. He was poised in a simple, easy posture on a plain cot, smiling gently. His eyes were open but his gaze was directed within. What divine luster glowed in those eyes! . . . He said, "So you've come."

"Yes, Sir," I answered. I stood for a while and then sat down. . . . I am still sitting there.[61]

Almost immediately, Nityananda began testing his disciple. Swami Muktananda would come and go from the valley; on his visits, he stayed in a hut behind the Vajreśvarī temple and walked the four miles over the fields to Ganeshpuri. In the crowd around Bhagawan Nityananda he remained in the background, content to watch his guru silently from the back of the hall. Of this time, Muktananda said:

For several years I kept coming and going from Baba's place. When I was there, I would become restless, so I would leave and go somewhere else for a while. The reason for this was ego and pride. Nityananda was a being who loved to insult others, and I was a person who was too proud. . . . Sometimes he would . . . pick up something, call someone close to him, and give him that. Whatever *prasad* he gave people was like a wish-fulfilling tree that would fulfill all their desires. I waited to see if I would receive anything. Nothing—not even a glass of water. Sometimes he would pick up something and say, "Come here," and I would go running. Then he would say, "Not you. I'm calling someone else." In that way, he would insult me in front of everyone again and again, and I would die. The bigger my ego was, the worse the insults became. This went on for several years.[62]

Swami Muktananda related how he would sometimes be kept standing for hours, even through the lunch hour, so that he would get his midday meal neither at his guru's place nor at his own. He later said that Bhagawan Nityananda was easygoing with his devotees, that is, with those who simply loved him and came for blessings. But when someone offered himself as a disciple, a spiritual apprentice with the desire and the capacity to attain the state of Self-realization that is the highest blessing the master is able to give, then Nityananda became very strict.[63] Swami Muktananda was being subjected to the time-honored training of a disciple. As an accomplished yogi, a scholar of many branches of yogic philosophy, a dedicated seeker of the truth, and a teacher with his own devotees, it must have been challenging for Swami Muktananda to remain in Nityananda's ashram, where he was tested often and given little overt respect by other disciples of his master. Yet Muktananda, proud and independent as he was, submitted himself completely to his guru.

There was a time when people in Ganeshpuri asked me where Muktananda Swami was, how he lived, and how he spent his days. I would conceal myself to that extent. I would not even wear saffron clothes while going to Ganeshpuri. I would roll up my saffron clothes in a bundle and go to Ganeshpuri incognito so that I would not be noticed by people there. . . .

I led my life around my guru, Nityananda, without showing off my knowledge. I behaved as though I were a great fool. I never let anyone know about all that I had received. Even though I went there I wouldn't sit too close to him. I would sit far away but where I could still see him. I learned everything from what he was teaching other people, what he was telling other people.

I wouldn't speak to anyone; I wouldn't make friends with anyone. Some people used to say I had a lot of pride and some people that I was a great fool. In this way, I received two kinds of degrees. I lived with those two degrees in Gurudev's ashram. This is absolutely true and this is the way one should live.[64]

His love for Nityananda, as his later writings demonstrate, had become the most powerful force of his life. In 1980 he wrote:

> My attainment is Gurudev. My sadhana is Gurudev. By the churning of milk, butter is produced. Similarly, joy arises through the churning of the love between the Guru and the disciple. . . . Only when I lost myself in the ecstasy of Nityananda did I realize who he was. He is the nectar of love which arises when everything, sentient and insentient, becomes one."[65]

To lose himself in Nityananda's ecstasy became his goal. He meditated on his guru,* carried his picture everywhere, obeyed him implicitly—even to the point of sitting down in his presence only when he was asked to do so.

Devotion, humility, and surrender are the traditional requirements of a disciple. Yet as Swami Muktananda often said, when he loved Nityananda and surrendered to him, he did not feel that he was offering his devotion to an individual as such. "When we use the word *guru*," he said, "we should not confuse the Guru with the human form. We should find out who a Guru really is. The Guru is pure Consciousness." He added, "The Guru is the grace-bestowing power of God. The Guru is not a particular body; he is the supreme grace-bestowing power of God functioning through that body."[66] In the same way, he often said that when he obeyed and surrendered himself to his guru, he did it not with the feeling that he was obeying and surrendering to a fellow human being but that he was surrendering his small self to the great Self, the supreme Self. Muktananda identified his guru's enlightened consciousness with the pure consciousness that Vedānta calls

---

*In *Play of Consciousness*, in the chapter entitled "My Method of Meditation" (pp. 55–68), Swami Muktananda describes his method of meditation, which he derived from a text called *Jñāna Sindhu*. He would mentally install Bhagawan Nityananda in every part of his body and meditate on his body as the body of Nityananda. Eventually, he wrote, he experienced such intense identification with Nityananda that he would experience Nityananda's inner state of equal vision and would even find himself speaking like Nityananda.

Brahman, the source and substratum of the universe. Therefore, when he identified himself with his guru, when he meditated on his guru, he experienced not a merging into a separate person but a merging into his own higher consciousness.

INITIATION

On August 15, 1947, in a gesture that was to prove pivotal to Muktananda's own development as well as to the future of the Siddha Yoga movement, Bhagawan Nityananda gave Swami Muktananda shaktipat initiation. According to Muktananda's account, he did it in a fashion that departed radically from his customary style of bestowing blessings. "Baba usually transmitted his grace by a seemingly casual look or gesture," Muktananda wrote in *Play of Consciousness.* On this occasion, as if to signal his own respect for Muktananda as a seeker and a future successor, Nityananda chose to perform what amounted to a formal ritual.

Swami Muktananda described in *Play of Consciousness* how his guru gave him the spiritually significant gift of wooden sandals from his own feet, and then performed worship of these sandals. Traditionally, since energy is considered to flow from the crown of the head to the soles of the feet, the sandals of the guru are considered to contain the guru's energy in its most concentrated form. So the gift of the guru's sandals is equivalent to the gift of the guru's spiritual energy. Nityananda then looked into Muktananda's eyes, and as he did so, Muktananda saw a ray of molten blue and gold light flowing from his guru's eyes into his own. "Its touch was searing, red hot, and its brilliance dazzled my eyes like a high-powered bulb. . . . I stood there, stunned, watching the brilliant rays passing into me. My body was completely motionless."[67]

Finally, Nityananda initiated him into the secret of the *Oṃ Namaḥ Śivāya* mantra, explaining how it should be repeated:

> All mantras are one. . . . All are *Om. Om Namah Shivāya Om* should be *Shivo'ham. Shiva, Shiva* should be *Shivo'ham.* It should be repeated inside. Inside is much better than outside.[68]

Bhagawan Nityananda, in his cryptic manner, thus instructed Muktananda that the mantra should be repeated with a feeling of identity with the deity of the mantra—the feeling of *Śivo'ham,*" "I am Śiva," and the awareness of the mantra being repeated inwardly. It was, in fact, a perfectly traditional initiation into higher awareness, combining several methods of initiation—transmission of power through a look, the giving of a mantra, and instruction in the teaching of the tradition. Swami Muktananda had no doubt that he had received the spiritual gift for which he had been searching. In later years, he would celebrate this day as his *divyadīkṣā,* "divine initiation," and the custom of celebrating the day of receiving shaktipat initiation from the guru would become a tradition among Siddha Yoga disciples. By coincidence, Swami Muktananda's initiation took place on the very day of India's official independence from Great Britain. He later said, "On the very same day that Lord Mountbatten said, 'India has become free,' my Sadguru, my Gurudev, told me that I had also become free."[69]

Nityananda's transmission uplifted Muktananda's state instantaneously. As he tells the story in *Play of Consciousness,* Muktananda placed the sandals on his head and began to walk down the road to Vajreshwari. "Love for the Guru and a feeling of oneness with him rose within me again and again. . . . I felt waves of emotion, and on these waves I felt my identification with Nityananda grow and grow."[70] As he reached the site of the present Gurudev Siddha Peeth ashram, his vision shifted, and he began to experience pure oneness, the intuition of the presence of God in everything. He saw everything around him filled with innumerable shining blue sparks of light. With his eyes open and closed, he was seeing the light of consciousness everywhere.[71] According to Abhinavagupta's *Tantrāloka,* Swami Muktananda was experiencing one of the classical symptoms of strong shaktipat: the emergence of *pratibhājñāna,* spontaneous knowledge that arises from within.[72]

SADHANA OF THE AWAKENED *KUṆḌALINĪ*

Confusion and Doubt

Shortly after Swami Muktananda's initiation, Bhagawan Nityananda told him to return to Nashik District and perform sadhana (Sanskrit, *sādhana:* "the practices leading to enlightenment") near Yeola, in his hut in a sugarcane field outside the village of Suki. But when Muktananda sat for meditation there, he discovered that his exaltation of the previous days had disappeared. Instead, his mind wandered restlessly, his spirit was agitated, and his body ached. Describing the experience once in an interview, he said that as he sat for meditation his legs suddenly moved into *padmāsana,* the "lotus posture," and his tongue curled up into his inner nasal passage. "I looked around me," he said, "and the whole sugarcane field nearby was on fire. I saw fire everywhere. I tried to get up and run away, but I couldn't because my legs were locked in lotus position."[73] In *Play of Consciousness,* Muktananda related this experience in greater detail:

> All around me I saw flames spreading. The whole universe was on fire. A burning ocean had burst open and swallowed up the whole earth. An army of

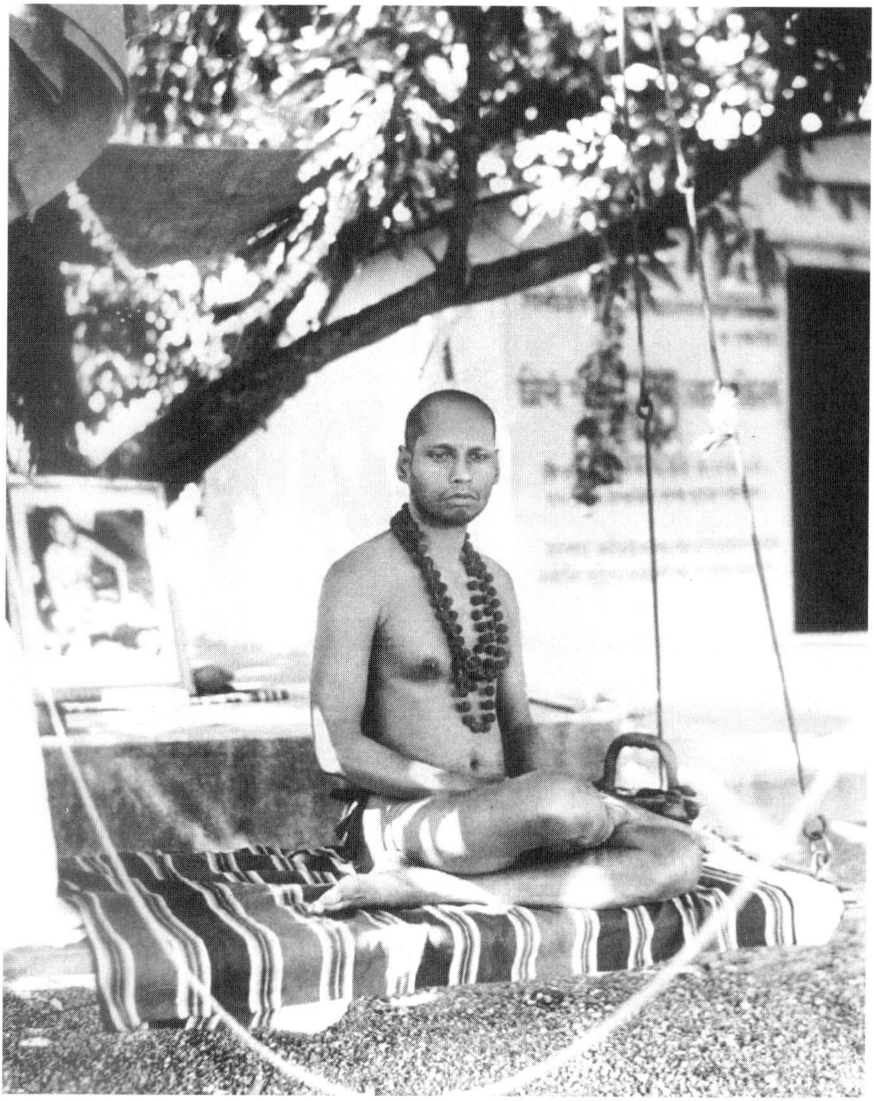

Fig. 5. Muktananda in front of his meditation hut in the village of Suki, 1955

> ghosts and demons surrounded me. All the while I was locked tight in the lotus posture, my eyes closed, my chin pressed down against my throat so that no air could escape. Then I felt a searing pain in the knot of nerves in the *mūlādhāra,* situated at the base of the spine. My eyes opened. I wanted to run away, but my legs were locked tight in the lotus posture. . . . I was quite aware that everything I was seeing was unreal, but I was still surrounded by terror. . . .
>
> Now, I saw the whole earth being covered with the waters of universal dissolution. The world had been destroyed, and I alone was left. . . . Then, from over the water, a moonlike sphere about four feet in diameter came floating in. It stopped in front of me. This radiant, white ball struck against my eyes and then passed inside me. I am writing this just as I saw it. It is not a dream or an allegory, but a scene which actually happened—that sphere came down from the sky and entered me. A second later the bright light penetrated into my *nādīs.* My tongue curled up against my palate, and my eyes closed. I saw a dazzling light in my forehead and I was terrified. I was still locked in the lotus posture, and then my head was forced down and glued to the ground.[74]

This dramatic experience began a period of spontaneous inner and outer purification, the effect of *kuṇḍalinī-śakti* manifesting in the body of an aspirant who had prepared himself for this awakening by many years of yogic practice. *Kuṇḍalinī-mahāyoga,*[75] as it is called—the spontaneous inner process that begins when *kuṇḍalinī* is aroused by a siddha guru—was taking place within Swami Muktananda.

Some modern texts on shaktipat point out that intense and sometimes frightening visions may occur immediately after a strong experience of shaktipat, as long-buried karma, psychic blockages, and the residue of deeply hidden impressions (*saṃskāras*) and inner impurities are dredged up to be expelled from the unconscious.* *Kuṇḍalinī* theory explains this by saying that as the awakened force moves in the subtle body (*sūkṣma-śarīra*), it removes the "impurities" that clog the energy channels (*nāḍīs*) there and dispels the accumulated conditioning that prevents one from seeing the inner light. The Śaiva sage Abhinavagupta claims that shaktipat actually removes *āṇavamala,* the "impurity of individuality," the primal sense of being a small (*aṇu*) or limited individual that Śaivite philosophy regards as the primary "veil" separating the embodied soul from the knowledge of its oneness with God.[76]

---

*In his *Devatma Shakti,* Swami Vishnu Tirtha Maharaj devotes three and a half pages of description to "some characteristic symptoms "of awakened Kuṇḍalinī," among them: "When your body begins trembling, hair stands on [its] roots, you laugh or begin to weep without your wishing, your tongue begins to utter deformed sounds, you are filled with fear or see frightening visions, . . . think that the Kundalini Shakti has become active." (Rishikesh, India: Swami Shivom Tirth, 1974, pp. 102–103.)

Muktananda's visions—the fire, the burning ocean, screaming figures, the sense of cosmic dissolution—can be seen as emblematic of this process. This was in fact how he was later to describe it, saying that the visions of fire symbolized the burning of his accumulated karma and impurities and, ultimately, of his sense of limited individuality.

At the time, however, he understood nothing about the effects of shaktipat initiation. Nothing could better indicate the remarkable secrecy that surrounded this process than the fact that such a well-read, widely traveled, and experienced seeker as Muktananda should have known nothing about the results of shaktipat. He was not aware that the awakened *kuṇḍalinī* dredges up and expels long-buried fears and emotions, desires and passions. Nor did he know that when this spontaneous process of *mahāyoga* begins, meditation comes on spontaneously, the body may find itself taking yogic postures without any conscious volition, and all manner of inner experiences, each with its own significance, may arise through the work of *kuṇḍalinī*. So he interpreted his experiences as signs of madness, or as the fruits of some long-buried sin arising to torment him. "It was one of the most painful times in my life," he wrote in *Play of Consciousness*.[77]

Over the next several months the experiences continued. One day a local saint, Hari Giri Baba, who had long been a mentor to Muktananda, arrived at his doorstep in a horse-drawn carriage. When Muktananda told the saint what was happening to him, Hari Giri Baba assured him that this process was beneficial. He said, "You are in a good condition. Things will be very good for you. You will become a god. You've got a beneficial fever. Through coming into contact with it, many people will be cured of their sickness and suffering."[78] Nonetheless, Muktananda was so disturbed by the experiences he was having that he decided to leave Suki and continue his sadhana in a place where no one knew him. After a few days of walking, he found himself in a place called Nagad, where a farmer offered him a hut. In a cupboard of that hut, Muktananda found a book that described exactly what was happening to him and explained that all these experiences were the work of the awakened *kuṇḍalinī*.* Eventually, Bhagawan Nityananda also sent Muktananda a message of reassurance, echoing Hari Giri's words that everything was going well for him.

Muktananda wrote in *Play of Consciousness*:

> Our saints, such as Jnaneshwar Maharaj, Saint Tukaram, and Janardan Swami, have described these experiences in their poetry, but in veiled language. . . . However, there are all sorts of experiences that come to devotees of

*Swami Muktananda wrote in *Play of Consciousness* that he studied modern compilations such as *Mahāyoga Vijñāna, Yogavāṇi,* and *Shaktipāt* as well as Śaivite scriptures in order to understand the workings of *kuṇḍalinī* within himself (pp. 114–115).

> Siddha Yoga which you neither hear nor read about. If you do happen to find such an account, it is usually in secret language, and you don't find a seeker who has perfected his sadhana who can tell you the meaning. For this reason, many aspirants do not understand the wondrous process of this amazing sadhana. Their minds become frightened, and they give up their practice.[79]

Years later, remembering this time of confusion, Swami Muktananda wrote extensively of the experiences that had followed the awakening of *kuṇḍalinī*. He described them vividly and with unprecedented frankness, he said, in order to reassure seekers who might be having similar experiences. In *Play of Consciousness*, he described how his body went through physical movements, including spontaneous *haṭhayoga* postures; the rapid and painful rotation of the eyeballs that happened as the Kuṇḍalinī purified them; the mental anguish that surfaced as his deeply rooted tendencies were flushed out and expelled; the periods when some latent disease would overcome his body. At the same time, he described beautiful subtle visions, experiences of inner lights, profound feelings of bliss, darshans of different forms of God. He spoke of how in meditation he traveled to other worlds, saw realms of light—including a subtle plane where the siddhas live in bodies made of consciousness. He experienced the vision of the *nīlabindu*, the "blue point" or "blue pearl," a tiny point of blue light that saints of the tradition have called the "light of the Self" or the "house of the Lord" within the human body.[80]

Self-Realization

As he recounted in *Play of Consciousness*, it was nine years before Swami Muktananda reached the goal of the inner journey that had begun with his initiation. Then the experience of oneness with the absolute, which he had touched many times along the way, became his permanent experience. From that time on, he wrote, he saw all the forms of the world, all creatures and objects, arising and subsiding within an ever-present field of blue light that appeared as the substratum of his experience.

> I still meditate now, but I have a deep certainty that there is nothing more for me to see. . . . [I]n the outer world I still see that same Light of Consciousness, whose subtle, tranquil blue rays I had seen spreading everywhere after the three visions. . . . [described earlier in his account of his experience of Self-realization]. It has never gone away. When I shut my eyes, I still see it shimmering and shining, softer than soft, . . . finer than fine. When the eyes are open, I see the blue rays all around. Whenever I see anyone, I see first the blue light and then the person. Whenever I see anything, I see first the beautiful subtle rays of Consciousness, and then the thing itself. Wherever my mind happens to turn, I see the world in the midst of this shining mass of light.[81]

He had attained the state that the poet-saint Kabīr calls *sahajasamādhi*, the "natural state of absorption" or open-eyed meditation,* and that Kashmiri Śaivism describes as *unmīlana samādhi*, the "unitive absorption," a state in which the unitive vision is no longer confined to indrawn meditation but has become an ongoing, ever-present experience.[82]

At that time, Swami Muktananda was living in a town called Chalisgaon, not far from Yeola. There, during the four-month rainy season, he was practicing intense austerities, living on one handful of *mung* beans a day, and maintaining a vow of silence. During that period one of Muktananda's devotees, Rajgiri Gosavi, an officer with an insurance company, traveled with a friend from Chalisgaon to Ganeshpuri for Nityananda's darshan. The two men were standing in line outside the ashram when a man came out of the gate shouting, "Where are the two devotees from Chalisgaon? Baba wants them." Gosavi and his friend found their way through the crowd and were taken to Bhagawan Nityananda. Bhagawan said to them, "Hunh, hunh, hunh. . . . Chalisgaon. . . . That Muktananda Swami, Muktananda Swami."

Nityananda said, "Why does he [Muktananda]. . . eat raw mung? Why does he burn his stomach? He has become perfect Brahma. . . . He has given up his human body. He has become perfect Brahma." Then Nityananda stood up and in front of everyone began to sing and dance with his arms outstretched: "Swami Muktananda, Swami Muktananda, Swami Muktananda, Swami Muktananda! He is the greatest of all. Hey, he has become supreme Śiva. He has become the supreme Lord. He has become Śiva. Oh, he has become Paramahamsa. Oh, he has become Paramahamsa!"**

Bhagawan Nityananda continued to sing Muktananda's name. Then he said to Gosavi and his friend, "Why did you come here? What is here? Everything is there. . . . He became perfect. All *śakti* was given to him. His name will become so great in the world, so great, so great, so great. In every nook and corner, in every house, he will be honored. He has become Paramahamsa." Again he started dancing.[83]

Muktananda Settles in Ganeshpuri

Soon afterward, Bhagawan Nityananda sent a message asking Muktananda to come and live near Ganeshpuri. A three-room hut already existed in

---

*In one of his songs Kabīr writes, "I have attained supreme knowledge; I am absorbed in the bliss of Sahaja, I have earned eternal repose." (V. K. Sethi, *Kabir: The Weaver of God's Name*, p. 492.)

***Paramahaṃsa*, "supreme swan," is a name given to a perfected yogi, a siddha; the name refers to a mythological bird who is said to have the ability to extract pure milk even when it is mixed with water. In the same way, the perfected yogi is said to have the power to draw the experience of God from the world of duality.

Gavdevi, built on Nityananda's instructions a few yards from the place where Muktananda had had his experience of *samādhi* the day he received shaktipat initiation. He had been invited by Nityananda to stay in this spot when he visited the area; now that invitation was a command. A ritual attended the installation of Muktananda in the place that was later to become the "mother ashram" of Siddha Yoga. The story behind it is typical of the mysterious ways of Bhagawan Nityananda.

During 1956, a rumor had begun going around that soon Bhagawan Nityananda was going to take *mahāsamādhi,* that is, that he would leave his physical body.* Some of the devotees asked Bhagawan if the rumor was true, and he said, "Yes." The devotees asked if they could build a temple in his memory and place a statue in it. Bhagawan agreed and instructed a group of devotees to supervise the construction of the temple behind the three rooms that had already been built for Swami Muktananda in Gavdevi. When Bhagawan Nityananda's statue was ready, it was brought to him for approval. Bhagawan Niytananda said "Give *jalasamādhi* to the idol." *Jalasamādhi* is an obscure practice in which a yogi deliberately ends his physical life by immersing himself in water while in a meditative state. Nityananda, the devotees later speculated, told them to dispose of the statue in this way in order to fulfill his earlier statement that he was about to take *mahāsamādhi.* The devotees asked Nityananda which form of God should be installed in the temple. He replied, "Muktananda." So a special ceremony was held, "installing" Swami Muktananda in the room built as a temple. That room became Swami Muktananda's living quarters, and many years later, his *samādhi* shrine.

Many devotees saw this incident as Nityananda's way of stating publicly that Muktananda was his successor in the lineage. In a clear though symbolic fashion, Nityananda with this gesture was installing a living successor rather than offering the devotees a stone idol to worship after his passing. According to Indutai Thia, an old devotee of Bhagawan Nityananda's from Ganeshpuri village:

> Bade Baba told all of us in Ganeshpuri: "Swami Muktananda is going to become very great. Swami Muktananda is going to become very great. The ashram is going to become very big and beautiful, and a lot of people from abroad, from America, from London, from Europe, are going to come and live there. And all the little hills around are going to be built into buildings."[84]

---

*Yogic tradition holds that when a Self-realized yogi's body dies, his consciousness actually merges permanently with the absolute consciousness (Brahman). Hence, the death of such a yogi is called *mahāsāmadhi,* the "great absorption."

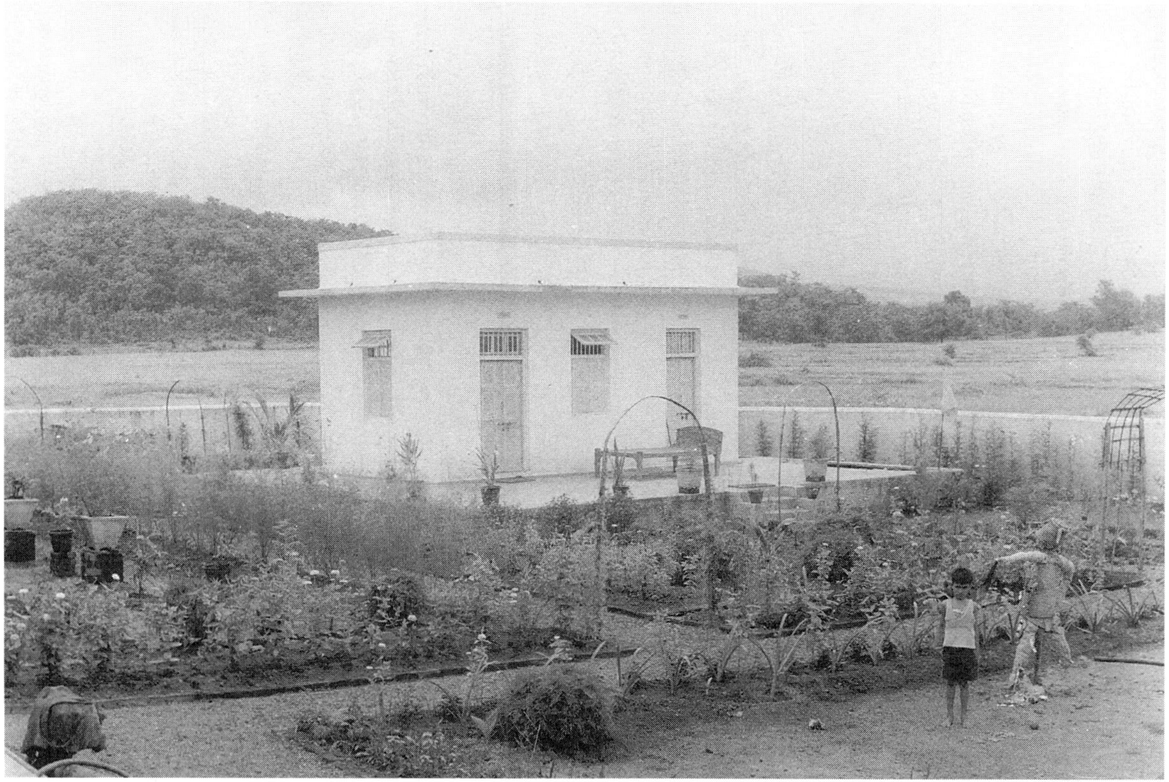

Fig. 6. The rooms built as a temple at Gurudev Siddha Peeth, then the Gavdevi Ashram, facing a rose garden, planted and tended by Swami Muktananda, ca. 1958

Other Disciples of Bhagawan Nityananda

Nityananda had several other monastic disciples to whom he had given ashrams. One, Jananada Swami, had been asked by Bhagawan Nityananda to take charge of the Kanhangad caves ashram that Nityananda himself had built many years before. Jananada Swami maintained this ashram until his death in late 1982.* Another, Swami Dayananda, known as Shaligram Swami, had a group of devotees in a nearby town and used to visit Bhagawan regularly; he would come riding in a palanquin, with his devotees chanting around him. Vasu Shetty and several other devotees remember an occasion when Dayananda and his followers visited Nityananda bringing many offerings, including a load of furniture. Nityananda told them to take it all to Swami Muktananda's place. "Darshan will be at Muktananda's today," Nityananda said. "Muktananda Swami is now *pūrṇa, pūrṇa, pūrṇa*" ("complete" or "perfect"), which Kaup Shetty, another devotee, understood to mean that Muktananda had become a fully illumined being. Dayananda Swami accordingly proceeded to Muktananda's small ashram and presented to him the tables and bureaus he had intended for his guru, then prostrated himself in a gesture of respect before Muktananda. From all reports, Swami Muktananda received him with great honor and humility; yet devotees saw this as an important indication of the unique position Swami Muktananda held in Bhagawan Nityananda's estimation.[85] Dayananda, who died in May 1961, is buried in the village of Ganeshpuri.

Early Days in Swami Muktananda's Ashram

In later years, Swami Muktananda hinted at the austerity he experienced during the early days of his ashram. For a man who was used to wandering and never liked to stay in one place too long, just remaining in a small ashram was in itself an austerity. "Three devotees used to visit me every Saturday," he once said. "They brought a loaf of bread and coffee powder, and I lived on that for the whole week. That was the way I did my austerities."[86] The fruit of that austerity, he used to add, was that in later years his ashram lacked for nothing. Venkappanna Shriyan, one of

*During Nityananda's lifetime, Jananada Swami had treated Swami Muktananda with marked hostility. A few months before Swami Muktananda's own death, he got word that Jananada Swami was seriously ill with diabetes and had asked to be brought to Ganeshpuri for a final darshan of Nityananda's *samādhi* shrine. Muktananda paid for Jananada Swami's journey, and received him with great honor in his own ashram before escorting him to the village of Ganeshpuri. In fact, Muktananda walked ahead of Jananada Swami's car, keeping curiosity seekers away with his own hands, and later arranged for the swami to be treated by his own doctor, a physician from Bombay. At that time, he told a group of his devotees, "No matter how someone treats you, you should always give them your love and respect." Jananada Swami outlived Swami Muktananda by a few months. (From an interview with Pratap Yande, March 25, 1989).

Swami Muktananda's earliest devotees, who visited him every weekend, once described how during monsoon the bread would often develop mold; Muktananda would cut off the mold and eat the bread anyway. Nityananda apparently never sent food or money to his disciple. According to Venkappanna, wealthy devotees would sometimes ask Bhagawan Nityananda, "Muktananda doesn't have anything, no money, no food—should we help him?" Bhagawan Nityananda would say, "He doesn't need your help. He won't be supported by you. He has another source. What do you think he is? Do you think there is any difference between him and me?"[87] He was hinting that Muktananda's ashram would develop on its own, through the will of God—and perhaps Nityananda's hands-off approach was a way of demonstrating his confidence in his disciple.

Early visitors described the ashram as idyllic—quiet, peaceful, and fragrant with the roses that Swami Muktananda grew in the small garden near his rooms. Visitors to Ganeshpuri took to stopping by to visit the swami, whom they found friendly and approachable. Bhagawan Nityananda used to send many of the well-educated devotees to meet him, and when people had serious questions about meditation or the scriptures, they were often referred to Chhota Baba, "little father," as Muktananda was increasingly known; Nityananda being called Bade Baba, "big father."

Swami Muktananda as a Disciple

Pratap (Dada) Yande, a government aide who met Swami Muktananda in the late fifties and became instrumental in the development of his ashram, used to say that he had never seen any disciple so humble as Muktananda. Yande recalled that Swami Muktananda would never sit down in Nityananda's presence or try to come close to him unless he was invited, and his entire demeanor before his guru was like that of a child in the presence of his father. For this reason, most of Bhagawan's devotees assumed that Muktananda was still a seeker, even though many noticed that Bhagawan Nityananda treated him with unusual respect and would often talk to him for hours.

The author of *A Search for the Self* wrote:

> Once you accepted that Baba [Muktananda] was a Self-realized soul, an obvious question was raised concerning his relationship with Bhagavan. If Baba was Self-realized, he was a master in his own right and so it was not obligatory for him to remain with Bhagavan Nityananda. Why did he choose to do so?
>
> Once I ventured to ask him [Baba Muktananda] this question. He replied, "It is not befitting (sic) a true disciple, no matter how great the spiritual heights he may have attained, to separate from his Guru. Such an act would show ingratitude towards the Guru for what he had given to the disciple. On

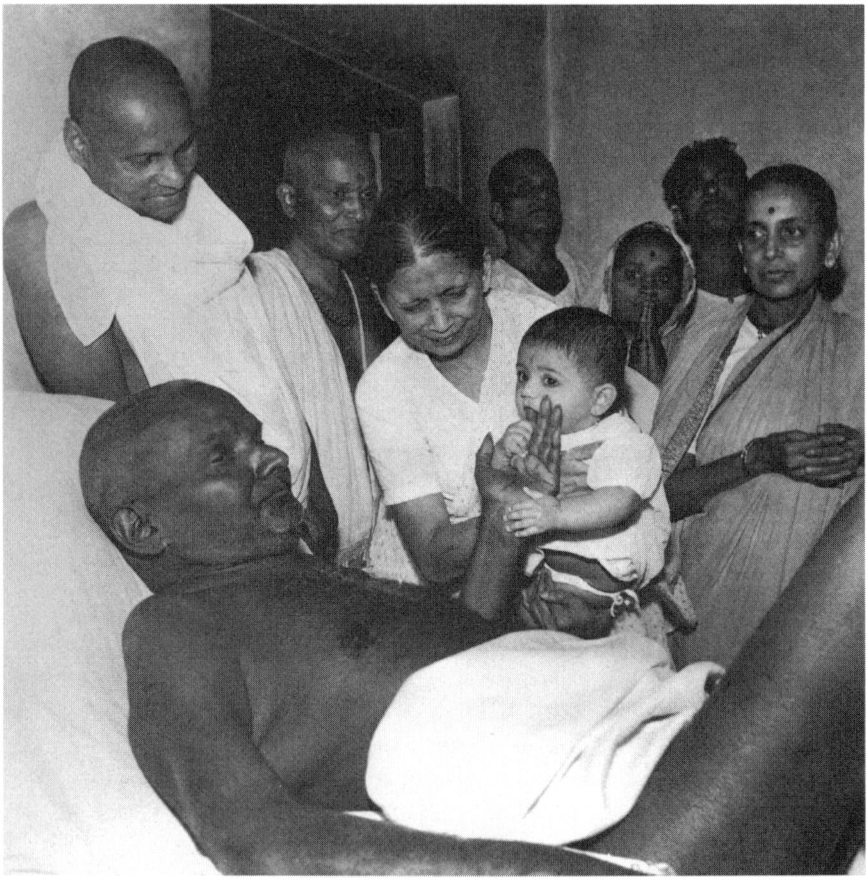

Fig. 7. Swami Muktananda with his guru, Bhagawan Nityananda, during darshan in Kailas Bhavan in 1959

the other hand, unlimited benefit lies hidden in the blessings of a Guru who is pleased by the disciple's humble devotion."[88]

THE PASSING OF THE LINEAGE: NITYANANDA TO MUKTANANDA

In August 1961, Nityananda died, or in the language of yoga, took *mahāsamādhi.*

Before leaving his body, Nityananda called Swami Muktananda to his bedside. According to Muktananda's account, Nityananda stroked Muktananda's head, then put his hand into his mouth. Muktananda sometimes said that he felt Bhagawan's hand go all the way down his throat. In that gesture, Muktananda related, Bhagawan Nityananda transferred to Swami Muktananda the power of the siddha lineage.

In an interview with author Lex Hixon in 1980, Muktananda described this experience:

> SM: The day before he left his body, he called me to him. He stroked my head for a long time. Then he put his hand into my mouth and transmitted something to me.
>
> LH: If you were already perfect, what was it that he gave you?
>
> SM: When a rich man is about to die, he prepares a will stating that his earnings should go to his son. In the same way, a Guru has a bundle that has been passed through the lineage, and usually when he is about to leave his body, he gives it to his disciple. . . .
>
> LH: Does the Guru give this final gift to his main successor or to several disciples?
>
> SM: He gives perfection to many, but he gives the final bundle to only one.
>
> LH: Would you describe what it felt like to have that final treasure placed inside you?
>
> SM: There are no words for that experience. To understand it you would have to live with me and learn the language that could describe it. In that language there is only stillness. You experience perfection when you are already perfect, and you lose yourself in that perfection. It fills you completely. You experience your all-pervasiveness, and your individuality is destroyed.
>
> LH: Did Bhagawan Nityananda ever give you an indication that you would be the instrument to spread the tradition of Shaktipat to so many countries?

SM: Yes, he told me that the day before he left his body.

LH: What, precisely, did he say to you?

SM: He said, "The entire world will see you one day." Some of the other things he told me are very secret. Such things are revealed only to the disciple on the final day.[89]

Everything that occurred in the passing of the lineage (*paramparā*) between Bhagawan Nityananda and Swami Muktananda took place in private—which is not at all unusual in Indian lineages. Ramakrishna Paramahamsa passed on his spiritual heritage to his successor, Swami Vivekananda, in an equally private fashion, and there are other examples in the literature of similarly hidden transmissions.[90] Nonetheless, this gesture of thrusting his hand down Muktananda's throat can be called a ritual gesture conferring a higher form of *dīkṣā,* initiation.* According to certain Śaiva traditions, there can be no succession without such an initiation, which formally creates the next link in the chain of transmission between guru and disciple and in which the guru formally invests his disciple with the unique powers needed by one who is to act as a shaktipat guru. The *Kulārṇava Tantra* lists many of these powers, including the capacity to empower a mantra so that it becomes a vehicle for shaktipat, to give shaktipat and control the working of *kuṇḍalinī* in a disciple, to remove the karma that blocks a disciple's progress, and to bestow direct experience of the absolute.[91]

Such a transmission of the guru's power is invisible and subtle. A witness cannot actually see what is transmitted, any more than an outsider can see what goes on when the guru gives shaktipat. All that is observable is the result: the appearance of the guru's powers in his chosen successor. In 1961, no one except Swami Muktananda himself knew that such a transmission had taken place. He later said that he had had complete faith that if his guru intended him to develop an ashram and a public mission, it would all happen on its own.[92]

SWAMI MUKTANANDA'S MISSION

"In the beginning I was very much against having an ashram. . . . But the Guru's will is more powerful than man's wish, than man's oath. In the beginning, first of all, it was he who built this house for me and told me to live

*It can be compared to the initiation described in the Śaiva texts as *putraka dīkṣā,* literally the "son's initiation," in which the guru initiates the disciple as his successor, or spiritual descendent.

here. So I began to live here and it began to grow."[93] This statement expressed a view that was basic to Muktananda's understanding as well as to the character of his movement. "In Kundalini Maha Yoga, only the grace of the Guru, only the command of the Guru matters,"[94] wrote Muktananda in *Play of Consciousness.* A disciple following his guru's intention could expect protection and success—if success was his guru's will. So Muktananda trusted that if his guru wished to use him as an instrument to transmit the grace of the lineage, that Nityananda himself would take care of everything. He always credited the growth of his work—the expansion of his ashram, his travels abroad, the coming of Western disciples, the founding of Western ashrams, and the publication of books—to his guru.

Swami Muktananda's writings indicate that he had received a mandate from his guru not only to give shaktipat but to bring an understanding of shaktipat and its significance to a wider public. The form of this mission evolved organically and gradually during the nine years between Nityananda's death and Muktananda's first trip to the West. During those years, foundations were laid for the structure and discipline of the ashram, as well as for the spiritual practices that Swami Muktananda would later take around the world. All these forms reflected Muktananda's own character: his concern with independence, his orderliness and rigorous personal discipline, his devotional approach to spirituality, and the inclusive, democratic spirit that was intrinsic to his Self-realized state.

Laying the Foundations

Fundamental to the structure of the emerging movement was Shree Gurudev Ashram, later known as Gurudev Siddha Peeth and referred to as the "mother ashram" of Siddha Yoga. In March 1962, eight months after Nityananda's death, Muktananda appointed trustees and made his ashram a charitable trust "devoted to the continuation of the spiritual heritage of Bhagawan Nityananda." In the trust deed of the ashram, Muktananda carefully delineated the guidelines for its purpose and activities. That document contains what could be called the core principles of the Siddha Yoga movement:

> The purpose of the ashram is *parasparo devo bhāva* (seeing God in others), *sarva duḥkha nivritti* (the elimination of all suffering), and *paramānanda prāpti* (the attainment of supreme bliss).

The trust deed also established the qualifications for the spiritual head of the organization and successor to the *gaddi*, the "guru's seat," making it clear that from the beginning Muktananda intended that his lineage should continue. In fact, he had already begun giving hints as to who his successor would be. According to Venkappanna Shriyan, Swami Muktananda began

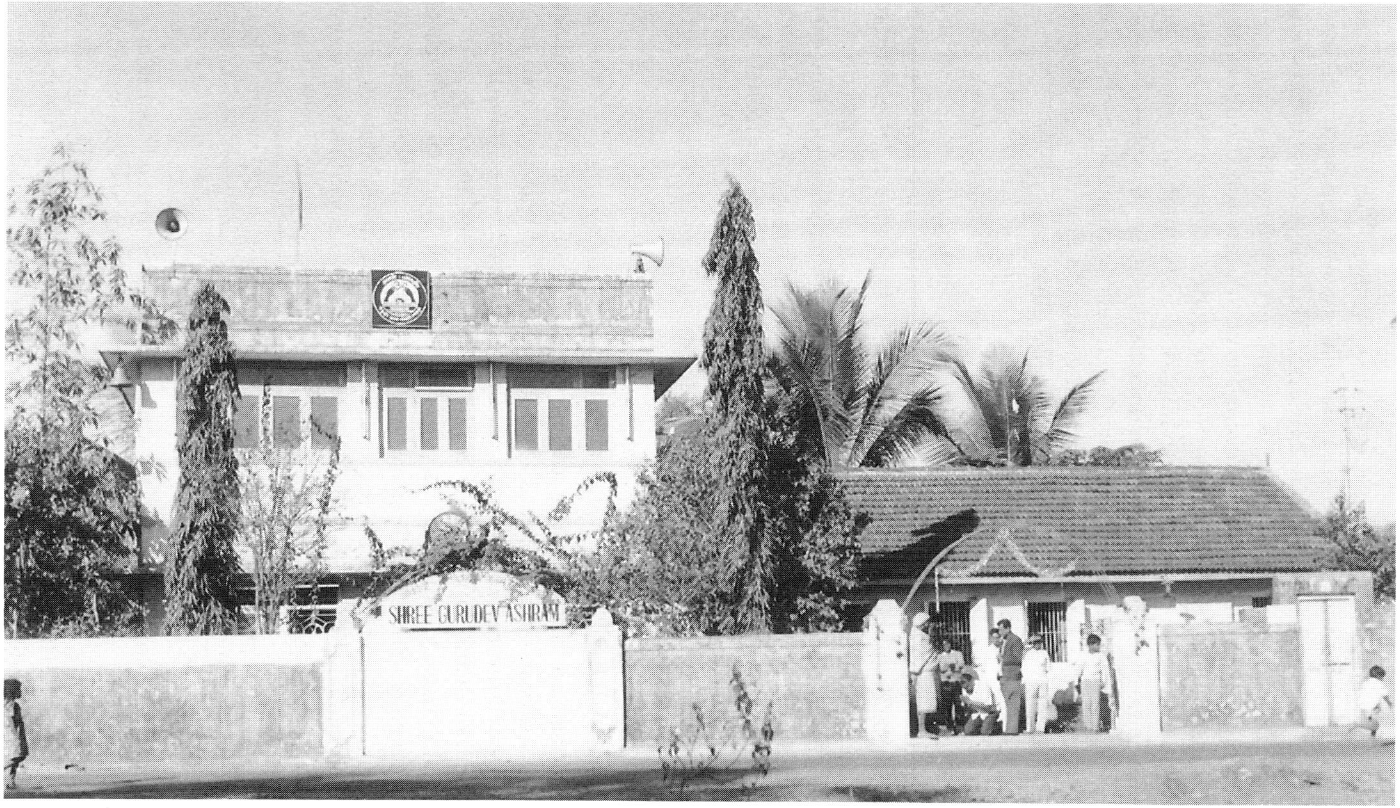

Fig. 8. After several years of growth, Shree Gurudev Ashram in the mid-1960s

speaking in the mid-1960s about the unique destiny of the child who would grow up to be Swami Chidvilasananda. At the time, however, no one thought much about it. There were more pressing issues—for example, the growth of the ashram itself.

In 1964, Swami Muktananda laid out for the ashram trustees the principles that would govern his ashram—indeed, his entire spiritual mission:

> True happiness is achieved only through the knowledge of the Self. . . .
>
> The purpose of religious institutions is to impart this knowledge and enable people to experience it. These institutions do not belong to any one individual—neither to me nor to you nor to any swami. [They are] open to anyone who has a love for knowledge of the Self."[95]

These were not, as Muktananda was to prove later, merely idle words. Shree Gurudev Ashram became one of the few traditional-style ashrams in India where Western seekers were not only welcomed but allowed to participate in the ashram routine. Its openness symbolized the fundamentally democratic attitude that is a basic characteristic of Siddha Yoga as a movement—summed up in Muktananda's 1981 statement: "Siddha Yoga belongs to everyone."[96]

Throughout the mid-sixties, as Swami Muktananda traveled in India, more and more seekers began to be drawn to him. However, in these years, only a few people lived in the ashram. Venkappanna Shriyan, who had moved there in 1960, managed the ashram and (with Swami Muktananda himself) did most of the physical work of maintaining it. Venkappanna recalls these early days, when the physical layout of the place began to take shape, as a time of intense effort. In the beginning, the facilities were primitive. For years, the ashram had no electricity, no bathrooms, and no cooking facilities besides Muktananda's small gas burner. Muktananda himself used to cook for and serve a few devotees. Others took their meals in a neighboring tea shop, and later at the home of Pratap Yande, who had a weekend cottage just outside the compound.

In 1963, fifteen acres were added to the original three. The new land, a former grazing ground infested with snakes, was barren; local villagers had cut down every single tree for fuel. Under Swami Muktananda's direction and careful supervision, it was cultivated, becoming meditation gardens with a thick plantation of mango, coconut, cashew, bamboo, banana, and eucalyptus trees. Sometimes, he would give hints as to the future of the place. Pratap Yande remembers Muktananda telling him that seekers would come from all over the world, that the ashram would become like a spiritual university, and that both Sarasvatī, the goddess of wisdom, and Lakṣmī, the goddess of wealth, would reside there.[97]

A Gentleman Yogi

It was at this time that the first glimmerings of Swami Muktananda's unusual destiny began to manifest. Muktananda's early mentor, Hari Giri Baba, had said of him, "He is a *mahārāja.* One day the entire world will be at his feet."[98] From now until the end of his life, devotees would show their respect for Muktananda by offering him gifts, by insisting that he sit on seats of honor, and by relating to him with increasing reverence. This is, of course, the norm in the Indian tradition, where "Mahārāj" (great king) is a standard term of address for yogis and *sannyāsīs*, perhaps in recognition of their mastery over the kingdom of spiritual blessings. In their gratitude for the spiritual generosity of saints, devotees often offer their gurus regal seats, clothing, and other forms of wealth. Indeed, they are enjoined to do so by various scriptures.[99] Bhagawan Nityananda had been surrounded by the offerings of many devotees, and now these were beginning to come to Muktananda.

Swami Muktananda used to explain the prosperity that now began to cling to his ashram by saying that when a yogi is in his last life, all his previous karma must bear fruit. If he has a great deal of merit accumulated from past acts of generosity, then that will return to him in the form of offerings. Moreover, despite the fact he himself had practiced immense austerities, Muktananda never advocated physical austerity for its own sake. He encouraged his devotees to live according to the dictates of their personal destiny, honoring whatever wealth and beauty came to them as God's bounty. His yoga was never world-renouncing; like the sages of Kashmiri Śaivism, he saw the world itself as divine, a manifestation of God's dynamic power, God's *śakti.* The real mark of a yogi, in his view, was that he could accept whatever came to him without attachment or aversion, always maintaining his yogic discipline, never allowing the world to pull his awareness from the Self. In an important chapter of *Play of Consciousness* called "The Secret of Renunciation," Muktananda wrote that one who is immersed in God lives in the world without being affected by it, neither turning away from enjoyment nor becoming attracted by it.

> The enlightened man, since he has the merit accumulated through countless births, will go through life supported by beauty and material wealth, but in spite of these things he will not be born again, and he will not be trapped by worldly enjoyments. A yogi like this lives ecstatically, turning sensuous enjoyments into pure yoga. He finds his delight in the Self, not in the senses.[100]

The "wealth" around Muktananda was modest compared to many temples and ashrams and never accrued to him personally. He himself lived with utmost simplicity, in rooms decorated with photographs of his guru. Devotees who served him as attendants or cooks have revealed how he ate—breakfasting on bitter melon, and lunching on a small handful of vegetables with a chapati, the flat bread of India. He wore the clothes that were laid out for him, and left to himself was likely to turn up in a crumpled collar or a vest with its buttons in the wrong buttonholes. The offerings of his devotees and disciples were used in his ashram or were given away. Nonetheless, he liked to refer to himself as a "gentleman yogi," noting that his bright orange silk clothes and the hats, sunglasses, jackets, and sweaters he wore presented a strong contrast to his own guru's near-nakedness. He spoke lovingly of the beauty of his ashram, with its abundant fruits and flowers, and the marble central courtyard that devotees built in the late 1960s. To him, all that gave further evidence of his guru's blessings—blessings that he taught his disciples were never to be taken for granted or misused.

"Baba was intolerant of any kind of waste," recalled Nirmala Thakkar, who took care of finances in the ashram for many years.

> He hated waste more than anything; he considered waste a sin against God, so he threw nothing away. A use had to be found even for the lemon peels and the skins of the guavas, and all leftovers were creatively recycled. If he saw a light left on or water left running, he would become very angry. In those days, the light bulbs were only fifteen watts, and only to be used when absolutely necessary. But years later, when there was plenty of water and electricity in the ashram, Baba was just as adamant as ever over waste. . . .
>
> Once he began to speak to us at great length. What he said was so moving that I don't think I will ever forget it. He said, "Do you realize that here in India people take food from their own mouths to give donations to this ashram? Here people don't eat themselves so they can give the ashram food. They have almost nothing, but the little they do have they give to us. Every single rupee given to this ashram is worth more than gold. It should be treated with that much respect."
>
> Later we discovered what had caused Baba to say this. While on his morning walk he had discovered some papers that had been thrown out. They had been written on only one side; the other side was blank. Half of each sheet had been wasted.[101]

Swami Muktananda's attitude toward the ashram's resources extended to every aspect of ashram life. He used to make daily rounds, and was likely to turn up at any moment in the offices, the kitchens, or even the dormitories—to make sure that no one had left on a fan or an unnecessary light. His attitude toward waste of physical resources was matched by his attitude toward waste of the *śakti.* Though he never advocated austerity for its own sake, he continually reminded his devotees that only personal discipline would allow them to hold the spiritual energy, the *śakti,* they received.

The Lion of Ganeshpuri: Muktananda as a Guru

As the sixties went on, and more and more seekers visited the ashram, the place expanded to accommodate them. Throughout these years, Swami Muktananda traveled all over India, visiting holy places. In this, he told devotees, he was obeying an inner command from his guru. (He often said that he would never make a move without such an inner message, usually received in meditation or dreams.) Occasionally he would spend some weeks in Bombay and New Delhi, staying in the homes of devotees and holding satsangs (Sanskrit, *satsaṅga*: "spiritual gathering"). A number of well-educated and articulate seekers began to find their way to the ashram—men and women who found it natural to write about their impressions of Muktananda. It is their reminiscences that form our picture of life around him.

"He has the voice of a king, the gait of a panther and the laughter of a child," wrote a New Delhi professor who met Muktananda in the mid-1960s:

> He is alert, active and ubiquitous: whether it is the manuring of paddy fields, . . . the planting of the trees, the tending of the cows, the digging of a well or construction of a building, there is hardly an operation in the Ashram to which he does not attend personally. And yet for several hours in the morning and in the afternoon, he is present in the Ashram hall to receive an endless stream of visitors. . . .
>
> The conversation ranges leisurely and freely over the location of a particular village, the condition of the crops, the health of the family. . . . The casual conversation suddenly takes a serious, even a philosophical turn; it is at such moments that one can hear the most fundamental problems of life expounded in simple, almost homely language. . . . There is no attempt to impress or awe the visitor or to preach at him. Indeed the visitor's last memory . . . is often the echo of Babaji's delightful laughter.[102]

In all the devotees' descriptions of Muktananda in those days, we find this same fascination with his multifaceted personality and similar experiences of his charisma. Another early devotee, a self-confessed religious skeptic, wrote of his early experience:

> I was pulled towards Baba, as it were. . . . I returned home; but Baba was the only thought in my mind. At night, I dreamt of Baba. . . .
>
> [The next day, I returned]. On seeing me, he bade me to sit—with a loving smile, the like of which I had never seen all my life. I touched his feet and started crying like a child. I could not stand the radiance of his radiant face. . . . Baba touched my head and embraced me. I do not remember to have received such a warm embrace even from my mother.[103]

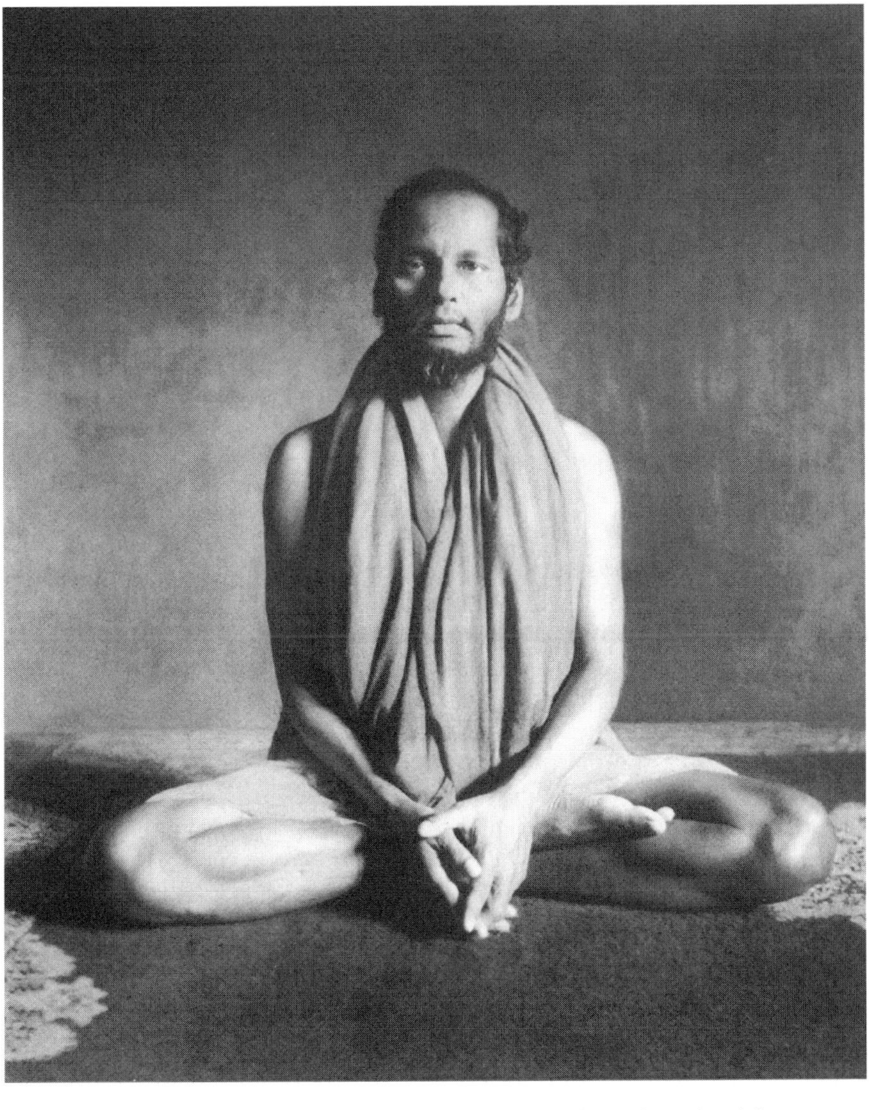

Fig. 9. Swami Muktananda, in his meditation room at Shree Gurudev Ashram

"He has opened the portals of my heart," wrote a South African woman in a rush of devotion in 1968:

> How did he do it? What power and mystery is there in him to so transmute the devotee that all barriers, all prison-bars of ego melt before his divine touch! . . . Who is Muktananda? How can I describe him to you? Come, take this hand, let's go to him, and, when his eyes fasten on you, your soul will start dancing, shackles of innumerable past lives will loosen and fall from you like the cocoon from a butterfly, revealing the true nature of your divine inner core.[104]

In those days, as in Bhagawan Nityananda's time, darshan—sitting silently in Muktananda's presence—was itself the main vehicle for the transmission of teachings. "One has just to remain in his presence; the longer the duration, the quicker is the progress," wrote a devotee from New Delhi:

> Most [questions] are answered silently. . . . However, when a discussion with a seeker does take place, Swamiji offers in his delightful style a feast of explanations and illustrations from the scriptures, from writings of saints, and from his own experiences.[105]

Sometimes Swami Muktananda would read from the *Bhagavadgītā*, or answer questions—answers that were transcribed by a devotee and later published in Gujarati, Hindi, and English in a book entitled *Paramartha Katha Prasang* ("Spiritual Conversations on the Highest Truth").

Many of these early articles note the breadth of Muktananda's knowledge, not only of yoga, but of Vedic ritual, the scriptures of Vedānta, astrology, and Āyurvedic medicine. Muktananda had begun to speak of Kashmiri Śaivism, referring to the *Śiva Sūtra*s and Kṣemarāja's treatise, the *Pratyabhijñāhṛdayam,* "Heart of the Doctrine of Recognition," which he said described better than any other texts he had read the siddhas' experience that the universe is composed of conscious energy (*citi-śakti*). "We sensed," wrote a woman who often spent weekends in the ashram, "that when he quoted from the descriptions of these texts, he was also describing his own experience."[106] Moreover, like the sages of Śaivism, he constantly reminded his students that a worldly life is not antithetical to God. Meditation, he told a devotee, is the key to experiencing the delight of the world. "Through meditation man can make the world his greatest friend," he wrote in *Play of Consciousness.* "Without meditation on God, this world is full of suffering and pain.[107]

I Make Gold out of People: Manifestations of Shaktipat

Just as Swami Muktananda's teachings were delivered informally, shaktipat continued to be transmitted in the same casual fashion favored by

Nityananda. "At that time, shaktipat was not something that was formally 'done,'" recalled Swami Sevananda, who came to the ashram in the mid-sixties as an officer of East African Airways and later became Swami Muktananda's full-time attendant. "You would come, and you would do your sadhana, and whenever you received, you received. At that time, when someone would receive shaktipat it would be the talk of the ashram. It was like a celebration, 'Oh, so-and-so received shaktipat.' It was considered the most auspicious of auspicious things."[108]

The ashram newsletters and magazines record many different incidents of *kuṇḍalinī* awakening. Swami Muktananda himself, commanded by his guru to write and speak about his experiences, had departed from the traditional yogic custom that spiritual experiences be kept secret. In a move that may have been partly motivated by his overriding mission to bring knowledge of shaktipat to the world at large, he also encouraged devotees to write and speak to each other about their own spiritual experiences. (In later years, Swami Chidvilasananda was to emphasize this even more strongly, saying that to remember and speak about one's spiritual experience helps a practitioner keep the experience alive.)

Guruvani (later known as *Shree Gurudev-Vani*), an annual magazine first published by the ashram in 1964, became the medium through which devotees shared their experiences. Their stories reveal the character of spiritual experience in Siddha Yoga: arising spontaneously, and connected directly to grace, the transmission of energy, from the guru.

Few of the seekers who came to the ashram were practiced meditators. Yet when they sat around the little rose garden or the tiny satsang hall, they would find themselves literally falling into meditation. An Indian civil service officer, B. P. Dalal, wrote:

> [A] strange drowsiness gets hold of you. . . and gently and imperceptibly as you [sit] around Baba, . . . your thoughts gradually cease; and before you are aware, you are in *dhyan*! [meditation]. . . . [I asked him] why did I get intense headaches and feel tired to exhaustion after my previous unguided efforts? Because, I was trying too hard, [Muktananda explained]. Without grace, all effort is futile. . . .
>
> And yet on my second visit, some months later, I find myself passing naturally from a relaxed state, into drowsiness, the slowing down then stoppage of the mind, and finally without knowing it, naturally and imperceptibly, I am in *dhyan*![109]

Basically, as Swami Muktananda described it, he passed on meditation by a process of contagion. He often said that the subtle vibrations of the thoughts, feelings, and activities that occur in a place remain in the atmosphere and that in a place where people have meditated, it is especially easy for others to "catch" meditation.* The reports of the visitors in those early years of the ashram bear this out. He might tell a visitor, "Sit for meditation," giving no formal instruction other than the mantra; in time, the person would pass into a deep state. Early visitors would meditate around Muktananda's bedroom in the evenings, where some devotees say they had some of the most profound inner experiences of their lives. Occasionally, a visitor would be invited to meditate in Muktananda's own meditation room; on one such occasion, B. P. Dalal heard the mantra *Oṃ Namaḥ Śivāya* emanating from the walls. Muktananda called that room his treasure-house. "That's where my wealth is," he once said. "I'm not talking about money. I'm talking about the wealth of my sadhana."[110] Many who meditated there attested to the power of the place.

For example, there was the young woman doctor from New Delhi. Her father, a devotee, had sent her to the ashram when she told him that without a direct experience she wouldn't believe in God. She related how when she first approached Swami Muktananda, offered him her garland, and told him who she was, he gave her only the briefest acknowledgment before turning back to his conversation. The doctor waited for Muktananda to give her some spiritual instruction but none came. Not that day, nor the next, nor the day after that did he speak to her or acknowledge her presence—in spite of the fact that there were no more than four or five people in the ashram at that time.

Finally, after three days, Swami Muktananda asked the doctor, "What brought you here?" She answered, "Nothing. There is nothing I want. I just wonder whether I could experience for myself the ecstasy of God." Muktananda turned to someone sitting next to him and said jokingly, "Oh, she doesn't want anything. She just wants to see the *giver* of everything!" Several days later, as she was sitting in the semi-darkness of the meditation veranda, she felt a strong hand on her arm. She looked up. Baba was pulling her toward the inner door, the door to his own meditation room. She said

---

*Muktananda taught meditation as the primary path to spiritual experience, and saw as its goal the state of liberation from suffering and oneness with God that the Indian sages call "*mokṣa*." He defined meditation both as a process and as a state. As a process, he said, it is the act of sitting quietly and turning your attention within. As a state, it is the experience of being in contact with the inner Self. Though he described this experience in various ways, to define it he often referred to the Upaniṣadic description of the Self as "the one who knows the mind is thinking but is not thought by the mind." For meditation practice, he often recommended that the practitioner sit quietly, repeating the empowered (*caitanya*) mantra given by the guru. Focus on the mantra calmed the mind and allowed the guru's energy to suffuse the meditator's awareness. At that point, the various subtle experiences characteristic of Siddha Yoga meditation would often manifest—inner lights, sounds, feelings of spontaneous bliss or expanding consciousness, and much more.

that for a few moments she was frightened. Swami Muktananda simply opened the door to the meditation room, told her to sit down, and left her. As he closed the door, leaving her alone, she passed into an ecstatic state. "I can't describe what happened to me in there," she said afterward, struggling to explain the formless, wordless state of utter stillness that she experienced. She found herself dancing in ecstasy in the small meditation room, and when Swami Muktananda came to take her out, she fell on her knees to thank him. He laughed and said, in reference to the subtle inner refining process of the awakened *kuṇḍalinī*, "We have a furnace of meditation here. We put people in and burn their karma and convert them into gold. I have a gold mine here. I make gold out of people."[111]

Spiritual awakening, Swami Muktananda wrote in his book *Ashram Dharma*, occurs automatically in the environment of a siddha:

> Wherever a great saint dwells, he endows that place with the character of his profound inner state. In fact, each abode of a Siddha bears the impress of his unique state. His Shakti envelops the place—sporting, manifesting itself, and generating ever-new bliss which never dies. . . .
>
> Partaking of the water, food, and fruits of such a sacred place, even smelling its flowers, awakens the spiritual energy in a human being.[112]

He had written that in Bhagawan Nityananda's presence, spiritual power was transmitted continually; scholar M. P. Pandit later said of Muktananda himself, "What makes him remarkable is that he is giving shaktipat twenty-four hours a day."[113]

A Life of Discipline Is a Life of Nectar: Development of the Ashram Schedule

As more seekers came to the ashram, a more formal structure began to emerge. Swami Muktananda began gradually to create his own version of a *gurukula*, the center of spiritual study and practice that he had first encountered in the ashram of Siddharudha Swami in his youth and that existed in many other ashrams in India. Though he rarely expected special disciplines of his householder devotees, simply counseling a moderate lifestyle and daily meditation, those who lived in the ashram were expected to throw themselves into practice and service.

The ashram day began at 3:00 A.M. with meditation, and progressed through a strictly enforced routine of chants and ashram *sevā*—all designed, Muktananda said, to ensure that the residents and visitors were constantly engaged in spiritual practice. Along with meditation, chanting and *gurusevā* were the core of the program; Swami Muktananda regarded both of these as central purificatory practices. "Chanting purifies all seven constituents of the body,"* he used to say,[114] and in his introduction to the ashram chanting book, *Swadhyaya Sudha,* or *The Nectar of Chanting,* he wrote: "The supreme and everlasting happiness that [one] longs for lies in inner purity alone. *Swādhyāya* [study and recitation of scriptures] is a subtle tonic that nourishes the inner being, imparts spiritual strength and purifies the mind and heart."[115]

By the late sixties, Swami Muktananda had introduced daily recitations of three scriptural texts—the *Viṣṇusahasranāma,* the *Śiva Mahimnaḥ Stotram,* and three chapters from the *Bhagavadgītā.* In 1972, he replaced the *Bhagavadgītā* with a chant that has remained the main scriptural text of Siddha Yoga: the *Gurugītā,* "Song of the Guru."** Muktananda found this philosophical poem on the guru-disciple relationship quoted within the *Gurucaritra,* a medieval (ca. 1500) hagiographic text on the primordial guru, Dattātreya, from the Maharashtrian yogic tradition.[116] Muktananda himself had chanted it privately for many years. The *Gurugītā* became the core of the ashram morning recitation.

Raul Roig, later Swami Shantananda, a Puerto Rican art history student and spiritual seeker who first came to the ashram in 1972, said: "It was the ashram program that most impressed me. I'd been traveling in India for a while before I came, and I'd been to many ashrams, but I'd never been to an ashram where the discipline was so strong. After you'd followed that routine for a while, you really did start to experience a still mind."[117]

Following the routine was not optional; in those days no one could stay in the ashram without attending all the programs. "Baba used to like military discipline," said Swami Sevananda. "He was famous for it."[118] Swami Muktananda believed implicitly in the value of regularity in practice; he often said that his own discipline had made it possible for him to attain everything in spiritual life, and he expected equal seriousness from his students. He himself set the example. Until his death in 1982, he rose each day at 3:00 A.M., bathed while reciting mantras, performed worship (*pūjā*) to the photographs of his guru, then meditated until it was time for him to attend the *Gurugītā* chant or, in later years, take his morning walk. He ate little—a handful of cooked vegetables, a little rice, and a chapati was his usual lunch—and always at the same hours. His days were spent in teaching, meeting devotees, and attending to ashram business, his evenings given to meditation and remembrance of God. He was absolutely punctual—those who

*The seven constituents of the body are the five physical elements (earth, water, fire, air, and ether) along with the senses of perception and the mind.

**A verse in the *Gurugītā* says that this text came originally from the *Skanda Puraṇa,* a scripture from which substantial portions have been irrevocably lost. Swami Muktananda can be credited with bringing the *Gurugītā* out of obscurity. After he began chanting it publicly, other spiritual groups discovered and incorporated portions of it in their practice.

served him remember that if he ever came late for a program or an appointment, it was because one of his attendants had mistaken the time. "A life of discipline is a life of nectar," he wrote in his book *I Have Become Alive.*[119]

The discipline also served a protective function. Curiosity seekers and tourists as well as genuine seekers used to wander from ashram to ashram during the late sixties and early seventies. Since accommodations at Swami Muktananda's ashram were free, and since his reputation was beginning to spread along the spiritual grapevine, the strict schedule helped discourage visitors who lacked a strong spiritual motivation. Said an editorial in *Shree Gurudev-Vani* in 1969:

> Baba emphasizes discipline in Ashram life to ensure that it enhances its dignity as a place of pilgrimage, that the divine shakti conducive to spiritual unfoldment is preserved and that its peaceful atmosphere with its soothing effect on the mind remains unpolluted. Discipline thus maintains the sanctity of our ashram and keeps all unholy elements away.[120]

The ashram rules were posted on a notice board just inside the gate, and they ranged from "talk little and softly when necessary" to "maintain propriety in dress and conduct"; from "do not consume liquor or tobacco in any form" to "always remember that you are Shiva." Here was a hint of Swami Muktananda's style of teaching: an insistence on absolute purity of lifestyle, combined with an equally rigorous insistence on the state of oneness with God that was the goal of it all.

"Baba made it seem the most important thing in the world that you were up at three o'clock in the morning," reported Carol Friend, who came to the ashram as a young woman in 1971. "It was inspiring. I felt that if he cared so much about my practice that he was willing to shout at me to attend a chant, then there must be something in it—the least I could do was take it as seriously as he did. The importance of keeping a discipline has stayed with me all these years since."[121]

Muktananda kept up his guru's tradition of fiery instruction. Many people who lived in his ashram still speak with relish of Swami Muktananda's dramatic style of making sure that people did their practices with focus. It usually took the form of strong words, sometimes punctuated by the gesturing of his upraised stick, which he called *chhoṭā-gurujī*, the "little guru." Helen Argent, an Australian who came to the ashram as a young woman in the early 1970s, described the effect of one of Muktananda's dramatic scoldings:

> We'd be having the *pūrṇahūti* [finale] of a long chant, and people would be chanting, shall we say, a bit lackadaisically. Then Baba would come in. He would sweep into the hall and immediately begin to shout: "Why is the harmonium there? Tell those singers to move closer!" Within seconds, he'd

> have totally captured our attention. Before, we might have been spacing out, our minds wandering. But now we were riveted, completely focused on the chant. Then he'd throw his head back and begin chanting ecstatically—and we'd get swept up into that same state.[122]

Like Argent, many other students noted that Swami Muktananda's fiery words (students used the term "Baba's Rudra *bhāv*," in honor of the fierce form of Lord Śiva) were, like his own guru's, a calculated display put on for the purpose of teaching, inspiring or keeping order, breaking through a disciple's mental fog, or pointing out manifestations of ego. Swami Prajnananda used to tell the story of how she once heard Baba shouting at the kitchen workers. A few minutes later, she looked up to find Baba standing before her. "How was I?" he asked, chuckling. No trace remained of the apparent anger he had been manifesting only a moment before.[123] Swami Chidvilasananda once spoke of an occasion when he had scolded a certain devotee. Afterward, he said to Chidvilasananda, "That man is so good. I had to correct him. I couldn't let him go on being the victim of that tendency."[124]

That Girl Is a Blazing Fire: Swami Chidvilasananda's Early Sadhana

As the ashram grew, the young girl who was to become Swami Muktananda's successor was growing also. Her name was then Malti, and she was the oldest child of a couple who had been devotees of Swami Muktananda since the 1950s.

Malti's father, a restaurateur, and her mother came originally from South India. Muktananda had not only actively encouraged their marriage but had traveled to the bride's hometown to attend the wedding. Family legend states that after the ceremony he had placed a coconut, symbolizing fruitfulness, in the folds of the bride's sari, as is customary in Indian weddings. The bride was nervous, and the coconut fell from her sari and rolled across the floor to Muktananda's feet. "That means the fruit of your marriage will come to me," he said.[125]

For the first few years of her life, Malti lived in a rural setting near Mangalore; then her family moved to Bombay. She was brought to the Ganeshpuri ashram when she was five, and said of her first meeting with Swami Muktananda: "Even as a tiny child, I had intense love for Baba and knew that I wanted to spend my life in the Ashram."[126] She and her family, including a sister and two brothers, traveled back and forth from Bombay each weekend, and Malti grew up in the ashram, learning the chants as well as the subtler lessons of equanimity and detachment. From the beginning she took her practices seriously. Even as a young child she kept a rigorous schedule that, by the time she was a teenager, included rising at 2:00 A.M. for

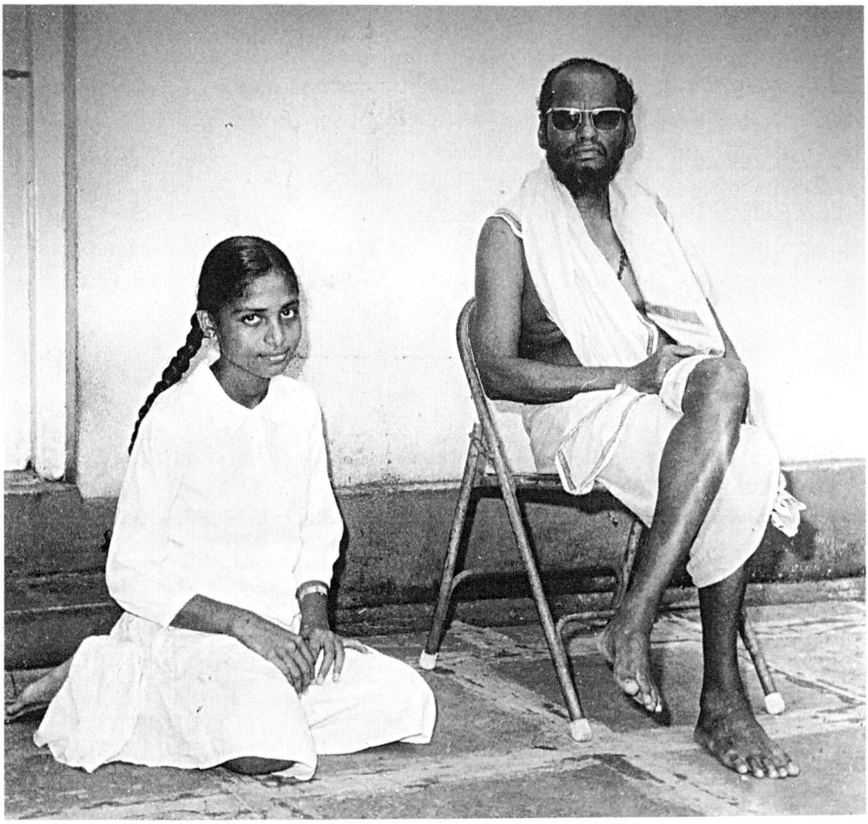

Fig. 10. Malti, with her guru, Swami Muktananda, mid-1960s

meditation and occasionally chanting for eighteen hours a day. One of her early memories was of a visionary experience she had the first time she heard the "Āratī" chant in the ashram. Listening to Upaniṣadic verses on the five elements, she experienced being transported to a world of fire, to a plane of air, and then to the sun. As each verse unfolded, she said she felt, "I am the fire . . . I am the air . . . I am the sun." Later, each time she heard the "Āratī" chant, she would return to this experience.[127] From the beginning, the ashram was the center of her life. "I was ecstatic when I was there," she said later. "Then I would cry my eyes out when I had to leave."[128]

In 1969, when Malti was fourteen, Swami Muktananda gave her formal shaktipat initiation. As she related in a 1982 article in an ashram magazine, *Siddha Path,* Muktananda told her to sit for meditation twice a day in the Dhyan Mandir but gave her no instructions. For several weeks she meditated unsuccessfully, while Swami Muktananda encouraged the other young girls at the ashram to tell her about their visions and other experiences. She wrote, "The calculated effect of all this was that in the course of those two weeks I developed an intense craving for meditation." Then, she wrote:

> One day while I was sitting in the meditation room, tears began to roll down my cheeks. . . . All of a sudden I heard footsteps and felt someone leaning over me. . . . The next thing I knew, Baba was whispering the mantra in my ear. The mantra felt like celestial water which was extinguishing the fire of my torment. Within a moment I felt incredibly good. Although I still had thoughts in my mind, I felt somehow transformed just by the sensation of the mantra in my ear. . . .
>
> The next day as I was sitting for meditation, Baba came in, smeared my forehead with sacred ash, then pinched the space between my eyebrows and pressed my eyes very firmly. He instructed me to sit on a particular cushion which I later found out was reserved for people who were being initiated. After I sat down he touched my head. I immediately lost all external consciousness and was aware of only one thing—a brilliant inner sun, shining with great intensity. Utterly transfixed, I kept watching its shimmering golden rays. It was bright yet cooling. I had completely lost all awareness of my body or where I was. Then from somewhere I heard Venkappanna calling my name and telling me to go eat my supper. A thought slowly took form in my head: "Supper? What does that mean?" I heard him calling my name over and over again. . . . When I finally opened my eyes, I saw that it was dark outside.[129]

When Malti lay down to sleep that night, the same brilliant sun appeared.

> I couldn't understand why there was so much light inside yet so much darkness outside. I wondered how I could sleep with all that inner light. I was afraid it would keep me awake.

She went outside and walked through the garden.

> Gradually I became aware of a new sensation. . . . I felt the earth slipping out from under my feet. I . . . grabbed the cement tree well on which I was sitting. But as I did so, I felt my hands sink through the concrete, which had suddenly become intangible as a cloud. I tried to lean against the tree for support, but there was no tree. I wondered what was happening. The only reality was the pain in my body and the inner radiance. I discovered that I couldn't walk back to my room because there was no ground. Every time I put my foot down I felt it sink through the earth. . . . At that point all outer forms began to undulate and finally disappeared. I was left with nothing that I knew or recognized. . . . Everything had disappeared except the pain and the brilliant light.

Malti somehow found her way back to her room. When she woke up in the morning the pain had gone and the world had returned to normal.

> I realized, however, that a revolution had taken place within me. Things looked different—they were brighter and more vivid, as if it had just rained.

During the months that followed, Malti meditated for hours every day, as the awakened *kuṇḍalinī* led her through a series of strong visionary experiences and yogic movements much like those that Swami Muktananda himself had experienced. Sometimes, she would wake up at night thinking that the lights were on in the room, so strong was the light she saw inside. Shyama Shivastava, a former English teacher from New Delhi who lived in the ashram and acted as Malti's tutor in those days, says that during that period Swami Muktananda concerned himself with every detail of Malti's diet and schedule, making sure that she ate food that fostered meditation, that her schedule was balanced, that she spent time with people whose company encouraged her spiritual growth.[130] During this time, too, Muktananda began to drop stronger hints about her future. "Baba would tell me who she was and what she would do in the future," said Venkappanna Shriyan. "Everyone didn't know about it, but Baba told me that Malti would be his successor."[131]

That same year, 1969, Swami Muktananda gave an indication of Malti's future role to the late Murlidhar Dhoot, at that time a trustee of Gurudev Siddha Peeth. Dhoot recalled:

> Baba was sitting with me and a few other devotees in the gardens of Ganeshpuri. Malti was standing a short distance behind him. Suddenly, Baba turned around and pointed to her. "You know," he said, "that girl Malti is a blazing fire. One day she will light up the entire world."[132]

Muktananda had pursued a solitary journey, often far from his guru's physical presence. Malti's destiny was to bring her into constant contact with her guru. Her life was molded by his intention for her as well as by what she described as her own growing desire for spiritual experience. From the first, her spiritual life was inextricably linked to her devotion for her guru and her conviction that his grace was responsible for all her experiences of inner illumination.

For example, in the *Siddha Path* article in which she described her shaktipat experiences, Malti wrote that at one point her meditation began to take the form of a deep, still state from which she would emerge refreshed and content. After a while, however, she began to wonder if something was missing, since she wasn't seeing visions—especially a coveted vision of white light. Then one day, standing outside Baba's window, she asked for his help:

> I mentally formulated the petition, "Baba, white light." Within two minutes Baba appeared at the window, looked up at me, and asked how my meditation was. I replied that it was very still and peaceful but that I never saw white light.
>
> He gave me a penetrating look and asked, "Do you want to see white light?" When I nodded excitedly, he said, "Come and meditate this evening and you'll see white light."[133]

That evening, in the meditation room, Muktananda touched her between the eyebrows. Within moments, she was in deep meditation, where she saw everything suffused with beautiful white light.

Later, she relates, she mentioned to Muktananda (who regularly inquired about her meditation experiences) that she would like to have physical *kriyās*, the purificatory movements of the body that are characteristic of certain phases of inner development.

> Again he touched me between the eyebrows, and my body instantly began to jerk and move about at the mercy of a force that I had come to identify as Shakti and which I associated inseparably with Baba. It was as though he had unleashed something that had long been pent up within me. I would sing, shout, jump around, and roll on the ground. I would dance wildly and ecstatically! Chanting would always intensify these kriyas. I would feel one with Shiva and the Goddess. I also had boundless physical strength. . . . I would sometimes go without eating for two or three days, but I never felt even the slightest bit hungry. There was so much light inside me that I always felt satisfied and nourished. . . . Sometimes the intensity of the kriyas would frighten me, but time and time again either I would hear someone explaining exactly what I needed to hear at that moment, or I would overhear someone reading aloud a relevant section from a book.

As time went on, however, she began to realize that none of these experiences were as important as the experience of devotional love. Like the *bhakta sant*s Tukārām and Mirabai, she began to pray for more devotion.

> The next time Baba inquired about my meditation I said, . . . "I don't have enough devotion. I feel dry inside."
>
> Somehow Baba seemed very pleased and said, "Ah-h." Very soon I became aware that waves of joy and love were beginning to well up from within. This was accompanied by a feeling of deep respect and reverence not only for Baba but for everything around me. I sensed that this was the true meaning of devotion—to feel love and respect for everyone and everything.
>
> Now I began to realize that I would never be satisfied until I attained Baba's own state. So I made one more request—I asked him for Self-realization. This time Baba said gently, "It isn't time yet. When the right time comes, that will also happen."

These experiences reinforced Malti's conviction that it was the guru's grace, the guru's spiritual intervention that brought spiritual development. Though strong-willed and independent, she demonstrated a devotion to her guru much like his own feeling for Bhagawan Nityananda. Other devotees remember evenings when they would hear her haunting voice, singing to herself Mirabai's songs of longing for God. They noticed how she threw herself into any task she did in the ashram and how seriously she went about fulfilling Swami Muktananda's instructions. "She could be playful and light," said a woman who met her during this period. "But when it came to sadhana or seva she was the most full-on person I had ever seen. I used to notice how she chanted. She would be lost in the chant. The rest of us might be looking here and there, but for her it was as if nothing else existed. Whatever she did, she did *totally*."[134]

Siddha Yoga Is the Yoga of Grace: Swami Muktananda's Early Writings

Swami Muktananda's articles (written in Hindi and translated into English by Swami Prajnananda and other devotees), began appearing in the mid-1960s. In 1966, his articles were collected into a small book called *Light on the Path*, which contained the first systematic formulation of his teachings on *kuṇḍalinīyoga*, the guru-disciple relationship, mantra, and the path of *gurubhakti*, "devotion to the guru." Muktananda's writings, like his instructions to devotees, consistently pointed toward guru's grace (*gurukṛpā*) as the means to attainment in yoga. As he often said, he had spent twenty-five years searching for God without success and had attained his goal only after receiving initiation from his guru; the path he taught was the path he himself had followed. *Light on the Path* contains Muktananda's first written use of the name "Siddha Yoga" to describe the path of guru's grace. "Siddha Yoga is not something that one 'does,'" he said in 1975. "The essence of Siddha Yoga is received through the Siddha Guru."[135] As the years went on and his movement expanded, he would use the name "Siddha Yoga"—which he

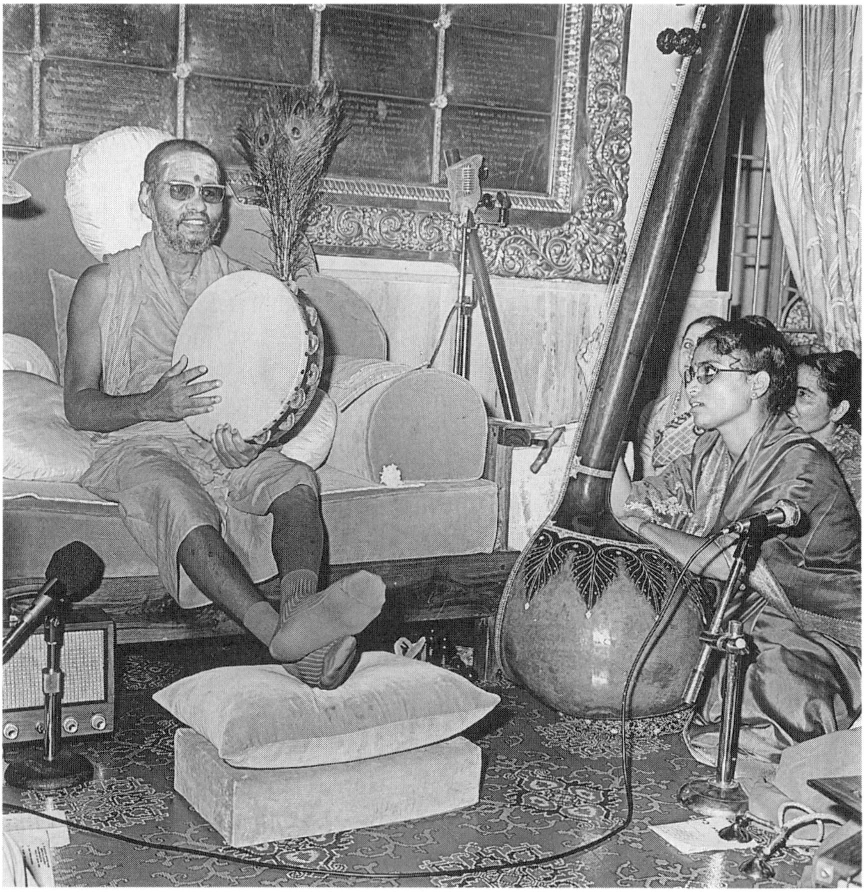

Fig. 11. Swami Muktananda leading a chant, in the Bhagawan Nityananda Temple in Shree Gurudev Ashram, with Malti, playing a tamboura, a traditional stringed instrument

initially defined as the spontaneous inner process that arises in a seeker who has received shaktipat from a siddha guru—more and more definitively to identify his specific formulation of teachings and practices.

To Swami Muktananda's devotees, all his writings would become scripture, defining their tradition and their practice. However, *Chitshakti Vilas,* published in English as *Play of Consciousness,* which Muktananda wrote in twenty-two days in 1969, is the primary definitional text of the movement. Often read by students of yoga for the vividness and clarity of its description of the experiences attending the awakened *kuṇḍalinī,* the book also laid out Swami Muktananda's essential teachings on spiritual practice, the experience of Self-realization, and especially the role of the guru and the nature of *kuṇḍalinī.* The significance of its place in his mission cannot be overstated. (For a chronological list of books by the Siddha Yoga gurus, see appendix 1.)

Swami Muktananda explicitly said in his introduction to *Play of Consciousness* that he wrote it at the request of his devotees, who had asked for an account of his spiritual experiences. He acknowledged in the book that such experiences are traditionally kept secret. "I have revealed them," he said, "at the command of my Guru and for the sake of students on the Siddha path." Writing *Play of Consciousness* was thus one of Muktananda's most important departures from tradition. As always when acknowledging such innovations, he stated several times in the text that the writing was done not through his own will or any conscious desire. It happened, he said, through the awakened Śakti herself.[136] "Everything in this book is the work of Chiti [consciousness]. It is Chiti's gift, and Chiti's creation," he said in his preface. "Siddha Yoga belongs to Goddess Chiti."[137]

As if to bear out Muktananda's statement, many seekers over the years have actually received shaktipat while reading *Play of Consciousness,* as if the text itself were imbued with Muktananda's spiritual energy. One young seeker, who began reading the book on a bus in Chicago in 1973, passed into meditation right on the spot, coming to ordinary consciousness only when the bus driver told her that they had reached the end of the line. Swami Chidvilasananda, who was among the small group of devotees around Muktananda during the time he was writing the book, recalls that when portions of the book were read out to them, they too would pass into meditation. At night, after hearing a portion of the book, she would find herself unable to sleep because she would see so much light when she closed her eyes.

When You Stand Next to a Fire, You Get Warm: Swami Muktananda's Tours

By the late 1960s, Swami Muktananda had become respected all over India as "the sage of Ganeshpuri," a modern exemplar of the ancient tradition. He had thousands of devotees and admirers. Yet the most dramatic phase of his public mission had not yet begun. The world-mission his guru had predicted would manifest in 1970, with Muktananda's first trip to the West.

The seeds of Siddha Yoga's Western expansion had been sown in the early 1960s, when the first Western seekers began coming to the ashram. One of these was Albert Rudolph, known as Rudi, who dealt in oriental art and taught meditation in New York's Greenwich Village. Rudi was a well-known figure in the small world of New York's Hindu-based spiritual movements. He had been a devotee of Bapak Subuh, the Indonesian teacher and founder of the charismatic Subud movement, and after leaving Subud, found his way to Bhagawan Nityananda in 1960. Nityananda sent Rudi to Muktananda. Soon, Rudi began paying yearly visits; having received shaktipat from Swami Muktananda, he also began teaching a form of spontaneous meditation based on *kuṇḍalinī* awakening. It was Rudi who first invited Muktananda to the West, and ultimately arranged Muktananda's 1970 visit to New York.*

The influence of Eastern spirituality on Western thought had been growing since the early nineteenth century, when Schopenhauer in Germany, and Emerson, Thoreau, and Hawthorne in America, were drawn to early translations of the Upaniṣads and recognized the depth of ancient India's wisdom. In 1859, the German Sanskritist Max Müller began translat-

*Swami Muktananda gave Rudi the name "Rudrananda," yet never formally initiated him into *sannyāsa*. Rudi nonetheless used this name for the remainder of his life; he wrote of his contact with several different masters, including Swami Muktananda, in his book *Spiritual Cannibalism.* After Rudi's death in a plane crash in 1973, several of his disciples continued a friendly relationship with Swami Muktananda. Muktananda gave initiation into *sannyāsa* to two of Rudi's disciples, who became known as Swami Chetanananda and Swami Shambhavananda. Though Rudi's disciples sometimes acknowledge a connection to the Siddha Yoga lineage, their main focus is on Bhagawan Nityananda.

ing some of the Indian sacred books. The study of Sanskrit became an important minor discipline in the German academy, and the influence of these texts began to touch poets like W. B. Yeats as well as the early Theosophists, Madam Blavatsky and Annie Besant. In the late nineteenth and early twentieth century, more and more Westerners found their way to India to seek out holy men and live as yogis. It would take far too long to describe the different spiritual currents that flowed from East to West during these years,[138] so here we will mention only a few of the teachers who directly impacted future Siddha Yoga students, or who were important influences on the spiritual climate of the early 1970s.

Perhaps the most significant Indian teacher to travel West in the early years was Swami Vivekananda, the disciple of the Bengali saint, Ramakrishna Paramahamsa. In 1893, this "Hindoo monk," as the press called him, galvanized the American public with his stirring lectures on the universality of all religions at the World Parliament of Religions in Chicago. Vivekananda taught in England and France, gathering a small but articulate band of Western devotees. He left behind him the Vedanta Society, with early outposts in New York, San Francisco, and London, manned by a succession of gifted swamis of the Ramakrishna Order. These swamis taught the Indian scriptures to several generations of intellectuals and seekers, including Aldous Huxley and Christopher Isherwood, besides publishing accessible, popular translations of the Upaniṣads, the *Bhagavadgītā*, Patañjali's *Yoga Sūtras*, and other texts, and creating ashrams where traditional forms of Hindu worship and devotion were practiced. Moreover, by popularizing the life of their guru, Ramakrishna Paramahamsa, they helped kindle in Western seekers an awareness of the transformation possible through contact with a Self-realized master.

Another great saint to visit the West was Swami Rama Tirtha, a brilliant mathematician-turned-renunciant monk who had arrived penniless in San Francisco in 1906. Later, Swami Rama Tirtha lectured so impressively on practical Vedānta that he captivated seekers and nonseekers alike, and even found his way to the U.S. White House, where he met President Theodore Roosevelt.

However, it was arguably the publication of Paramahamsa Yogananda's *Autobiography of a Yogi* that created the most widespread interest in the practice of yoga and in the power of the guru-disciple relationship. Filled with accounts of the extraordinary powers of the holy men Yogananda had known, and with entrancing memoirs of his own relationship with his guru, this book made yoga seem both attractive and accessible. Yogananda's Self-Realization Fellowship, founded in the 1920s, sponsored a correspondence course that allowed his disciples to practice his *kriyāyoga* systematically, through weekly home lessons, and in the 1960s and 70s became an early influence on many would-be yogis who later found their way to living teachers.

In the late 1950s and early 1960s, disciples of the well-known saint Swami Sivananda of Rishikesh began traveling to the United States, Europe, and Canada, establishing their own traditional yoga institutions under their guru's rubric, the Integral Yoga Institute. Swami Satchidananda, with his long white beard, became a familiar figure on lecture platforms during the 1960s. His guru-brothers, Swamis Vishnudevananda (who did much to popularize *haṭhayoga* in the United States and Canada) and Swami Venkatesananda (who taught mainly in South Africa), were less well-known but equally successful in making the traditional teachings relevant to Western seekers.

Yet it was left to Swami Bhaktivedanta and Maharishi Mahesh Yogi to define Indian spirituality in the popular mind, at least during those years. Both came to the West in the 1950s, Bhaktivedanta to establish the International Society for Krishna Consciousness, (popularly known as "the Hare Krishnas"), which attempted to establish orthodox Vaiṣṇavism as a broad-based religion. Maharishi Mahesh Yogi (known as Maharishi) took a deliberately nondevotional approach. His Transcendental Meditation ("TM"), with its scientific studies of the effect of meditation on physical and mental health, became enormously popular and brought the notion of secret mantras and spiritual initiation into public consciousness through the press and the brief involvement of entertainers like the phenomenally popular Beatles. These two very different organizations became identified in the public mind as the main poles of Hindu-based spirituality in the West.

As the 1960s drew to a close, yogis, gurus, and teachers of meditation from many different sects and of various levels of spiritual attainment had begun journeying to the West. At the same time, Western seekers in unprecedented numbers roved through India, looking for ashrams and gurus who could open their third eye, tell them the secret of life, show them God, and give them a revelation of their higher purpose.

It was inevitable, given the spiritual climate of those days, that Swami Muktananda's Western admirers should have pined to introduce the siddhas' *śakti* to the West. Swami Muktananda himself must have sensed where his destiny lay; after all, his guru had told him that he would one day be known all over the world. "My Baba gave me so much *śakti*," he told Venkappanna in the early sixties. "Right now I hold the *śakti* in my closed fist. When I open it, the world will be astonished."[139]

A LION IS ROAMING THE WORLD: SWAMI MUKTANANDA'S 1970 TOUR TO THE WEST

The signal to open his fist arrived in May of 1970. Said an article in *Shree Gurudev-Vani*:

Baba's foreign devotees had been inviting him to their countries for many years. . . . But each time, Baba had maneuvered himself out of it with characteristic dexterity, leaving everyone guessing whether he would ever undertake a foreign Tour. And then all of a sudden one day [May 12, 1970] he declared that he had received his Guru's message to go abroad, not to sell new techniques, not to enroll more and more people in the list of his followers, not to teach physical yoga, but to enable his Western devotees to realize their own Divinity, to overcome miseries and to attain supreme bliss and peace.[140]

When Swami Muktananda went abroad, he was sixty-two years old, the age when most people are thinking about retirement. He spoke only Indian languages and knew only a few dozen people in the West. Many of his own devotees in India felt skeptical about what he could accomplish. As he embarked on his journey from the Bombay airport, he told the crowd of devotees and well-wishers who had come to see him off:

To be frank, I am also feeling surprised at what is happening. When people ask me, "What will you do there? What will you say?" I tell them, "I will do whatever God wills me to do. I will say whatever God wills me to say."[141]

Muktananda's first world tour lasted for three months and took him to Italy, France, Switzerland, England, the United States, Australia, and Singapore, with long stays in New York, Los Angeles, and San Francisco. (See appendix 2 for the full itinerary.) In this brief trip, we discover many of the significant characteristics that devotees would notice and record on his subsequent tours. First, there was the fact that Swami Muktananda saw himself purely as an instrument—he consistently said that his guru and God were the authors of whatever happened on the tour. Second, devotees noticed that he never needed to ask for help—people who could help his work seemed to turn up on their own, often in advance of his coming. Third, though Muktananda clearly learned from and adapted to his new environment, he never compromised the path he taught or the practices he considered essential. This would become increasingly apparent, devotees of that time relate, as Swami Muktananda came in contact with Western and Westernized teachers, psychologists, and creators of different self-help movements and therapies. Said Don Harrison, an American businessman who traveled with Swami Muktananda and helped manage the 1970 tour:

What I always saw was that he gave his love and support to all these people—especially those who came close and offered their service. But you never felt that they were influencing him. It was always the other way around. His energy was always the most powerful in the room. You saw how he lifted other people up to his level rather than going to their level.[142]

As Harrison shepherded Muktananda and his party of five through Europe, New York, and California, he noted the ease with which Muktananda interacted with the Westerners he met.

> From the beginning Baba just met people through the heart. It was very spontaneous. Baba would just sit and chant and hang out with people. Someone would invite him somewhere and he would go. There was a sense that things were just unfolding in this very spontaneous way.

These unpretentious gatherings—in Paris and Rome, they often included only ten or fifteen people—had their own impact. One particularly vivid example is the experience reported by Michael Mauger, an English film editor whom one of Muktananda's London devotees invited to drive the saint from the airport. As he shared in a 1976 BBC documentary on Muktananda, *The Guru's Touch,* Mauger knew nothing when he first met the swami except that he was a saint from India. That night, after dropping Swami Muktananda off, Mauger woke up in the middle of the night flooded with a feeling he described as "cosmic bliss." He sat up in bed, where to his immense surprise he found himself performing complex and graceful gestures (*mudrās*) with his arms—movements that went on until dawn. As soon as he decently could, he leapt into his car and drove to the place where he had dropped the swami off. "What's happening to me?" he asked Swami Muktananda. "This is called shaktipat. It's very good," Muktananda said. "But why me?" the filmmaker asked. "I haven't done anything. I'm not even a believer." Muktananda laughed. "When you stand next to a fire, do you have to be a believer in fire to get warm?" he asked. "You're a good man, and the *śakti* liked you!"[143]

Mauger's story typifies the flavor of Muktananda's first world tour. Ram Dass, the former Harvard psychologist Richard Alpert, who accompanied Muktananda through California and Australia, described another such experience:

> In one instance I watched people who had merely loaned their house to Babaji, but who had no conscious spiritual aspirations, become entirely transformed in the direction of their lives through contact with Babaji over a period of just a few days. A reporter who came only to interview him at an airport ended up sitting each morning before him while the blessing of Shaktipat worked its magic upon him.[144]

"There were no explanations at that point," Harrison recalled. "Baba was speaking on *kuṇḍalinī* and on the Guru, but they weren't formal lectures. He never said, 'I'm the Guru.' Or 'I'm now going to awaken your *kuṇḍalinī*.' Things just happened. Later on you found out why."[145]

At first those who met Swami Muktananda on that tour tended to be part of the relatively small circle of spiritual seekers who had a long-term interest in Indian teachers or teachings. It did not take long, however, for the circle to expand. According to Ron Brent, who helped to organize the tour, as word got out that Muktananda was in America, various spiritual teachers and yoga groups offered help. "It was a very ecumenical thing," Brent said. "Different organizations offered the use of their facilities. Nearly everyone was excited that Baba was here and wanted to lend a hand."[146]

The most prominent contributor to Swami Muktananda's work during the American phase of his tour (which then, as later, comprised its major portion), was Ram Dass. Ram Dass was then at the height of his fame as a spiritual catalyst for American youth. His book, *Be Here Now,* had become a best-seller among the newly fledged seekers of those years, his tapes on yoga philosophy were played on university radio stations from coast to coast, and he had just completed a national series of lectures about his experiences with his own guru, Neem Karoli Baba.* Many had gone off to India to look for a guru as a result of hearing Ram Dass lecture.

Invited to one of Swami Muktananda's early meditation retreats in the Catskill mountains, just a few weeks after his arrival in New York, Ram Dass came simply to pay his respects. Yet, as he told the story later, when he sat with Swami Muktananda he fell into a state of deep peace and stillness. He felt that he had "come home." It was a feeling, he said, that he had experienced only in the presence of his own guru. "When I was questioned as to what I thought of Babaji, I could only say, 'He is the real thing.' They asked me how I knew, and I could only point to my heart—for I knew it as the place beyond knowing."[147] A few days later, Harrison suggested that Ram Dass spend some time traveling with Muktananda. Though he had his own guru and never became a disciple of Swami Muktananda, Ram Dass decided that he had an obligation to let other seekers know about Muktananda's presence in the United States. He wrote, "Here were all these people who thought you had to go to the Himalayas to find a guru. And here was a genuine spiritual master, right here in New York City. Didn't I have a responsibility to share him with all the other true seekers in America?"

Ram Dass volunteered to do advance work in preparation for Swami Muktananda's tour. He traveled ahead of Muktananda to Boston, Los Angeles, and San Francisco, setting up programs and inviting "his" people to meet Muktananda. Says Brent, "Word began to spread that there was a genuine guru in America, one of those spiritual giants like the masters you read about in books." Several hundred people at a time—mostly youthful and long-haired—began turning up at Muktananda's lectures. It was a small foretaste of what would eventually become the "mass" character of Muktananda's mission.

---

*An *avadhūta* whose ashram in the Himalayan foothills became a mecca for many of the young seekers of the 1960s and early 1970s, Neem Karoli Baba died in 1973, leaving no successor.

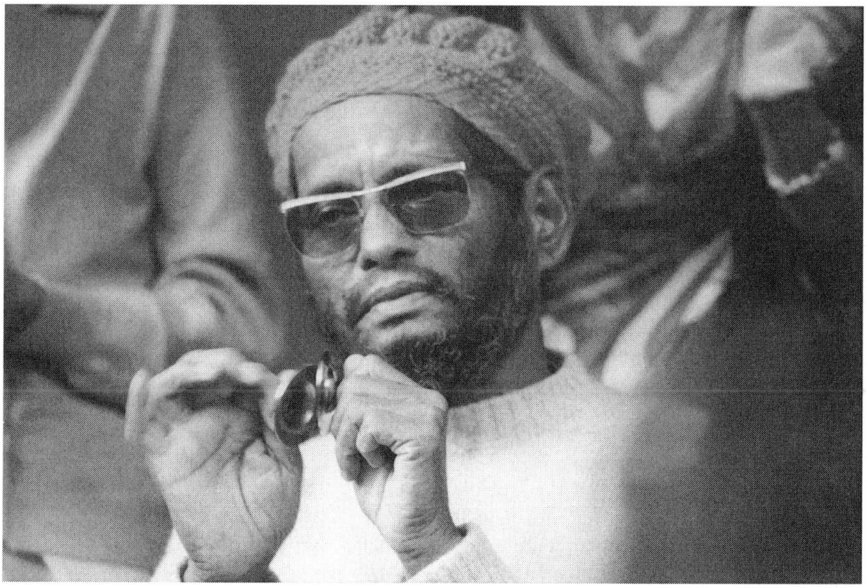

Fig. 12. Swami Muktananda on his first world tour, 1970

The programs were simple, held at places like the Universalist Church on Fifth Avenue in Manhattan, or the Unity Church in Boston, or at the homes of Swami Muktananda's hosts in the different cities he visited. Melbourne devotees remember a house in the suburb of Kew where everyone crowded companionably into the living room to meditate with Swami Muktananda in the early mornings, and where one devotee received shaktipat when Muktananda's silks brushed his shoulder as the guru walked by. During the public programs, Swami Muktananda would sit on a stage with a few musicians around him and would begin by leading *Govinda Jaya Jaya* or *Gopala, Gopala*—chants that were familiar among the Hindu-based spiritual movements in Australia and America. Ram Dass wrote:

> Midst flowers, flashbulbs, drums and song, Baba worked his magic. Whether his topic was Vedanta, Bhakti, Kundalini, or the Guru, he charmed and drew out each audience—with the music of his voice, the dance of his hands, the liquidity of his facial expressions and the inner cosmic chuckle.[148]

Most people found Swami Muktananda quite different from anything they expected. Steven Auerbach, a student who met him at a meditation retreat at Rudi's Catskill Mountain ashram in Big Indian, New York, during Muktananda's first weekend in America, said:

> I thought a guru would be a very calm, still, peaceful being—maybe a little old man with a blanket. Here was this dynamic person wearing orange silk and a ski cap and these very hip-looking dark glasses. He was always moving, never still—so much energy coming out of him. This was like no one I had ever seen before.[149]

As in Ganeshpuri, there were no formal ceremonies of shaktipat initiation. "I remember once being in a room with Baba and three or four other people," recalled Harrison. "Everyone was in deep meditation. A woman who had been sitting there with Baba said, 'How do I get initiation?' Baba just said, 'When it's your time, it happens.'"[150] For most of the seekers who met Swami Muktananda during this time, the awakening happened quite spontaneously, often during a lecture or a chant. Said Steven Auerbach:

> During one of his programs in Manhattan, he was giving his talk and suddenly I couldn't see him. I could only see a mass of blazing blue radiance sitting there. I was amazed by this. Then I noticed that out of that light was coming rays of light that were penetrating into the chest of every person in that room. I was looking at this, intrigued and amazed. I noticed then that there was a ray of light coming into me. I noticed my eyes were totally indrawn. I was taken into the center of that light and realized that this was the essence of his message. It was so beautiful to see that his message wasn't "Look at me, I am great." It was "Look at yourself." I knew the essence I saw in him—that power-

ful, tremendous radiance—was the heart of the truth of my own being. So I stayed around him as much as I could.[151]

Auerbach experienced other phenomena that would become familiar to subsequent generations of Siddha Yoga students. He found himself being pulled to meditate, even waking up at 3:00 A.M. with the desire to sit for meditation. A young legal secretary, who met Muktananda at the same time, relates that she spontaneously let go of a fifteen-year smoking habit, became a vegetarian overnight, and found herself drawn to go to India with her new guru. Experiences like this helped to spur the legend that grew up, at least in the American spiritual community, of Muktananda as an orange-robed sage who, in the jargon of the time, "zapped" people with powerful spiritual energy and gave them experiences that changed their lives. "What can you say to a man who knows your mind before you open your mouth?" wrote Australian journalist Don Sharpe in the Melbourne *Sunday Observer*. "What can you do except smile in acknowledgement of his power and rock with innocent laughter? To talk about Swami Muktananda is to reveal the boundaries of your rational mind."[152]

After his brief stop in Melbourne (planned as a rest stop, but soon evolving into a series of informal meditation retreats that brought together the nucleus that later became a flourishing Australian Siddha Yoga community), Swami Muktananda returned to India in December. He had been away only a few months. Seeds had been planted that would later bring hundreds of seekers to Shree Gurudev Ashram and form the beginnings of what would become the worldwide movement. One admirer, in a paean printed in one of the ashram magazines, wrote, "A lion is roaming the world—the Lion of Ganeshpuri. And wherever he goes he frees people to love God, to have faith in their own Divinity."[153]

Living Like Yogis

From 1970 until Swami Muktananda left on his second tour in 1974, a small stream of Americans, Europeans, and Australians passed through Shree Gurudev Ashram. Some of them were spiritual tourists traveling in India, lured by reports that Swami Muktananda's ashram was a hothouse for spiritual experience. Others had met Muktananda briefly in the West. In their *Shree Gurudev-Vani* articles, written in the fervent devotional style that was a hallmark of the Siddha Yoga culture in those days, they related the tales of their seeking, their desire to meet and live with a guru, like yogis in the books they had read. Mostly young, footloose, and middle-class, they were in a position to commit themselves to a full-time ashram life. They were also vastly ignorant about both Muktananda's tradition and the ways of Indian culture. To address this, Muktananda instituted formal sessions of questions and answers, held twice a week in the ashram courtyard, during which he formulated many of the teachings that were to be the underpinning of Siddha Yoga culture and theology.

Swami Chidvilasananda speaks of how, in the beginning, many of the Indian devotees worried about the presence of Western seekers, thinking that these foreigners would take their guru away. Muktananda, however, not only welcomed the Westerners but went out of his way to create cultural bridges. He took his Western students on his trips around India. He praised their dedication to yoga and their willingness to perform humble tasks in the ashram, describing to the Indian devotees the careers and respectable family backgrounds these young people had left behind.

He also intensified the strictness of the ashram discipline. During these years, the structure of the ashram day, built around chanting and ashram work, solidified into a monastic routine of activities ranging from silent meditation and devotional chanting to active engagement in *gurusevā*, which could take the form of office work, gardening, cleaning, and similar tasks. The ashram rule required strict celibacy and vegetarianism, and ashramites were discouraged from going to Bombay, from reading magazines and novels, and even from indulging in merely social conversation. Gauri Hubert, who stayed in the ashram between 1971 and 1973, recalled:

> So many of us had lived the typical sixties lifestyle before meeting Baba. The life around Baba was so different. It was like living in a pressure cooker. There were none of the usual outlets, and a lot of us were going through heavy purification. So you came face-to-face, day after day, with your own stuff. Sometimes you felt unbelievably blissful. Sometimes, you felt as if your whole soul was being reamed out from within. The purification process could be intense, but at the same time it was the most exciting experience I'd ever had.[154]

Throughout these years, Swami Muktananda continued to tour in India, often holding meditation retreats where several hundred people would meditate together, listen to his lectures, and often receive shaktipat. These retreats would become the prototype for the early, formal shaktipat programs on his second tour of the West.

ALL COUNTRIES ARE NITYANANDA'S— SWAMI MUKTANANDA'S SECOND WORLD TOUR

Nineteen seventy-four was a watershed year in Siddha Yoga, the time when Siddha Yoga began to emerge as a worldwide movement. Its vehicle was a structure that came to be known as "Muktananda World Tour," the name given to the agglomeration of people who traveled with Swami Muktananda on his second world tour.

Lasting from February 1974 until October 1976, Muktananda's second world tour took him to Australia, the United States (where he crisscrossed from coast to coast but spent long periods of time in California and New York), to England, Switzerland, Germany, and France. (See appendix 2 for the tour itinerary.) It transformed the base of the movement. Many crucial organizational structures were set in place during this tour. Disciples were trained and formal programs for giving shaktipat developed. These years saw the creation of a worldwide organization that included residential ashrams and meditation centers and allowed the transmission of the Siddha Yoga teachings and culture to an ever-widening group of students.

Most people who had met Muktananda on his first world tour had been conscious spiritual seekers, affiliated with one or another of the Hindu-based movements. During the 1974–76 tour, especially in the United States, the cultural base broadened to include many whose journey had led them through one of the new psychological or human development movements that were burgeoning in the Western world in the mid-1970s. One of these movements was *est* (Erhard Seminars Training), which ran a popular weekend seminar training developed by Werner Erhard.

Erhard was an acquaintance of Don Harrison, who by that time was managing a Siddha Yoga ashram in Piedmont, California, near San Francisco. In 1973, Erhard decided to travel to India, apparently hoping to meet an authentic spiritual master whom he could present to his *est* students as a model of a Self-realized being. Harrison suggested that he visit Ganeshpuri. Though Erhard never spoke specifically about his experiences, he clearly felt Muktananda's spiritual power and the fascination of his company. He offered his help in bringing Muktananda to the West. His offer was accepted: Erhard loaned Swami Muktananda's American devotees the money for five round-the-world tickets for Muktananda and his immediate party. Erhard also set up a series of lecture programs during which he introduced Swami Muktananda to thousands of *est* students in Honolulu, San Francisco, Los Angeles, Aspen, and Manhattan. Just as Ram Dass had played an important role in introducing Swami Muktananda to the first layer of Western disciples, Erhart and *est* provided a springboard that helped introduce Siddha Yoga into the mainstream of American consciousness. Yet just as Swami Muktananda remained independent of those whose help he appreciatively accepted during his first tour, so he remained independent of Erhard and the others who came forward to help facilitate this one.

Swami Muktananda Defines His Mission: The "Meditation Revolution"

Swami Muktananda inaugurated his second tour in February 1974 with a speech that has become a definitional statement in Siddha Yoga. Speaking before a crowd of several thousand at Bombay's Santa Cruz Airport, he said:

> Today, with my Guru's command and grace, I am going away from India for some time. Owing to our limited vision, we consider various countries as different. For God, all countries are His and all beings are His. In God's house there is no particular region or sect or faith. To Him all are the same.
>
> I am going abroad to initiate a revolution, a meditation revolution. As a result of this revolution, man will regain his prestige which has been tarnished. Man is suffering today, not only here, but throughout the world. The story of man today consists of breaking, burning and killing. That kind of revolution cannot succeed. Man is caught in evil because he has forgotten his true nature and the true nature of the world. Once he knows what he really is, love will flow among human beings.[155]

Swami Muktananda's vision of a "meditation revolution" became the philosophical foundation of the Siddha Yoga expansion. Its basis was shaktipat, which in these years he began offering on an unprecedented scale.*

An anecdote from the early days of the 1974 tour reveals something of how he saw his work at that time. In April 1974, shortly after his arrival in the United States, Swami Muktananda had unexpectedly walked into a meeting in which his translator, Jinendra Jain, and David Pierce, the American tour manager, were discussing their plans to create publicity for the tour. Muktananda told them, "I need no planning, no publicity. . . . I'm here on my Guru's command, not on my own. I can just walk down the street and give shaktipat to whoever comes. Just watch how it works."[156] Though in fact Swami Muktananda generally gave shaktipat in more protected environments, there are accounts of just such spontaneous transmissions—like the California man who related how he first met Muktananda at a bus stop on San Pablo Avenue in Oakland and experienced shaktipat on the spot.[157] Swami Muktananda gave shaktipat to people who met him in private interviews, to journalists, and even, in Miami, to the host of a television show while on the air. "You had a feeling," his attendant Swami Sevananda said later, "that Baba knew he had a lot to do and not much time to do it."[158]

Reading the excited reports of devotees of those years gives the impression of a movement expanding radically in an astonishingly short period of time. When Muktananda arrived in the West in 1974, there were just five Siddha Yoga meditation centers—London, Paris, Melbourne, New York, and Piedmont, California—and no overall organizational structure.

---

*Other saints, the fifteenth- to sixteenth-century *bhakta* Caitanya Mahāprabhu being the most notable example, had transmitted spiritual energy to large numbers of people. Swami Muktananda, however, was the first to do it internationally, as well as systematically. The difference was one of scale as well as intention.

When he left in 1976, there would be more than 150 meditation centers, three residential ashrams, and a worldwide volunteer organization.

The Traveling Ashram

The 1974–76 tour began in Australia, with a series of intimate sojourns in the homes of devotees. Programs were held on lawns and in living rooms in suburban Turramura or Kew, where Swami Muktananda taught not only his devotees, but visiting journalists, clergy, and even bevies of local schoolchildren. Commemorated years later in a video-taped documentary called *A Very Rare Occasion,* the Australian tour catalyzed a community that was to become the second-largest Siddha Yoga satsang outside India. However, it was after he arrived in the United States, where he stayed for two years, that Swami Muktananda began to make the organizational innovations that were necessary to support his work in the West. For this reason, much of this account deals with events and trends that began when Muktananda arrived in San Francisco.

It was an eventful period: Between April 1974 and April 1975, Swami Muktananda and his party spent long and short periods of time in such places as Oakland, Los Angeles, Seattle, Honolulu, Denver, Oklahoma City, Chicago, Ann Arbor, New York City, Washington, D.C., Boston, Miami, Houston, and Albuquerque. Rather than describing the events of this tour in strictly chronological order, we have chosen to deal thematically with the major trends and developments noticed by the people who observed Swami Muktananda during this time.

In his first months in California—from April through July of 1974, Swami Muktananda set the tone for everything that was to follow. He began by making it clear that though he was willing to adapt to the ways of the West, he intended to retain not only the essential teachings but also the full panoply of traditional rituals and practices. The tour managers tended to regard the traditional elements of the programs—the Sanskrit chanting, photographs of the loincloth-clad Nityananda, the waving of lights (*āratī*) to those photographs, and the ashram schedule—as mere "trappings" disguising the essential elements of meditation and shaktipat. Swami Muktananda, however, had no intention of allowing his essential message to be divorced from the formal structure he had created in his ashram. The forms, he often explained, held the *śakti. Āratī,* chanting, the worship of his guru, and the ashram schedule could not be abandoned simply because he had come west.

So the Muktananda World Tour became a sort of traveling ashram, which recreated the ambiance of Shree Gurudev Ashram wherever Muktananda happened to be. All tasks—from running the programs and arranging transportation to organizing the tour movements and negotiating contracts—were performed by volunteers as *gurusevā*. No matter where Swami Muktananda was, or how busy everyone was, meditation was held at 4:30 each morning. The *Gurugītā* chant went on—and everyone was expected to be there. Lights were waved to the picture of Bhagawan Nityananda.

The challenge for Muktananda's students was to maintain their connection to the rituals and practices that sustained their sadhana, while learning how to perform organizational and social tasks that many of them had never before attempted. From the moment of Muktananda's first program in the small Siddha Yoga ashram in the Piedmont hills in April 1974, the young seekers who had gathered around him found themselves feeding and housing hundreds of people, transporting equipment, and learning to express the teachings to people unfamiliar with Indian culture. "Most of us were kids," said Swami Maheshananda, who joined the tour as a nineteen-year-old Brooklyn College student and helped run the traveling ashram kitchen. "None of us knew how to do anything. Baba trained us himself. He taught the musicians how to play the instruments. He trained the speakers. He spent hours every day showing us how to cook Indian food. He showed the tour managers how to run an organization. He taught us how to live by a certain standard of excellence. That in itself was quite revolutionary for some of us." One ashramite remembered a morning during Swami Muktananda's stay in Piedmont, when he had the job of opening the meditation hall at 4:30. The student had been up late; he didn't arrive until 4:45. He found that Muktananda himself had opened the doors and was standing with a flashlight ushering people in. For the staff, the tour became a kind of spiritual school in which *gurusevā* was the major practice, and they received training not just in new skills but also in inner equipoise. "We had to learn to remember God while functioning at high-speed, with so much going on," said Maheshananda.[159]

Not the least of the challenges were the physical conditions of the tour. In the early days in California, when the first weekend retreats were organized, the staff got used to going to bed late and getting up early. Later, when the tour left California and began to move through the southwestern and midwestern United States, the schedule became even more demanding. The staff traveled in vans, cars, and a white school bus, trailed by an old Ford truck that carried, among other things, the foam mattresses on which the tour staff slept. Often they would run a weekend retreat in one city, then dismantle everything, drive all night to the next town, and set up the hall in time for morning meditation and breakfast. Accommodations in those days were sometimes casual; in Los Angeles, in 1975, the tour stayed in an old riding camp, where Swami Muktananda's quarters were adjacent to the paddock. "There were even a few times when you literally didn't know where you'd sleep that night," recalled someone who traveled with the tour for a time. "It was a constant experience of learning to trust in grace. Somehow, you were always taken care of. And somehow the dignity and the purity of Baba's presence would turn these Boy Scout camps into meditative environments."

Because there was so much to do, staff members often found themselves doing things they had never done before. "Psychologists became managers. Writers became cooks. Musicians found themselves organizing meditation retreats," said Peggy Bendet, a journalist who met Muktananda while interviewing him for a Honolulu newspaper, received shaktipat and joined the tour soon afterward. "You never knew what you'd be doing next, and that in itself was exciting. But it was the feeling of love Baba created, the sweetness of the atmosphere, that made it so lovely. For a lot of us on that tour, it was the best time we'd ever had in our lives."[160]

The Meditation Retreats and the Experience of Shaktipat

From the beginning, Swami Muktananda attracted many leading figures in what was colloquially known as the "consciousness movement."* Researchers, scientists, psychologists, Christian monks interested in meditation, ecumenical rabbis all trickled into his temporary ashram in the Oakland hills to ask him questions about science and consciousness, about their own experiences of *kuṇḍalinī*, and about the effect of meditation. Muktananda's prescription to all of them was, "Meditate." Though he occasionally gave visitors shaktipat by touch on the spot—the small room off the living room where he received guests was often filled with people whom Muktananda had just initiated, usually by touching them between the eyebrows—his main vehicles for shaktipat were meditation retreats held in country campsites, often in the mountains. The retreats allowed several hundred of the seeking and spiritually curious to leave their normal rounds, immerse themselves in Muktananda's environment, and enter more deeply into the experience he offered.

Each morning at Muktananda's Siddha Yoga Meditation Retreats, participants rose at 4:30 A.M. for meditation, ate a breakfast of oatmeal and milky Indian tea (*chai*), and chanted the *Gurugītā* together—on alternate days in an English verse translation. At the programs, Swami Muktananda lectured and answered questions, his talks liberally sprinkled with traditional stories from Indian scripture and folklore that often had his audi-

*This is an umbrella term that encompassed writers, scientists, researchers, and thinkers as diverse as Rupert Sheldrake and Ken Wilbur, and which in the 1970s was used to describe those with an interest in exploring Eastern teachings in a Western scientific context. The movement was described in Marilyn Ferguson's *The Aquarian Conspiracy: Personal and Social Transformation in Our Time* (Los Angeles: G. P. Tarcher, 1987).

ence rocking with laughter. During meditation, he sometimes walked among the seated rows of people, touching some between the eyebrows in a classical gesture of initiation. Then, all the participants in the retreat would line up for darshan, to be blessed by Swami Muktananda, who would touch them with a long wand of peacock feathers. This was an innovation designed to allow him to reach everyone without strain. It quickly became one of his trademarks.

"The Indian trappings turned me off at first," recalls Mac Littlefield, a computer scientist who had sampled most of the "growth groups" of 1970s California. "I left after the first visit thinking I would never come back again—all those chants I couldn't understand! Curiosity drew me back, and then I loved the feeling I had in those retreats. Even though the lifestyle was unusual for 1970s America—practicing celibacy and keeping early hours was not something common for the time—there was always a feeling of excitement. You never knew what would happen."[161] Like Littlefield, many were struck by the dynamic quality of these gatherings, the combination of disciplined rigor with rollicking spontaneity. Though the hours were long and the schedule monastic, a celebratory spirit reigned during Muktananda's darshans, and during the long, percussion-filled chants that proved a major attraction to many of the jaded seekers of those days. "I couldn't believe I could experience so much joy by sitting in a group of people and singing the same words over and over again!" said a young physicist after the crescendo of an all-night chant.[162] Sometimes, at those retreats, the entire room would turn into an ocean of sound. When the awakened *kuṇḍalinī* was manifesting strongly, or breaking through a meditator's inner blocks, or simply releasing some buried memory or long-suppressed feeling, people would sometimes shout out Sanskrit mantras, laugh, cry, or perform rapid yogic breathing.[163]

To judge by the published reports of those who encountered Swami Muktananda in those years, one of the common effects of Muktananda's company was an awakening of the capacity for joy. Kathleen Speeth, a psychotherapist who spent time around Muktananda in 1974, described this experience in an article published in the 1975 *Gurudev-Vani.*

> In the weeks that followed [meeting Swami Muktananda] I felt as if a siren, one that I had been aware of only in the deepest recesses of my consciousness, had somehow been silenced. That siren, continuously though subliminally sounding since my earliest childhood, was the voice of emotional pain. I realized that I had never been happy before.[164]

She went on to say, "For me this blissful overflow has been the beginning of a new emotional life."

Author Paul Zweig, who met Swami Muktananda in Manhattan in 1974, described his initial experience as a profound emotional release. Sit-

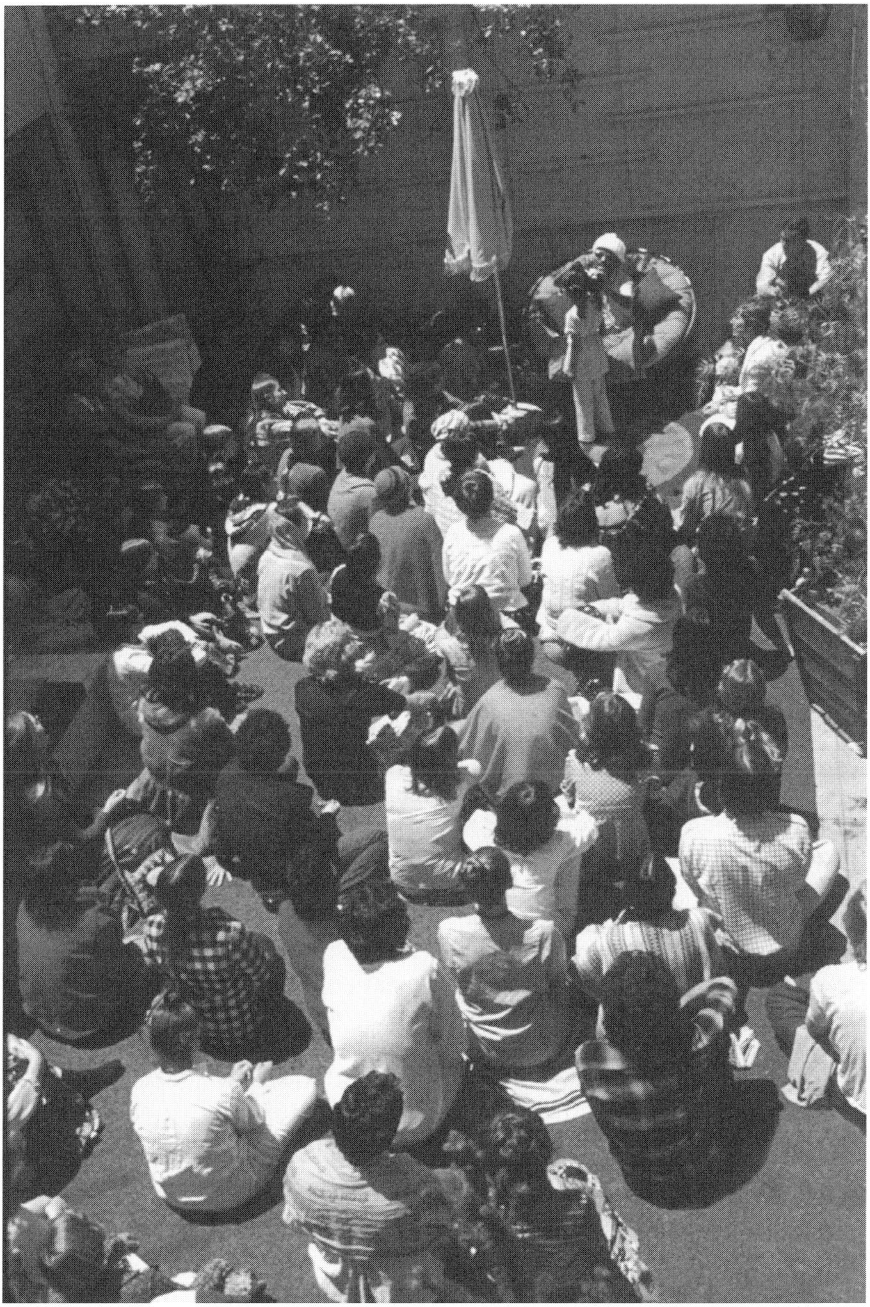

Fig. 13. Swami Muktananda in the courtyard of the Oakland Ashram during his second world tour, 1974–76

ting with a group of people, listening as a young woman asked questions of Muktananda, Zweig began seeing a silvery light:

> I became aware that I had to make an effort not to cry, yet it wasn't simply crying, for my body had become buoyant and warm. . . . My eyes seemed to be peering out of a deep, silvery tunnel, while the forms and colors of the room glided across their surface like paper cutouts. . . .
>
> With no transition I seemed to be seeing my life from a new angle. . . . All of us sitting in that room were on the point of crying out, for we existed far from the light. I had accomplished all sorts of things in my life. I had a position in the world; I wrote books, I was a discriminating person who cringed from the naive self-importance of these "kids." Yet nothing I had done meant a thing from the viewpoint of that light. . . .
>
> Until that very minute I had accepted mental pain as an ordinary part of life. I believed that my insufferable anxieties belonged to the fabric of existence; that in some way they were a good thing. This morning, sitting on a hard wood floor, looking at a dark-skinned Indian man with a large belly and an orange ski cap, a strange light had been driven into my gloom: the sickness can be cured, it has been cured. You are already free. I was experiencing the delirium of release.[165]

That sense of release, of transformation, of a new life beginning, is so characteristic of the experience of shaktipat that it can be found in the reminiscences of Siddha Yoga students from Swami Muktananda's day to the present. As Speeth's and Zweig's experiences imply, it is often accompanied by a paradigm shift that for many people transforms the perspective from which they look at their lives. Swami Muktananda taught—not just in words but through the experience his *śakti* conveyed—that the ultimate reality of life is not suffering but joy. In a cultural atmosphere dominated by deep divisions, by the violence and despair of the post-sixties world, Swami Muktananda chose to affirm the path of bliss.

Though radically unexpected and often initially difficult for his Western devotees to accept, Swami Muktananda's position was not a denial of the world nor was it due to a refusal to face the facts of life. On the contrary, anyone who spent time around Muktananda soon discovered that he was an arch realist; one lawyer devotee reported that when he discussed a case with his guru, Muktananda's suggestions were often more grounded than his own. Muktananda did not turn away from people in pain; devotees saw him weeping with an Australian mother whose child had drowned, and many devotees experienced his deep understanding of their sorrows. His stance was based on his own inner experience that God is immanent in everything and that God's nature is ecstasy. Swami Muktananda affirmed this position even when he himself faced physical suffering,* and he taught his students not to ignore pain but rather to recognize the bliss at the root of all manifestation.[166] "In the realized state," he once said, "you are happy when you are happy, but you are also happy even when you are in pain. The perception of suffering is ordinary perception; the enlightened perception is the perception of joy."[167]

Swami Muktananda's Yoga of Daily Life

At the same time, Swami Muktananda impressed the sometimes star-struck seekers of this period with his practical attitude toward the realities of day-to-day life. He taught freedom; to him that meant freedom from dependence on psychological crutches of any kind. Hence his emphasis on personal discipline. Not only did he stress the necessity of daily practice, good diet, and healthy exercise, he also expected his students to be self-supporting, free of debt, and able to live, as he often put it, with dignity and self-respect.

"What do you do?" he asked a young man who approached him in Los Angeles in 1974, dressed in flowing robes and a beatific smile.

"Nothing," the seeker replied. "Somehow, God seems to take care of me."

"Have some mercy on God and get a job," Muktananda said.[168]

His advice to meditators was similarly practical. When Kathleen Speeth came to ask for techniques to improve her practice, he said, "You look thin and pale. Meditate no more than an hour a day, and eat rich [that is, nourishing] foods."[169]

Swami Muktananda's teachings on dharma, "righteous behavior," based on the values of the Indian tradition, were powerfully transformative for young people caught up in the value crisis of those years. For many people who met Muktananda in the 1970s, the shift in their inner life was mirrored by behavioral changes: perhaps a resumption of neglected family duties, a renewal of broken marriage vows, a commitment to paying their debts, an ability to renounce habits like smoking and drinking. Nearly every night during the daily programs he held throughout this tour, someone would approach Muktananda in darshan to offer a packet of cigarettes or a whiskey bottle, in token of his or her resolution to give up these things.

---

*Swami Chidvilasananda once spoke of a time in the early days of the ashram when Swami Muktananda's *rudrākṣa* bead necklace got caught in the rope of the well, which pulled the rough beads so tightly into his neck that they left a deep gash. Muktananda had to wait for half an hour before someone found him; when he was discovered, he seemed perfectly content. Later he said that when his *mala* had gotten caught, he had had a vision of his guru standing before him. He said "His smile and his face were so bewitching that I didn't feel the passage of time or what was happening to my body." [Swami Chidvilasananda, "The Name Which Is Prayer Itself," *Darshan* No. 7–8 (July-August 1987), p. 130].

Muktananda greeted these people enthusiastically. "I want to thank this person who has renounced poison," he would say, holding up the cigarette package or the whiskey bottle. "There is so much more intoxication in the name of God." Once, he handed someone the card containing the Siddha Yoga mantra *Oṃ Namaḥ Śivaya* and said, "Smoke this."[170]

Siddha Yoga Sadhana and the Process of Purification

Though the primary function of the 1974–76 tour was the transmission of shaktipat, much of Swami Muktananda's work with his disciples revolved around issues of sadhana—the practices they did to hold and expand the awakened *śakti.* Most devotees quickly found out that shaktipat was not simply a thrilling experience, nor was it a magic pill that removed all their troubles. In short, though the awakening of the *śakti* conferred a capacity to meditate and a strong impulse toward spiritual life, it did not wipe away the necessity of spiritual effort.

That was what Penny Clyne, who met Swami Muktananda in 1974 and became a deeply committed practitioner of Siddha Yoga, remembered:

> There was a common experience that we had in those days. With shaktipat there would often be a profound experience of your own divinity, incredible happiness, and a desire to serve humanity. It was like a glimpse of the goal. Then you'd come down, so to speak, and find out that to hold that experience you had to work. Purification had to be done. But that initial experience was so powerfully attractive that you would get inspired to go for it, to meditate and give yourself to spiritual practice. And the awakened energy would impel you along, keep giving you experiences, keep changing you.[171]

Often when Swami Muktananda would come to town, the seekers who met him would go through a period of excitement, an almost romantic immersion in the new-found wonders of their own inner world. Then he would leave, and they would be left to integrate their new-born sense of spiritual power, love, and purpose into their daily lives. Most people required periods of adjustment, as they reexamined their work, family, and social life in the light of this nascent spiritual awareness and tried to fit it all together. Moreover, since a major aspect of sadhana with an awakened *kuṇḍalinī* involves spontaneous purification, seekers sometimes faced long-buried inner tendencies thrown up by the awakened *śakti* in order to bring them to awareness and expel them. Penny Clyne said:

> What separated the committed Siddha Yoga students from the trippers was the willingness to stick around and do sadhana and let the process unfold. Sometimes because the experience seemed so magical at first, people would expect Baba to wave a magic wand and take away their difficulties. If this did

not happen, they might blame Baba or feel that Siddha Yoga had failed to live up to its promise. But if you stayed with it, you'd find that deep, lasting transformation would happen. Little by little, instead of identifying so much with my emotions, I began to identify with that part of myself that can witness the emotions and go beyond them. But that process happened right in the middle of my family life. For me, sadhana was all about how I reacted when my husband left the newspaper on the floor or when my son acted like a typical adolescent.

Swami Muktananda as an Expounder of the Science of Kuṇḍalinī

Swami Muktananda's writing and teaching during this period addressed these issues, spelling out for new students the practices and attitudes that would allow them to integrate their daily duties with their meditation practice, and helping them understand the process of purification that shaktipat had initiated.* He was familiarizing his students with the experiences of the awakened *kuṇḍalinī,* as well as with the essence of scriptures like the *Bhagavadgītā* and the *Śiva Sūtras*, the lives of saints, and the mystical poetry of India.

Reading transcripts of these talks and interviews, we can see how much of Muktananda's work in the West involved dispelling popular misconceptions about *kuṇḍalinī* and spirituality. Interest in *kuṇḍalinī* was growing among Western seekers, but so was fear of its effects, especially since some of the popular books on the subject described the awakened *kuṇḍalinī* as potentially dangerous for unwary seekers. Baba Muktananda taught that *kuṇḍalinī* awakening is safe and productive when it occurs through the grace of a guru who has himself completed the spiritual journey. "It is not enough for the *kuṇḍalinī* to be awakened," he often said. "It must rise to the sahasrara and become established there."[172] This, he maintained, becomes possible through the inner guidance of a guru.

Swami Muktananda was one of the few—perhaps the only—spiritual teacher in the West at that time who could systematically explain these movements and help meditators regulate them. As such, he was periodically sought out by frightened seekers whose own teachers were unable to help them understand their meditation experiences. Once, a well-known Indian teacher who taught *haṭhayoga* and meditation telephoned Muktananda to say that one of his students was having uncontrollable *kriyās*, yogic movements of the body. The teacher could not calm her. Muktananda had him put the student on the telephone; after he spoke to her for a few minutes,

*In 1978, Muktananda also asked a student, Ram Butler, to write the bimonthly *Siddha Yoga Correspondence Course*, which over the years has provided teachings for devotees who practice Siddha Yoga away from the ashrams.

her physical manifestations quieted. "A real Guru" he used to say, "is one who . . . is able to control the working of the Shakti in the disciple after he has awakened it."[173]

Organizational Development During the Second World Tour

Between 1974 and 1976, Siddha Yoga matured from a casual assemblage of disciples to a relatively well-known spiritual organization. Each ring of its growth process was marked by increased attention to explaining the teachings and the gestures of the Guru, by a growing formalization of the programs, and by the development of structures and institutions.

During this two-year period, Swami Muktananda gave birth to four major Siddha Yoga institutions besides the traveling ashram known as Muktananda World Tour. These were: 1) the Siddha Yoga Intensive, which allowed shaktipat to be given en masse over the course of a weekend; 2) the Western residential ashram; 3) SYDA Foundation, which would provide the organizational and financial infrastructure for the expanding movement; and 4) the Siddha Yoga courses and trainings, through which the teachings were disseminated to new students. Each of these institutions arose in response to the needs of the growing circle of students.

The Intensive Exists to Show You Your Own Self

The Siddha Yoga Meditation Intensive, which would become the major vehicle for the dissemination of shaktipat, came into being in Aspen, Colorado, in August 1974. Swami Muktananda and his aides had noticed that many people resisted leaving home to come to a meditation retreat. "So, for people's convenience, Babaji began to think of a weekend program that could be held in a hall, where people didn't have to leave town," said one of the people who helped organize the tour.[174] Muktananda himself chose the title—which he used to pronounce "Intense," because, as he said, the weekend Intensives gave an intense experience of *śakti.*

From the moment of its inception, the Intensive became the "official" Siddha Yoga shaktipat program—described in one informational brochure as "giving the kind of experiences that were previously available only to those who spent a long period of time in the ashram." On the surface, the program was simple—two eight-hour days in which Muktananda gave two lectures, answered questions, and led chanting and meditation, while trained disciples introduced the program, described their own experiences, and explained how things would work. "The whole Intensive gives shaktipat," said Swami Ishwarananda, a teacher of Siddha Yoga, in a lecture in 1985. "Just the way when you sit in an air-conditioned room you get cool, when you sit in the Intensive you receive shaktipat. It happens automatically, by osmosis through the Guru's will."[175] In fact, nowhere is the mystical dimension of Siddha Yoga more apparent than in the Intensive, where hundreds of people simultaneously can experience the transmission of spiritual energy and where many report dramatic inner awakenings.

In *The Guru's Touch*, a BBC film made in 1976 in London, we catch a glimpse of the atmosphere of Swami Muktananda's Intensives, where during each meditation session he would walk through the room brushing every person present with his peacock feather wand, awakening the *kuṇḍalinī* by touch. "Baba didn't need to give the touch," Swami Sevananda explained in an interview in 1988. "Shaktipat can just as easily be given through a mantra. In fact, usually it just happens spontaneously as people sit in the Intensive. But people felt that if he touched them, they had really received something."[176] It was the Intensive that would eventually allow Muktananda's "meditation revolution" to reach thousands at a time.

"Baba loved to hear about the experiences people had in meditation in the Intensives," Swami Sevananda said. "We would have sharing sessions, and Baba would watch. Once he said, 'I wonder if these people know what they are receiving. Yogis in the Himalayas do *tapasya* for thirty years without having the experiences these people have in a weekend.'"[177] Occasionally, just such a yogi would appear at one of the Intensives, to marvel at how this esoteric and rare initiation could be so available. "I've been studying spiritual books for forty years," announced a white-haired man at an Intensive in Miami in April 1980. "I've studied the Old Testament, the Bhagavad Gita. After all this, I've come to Baba. He seems to synthesize forty years of scriptural reading and philosophy. He makes everything clear, he confirms everything I thought to be true."[178]

Development of American Siddha Yoga Centers and Ashrams

When Swami Muktananda arrived in America in 1974, there were just two Siddha Yoga centers in the United States—one in an apartment on West 94th Street in Manhattan, another in a house in Piedmont, California. By 1975, mid-way through his tour, there were more than a hundred. Most were in private homes, where groups of devotees would meet to chant, meditate, and hear Swami Muktananda's teachings. Swami Muktananda himself brought many of these centers into being. He believed that Siddha Yoga spread naturally from one meditator to another, so in the early days, he would simply pick out someone who was having strong meditation experiences and ask that person to open a meditation center. He even authorized some of these early center leaders to give Intensives in his name, at which shaktipat would occur even though Swami Muktananda was not physically present. Ram Butler, one of those early center leaders, related his response when Muktananda first asked him to give Intensives. "Baba," he said, "what if nothing happens?" Muktananda replied, "Don't worry. You do your job, and I'll do mine."[179] Paul and Carolyn Zeiger, a professor and psychologist who were invited to open a center in Boulder, Colorado, took Muktananda at his word. They set aside Sunday nights for their meetings and held a program for whomever came. In the beginning it was just meditation; later it evolved into something more structured—with a *kīrtana* (a fast repetitive chant of one or more of the Sanskrit names of God) accompanied by drum and harmonium, a reading from Muktananda's writings, and a session of meditation. "We had it whether anyone showed up or not," recalled Carolyn Zeiger, whose center eventually became formalized and the nucleus of the Boulder Siddha Yoga community.[180]

At first, the centers were independent, decentralized units. Only when Swami Muktananda's tour settled in Oakland in 1975 was a serious attempt made to organize and centralize the centers and their programs.

The Oakland Ashram

"In 1975," recalled David Pierce, a California lawyer who served as tour manager from 1974 through most of 1975, "Baba told us that we needed a place for people to spend time with him. You have to understand that we'd been traveling nonstop for almost a year, holding programs in Boy Scout camps. A lot of people wanted to be with Baba. He was almost a Pied Piper for people. They would meet him and get overwhelmed by the feeling of love around him and want to come and live with him. Baba's policy was 'everybody come.' So we needed a place."[181] The Oakland Ashram was crafted by a volunteer staff out of the shell of the fearsomely derelict Hotel Stanford, in a down-at-the-heels neighborhood in Oakland. The place was filthy and run-down, and its transformation into an immaculate ashram became the prototype for many such renovations over the years. Siddha Yoga devotees, offering their labor as *gurusevā,* would turn numerous run-down hotels, residences, restaurants, and the like into modern facilities for Siddha Yoga programs; in fact, shortly after Muktananda arrived in Oakland, a group of Australian Siddha Yoga students visited the ashram and were inspired to create a similar urban monastery in Melbourne.

Oakland would eventually become the center of the largest lay Siddha Yoga community in the world. Beginning in 1975, devotees began renting or buying housing in the area around the ashram and invested time and money in upgrading both their own property and the public spaces. Swami Muktananda lived in the Oakland Ashram for ten months in 1975–76, and it was there that he initiated many of the organizational developments, including the Siddha Yoga courses and teachers trainings, the book publication departments, and SYDA Foundation, which would eventually provide the financial and organizational infrastructure for Siddha Yoga in the West. "Most of us were anti-organization types, as spiritual seekers tend to be," said Norman Monson, a trustee in the early years. "It was a real learning process to discover that instead of squashing the *śakti*, the foundation provided a more effective vehicle for Baba's grace."[182]

The Birth of SYDA Foundation

Taking the place of the temporary legal entity, Muktananda World Tour, which had handled financial matters since Baba had left India, SYDA—the initials mean Siddha Yoga Dham ("abode of Siddha Yoga") Associates—was designed in 1975 to become the administrative body for all of Siddha Yoga in the West. "I remember Baba saying that one of the reasons certain ashrams in India run into difficulty, or aren't able to sustain themselves," recalled Peter Sitkin, a northern California lawyer who served as legal counsel to the foundation and as a trustee, "was that not enough attention was paid to the practical details of operating the ashram or the spiritual community. There was almost an exclusive emphasis on the lofty teachings but without a solid foundation. Without a foundation you can't go to the higher floors of a building. I remember Baba saying that it was very, very important not only to have a structure but to really be in tune with every single detail."[183]

The original organizational structure was hammered out under Swami Muktananda's direction by a group of devotees, including Chicago attorney Ronald Friedland, who became the first president. SYDA Foundation included a board of trustees, a number of administrative departments, and a committee structure to oversee such areas as ashram publications and public relations. SYDA Foundation also helped to administer Muktananda's work with the *ādivāsīs* in the Tansa Valley, where he was continuing this aspect of his guru's efforts by building a high school in the town of Vajreshwari and several housing colonies for hitherto homeless tribal people. These projects were financed partly by Swami Muktananda's Intensives, which also allowed the ashram to contribute to local disaster relief projects.

The birth of SYDA Foundation marked a major organizational shift from a system in which most ashram decisions were referred directly to Swami Muktananda, to a departmental system with regulated channels of communication. The Siddha Yoga centers, which had to date been independent and as idiosyncratic as each individual who ran them, also fell under the governance of SYDA Foundation, which began now to set up standards, structures, and systems of accountability for the dissemination of teachings.

The Teachings Should Play in Your Blood: Trainings and Teachers

The first Center Leaders' Training, held in 1975 at a retreat in Arcata, California, established guidelines for nearly every aspect of Siddha Yoga satsangs, from the order of the program to the chords of the chants, from the items placed on the *āratī* tray to the points to be covered by the master of ceremonies in his welcoming remarks. Though the guidelines would shift many times over the years, they represented the first attempts to establish ways of doing things that were specific to the Siddha Yoga culture. "I was one of the people who was taking that training," said Karen Shiarella, a former college dean who headed the Siddha Yoga Centers' Office for many years. "I could see the importance of developing a system of education and regulation for those who would claim to speak in the name of Siddha Yoga so that the teachings could be disseminated in the way Baba had originally taught them." At the same time, Swami Muktananda continued to emphasize the spiritual core of the trainings. "The most important thing we got in those trainings was that learning was not just about acquiring information," Shiarella said. "At the end of every course, Baba used to say that it wasn't enough just to memorize what had been taught. He kept saying, 'You have to imbibe the teachings so deeply that they play in your bloodstream and come up when you need them.'"[184]

The attorney Peter Sitkin remembered that graduates of the training were given certificates, and he also recalled drawing up agreements between the foundation and the center leaders. "People made a formal commitment, by saying, 'Yes, I will be an appropriate representative of Siddha Yoga,'" Sitkin said in an interview in 1995. "It is so important that the people maintain that commitment. Otherwise, they would not be able to continue teaching on behalf of Siddha Yoga."

Not only prospective teachers were getting educated. A whole generation of Siddha Yoga students had begun to imbibe the rudiments of the Indian scriptures and culture. Formal study was new in Siddha Yoga ashrams; since Nityananda's time teaching had been informal and spontaneous. At the same time, even in the early days in Ganeshpuri, Muktananda had responded to his disciples' need for verbal guidance, confirmation of their experiences, and instruction in the philosophy and practices underlying Siddha Yoga. Now, in the programs he held almost nightly during his years in the West, Swami Muktananda would answer thousands of questions about spiritual life and make himself available for personal questions to whoever came before him in darshan.

In Oakland in 1975, during the nightly programs that became the nucleus of life in the first Western Siddha Yoga *gurukula,* Muktananda began teaching Kashmir Śaivism, the monistic philosophical system that had originated in northern India in the late eighth century yet had remained relatively unknown even in the rest of India until the mid-twentieth century. Swami Muktananda had been speaking from these texts for many years; he often said that he had become interested in them because Kashmir Śaivism above all other systems describes the world the way he saw it—as a manifestation of divine energy, a play of divine consciousness. In keeping with that perspective, he taught Kashmir Śaivism to his Western disciples primarily as a conceptual framework for their practice. The Śaivite view that the world itself is God, that all forms are both *created by* and *permeated with* the dynamic power (*śakti*) of God, provided the philosophical basis for his instruction to disciples to see the divine presence in everything around them. Swami Muktananda rarely presented a systematic approach to Śaivism (although he did encourage his disciples to study and later to teach the philosophical and technical aspects of the system). His interest in Śaivism was practical: To him, it was a means of guiding his students towards the understanding of their oneness with the divine reality he saw in everything. As one American student noted, "Baba uses the concepts [of Kashmir Śaivism] as a means for people to do sadhana. He does not care about proving principles or theories. He takes them ready-made and asks us to put them into use in our lives. . . . Baba does not try to prove that everything is God. He sees everything as God, and we can see that he sees it that way. He says, 'See everything as God! Do it! Don't merely talk and think about it. Do it!'"[185]

When Muktananda taught Kashmir Śaivism, moreover, he did more than simply explain the concepts. "There was a spiritual power in his words that literally enlivened the teaching," said Harold Ferrar, then a literature professor who came into contact with Śaivism through Swami Muktananda's teaching. "When he was speaking of how the world is Consciousness, or talking about how everything comes out of God, the words would set off an experience inside me, sometimes a realization, or even a full-blown vision of oneness. Listening to him was literally mind-expanding."[186] The power Swami Muktananda infused in these words seemed to touch not only his own students, but even casual spiritual seekers who came in contact with him during those years, or read his small book of commentaries on the aphorisms of Kashmir Śaivism, *Siddha Meditation*. Muktananda not only taught Kashmir Śaivism himself; he was instrumental in bringing the texts to the attention of a wider public. When Jaideva Singh had completed his groundbreaking translation of Kṣemarāja's *Pratyabhijñā-hṛdayam*, Muktananda asked the prominent New Delhi publisher, Motilal Banarsidass, to bring it out and later to publish Singh's English editions of the *Śiva Sūtras*, *Spandakārikās*, and *Vijñānabhairava*. Several of these editions carried next to their title pages a statement of benediction from Swami Muktananda.

During 1975, Muktananda authorized some of his senior disciples to set up the first Siddha Yoga courses, including a two-week survey course that explained the basic teachings through lectures and discussions on *kuṇḍalinī*, mantra, the guru-disciple relationship, Vedānta, Kashmir Śaivism, meditation theory and practice, and the nature and purpose of yoga and spirituality. It had become obvious, as his following grew, that he could not physically deal with everyone who was coming to him, or answer everyone's questions, or travel more extensively than he was already doing. So Muktananda began to train teachers and give them authority. Certain of Muktananda's disciples, those with communications skills or previous experience as teachers, began to emerge as Siddha Yoga "professors"—as Muktananda sometimes jokingly called them.

"Baba empowered us to speak in his name," recalled Swami Shantananda, who was one of the first of these teachers. "Certain of us would travel around, giving Intensives—we would even give the touch. It was very exciting for us, because we discovered that all we had to do was follow Baba's instructions and the *śakti*, Baba's spiritual energy, would flow through us and people would have spiritual experiences. It all happened through Baba's will, his *saṅkalpa*. We were instruments, so to speak. For us it was a demonstration of the power of the Guru's intention."[187]

These disciples would help spread Muktananda's message to thousands of people who never met him personally. Moreover, they demonstrated that the *śakti* of the Siddha Yoga lineage could flow through many channels. Once Muktananda had created vehicles like the Intensive and authorized the giving of shaktipat there, the process seemed to work whether he was physically present or not. Many people experienced *kuṇḍalinī* awakening at Intensives given by his disciples in India and Europe even while he was in America. Swami Muktananda used to say that one could receive shaktipat through an authorized disciple of a siddha guru; it was the guru's intention, not his physical presence, that made shaktipat occur. Nonetheless, he always cautioned seekers to remember that the source of the *śakti* was the guru, and ultimately God.

Siddha Yoga Lifestyle

By the end of 1975, a sociologist of religion would have found it easy to discern a recognizable Siddha Yoga lifestyle. A student of Siddha Yoga typically devoted from ten minutes to three hours a day to meditation, and many practiced repetition of the main Siddha Yoga mantra, *Oṃ Namaḥ Śivāya*, during the day, often while walking, cooking, or performing routine tasks. Some attended Siddha Yoga centers and supported those centers by offering service there; others preferred to keep their practice more private; and there were some who pursued the practice of Siddha Yoga while continuing to follow their own Christian, Jewish, or other religious traditions. Though most Siddha Yoga students lived ordinary "worldly" lives, pursuing careers and raising families and visiting the ashram for a few weeks or a few days each year, a group of several hundred spent as much time as work and family allowed with Swami Muktananda (and later Swami Chidvilasananda). As the organization grew, many of these people came to live as residents in the Siddha Yoga ashrams around the world. This population would periodically change, as people who had spent time in the ashram returned to raise families or pursue careers, while others took "sabbaticals" from their professional lives to spend a year or two in the ashram. A Siddha Yoga community, with its own culture, its own terminology, and an enormous shared body of experiences had taken form and was to continue to expand through the 1980s and 1990s.

THE PREPARATION OF MUKTANANDA'S SUCCESSOR: MALTI BECOMES TRANSLATOR

In Oakland, in 1975, an event took place that would have far-reaching implications. Muktananda's translator, Jinendra Jain, left the tour to get married, and Muktananda chose Malti to replace him. Up to that time, Malti had remained in the background, a quiet, dedicated young woman who assisted Swami Muktananda at darshan, took notes on his talks, and occasionally translated for him in private meetings with devotees. Now, though she knew little English, she was thrust into the most public of roles. Her on-the-job training as a translator began with an intensive English course, daily study with Katherine McCormick (later Swami Kripananda), a professor of Spanish literature at San Jose State University who came to live in the ashram full-time.

The translator was of necessity the main intermediary between the Hindi-speaking Muktananda and his English-speaking students. So Malti's new role put her in a position to imbibe directly the entire range of Swami Muktananda's teachings and his methods of working with students. Barbara Hamilton, who served as Malti's secretary between 1979 and 1982, observed in an interview in 1989, "Baba spoke a potpourri of languages, pulling words from one dialect or another and mixing them all together. And, as if that weren't challenging enough, he would often speak in incomplete sentences or leave phrases dangling. She had to penetrate the essence of what he was saying. Her translation wasn't just an academic transposition of words from one language into another. . . . [I]t relied on her fine inner tuning to the heart of what Baba was communicating."[188]

The essence of the training she received was an attunement to the subtle hints and messages given by her guru. Swami Muktananda always said that when a disciple's mind becomes inwardly united with the guru's, the disciple's inner state gradually becomes purified and uplifted by the guru's own elevated state of consciousness. This act of turning toward and "becoming one" with the guru's inner state is the essential mystical strategy of the path of discipleship, in which a disciple contemplates and meditates on his or her guru with the understanding that the guru has become one with God.

Swami Chidvilasananda has often spoken of how she learned that attunement through the daily process of assisting Swami Muktananda in his interactions with students:

> In darshan, [where several hundred people came up in the course of several hours] I would translate for the people asking questions, and I would also need to stay aware of everything that was going on. Baba would communicate with me, but usually it wasn't with words. He would speak with his knees. His knee would move in a certain way and I would need to know that he wanted the audio person to change the tape. Or his elbow would move, and it would mean, "Ask that person to sit down."[189]

To stay abreast of all this required her to develop subtle awareness and the ability to flow intuitively with a fast-moving situation.

Mercedes Stewart, an Australian woman who was then a teenager, remembered the first several times she assisted Malti during Swami Muktananda's nightly darshans:

> Everything seemed to be happening so fast. So you had to be watching all the time. On my second night I got so nervous, I was sitting there and wringing my hands. [Malti] turned to me and she said: "You don't need to pretend to be frightened." When she said that, I felt like this whole façade that I had sort of shattered and fell to the ground. I didn't know I was pretending to be frightened. I thought I *was* frightened. But as far as she was concerned, fear was unreal. What she really showed me in that moment was that I had a choice as to how I handled pressure. From that moment on, no matter what happened, I tried to keep a steady posture, because I could see that was what she did."[190]

As this exchange shows, Malti quickly became both an example and a teacher to other devotees. Helen Argent recalled:

> She was the model. One thing we always saw was that no matter how much she had to do, she was so dedicated to her practices. I remember when the tour stayed at my parents' house in Sydney, no matter how early I got up in the morning, she would be there on the porch, deep in meditation.[191]

Little by little, she would become increasingly involved with Swami Muktananda's other students. She corresponded with people all over the world, helped them clarify their questions, brought them to meet Muktananda, listened to their difficulties. At Muktananda's direction, she began to develop an intimate understanding not only of spiritual but of administrative issues. In contrast to Muktananda, who had pursued the indrawn path of meditation, Malti's was primarily a path of service. Said Barbara Hamilton:

> What became immediately clear to me was that [Malti] served Baba all the time. . . . Her time was Baba's time. Her deadlines were all related to his daily

> schedule. . . . For her, everything . . . [was] measured by her relationship to Baba. This isn't just a metaphor. This stance was second nature to [her]. Her devotion was not just emotional; her whole life proved it. Many of the devotees thought that, given the opportunity, we could have that kind of devotion. But from my own experience, this isn't necessarily true. . . .
>
> [H]er devotion to Baba was so intense, it gave her such momentum, that it propelled her through obstacles and beyond problems. The unity between her and Baba was profound.[192]

"Even when I wasn't in charge of things, Baba always expected me to be responsible," Swami Chidvilasananda said in later years. "If someone made a mistake, he would ask me, 'Why didn't you let them know how to do it?' He taught me to think of his work as my own work."[193]

Malti's training, though unusually rigorous, was similar in some ways to the training that many of Swami Muktananda's other disciples received. Their practice of *gurusevā* allowed the insights of meditation to translate into daily life and provided an arena through which Swami Muktananda taught them the basic principles of yoga as skill in action. One way he often did this was by creating high pressure situations, in which a disciple would feel impelled to accomplish tasks quickly and well. "It forced you to concentrate, and it developed all kinds of other qualities—flexibility, for instance, and follow-through," said Peggy Bendet.[194] Swami Maheshananda, who worked for many years in the ashram kitchen, recalled how Muktananda would visit the kitchen daily and how he made each task there an occasion for lessons on one-pointedness, focus, and equanimity:

> He expected us to be completely alert and on our toes—and believe me, that wasn't easy, since the *śakti* around him was so thick that you were constantly fighting the temptation to fall into meditation. If you spaced out or forgot something, he would call you *jaḍ*, which is Hindi for "inert." Once he had us all bent over a pan, teaching us how to make the "magic," the flavoring for Indian dishes. He had told us to brown the mustard seeds until they popped, and we were all listening to hear the sound of mustard seeds popping. All of a sudden, he shouted, "There it is! *Jaḍ*! You all missed it! That was the moment—the moment of yoga. If you can't be one-pointed in the moment, what can you accomplish?" I've never forgotten that.[195]

"Over the years I came to understand that Baba saw us all as equals, as expressions of the divine power," said Swami Shantananda. "Essentially, when I did seva, I felt Baba become my friend and support. From time to time he would work with you . . . and you would get close to him on the inside."[196]

In fact, Swami Muktananda's final message to his American students, before leaving in 1976, was an expression of how he viewed those whose service supported his work:

> I do not look upon you as my devotees or disciples. I consider you all sisters and brothers in the family of my Nityananda Baba.
>
> You are all pure souls. You were born pure. Your perfection was already with you. Each of you was a flame of that pure Self. Being of the family of Nityananda like me, you have joined me to do his work. This is my understanding.[197]

BRINGING THE WEST TO THE EAST: SWAMI MUKTANANDA IN INDIA (1976–78)

In 1976, after a six-week visit to Europe that laid the foundation for what would became a network of ashrams and meditation centers in England, France, Germany, Switzerland, and Holland, Swami Muktananda returned to India. At that point, he began the process of turning his culturally disparate collection of devotees into a genuine international community. Seekers in the ashram—multi-racial, multi-national, spanning major chasms in terms of age, class, and social values—found themselves part of a spontaneous experiment in cultural integration. As in the *hajj*, the pilgrimage to Mecca in the Islamic tradition, differences of race, culture, and social class were put aside. People who might otherwise never have met came to accept and like each other.

"The whole basis of it was Baba's teaching of respect," said Swami Sevananda. "Baba used to say, 'In my ashram, everyone has to get along with everyone else.' Even the dogs had to get along. He would simply not put up with people quarreling or undercutting each other. He didn't just teach, 'See God in each other.' He expected people to live it. Of course, people did get jealous and angry—people are people after all. Baba was patient. But Baba had an ideal, a vision. He used to say, 'This ashram is Vaikuntha, heaven. Don't bring the ways of hell into it. Never look on each other with anger or resentment or an eye to see differences.'"[198]

Swami Muktananda had his own ways of dealing with disharmony. In 1978, an American football star with a well-deserved reputation for volatility was residing at the ashram and soon had opened hostilities with another student, an ex-Marine with an equally hair-trigger temper. The two of them came to blows one day in a corridor outside the ashram kitchen. The next morning Muktananda walked into the kitchen and took them both by the ear. "You would have had to see this to believe it," said Swami Maheshananda, who witnessed the scene. "Baba was five-foot-seven inches tall, and these guys were over six feet. But he was the only person either of them had ever listened to, so they let themselves be dragged over to a corner, and stood up face-to-face. 'Now shake hands,' Baba said. There was an almost audible growl from one of the men. 'Shake hands,' said Baba.

Reluctantly, the two shook hands. 'Now hug each other,' Baba said. They looked at him in wide-eyed disbelief. 'Hug each other!' The two men awkwardly embraced. Baba was still not satisfied. 'Now kiss each other,' he said. At this, both of them looked at Baba, and at each other, and then they gingerly went for it. As they kissed each other stiffly on the cheeks, Baba embraced them both and started to dance."[199] The two men never fought again.

TAKE *SANNYĀSA* FOR THE SAKE OF THE SELF: THE FOUNDING OF AN ORDER OF MONKS

In April 1977, a few months after his return to India, Swami Muktananda took a major step in the development of Siddha Yoga. He initiated a group of Western and Indian disciples into the Sārasvatī Order of *daśanāmi sannyāsa,* the tradition of renunciant monks founded by Śaṅkarācārya. "Creating *sannyāsis* was very much a part of Baba's vision of Siddha Yoga as a worldwide teaching mission," said Swami Shantananda. "My sense was that he intended to found a teaching order, similar to the Ramakrishna Mission or the Divine Life Society. Not all the monks were teachers, but he definitely considered teaching one of the main functions of the swamis." Between 1977 and 1982, Muktananda performed four *sannyāsa* ceremonies. The first one was only for men. In 1978, 1980, and 1982, he also initiated women. By 1982, its peak, the total number of *sannyāsīs* in the organization was sixty-five, of whom fourteen were women.[200]

The Decision to Take Sannyāsa

In an interview in 1987, Swami Shantananda told the story of how Swami Muktananda, with his characteristic mixture of seriousness and play, invited him to take *sannyāsa*:

> Baba asked me, "What do you want to become?"
>
> I said, "What do you mean, Baba?"
>
> "Well, do you want to get married or do you want to be a swami?"
>
> For a moment I was speechless, I didn't know what to say. Finally, I said, "Baba, I feel fine the way I am right now."
>
> "But you're nobody," Baba said. "You have to become somebody. So, if you want to get married, you can do that. If you want to be a swami, that's fine too."
>
> Again, I was completely speechless. I managed to muster a few words. "Baba, I'll let you make the choice for me," I said.
>
> Baba said, "Very good! In that case, you should be a swami. And your name

will be"—he leaned back and thought for a second—"Swami Shantananda ['the bliss of peace']. And your work will be to teach Siddha Yoga. You will travel to different parts of the world, teaching, and also you will run the ashram in Oakland."

He took a chocolate and gave it to me . . . with great sweetness and gave me a kiss on the cheek. "Now you can go."[201]

Shantananda then went through a year of reflection, doubt, and questioning before he made the final decision to take *sannyāsa*, at which point he informed Swami Muktananda of his commitment. "Baba's telling me to choose between *sannyāsa* and marriage was a way of getting me to find out what my real vocation, my role in life should be," Shantananda said. "It wasn't that he made the decision for us. On the contrary. One of our main teachers was invited by Baba to take *sannyāsa* at the same time I was. In a meeting before the ceremony, Baba asked him, 'Do you really want to do this?' The man—trying, I think, to conform to an idea he had about how a disciple is supposed to act—said, 'If that's what you want, Baba.'

"Baba said, 'It's not a matter of what Baba wants. You don't make a decision like this because you think that someone else wants it. Baba doesn't want anything. Baba is happy in his own Self. What do *you* want?' This was a most significant moment for all of us, both as *sannyāsīs* and as disciples. Baba always taught that obedience to the guru should not be blind, that having a guru is not an excuse for giving someone else the responsibility for your life. He would indicate a direction that he felt would be right for you, but he never wanted you just to adopt it without real contemplation and truly make it your own."[202]

The Siddha Yoga swamis took vows of renunciation that included the promise of celibacy. They vowed to abstain from earning money, marrying, or engaging in other worldly pursuits, and to live with simplicity, humility, and purity. Their vows are the ones traditional to the *daśanāmi sannyāsīs*; the mantras they recited state the intention to renounce "the pleasures of all three worlds" for the sake of the pure experience of the absolute, to give up identification with the body, and to dedicate their lives to serving humanity and attaining knowledge of God. Muktananda had them initiated in a two-day ritual that included a ceremony of *brahmacarya dīkṣā*, "initiation into the student stage of life" (which traditionally must precede *sannyāsa*), conducted by brahmin priests, as well as a *homa*, "fire ritual," and river ceremony conducted by a *mahāmaṇḍaleśvar*, an official of the order of *sannyāsīs*.

It is worth noting that in contrast to some other contemporary Indian teachers who created orders of *sannyāsīs* that had legitimacy only within their own movement, Muktananda consciously did everything he could to make sure that his monks could be recognized by the wider community of traditional *daśanāmi* swamis. Rather than preside over the ceremonies himself (as he was quite entitled to do), he invited a *mahāmaṇḍaleśvar*, the head of Jyotir Matha in Haridwar, to perform the rites, thus investing his order with the imprimatur of an authority outside Siddha Yoga. Muktananda also made it clear that no one could be considered a Siddha Yoga swami who did not go through the process that included a ceremony of *brahmacarya dīkṣā* conducted by brahmin priests, as well as the traditional *homa* and river ceremony conducted by a *mahāmaṇḍaleśvar*.

The Ceremony

The swamis performed their own funeral rites as well as the funeral rituals for their parents, thus freeing themselves of one of the main filial obligations of traditional Hindus. After performing these rituals, a *sannyāsī* considers himself to have died to his former life, and traditionally avoids his home, friends, and relatives for at least twelve years. This rule, however, was modified for the Western monks of Siddha Yoga, whose families had no cultural framework for understanding the tradition; Western Siddha Yoga *sannyāsīs* are encouraged to maintain cordial relationships with their families.

At the end of the all-night initiation ceremony, the *sannyāsīs* immersed themselves in a river, throwing away the clothes they had worn in their former estate, while intoning mantras of renunciation. The new monks then put on orange robes, and gathered to receive the names characteristically given to members of the Sārasvatī Order.* Swami Muktananda himself gave a final initiation to all of them. "The main purpose of this initiation is to know your own Self," he told the swamis in 1977. "Some people take sannyas when they get fed up with work, some people when they fail in school, some people when they have a quarrel with their family. And if you take sannyas for those reasons, then the result is also of that quality. . . . But if you take sannyas for the sake of knowing the Self, then the result is really great."[203]

The swamis were to play an increasingly significant role in Muktananda's third tour—doing much of the teaching, running ashrams in different cities, and eventually being sent to tour in India, Europe, and Australia on his behalf. Moreover, their existence came to have an enormous impact on the social order of Siddha Yoga, since the existence of a monastic alternative to ordinary household life caused numbers of Siddha Yoga students to consider, at least for a time, the option of dedicating themselves to a monk's life.

---

*The monks of the Sārasvatī Order take names ending with *ānanda*, "bliss."

THE ISSUE OF SUCCESSION (1977)

Swami Muktananda seems to have known since 1975 that his body would not withstand the pace of constant travel and wide-scale shaktipat for many more years. The outpouring of physical energy this entailed was taking its toll. Swami Sevananda said later:

> He knew his mission, the number of people to whom he had to give shaktipat. So he had to do it in the minimum amount of time, and the more freely he gave, the more karma he took on. Someone had to balance those karmas. It's said that shaktipat takes place when there is a balance among the karmas. In the traditional course of things, when there is time, a person would do sadhana and his mind would get purified, and then the guru would give him shaktipat. But since Baba made the time of purification so short, he himself would take the people's karmas. He would burn them up in the fire of his meditation, in the fire of his yoga. But the body had to take it on. He would say, when something would go wrong with his body, "This has nothing to do with the body. It's just a karma I took." He would lose two pounds every time he gave an Intensive.[204]

In 1977, during his birthday celebration at Shree Gurudev Ashram, Muktananda suffered a major heart attack. He said later that during the heart attack, he left his body and found himself in Siddha Loka, the subtle plane he had written about in *Play of Consciousness*, where, he always said, siddhas exist in forms made of light.[205] He said:

> When I got there, my Guru was waiting for me. I sat with my Baba for a while, and then my Baba said, "Go back, you have more work to do." When Shree Guru's car is standing in the road, not even the lord of death can pass.[206]

The near-fatality gave the issue of Swami Muktananda's succession great importance. "It was obvious to many of us that it would have been difficult for Siddha Yoga to survive as an organization if Baba had left at that point," said Swami Shantananda. "He was the only one who had the power to keep all of us together. It could have been like what happens in so many spiritual groups when the guru dies. People would have been cut adrift.[207]

"We were especially concerned," Shantananda remembered, "because we realized something might happen to Baba and he had never announced who he wanted to succeed him."

In fact, Swami Muktananda had already indicated his choice. Several of the Indian devotees, including Venkappanna Shriyan, Shyama Shrinivasta, the ashram trustees B. D. Nagpal and Murlidhar Dhoot, and others often had heard him speak of his intention. "There was really never any doubt about who was going to be Baba's successor," recalled Swami Sevananda, who at the time was Swami Muktananda's personal attendant. "Baba didn't hint at it; he said it. He said it so many times: 'Malti is the one.' I remember one time when a devotee, a very fine artist, was visiting Baba. Baba pointed to Malti and said, 'She is going to be my successor.' Later I told the man, 'That is just for you. You shouldn't go telling everyone.' But among a certain group of people, there was no doubt. Baba said it many times to each one of us. It was an open secret."[208]

Malti herself had been told many times. When Australian journalist Christopher Forsyth asked her in a 1982 interview if she had known of her guru's plans for her, she described two of these instances:

> [Baba] tried to talk to me about the administration of this ashram when I was fifteen years old.... After that, he would prod me from time to time. He would tell me little things here and there to see how much I would take in. The only thing he asked me to promise completely was that I would offer my life to this ashram, that I would give my life to him. I did make that commitment.
>
> Once when we were driving in Switzerland [in 1976], Baba asked me out of the blue, "Do you feel fully that you will offer your life to me, to the Ashram? Will you carry on my work even after I leave this world?" I did not want to look at his face. I looked out the window. I was watching the meadow and the beautiful cows. Then . . . I looked back at Baba. I said, "Yes," and nodded my head.[209]

Soon after his recovery, Muktananda began making plans to visit the West for the third time. This tour would last three years. A few months before his departure, he gave to Malti's fifteen-year-old brother, Subhash, initiation into *brahmacarya.* Then he invited Subhash to accompany the tour. Subhash began receiving extensive training in the scriptures and as a speaker. In 1980, in Los Angeles, Swami Muktananda gave Subhash *sannyāsa* initiation and the name "Swami Nityananda," after his own guru. At that time, it began to be speculated that Subhash was also being prepared as a successor to Swami Muktananda.

SWAMI MUKTANANDA'S THIRD WORLD TOUR

The Western sojourn that began in 1978 was a far cry from the tours of the early seventies. To begin with, Siddha Yoga now had an organization, ashrams, and a sizable body of seasoned practitioners. Moreover, the style of the tour was far less peripatetic. Instead of traveling from place to place, Muktananda and his company would remain for several months in a single

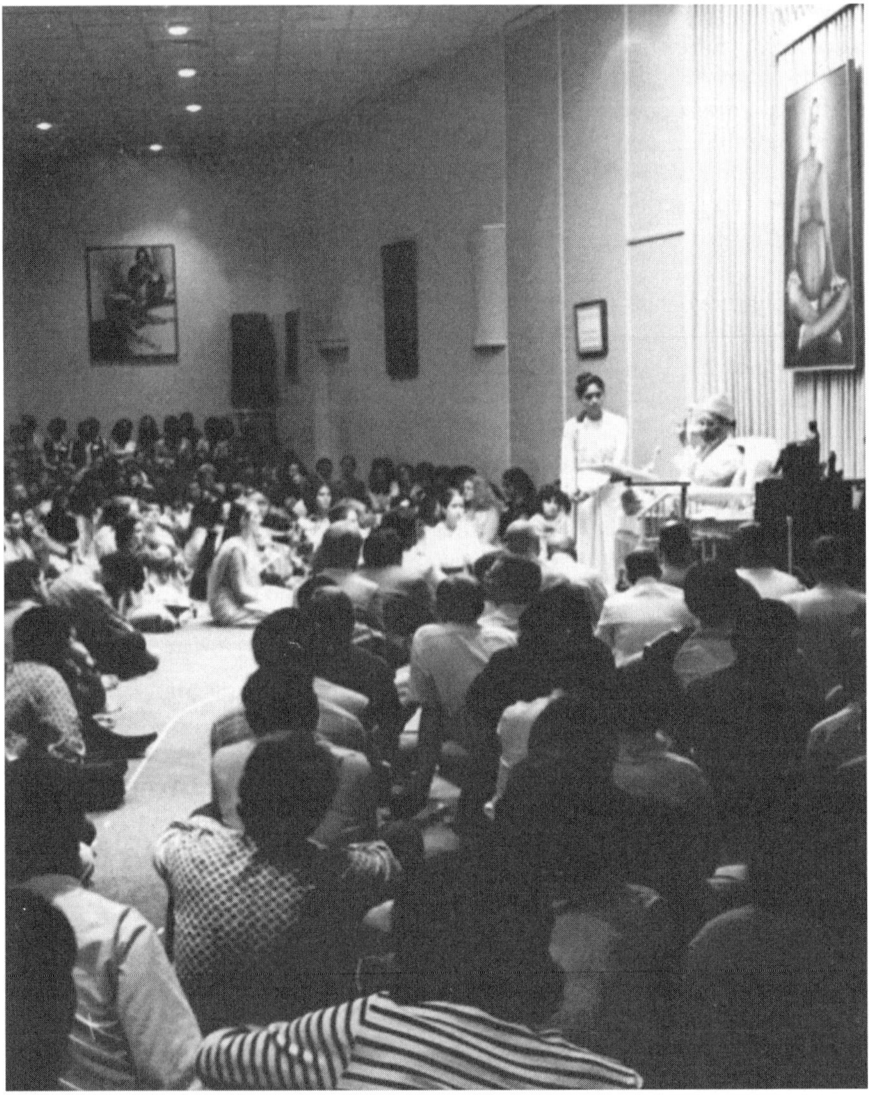

Fig. 14. Muktananda speaking on his third world tour with Malti translating

location, each time setting up an ashram where students could live the *gurukula* lifestyle. In Melbourne, in Oakland, in a newly permanent headquarters that sprang up in South Fallsburg, New York, and in such temporary headquarters as a beachfront hotel in Miami and a huge tent erected in a parking lot in Santa Monica, California, Swami Muktananda created environments where several hundred people at a time could live and practice with him. (See appendix 2 for his itinerary.)

The three years between 1978 and 1981 were arguably the peak period of Swami Muktananda's public work. He appeared on television in Australia and the United States, gave large public lectures at places like Carnegie Hall in New York and the Palace of Fine Arts in San Francisco. Conferences on meditation brought artists, actors, psychologists, doctors, lawyers, and businessmen to the ashrams in Australia, California, and New York. He founded a major program, the Siddha Yoga Prison Project, to carry Siddha Yoga meditation to prison inmates. Eight of Muktananda's books were published and translated into a number of European languages. New courses and trainings were developed. New centers and nearly twenty residential ashrams sprang up, including ashrams in Melbourne, Sydney, Paris, and Barcelona, as well as Siddha Yoga's main organizational headquarters in South Fallsburg, New York. Thousands of seekers attended Intensives and retreats. Significantly, all this took place in an atmosphere that had seldom been less hospitable to gurus and spiritual groups.

Cults, False Gurus, and the Culture of Suspicion

Muktananda's previous trips to the West had been undertaken during a period of unprecedented openness to Eastern teachings. By 1978, the climate had changed. There were several apparent reasons for this. One was the negative press generated by some of the so-called new religions that had come to public attention during the seventies. Certain groups were said to favor religious practices that isolated their devotees, exhausted them, and consumed their emotional and financial resources. When press stories appeared that alleged financial mismanagement as well as exploitation and intimidation of members and ex-members among some of these groups, the issue of "cults" became a matter of serious public attention. Concerned parents occasionally resorted to "deprogrammers," who in some cases forcibly removed young people from the religious groups to which they had given allegiance and subjected them to brainwashing techniques designed to remove the "programming" of alien religious traditions. The press strove to give exact definitions to the word *cult,* a word that cultural observers noted was often applied to any movement with roots outside of established Western religion.

Muktananda was quite aware of this trend. "These days, the Guru market is booming," he said in a talk given in 1979 and later collected in his book *Where Are You Going?* "But . . . opposition to Gurus is also on the rise. Because of the behavior of false Gurus—those who call themselves Gurus without having had a Guru of their own—some people become very upset whenever they hear the word '*Guru.*'"[210]

In November 1978, a few weeks before Muktananda's arrival in California, the public fear and opposition to religious cultism received dramatic confirmation when followers of Jim Jones's People's Temple committed mass suicide in Guyana. When Muktananda arrived at the San Francisco airport, he was met by reporters who asked him point-blank, "What do you think of Jim Jones? Is Siddha Yoga a cult?" Muktananda, who loved nothing better than a challenging question, took the opportunity to speak about the difference between true and false gurus. "The government . . . should visit every ashram," he said briskly. "They should talk to everyone there to see that these gurus are giving good teachings, that they are leading pure lives, that they are uplifting people and not drowning them. You should never have blind faith in anyone. The followers of a spiritual leader should always test him. Is he following good discipline? Is he leading a good life? Is he pure? Is he clean?"[211] He went on to talk about the responsibility of a disciple, a theme that he was to amplify both in his lectures and in his book *The Perfect Relationship*, where he made use of the criteria cited in the *Kulārṇava Tantra* and other texts to describe the differences between true and false gurus and disciples.[212]

To those who wondered how they could know if a particular guru is true, Swami Muktananda offered one piece of advice: "If by the influence of a yogi your inner consciousness evolves and you become transformed, then it means that you are spending time with the right one."[213] He used to say, "Through association with a Guru one must experience transformation within. Otherwise, what's the point of going to the Guru?"[214] Many of his public statements on this tour would address the issue, reiterating again and again that a guru should transform one's undesirable qualities, that he must awaken one to the experience of inner Self.

An Ashram in the Catskills

The major institution to emerge from Swami Muktananda's third world tour was Shree Nityananda Ashram in South Fallsburg, New York, named after Muktananda's guru.*[215] The Gilbert Hotel, which like many other Catskill resort hotels had fallen on hard times, became the nucleus of a complex that would eventually expand to include two other former hotels

*The ashram in South Fallsburg, New York, was renamed Shree Muktananda Ashram in 1983 by Swami Chidvilasananda, in honor of her guru's legacy.

in the neighborhood, as well as a lake, gardens, and woods spread over more than a hundred acres of land in the South Fallsburg area.

In the summer of 1979, Siddha Yoga students assembled from all over the world for what would become a yearly tradition: the summer retreat in South Fallsburg. These retreats became the setting for the international Siddha Yoga community to define itself, to take form. Several thousand people could experience living in an ashram, following a discipline, performing spiritual practices in a supportive environment.

From the beginning, the retreats were filled with activities—Swami Muktananda's evening programs of lectures, question-and-answer sessions, and darshan; courses in Siddha Yoga philosophy and the background scriptures of the tradition; trainings for teachers and leaders of Siddha Yoga centers; long chants; programs for children; conferences; as well as the ongoing daily practices of chanting, meditation, and ashram service. Programs were regularly translated into French, German, Dutch, Spanish, Portuguese, Hebrew, and other languages.

At the same time, Swami Muktananda continued to tour. Between 1978 and 1981, he spent approximately six months of the year in South Fallsburg, and the remaining time in places like Oakland, Los Angeles, Miami, and Boston.

Now I Know My People Can Do My Work: Malti's Developing Role

In 1980, during a six-month stay in Miami, Swami Muktananda gave the first public hint of Malti's future role. One Sunday evening, Baba pointed to her and said, "Tonight let Malti speak instead of me. She has been translating every day and I wonder what she has learned from me. So, I want to find that out." Malti stood up and said, "He wants me to speak. Yet what's the use of lighting a lamp when the sun is shining? What's the use of offering a handful of water to the ocean? However, the command of a Siddha can never be disregarded."[216] She spoke on the *Śiva Sūtras*, one of the foundational texts of Kashmir Śaivism. When it was over, Muktananda said, "Now I know that my people can do my work." For the next eighteen months, Malti spoke every Sunday evening, while Swami Muktananda looked on. These talks became a major aspect of her training in the foundational scriptures of Siddha Yoga—especially those drawn from Kashmir Śaivism. She was expected to know by heart the *sūtras* of several of the major texts of Śaivism, and often he would call on her informally for an impromptu commentary on one of them.

Barbara Hamilton recalled:

> Sometimes, when they were in the elevator on the way to the program, Baba would give her a Sanskrit *sutra* and say, "Add that sutra to your talk tonight."

> So she would have to memorize the sutra, having heard it only once, and reconceive her talk in her head in the few minutes remaining before she spoke. It wasn't easy, but it was an exhilarating process to observe; she got more and more inspired as the talks progressed.[217]

Later Swami Chidvilasananda would tell the story of how Swami Muktananda once asked her to explain to him the meaning of the *Śiva Sūtra, vitarka ātmajñānam,* which Jaideva Singh had translated as "Full conviction of one's identity with Śiva is what is meant by knowledge of Self."[218] She said, "Well, if you have the knowledge of the Self, if you have the awareness of the Self, then you have conviction." Muktananda shook his head. "That is good. But what does it *mean*?" he asked. Like a Zen master's koan training, this interrogation went on for several days. She would offer an interpretation, and he would reject it, asking her, "What does it *mean*?" As the days went on, his question plunged her into an increasingly intense process of *vitarka,* which also means "inquiry." One day, she said, as she stood before Muktananda, the process and the *sūtra* simply merged into one. Her entire body began to vibrate, and a powerful experience of oneness washed over her. Muktananda said, "*Vitarka ātmajñānam*"; but now it was no longer a question. *Vitarka* had brought an experience of her identity with divine reality.[219]

Barbara Hamilton recalled Malti's schedule during that time:

> Every day she got up at three o'clock, went for a run, meditated, served Baba his breakfast, went to the *Gurugītā* and the *Rudram* [ashram chants that were recited daily], translated for [Baba's] private meetings with students, prepared talks on the *Śiva Sūtras* for the evening programs, studied, served as translator at the evening program, had dinner, got back to her own room around 8:30, delivered messages from Baba to people, and did her own correspondence and whatever administrative chores Baba had given her. Then she would write news of the tour to people in Ganeshpuri. She didn't just do what she had to do; she did more than she had to do, especially by communicating tirelessly with people.[220]

In a poem written in 1985, Swami Chidvilasananda described some of the subtler aspects of her spiritual training with Swami Muktananda:

> When he gave me Shaktipat
> He began his conscious work on me.
> He revealed the truth in many ways.
>
> Of course, I was not always aware
> Of what was being thrown in my path—
> Sometimes it was love, sometimes it was envy,

Sometimes it was harsh words, sometimes it was sweetness,
Sometimes utter bliss,
Sometimes the feeling of eternal life,
And sometimes a sense of life's fleeting nature.[221]

The poem suggests how Swami Muktananda made use of the different situations of her life to teach Malti to maintain equanimity through the challenges that came her way. She went through many tests: the projections of other students, the demands of people who wanted to use her to get closer to Muktananda, the flattery of would-be supporters, the criticism that inevitably comes to anyone whose service touches so many people's lives, and Muktananda's own direct "work on her ego," as the Siddha Yoga phrase describes it. All this, as Muktananda often intimated, was designed to teach her patience and detachment in the face of life's fluctuations. Asked how he managed to live surrounded by so many people, Muktananda had once answered, "I do not live in the midst of people; I live in the midst of God."[222] He often said that a siddha's awareness of God's presence is so strong that he sees only the divinity in everything and everyone, and that he expected his disciples to learn how to maintain their meditative awareness no matter what they were doing. He once asked Malti, "Do you practice the stilling of the mind?" She said, "Yes, I do." He said, "Just make sure you don't lose that stillness no matter what you're doing. . . . When you're doing the outside work, make sure that you are able to apply your inner state to that work. Only then is that work important. If you do the work without the inner state, it is dust."[223]

Along with spiritual training, Swami Muktananda gradually gave Malti more and more administrative responsibilities. In 1981, she was placed on the Board of Trustees of SYDA Foundation as well as of Gurudev Siddha Peeth Ashram Trust in India, and soon afterward he made her executive vice-president of SYDA Foundation. She sat on the committee that supervised ashram programs, acted as advisor for all ashram publications, took a hand in tour management, oversaw the meditation halls and the darshans where students came to meet Muktananda, and helped them ask him their questions. That same year, at a worldwide conference for Siddha Yoga center leaders, he spoke of preparing for the great work of the future. ". . . Your Siddha Yoga will spread throughout the entire world," he told them. "Now, it seems that you are doing a lot of work, and truly, your work has been great. But in the future, the work you are doing now will seem like nothing. So now, you should start expanding your hearts so that you can prepare yourselves for the great work that is to come."[224] None of them realized that he would not be there for that future work. Few of his students were ready to admit that Swami Muktananda was preparing to leave the world.

Everything Happens Through His Grace: The Passage of Power

Swami Muktananda had often said that he intended the core of his path—the bestowal of grace, the teaching based on his own distillation of fundamental yogic doctrines, and the discipline he advocated—to remain unchanged. To guarantee that the Siddha Yoga teachings and practices would be preserved in their essential integrity, it was imperative that he choose the one who was to succeed him, and that he make that choice formal. As the seventies drew to a close, Swami Muktananda began making moves that would settle the issue of his succession. In the mid-1960s, he had formally laid out the requirements for a Siddha Yoga guru, based on statements in the scriptures. Among the criteria were the requirements that the guru be a *naiṣṭika brahmacārī*, a dispassionate lifelong celibate, and that the guru be Self-realized, learned in scriptures, and able to give shaktipat as well as to control the awakened *śakti*.

'He Has Just Entered My University'

In 1981 on Guru Pūrṇimā, the full-moon day traditionally dedicated to honoring the guru, Swami Muktananda made a surprising announcement. At the end of a long darshan, with striking nonchalance, he said, "In my talk, I forgot to say one thing: this person will be my successor." Then he put a garland over the head of eighteen-year-old Subhash Shetty, now Swami Nityananda.[225]

This dramatic moment began a succession process that would take several years to fully unfold. Here are the major events in the process.[226] Six months after naming Nityananda, Swami Muktananda officially named Malti as co-successor. In April 1982, she received initiation into *sannyāsa* and was given the name Swami Chidvilasananda. The two successors were formally anointed by Muktananda in May 1982, and assumed responsibility for the movement on Swami Muktananda's death in October of that year. Three years later, in October of 1985, Swami Nityananda resigned from the guru's seat, after having demonstrated that he did not wish to fulfill the responsibilities of the position. He released himself from his duties both as a guru and as a monk in a public ceremony prescribed and performed by a *mahāmaṇḍaleśvar.* Swami Chidvilasananda then became the sole head of the Siddha Yoga lineage and sole guru of Siddha Yoga's students. Nityananda later asserted a claim—repudiated by Siddha Yoga's students—that he still considered himself a bonafide successor to Muktananda.

Despite this controversy and the occasional glare of publicity that accompanied it, Siddha Yoga continued to thrive and grow. However, the succession process provoked intense questioning for Siddha Yoga students. Many wondered how such an apparently untidy situation could flow from the will of an enlightened master. Why, students asked, had Swami Muktananda put Nityananda on the seat if he could not hold it? Was it possible for a guru to fall?

Though by their very nature, such questions are not susceptible to definitive answers, over the years students have advanced several different theories and explanations. Many long-term students experienced the entire sequence of events as a valuable demonstration of certain spiritual principles. Muktananda had always maintained that disciples should observe a guru very carefully before accepting him. He had often reiterated the scripturally sanctioned criteria of a true guru—that he should have attained the enlightened state, that he be a disciple himself, that he live his own teachings, that he have the capacity to transform a disciple's inner state of awareness. The situation that unfolded during the succession process challenged Siddha Yoga students to observe, to test, to learn from experience how to discern the qualities of a spiritual guide.

Those familiar with the history of other spiritual lineages have also pointed out that it is not unusual for a spiritual master to name more than one successor and then allow the "true" successor to prove title to the seat.[227]* Since tradition holds that a siddha guru is far more than the formal head of a lineage, any successor in a siddha lineage must eventually demonstrate his or her entitlement (*adhikāra*) to the position by revealing the inner state of Self-realization as well as the other qualities of a true guru. "The true successor must reveal his own light," explains a traditional text. According to this view, Nityananda had been given a unique spiritual opportunity, and simply proved unable or unwilling to meet the challenges it presented.

In fact, this last viewpoint is consistent with one of Muktananda's main qualities as a teacher: his almost prodigal generosity in offering spiritual

*In fact, such a situation had occurred relatively close to home. Swami Muktananda once told Venkappanna that after the *mahāsamādhi* of Siddharudha Swami, his former mentor, two disciples had emerged as his successors. According to devotees in Siddharudha's *maṭh,* both disciples had been given commands by their guru, but one persistently ignored Siddharudha's instructions. In time, this disciple found himself unable to continue in his position, while the one who had upheld his guru's teachings became the sole head of the lineage.

gifts to those whose lives intersected his. Not the least of these gifts was the regard with which he held his students. "Baba had such a benevolent vision of us," said a close disciple. "He looked at a person and saw the greatest possibilities that person was capable of. For example, he always told us that we could achieve Self-realization in this lifetime—something that many of us would never have dared to imagine for ourselves. Being a true disciple of his meant being willing to live up to that vision. If you could accept his vision of you and follow the path that would allow you to actualize it, his grace would turn you into something much greater than you would ever envision for yourself."[228]

Many of his disciples have described their own experiences of being "empowered" by Muktananda's regard for them, of being given responsibilities or challenges that required that they transcend their own sense of limitation. If they were willing to step into the challenge, he would pour into them the tremendous force of his spiritual energy, and inner growth would occur. Some people found the intensity of Muktananda's spiritual generosity too overpowering to accept or even appreciate. Others would revel in the initial experience he offered, then find that they did not wish to live the disciplined life required to maintain it. And there were those who accepted his generosity according to their capacity and allowed it, to a greater or lesser degree, to shape their lives. For his students, the ability to hold Swami Muktananda's gifts depended in no small measure on their willingness to affirm and grow into his vision of them as potential siddhas—beings able to live in the joy that lies beyond the experience of the senses. Many felt that the events following the succession indicated that Nityananda had not fully embraced his guru's vision for him.

Like Malti, who was eight years his senior, Nityananda had essentially been brought up in the ashram, even though his schooling and family life took place in Bombay. He was a good-natured, easygoing young man who loved to chant and enjoyed playing the *mṛdaṅg*, a long double-headed drum. He was also, by the testimony of those who knew him over the years, disarming and lovable, though some felt that he lacked Malti's mystical bent, and noted that he often joked about not having spiritual experiences.[229] Many Siddha Yoga practitioners felt great affection for him. Moreover, the fact that Nityananda had been given the *sannyāsa* name of Muktananda's own guru was not lost on the devotees.

Nonetheless, from the beginning, observers noted that questions surrounded his succession. The night after announcing it, Muktananda began his evening lecture by saying: "[Yesterday] at the end of my talk I said something. I said, 'This fellow will be my successor,' and everyone started to cry. . . . So I want to let you know that this doesn't mean I am going to leave this world!" At that, everyone rose and began to applaud. Waving them to their seats, Muktananda said, "I've chosen him, true. What this means is that he has been admitted to my university. It's up to him whether he's going to pass or fail." Then he told the assembled devotees, "You have to have some discrimination, too."[230] To thoughtful listeners, Muktananda's statement sounded like a hint that the process might not be as simple as it appeared. "Looking back at that moment," said a Siddha Yoga swami who was present, "I realize that Baba was telling us, 'There's something for you to learn here. Watch carefully.'"[231]

In February 1982, Muktananda formally announced that Malti and Nityananda would share the guru's seat. At the same time, he began to invite students and dignitaries to be present at the ceremony planned for May 8, when he would formally anoint the two of them in a consecration ceremony called a *paṭṭābhiṣeka,* a ritual conducted by brahmin priests in much the same fashion as the traditional anointment of an Indian *rāja,* a king. The formality of Swami Muktananda's gesture indicated how far Siddha Yoga had become established as a movement since Bhagawan Nityananda's time.

'My Guru Turned Base Metal into Gold': Transmitting the Lineage

In late April 1982, one week before the ceremony that would install her as Swami Muktananda's successor, Malti passed through a three-day ceremony of *brahmacarya dīkṣā,* the initiation that traditionally precedes *sannyāsa dīkṣā.*

Swami Muktananda had previously given initiation into *sannyāsa* to many others. For everyone else, including Swami Nityananda, the complete rituals were performed over a twenty-four-hour period. However, Muktananda had said for years that he would give Malti a very special initiation into *sannyāsa,* and this ceremony, much of which he attended himself, signaled her unique position in his regard. During her *brahmacarya* initiation, she was given white robes to wear and her hair was shorn (another departure, as other women swamis in Siddha Yoga did not shave their heads). Swami Muktananda himself took part in the cutting of her hair.

"During this *brahmacarya* ceremony, we used to hear her chanting until very late into the night," recalled Helen Argent, whose room was next door to Malti's. "One day she told me that she had woken up in the middle of the night because she was seeing so much light in the room that she thought it was morning. That light didn't go away. It was clear that something was happening that went beyond any formal rituals."[232]

In a poem written on the third anniversary of the *paṭṭābhiṣeka,* Gurumayi Chidvilasananda herself described her experience during this time:

. . . At last the day arrived: April 26, 1982.
My Guru sheared off my hair;
He clothed me in a white sari,
And shot the dragon's fire at me.
Maha Shaktipat took place.

For days on end I walked in that light,
Slept in that light,
Ate in that light.
Everything within and without
Was bathed in white light.
No more questions, no more doubts,
No more of those things which had gnawed at me.
I was gone.
I don't know how I left;
I only know that grace took me away
And began to install *purno'ham*[233]

The final day arrived: May 8, 1982.
Not much remained to be killed.
There was only the physical body that had to be covered.
Not in a white sari, but in orange cloth—
The color of the fire which had been shot at me.

That morning I went to my Guru's room,
And did a full *pranam.*
I looked at him; he looked at me.
How many times can one melt
When one has already melted completely?
So much love, so much Shakti!
Did my poor body have enough strength
To contain this?[234]

The language in this poem bears close reading. When Swami Chidvilasananda speaks of "the dragon's fire," she refers to the fire of yoga, the awakened *kuṇḍalinī* energy, often experienced as an intense heat or as a flame or molten light that passes from the guru to the disciple in spiritual initiation. She calls it "Maha Shaktipat," indicating that this "great" initiation surpassed her previous initiatory experiences. One effect of the process was the dissolution, or melting, of her sense of separate identity—as she puts it, "I [meaning her limited ego] was gone." Instead of this small "I," the "I" that identifies itself with body, mind, and personality, she was experiencing the pure I, or *pūrṇo'ham*—the Self as pure divine consciousness, the witness-Self.

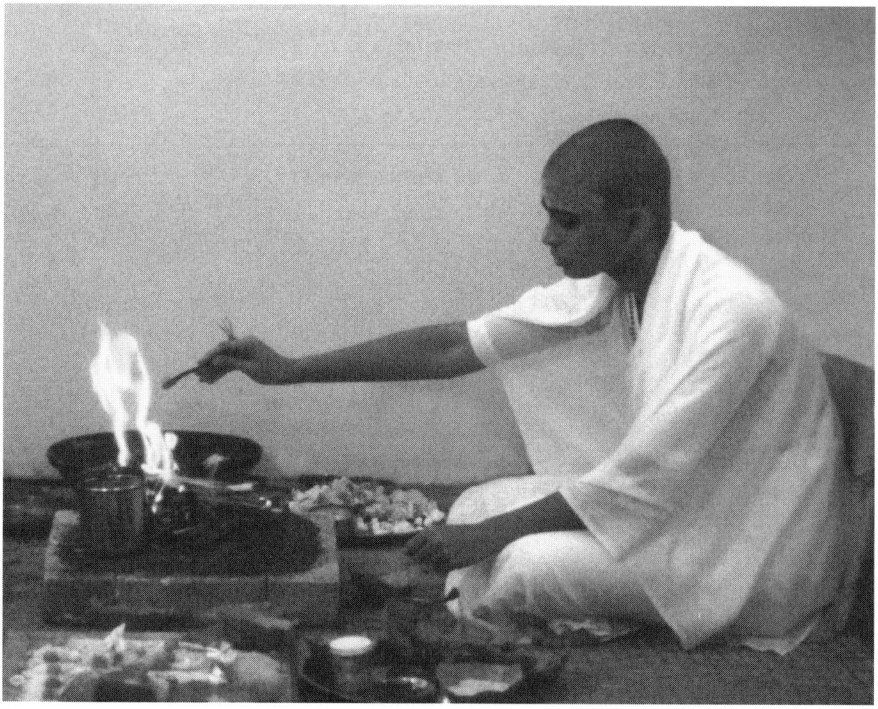

Fig. 15. Malti taking *brahmacarya dīkṣā* in preparation for *sannyāsa dīkṣā*, April 1982

The imagery in the poem, similar to the language found in the poetry of Indian saints like Kabīr, Allamaprabhu, and Akkamahādevī, as well as in the Zen tradition, conveys the shattering nature of the moment of final enlightenment—when the walls of the personality "melt," when the sense of individuality is "killed," when the small self is "shattered" and paradoxically the deeper Self, the true Self, is experienced in its wholeness. The last section of the poem describes the *paṭṭābhiṣeka* itself, which took place at the end of a five-day *yajña* (fire ceremony) conducted by a group of brahmin priests, in front of the five thousand students and well-wishers whom Swami Muktananda had invited to witness the occasion. It suggests the depth of experience from which Swami Chidvilasananda would draw to respond to the challenges she faced. She recalls:

> I took my seat in the Yajna Mandap [ritual enclosure] near the blazing fire.
> My Guru was seated on his throne,
> But in that place deep within me,
> Near the fire, he exploded
> And became everything in the universe for me.
>
> It thundered; it poured.
> The lightning bolts smiled.
> Was I shattered to pieces?
> Or was I in the process of becoming whole?
>
> Initiation occurs once in a lifetime,
> Although experiences are many and come at different times.
>
> This was when *purno'ham* was installed
> In place of Swami Chidvilasananda.
> The perfect I-consciousness, *purno'ham vimarsha,*
> Is the gift of the Siddhas.
> My Guru, out of his compassion,
> Turned base metal into gold.
> Whatever remains is his work of art.
> Everything happens through his grace.[235]

This passage describes an unusual congruence of inner and outer experience. While she sat before the *yajña* fire, Chidvilasananda had an interior vision of Swami Muktananda's form exploding, expanding to fill the universe. Simultaneously, in the outer world, the cloudless blue sky suddenly darkened with rain clouds, and an unseasonable thunderstorm broke over the ashram. Since rain is almost unheard of in western India in May, the dramatic effect of this sudden downpour was intense. In the Indian tradition, rain is considered to be a sign that a fire ritual has been successful. So it is understandable that when Swami Muktananda heard the rolling thunder and saw the sheets of rain, he raised his arms to the sky and cried out the Hindi words with which all auspicious events in Siddha Yoga are begun and ended: "*Sadgurunāth mahārāj kī jay!*" adding, "The clouds have come to welcome them!"[236]

The *paṭṭābhiṣeka* ceremony continued as Swami Muktananda poured consecrated water over the heads of his two successors. Finally he formally announced that he was passing the power of the lineage and retiring from his position. In a telling gesture, he had dressed his successors in brilliant orange silk, but put off the bright orange silk clothing that he normally wore, choosing instead to dress in crumpled, faded saffron cotton. By donning the traditional clothes of a mendicant *sannyāsī,* he was symbolically signaling his own retirement, the handing over of his spiritual kingdom.

However, the ceremony was by no means purely symbolic. As Swami Chidvilasananda's poem indicates, Muktananda in that moment had given her the experience of Self-realization—surely one of the few times in history that such a transmission has taken place before thousands of witnesses.

THE PASSING OF SWAMI MUKTANANDA

In late September 1982, Muktananda took his two successors and a small party of other students to Kashmir to visit some of the sacred places there. The week after his return, on October 2, 1982, Swami Muktananda died or—in the language of the scriptures—took *mahāsamādhi,* the yogi's final merging into the absolute.

Until the end, he went on giving shaktipat to students. All summer, he had spent several hours each evening giving shaktipat by touch to anyone who happened to be in the ashram's main meditation room. Night after night, the ashramites would crowd into the room, while he walked among them touching them on the head or between the eyebrows. He had paid special attention to the teenagers, reserving seats for the boys and girls around the door to his house each evening so they would be sure to receive his touch.

For a week before his passing, Muktananda walked around the ashram barefoot. On the evening of October 2, he went for a walk as usual, and made a point of speaking to almost everyone he saw. Then he came out to

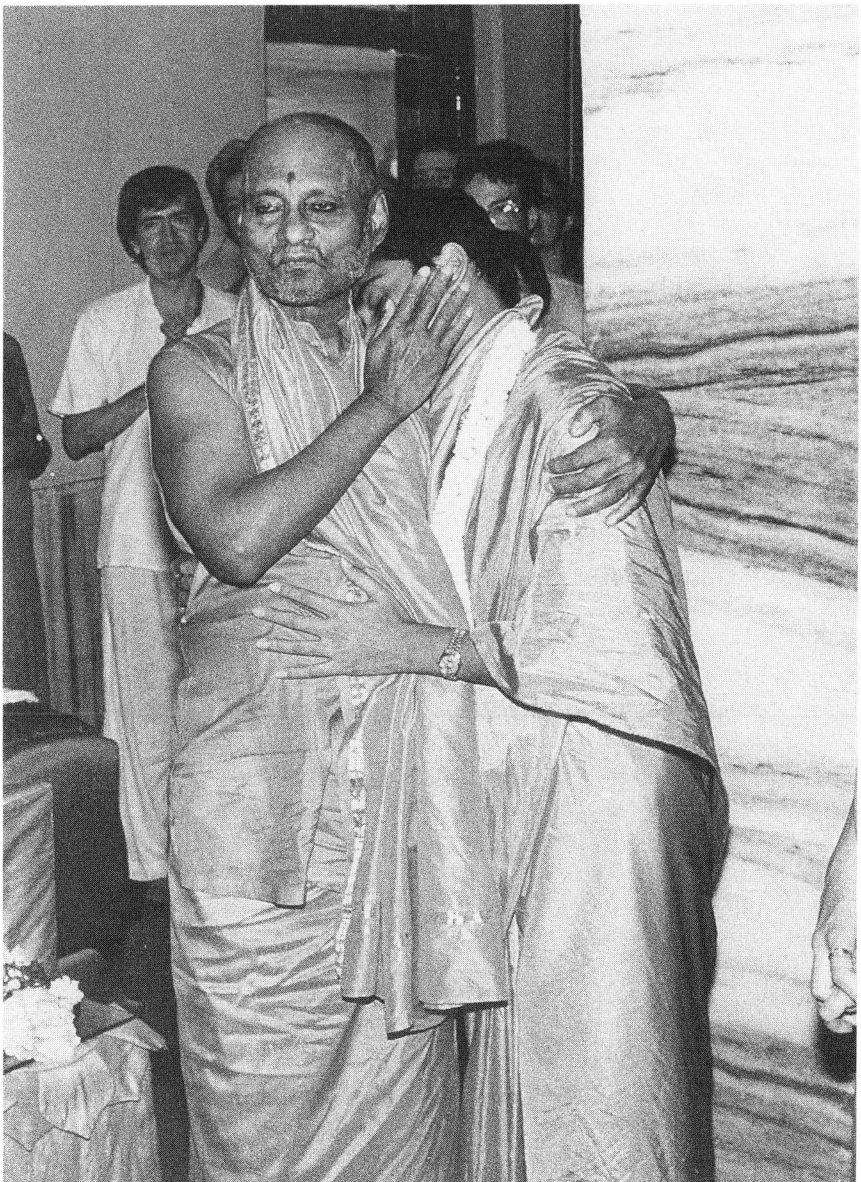

Fig. 16. Swami Muktananda bidding farewell to Swami Chidvilasananda, as she leaves Gurudev Siddha Peeth for her first meditation retreat as the guru, July 1982

sit on his seat in the courtyard, where the ashramites were watching a video.*

At around 9:00 P.M., he called for a woman from France, who had arrived in the ashram that morning with the express wish to receive shaktipat. She was brought to the meditation room. Muktananda touched her between the eyebrows, put her into meditation, then went upstairs to Swami Chidvilasananda's room. Looking at a series of photographs of Zipruanna, Hari Giri Baba, Shirdi Sai Baba, and other siddhas that Chidvilasananda had just placed around her altar, he said, "I'm glad that all the siddhas will be protecting you." Then he added, "I would never want to leave you."

Swami Chidvilasananda later said that at that point, he began reminiscing about his life, speaking of places he had been and people he had met. She noticed that he was speaking in the past tense. "Always repeat your mantra," he said as he left her. "Always have faith in me."[237] After that, Muktananda went to his room. According to his attendant, Swami Sevananda, as he was preparing for bed, "he mentioned that he was having some slight heart pains, but that it wasn't serious."[238]

At eleven o'clock, Sevananda heard the call bell over his bed ringing. This was very unusual. He rushed back into Baba's house. "I saw him lying on the bed looking very calm and beautiful. I called his name and then realized that he was gone. Baba had always told me, 'No one will be with me when I go.'"

Swami Chidvilasananda and Swami Nityananda were called. Despite their grief, they immediately began to direct the arrangements. Swami Muktananda's body was placed in an upright position on his meditation seat. Toward morning, as chanting rang through the ashram, the ashramites were called for a final darshan. While the stunned devotees filed through Swami Muktananda's room to pay their last respects, they heard the sound of hammers. The burial place was being made ready.

During the days that followed, tens of thousands of students, admirers, friends, and religious pilgrims poured into the ashram for the funeral ceremonies. Chanting went on in the ashram courtyard—the chant would continue for thirty days and nights—while the ashramites threw themselves into feeding, housing, and taking care of the visitors. The ashram schedule continued as always.

The shock and grief of the devotees was palpable—photographs of those days show the stunned, saddened faces of those who had loved Swami Muktananda. At the same time, many Siddha Yoga students spoke of experiences that convinced them that though the siddha guru Muktananda was physically gone, he would continue to guide them inwardly. A Siddha Yoga

*By coincidence, the video shown in Gurudev Siddha Peeth on the night of Swami Muktananda's passing happened to include a talk he had given on his own guru's passing.

monk, Swami Indirananda, described how she felt when she first heard that Muktananda had died:

> Incredible grief came up in my heart. Even in that moment I remember feeling how fortunate I was to have been loved so much and to have loved so deeply—and yet the pain was so profound. I remember wondering what life would be like, never smiling again. . . . And yet the next morning I found myself taking a walk through the beautiful gardens . . . and as I looked around, I was struck by this incredible golden light that was emanating from everything and everyone around me. In that moment, I heard Baba's voice very clearly inside of me, and he said, "Where do you think I've gone? Didn't I always tell you I'd always be with you? Didn't I always tell you I live inside of everyone and everything? Now you are having the experience."[239]

Again and again, in the reports of this time, we hear similar accounts of unexpected teachings or inner experiences. "What amazed me about this time was that I actually felt ecstatic," recalled David Kempton. "On the surface there was grief, but at the same time the love that kept welling up was so much stronger than the grief."[240] "All through the first weeks after Baba's death," said an Italian ashramite, "I would look at people's faces and see light pouring from them. I would look at the trees and see light pouring from them. I kept remembering something I'd read—that when a spiritual Master dies, his energy enters the hearts of his disciples. That was how I felt—as if he'd given me a gift of vision."[241]

Swami Muktananda's funeral rites began with the traditional *abhiṣeka*, the ritual bathing of his body. His body was then placed on an open vehicle and taken in procession to the village of Ganeshpuri. Several thousand people walked beside the vehicle, chanting *Oṃ Namo Bhagavate Nityānandāya.* Before the open doors of Bhagawan Nityananda's shrine, Muktananda's body faced his guru's *samādhi* shrine for the last time, while his successors placed their offerings around the statue. Then the procession wound its way homeward. At last, while the brahmins chanted, Muktananda's physical form was placed in the earth in a seated meditation posture, and covered with camphor, salt, and sandalwood. The site would become a shrine and a place of pilgrimage. During their visits, thousands have attested to the spiritual power that emanates from the shrine.*

---

*Hindu as well as Islamic tradition holds that after death the body of a saint should not be burned like that of an ordinary person but placed in the ground. At the burial site is built a *samādhi* shrine. It is said that the spiritual power of the saint also clings to the shrine, and pilgrims who visit these shrines often attest to experiencing blessings. One of the most famous shrines in western India is that of Sai Baba of Shirdi, who told his devotees before his passing, "The stones of my *samādhi* will speak to you." Thousands of pilgrims have left accounts of visions or blessings obtained by visiting the shrine at Shirdi or praying there; similar experiences are reported by visitors to Swami Muktananda's shrine.

THE PERIOD OF TRANSITION

The Accession of the Successors

Sixteen days after Swami Muktananda's passing, brahmin priests presided over a formal ceremony installing Swami Chidvilasananda and Swami Nityananda on the Siddha Yoga *gaddi*, the "seat" of the lineage. Already, they had stepped into their designated roles. As they organized the rituals, made decisions, dealt with the questions and condolences that were pouring in from over the world, the two gurus also made a point of meeting the students. Within days, darshan had again become a regular feature of ashram life.

One striking feature of this period was that despite the profound change that had occurred, the ashram routine never ceased. The order established by Muktananda would continue in the Siddha Yoga community through the months that followed, as students grieved for him, contemplated and tested their relationships to Muktananda's successors, and watched as the new gurus began a new era in Siddha Yoga.

It was a critical time, a time of soul-searching. As students who had placed Muktananda at the center of their spiritual life considered what it would mean to transfer their spiritual allegiance to the new gurus, many found themselves reevaluating their relationship with the guru and with Siddha Yoga. This was not always a simple process, since the inner bond with Swami Muktananda ran very deep. Indeed, for many of his students, Muktananda's death had the impact of the death of a beloved parent.

At the same time, Siddha Yoga as a path rests on the relationship with a living master, so many devotees wanted to continue under the guidance of the new gurus. Their ability to do so would rest entirely on their inner experience, on their capacity to establish a spiritual connection with Swami Muktananda's successors. "A Guru may create a successor," said Swami Shantananda, "but the disciples can't just adopt that successor as their own Guru unless they discover the light of the Guru in that person for themselves. Their allegiance has to be based on genuine experience over time, not just on an idea or a sense of surface loyalty. Otherwise they just give away their power and there's no spiritual growth."[242]

Muktananda had always taught that the guru is not just a physical body but an inner principle. When people tried to attach themselves to him as an individual, he would remind them forcibly that when we honor a spiritual master, we are honoring not the individual but the power of grace that pours through him. Yet few of his students had ever experienced the guru in any other form beside Swami Muktananda's. His passing forced many to confront this basic Siddha Yoga teaching for the first time.

"For me, that was the most remarkable thing about the whole process," said John Greig, an English investment banker who had first met Muktananda in 1971. "I had always experienced the grace and *śakti* of Siddha Yoga as being connected to Baba's person. I was in India when Baba took *mahāsamādhi*, and at first my support of his successors was based on my faith in Baba and in everything he had ever said about the living Master. It was clear to me that the *śakti* could be passed on. Later I began to recognize that the love and spiritual energy I identified as 'Baba' was indeed flowing through Gurumayi [as Chidvilasananda was soon to be known] and her brother. From this I truly understood that the Guru is *not* just an individual, that the Guru is the *śakti*."[243]

There were, the students said, definite signs. For some, it was simply that when they came into the presence of the new gurus, a feeling of love would arise, or they would feel a heightened energy or a sense of peace. Others had experiences in dreams or in meditation that gave them faith or a sense of connection to the successors. Several said that they had the feeling they were receiving shaktipat all over again.

Not everyone was able to make the connection to the new gurus. As often happens when a powerful spiritual leader dies, a number of full-time students, including some who had toured with Muktananda for years, left the movement. Among these were several senior swamis, men and women who had been the leading teachers in Muktananda's time. Though these swamis left for varied reasons, most wanted to return to worldly life or nurtured desires and ambitions that could not be satisfied in their present situation. A few became independent teachers, while others transferred their acquired teaching skills to the field of stress management or psychology. By the end of 1985, more than half the original corps of *sannyāsīs* had relinquished their vows; many of these had also left the movement.[244] Of those who stayed, some did so, at least initially, out of loyalty to Muktananda's memory and to their vows. Others, however, remained because they were experiencing the guru principle in the new gurus.

These varied reactions mirrored patterns seen in other spiritual organizations after the death of a charismatic leader.[245] They all contributed to the sense of prolonged transition that characterized Siddha Yoga in the years between 1982 and 1985.

TO KEEP SPREADING THAT INNER LOVE: THE EMERGENCE OF GURUMAYI CHIDVILASANANDA

By late 1983, the spiritual focus of most Siddha Yoga students had shifted. The locus of *śakti*, of guidance, and of connection to grace was in the new gurus. After 1983, Swami Chidvilasananda and Swami Nityananda frequently toured in India, Australia, Europe, and the United States, giving shaktipat and guiding students and the direction of the movement. Their tours brought a new generation of students. Moreover, for the "old" students who remained within the movement, their relationship with a new living master had become the center of their sadhana.

Many longtime students spoke of a sense of personal empowerment they felt as they witnessed Swami Chidvilasananda, whom they had known as a fellow disciple, demonstrating qualities they had seen in Muktananda. Said Janet Dobrovolny, a lawyer who lived in the Oakland Siddha Yoga community, "In Baba's time, I always felt that his state was completely beyond my reach. But when I saw it manifesting in Gurumayi, I began to think that I could attain it too, if I was willing to go for it the way she did."[246]

In Swami Nityananda, devotees saw an engaging deadpan humor and a boyish simplicity and sweetness. Those who were close to him found him natural, unassuming, and highly spontaneous; accompanying him on a two-week trip to holy places around Maharashtra in 1983, devotees enjoyed the informality of his company and the silent darshans that were his hallmark. In 1984, people began to call Swami Nityananda by the traditional title "Gurudev" and to address Swami Chidvilasananda as "Gurumayi."[247] By this time, Gurumayi's unique qualities as a teacher had begun to reveal themselves; not the least of these was a highly personalized concern for the lives of devotees. "I noticed that she really seemed to understand how much we had to struggle to do our spiritual practices in the midst of all the pressures of our worldly activities," recalled a devotee from Vicenza, Italy. "I remember being very touched once when she said, 'People go through so much in their worldly life, and that in itself is a great yogic austerity if you do it with the right understanding.'"[248] Other students were struck by her willingness to enter into their issues and concerns. When she toured, or during programs at the ashrams, she would often sit for six hours, without a break, giving darshan—during which she would answer questions, give blessings, and interact in some fashion with several thousand people, one after another.

Much of her teaching took place in these face-to-face encounters. Students like to share the story of the young man who came up to her during a darshan in New Mexico and asked, "Can you take away my suffering?"

Gurumayi replied, "I don't take away suffering. I show you the cause, and I help you remove it yourself." She held up a rose that someone had given her. "Look at this," she said. "Even though the thorns are there, the rose is beautiful. Even though suffering is there, life has its own beauty. You don't suffer because there's suffering in the world. You suffer because you embrace that which causes suffering." The young man reached out his hand to touch one of the thorns, and Gurumayi moved his hand away. "It's sharp," she said. "It will hurt you." Then she laughed. "You see," she said, "the suffering didn't go to you. You went to the suffering."[249]

"I always felt that she was trying to give as many people as possible the experience of what the Guru-disciple relationship is about," said a woman who traveled with Gurumayi for many years. "It's about change, transformation, getting out of your old stuck ways."[250]

Disciples who traveled with Gurumayi and lived in the ashrams have spoken of moments when she engaged directly with their weaknesses or negative tendencies. Said Robert Kemter, an Australian lawyer who spent several years in Gurudev Siddha Peeth, "You felt that she was willing to see you through the process of inner change, even if it took years."[251]

Kemter described an exchange he had with Gurumayi in the ashram in 1986 that he claimed initiated a lasting change in his interactions with others. The incident, a classic illustration of the transformative power of an encounter between guru and disciple, arose in connection with his seva, his ashram service.

> In business negotiations, I had a very fixed idea of the result I wanted and a limited repertoire of ways to bring that about. So my dealings with people rarely evolved as I thought they should, and I would get frustrated about this and angry. One day I had an unpleasant exchange with someone. It got back to Gurumayi, who spoke to some people about this tendency of mine. I had heard all of this by the time I next saw her. She was walking through the ashram office, and when she saw me, she called me over and asked, "Did you hear what I said about you?" I said, "Yes, Gurumayi."
>
> In that moment, I felt a little anguished and disheartened. I knew that this was a real issue in my business dealings, and I felt powerless to do anything about it. Then Gurumayi took a step closer, so that she was standing directly in front of me, and she looked at me with such total love—it absolutely melted me. She put her hand on my heart, and she said, "You have to listen in *here*."
>
> Something monumental happened in that moment; some permanent change took place. I was filled with love, and the next day I was operating in a different way. I found that when I listen to my heart, things would begin to unfold differently than I expected, and I could move with them—and then the right result would come but in a way I hadn't predicted.

Kemter added that this experience of the power of the guru was just one incident in a process that went on for years, shifting his inner sense of himself as well as his outer behavior. He said, "It isn't only that Gurumayi demonstrated that she cared for *us*. She consistently went out of her way to teach us to be more loving and respectful toward other people."

The message in her words to Kemter was Gurumayi's most often-reiterated teaching, one she began making early in her tenure as the guru and has repeated again and again, over the years—that love is the core experience of spirituality. "We are not out to conquer the world or to convert people," she said in a program in Hawaii in 1984. "There is one thing we want to do—to keep spreading that love as much as possible. . . . Let us spread that one thing that is so sweet, so tender, and so tangible—love. Not a love filled with emotion, crisis, and human temptations, but a love that is pure and can take us where we really want to go, a love that can touch the heart, where God dwells."[252]

Her work with Kemter and others was intended, she said during this period, to help her students peel away the subtle barriers that stood in the way of their steady experience of that love, the encrustations of what the yogic scriptures describe as *ahaṃkāra*, the ego, the false, limited self. As many have noted, the love she described was not to be confused with personal attachment. In this period, she sometimes described her own experience of spiritual love as a fire that had burned away her own limitations. It had left her, as devotees would note over the next few years, in a state of inner equipoise that seemed unshakable. It had also given her a deep bond with her disciples. Students noticed that around her they felt known in a deep way, as if there were a powerful inner link between them—again, as there had been with Muktananda.

A student named Mary Adams shared an experience of how this bond could manifest:

> I hadn't seen Gurumayi for days, and I was missing her intensely. One night I couldn't sleep, so I came downstairs and sat in the small courtyard just outside Baba's *samādhi* shrine. I was thinking of her, missing her, wishing I could see her. All of a sudden, the window opened, and Gurumayi looked out. She said, "Oh, you're still awake! You should get rest." Then she gave me a sweet smile, and she said, "How can I sleep when you're calling me like that?"[253]

During this time, Swami Chidvilasananda described her own experience of the subtle communication between her students and herself:

> It doesn't matter how far away you are. You come in my dream, or you come in my thoughts, or all of a sudden, I hear you calling my name."[254]

By the end of 1983, both of the gurus had their own staff. In general, they toured separately, coming together in South Fallsburg or Ganeshpuri for major celebrations, such as Swami Muktananda's *mahāsamādhi* anniversary. Students were aware that the public styles of the two gurus were quite different—hers engaged, his more impersonal; hers stressing discipline, his more easygoing.

By early 1985, in fact, some of the longtime practitioners were beginning to view Nityananda's nonchalance less as an issue of teaching style than as a symptom of what they saw as his discomfort in his role as guru.

Nityananda Leaves the Guru's Seat

As early as 1983, Nityananda had demonstrated what some people considered a rather laissez-faire stance toward both the Siddha Yoga organization and his position as a guru. Students noticed that he would periodically speak both in public and in private about how he disliked being a guru. "You would hear him say, 'I watch people walking down the street, and I envy them because they're free,'" remembered Swami Ishwarananda, who traveled with him in Europe in 1983.[255] To Rebecca Pratt, his cook, Nityananda confided one day in 1985 that he hoped in the next few years to take a few people and live alone somewhere, away from the demands of the organization and its thousands of students.[256] Once in a public talk, after commenting on a spiritual teacher who had been removed by his own students, he said, "I am still waiting to find that perfect being who will one day dethrone me. And I will be so happy."[257]

In October 1985, during the celebrations of Swami Muktananda's third *mahāsamādhi* anniversary, a group of devotees privately questioned Nityananda about his lack of commitment to his role as guru, including the fact that he was not upholding his monastic vows.[258] Nityananda took a few days to reflect on his situation. Then he chose to resign from the seat of the guru as well as from his position as a *sannyāsī*. It was decided at that time not to make public the breaching of his vows, in order to allow him to leave the seat with dignity, to protect the privacy of the others involved, and to spare the feelings of the devotees.

Nityananda announced his retirement in a speech given at the end of an Intensive.[259] Afterward, Gurumayi reassured the devotees by declaring her own commitment to continue fulfilling her role as their spiritual guide. She said:

> I offered my life to my Guru, and he said, "Serve." So I want you to know that I belong to you all."[260]

Nityananda went through a formal ceremony, performed by the brahmin priest Bhau Shastri and the *mahāmaṇḍaleśvar* Swami Brahmananda Giri, to remove his *sannyāsa* vows. Since he had said that he preferred not to take back his original name, Subhash, he was given the name Venkateshwar Rao.

On November 10, before five thousand Siddha Yoga students assembled from all over India and abroad, brahmin priests and the *mahāmaṇḍaleśvar* conducted a ceremony anointing Gurumayi as sole head of the lineage. Nityananda participated in the ceremony, and then made a formal retirement speech, for the most part repeating what he had said in his earlier announcement.[261]

However matters did not end there. Several months later, in February 1986, a national magazine called *The Illustrated Weekly of India* printed an article based on statements by some of Venkateshwar's supporters that cast doubt on the reasons for his retirement. Soon after, Venkateshwar announced that he had changed his mind about retiring. He flew to Bombay, put on the orange robes of a monk, resumed his former *sannyāsa* name of "Swami Nityananda," and gave an interview to *The Illustrated Weekly* in which he asserted that his retirement had not been voluntary and that he still considered himself a successor to Swami Muktananda. The resultant publicity created great confusion among the devotees, and led the trustees of Gurudev Siddha Peeth and SYDA Foundation to issue a statement explaining the reasons behind Nityananda's retirement.

Gene R. Thursby, a historian of religion at the University of Florida, later described these events in *When Prophets Die: The Post-Charismatic Fate of Religious Movements*:

> The *Weekly* eventually printed a retraction and an apology, but in the meantime, the two reports and the questions they raised about behavior within the movement and about the circumstances surrounding the succession to Siddha Yoga leadership, damaged the reputations of the blameworthy and the blameless alike.
>
> Even though eventually withdrawn as groundless, for a time the stories reported in the *Weekly* had the effect of creating confusion among those who read them. . . . Because Venkateshwar reportedly claimed that he was a victim of intimidation, [the ashram] had to make public that he had resigned due to the shame of having broken his monastic vows, thereby having made himself unfit to guide others. It also made him unfit to continue to serve as head of the Shree Gurudev Siddha Peeth, the home institution of the Siddha Yoga movement and a public trust in India, because lifelong celibacy was a requirement of the office.
>
> In order to protect the legitimate authority of the guru's seat and office, there was a responsibility to address these charges. But what made it crucial to address and refute them was the charismatic function of the person of the guru. Swami Muktananda had defined the focus and the heart of the movement as "the yoga of the guru's grace." Therefore, the very foundation of Siddha Yoga is trust in the legitimacy, the power, and the special spiritual qualities of the guru. It is also the responsibility of the guru to test the devotee, as Muktananda had stated in his characteristically strong manner. . . . This phase in the succession from Swami Muktananda was a time of testing for Siddha Yoga and all of its devotees.[262]

Nityananda subsequently set up his own organization, unaffiliated with the Siddha Yoga movement. After 1986, he often traveled in the United States, India, Europe, and Australia, holding programs and conducting

Intensives in which he claimed *kuṇḍalinī* was awakened. He continued to assert his claim to be Muktananda's successor, and from time to time his viewpoint has found its way into the press. In 1986, after a group of Nityananda's devotees threatened to install him on the seat of the New Delhi Siddha Yoga ashram, an Indian High Court judge formally declared:

> After having gone through the rituals and ceremonies [of renouncing his position] and repeatedly reiterating that he was no longer interested in "Sanyas," and [having] abdicated his position voluntarily, it is not open to him to take a different stand at this stage.[263]

Aftermath

For several months, Siddha Yoga students devoted themselves to coming to terms with the retirement. Swamis and other teachers traveled in Europe, the United States, and Australia to meet with fellow students, inform them of the events, and answer their questions. While acknowledging the controversy and providing avenues for students to find answers to their questions, Siddha Yoga's teachers continued to emphasize the spiritual core of the movement—its teachings and practices—as the means for students to process their experiences of the transition. Students were encouraged to contemplate their inner experience in Siddha Yoga and their understanding of the guru's role in their lives, and to use the occasion to discover the spiritual lessons that can arise during times of intense change and crisis.

Many devotees have subsequently reported that for them, the contemplation of these events did indeed provide a fount of spiritual learning. "Baba always taught us that a yogi learns how to turn every situation into a spiritual opportunity," said one student, "and what I see is that for many of us, it was a time of coming to maturity, of taking responsibility for our own experience of Siddha Yoga. We learned how much we did care that this very precious heritage that Baba had given us got handed down the way he had taught it."[264]

"To me the events had some of the power of the [Indian epic] *Mahābhārata,* which is filled with lessons about destiny and the consequences of actions," said Swami Ishwarananda. "I learned a great deal in those years about the importance of following the dharma, the higher law. Even though the guru may give you a position and even a spiritual state, if you don't respect it and maintain the discipline that's required to hold it, it will slip away. That's true whether you are a teacher, a swami, or simply a devotee. I've never stopped contemplating this."[265]

Present-day Siddha Yoga has not only survived the upheavals of those years, it has in some ways been forged from their crucible. For many Siddha Yoga students who went through the transition period, the integrity of the movement may ultimately have been proved by Gurumayi's steadiness in upholding and expanding Muktananda's mission despite the tests and challenges of the time. "Baba had always said that a true Guru is not the plaything of his desires or emotions. As I observed Gurumayi guiding the movement through those fiery years of transition—despite the criticism of a number of Siddha Yoga students, the attacks of the press—I saw that she was constantly exhibiting that state that he had spoken of," said Swami Shantananda. "I saw she had this state of calm, clarity, and certainty. No matter what happened, her concern was to look for ways to uplift people. This was the point at which I became convinced that Baba had truly passed onto her the state of enlightenment."[266]

Let Every Action Be an Offering: The Mission of Gurumayi Chidvilasananda

In the years since 1985, Gurumayi Chidvilasananda has expanded her guru's work to such an extent that the present-day Siddha Yoga community includes many to whom the events of the movement's history are simply legends. For others, this period receded in importance as their own spiritual life proceeded, and as they participated in the practices, traditions, and rituals of Siddha Yoga life—which despite the expansion of the community, remained largely unchanged.

LIFE AS A *YAJÑA*

A love of celebration has characterized Siddha Yoga from the beginning, and one of the great celebratory moments in the life of the Siddha Yoga community is the finale of a *yajña,* a fire ritual. Gurumayi holds *yajña*s at least twice a year, either in Gurudev Siddha Peeth or Shree Muktananda Ashram, and the announcement of a *yajña* invariably attracts Siddha Yoga students from near and far. Months go into the preparation. When the *yajña* is to be held in South Fallsburg, brahmin priests come from India. In the big outdoor Shakti Mandap pavilion, amidst gleaming marble and glass, the ritual fire is kindled by brahmins clad in bright silks. The students gather to watch the fire and hear the mantras in a space made sacred not only by the ritual itself but by the years of chanting, meditation, and darshan that have taken place there.

Gurumayi, dressed in red robes, presides from a slight distance. At moments in the *yajña,* the brahmins will approach her—offering the flame for blessings, garlanding her, performing acts of worship. Her placement—observing yet subtly directing, a witness to acts performed by others, yet patently the inspiration of those acts—is a metaphor for her position in present-day Siddha Yoga. As Swami Muktananda did, Gurumayi consistently presents herself as a disciple, ascribing the fundamental teachings she offers as well as the success of her work to her guru. In 1996, in a typical exchange, when a visitor said to her during darshan, "Whatever you do here, it's working," Gurumayi responded by saying, "Baba's grace."[267] Yet to her students—even those students who began Siddha Yoga as students of Swami Muktananda—Gurumayi is very much at the center of their spiritual life. She has become the exemplar of what they hope to attain, as well as the source of grace, teaching, and spiritual guidance. Students have described her spiritual power as a steady transforming force, a subtle influence that uplifts and transforms, unlocks their inner world and sweeps away blocks in their inner and outer lives. Linda Johnsen, a journalist who visited the Siddha Yoga ashrams in 1993, described something of Gurumayi's public impact in a book on Indian woman saints, *Daughters of the Goddess:*

> Gurumayi's striking beauty rivets attention wherever she goes. . . . [H]er energy seems inexhaustible. Her grace, delightful wit, and respectful regard for the needs of each devotee have expanded Siddha Yoga's appeal beyond what even Muktananda achieved.[268]

The image of the *yajña* is central in Gurumayi's teachings. In *yajña,* the fruits of the earth are offered to God and then burned in a fire that sacralizes that offering, transforms it into essence, and takes it higher. In yoga too, actions are offered sacrificially—this time, to an inner fire that transmutes the yogi's effort into the experience of inner light and love, the experience of God. From statements Gurumayi has made over the years, it is clear that she regards her own life as *yajña,* an offering to her own guru and to her students. And to those who turn to her as a guru, she consistently offers the model of sacrifice as the secret for a fulfilling life. For several years, in the mid-1980s, she held courses in the ashram that explored the central theme of fire as a metaphor not only for yogic practice but for life itself. "Life is an offering" and "Let every action be an offering" are phrases that she often uses. "When you give yourself selflessly with no strings attached, then you are free," she said in 1987; "there is nothing holding you back. So you are privileged to experience your own joy, to explore your own God within."[269] If one overall ethical teaching could be said to characterize her ministry, it is the teaching of unselfish action.

The years since 1982 have seen an increasingly conscious attempt to mold the Siddha Yoga movement into a fusion of individuals and institutions that can embody that message. Through periods of physical expansion—the South Fallsburg ashram more than tripled in size during the late 1980s; through tours that took Gurumayi to Australia, Europe, and the Far East, and on caravans through the New England countryside; through organizational shifts and the comings and goings of thousands of students, Gurumayi's intention to create a community of people who live what they profess to believe has run through all her teachings and interactions.

Siddha Yoga in the eighties and nineties faced a far different set of challenges than in Swami Muktananda's day. Muktananda had come to the

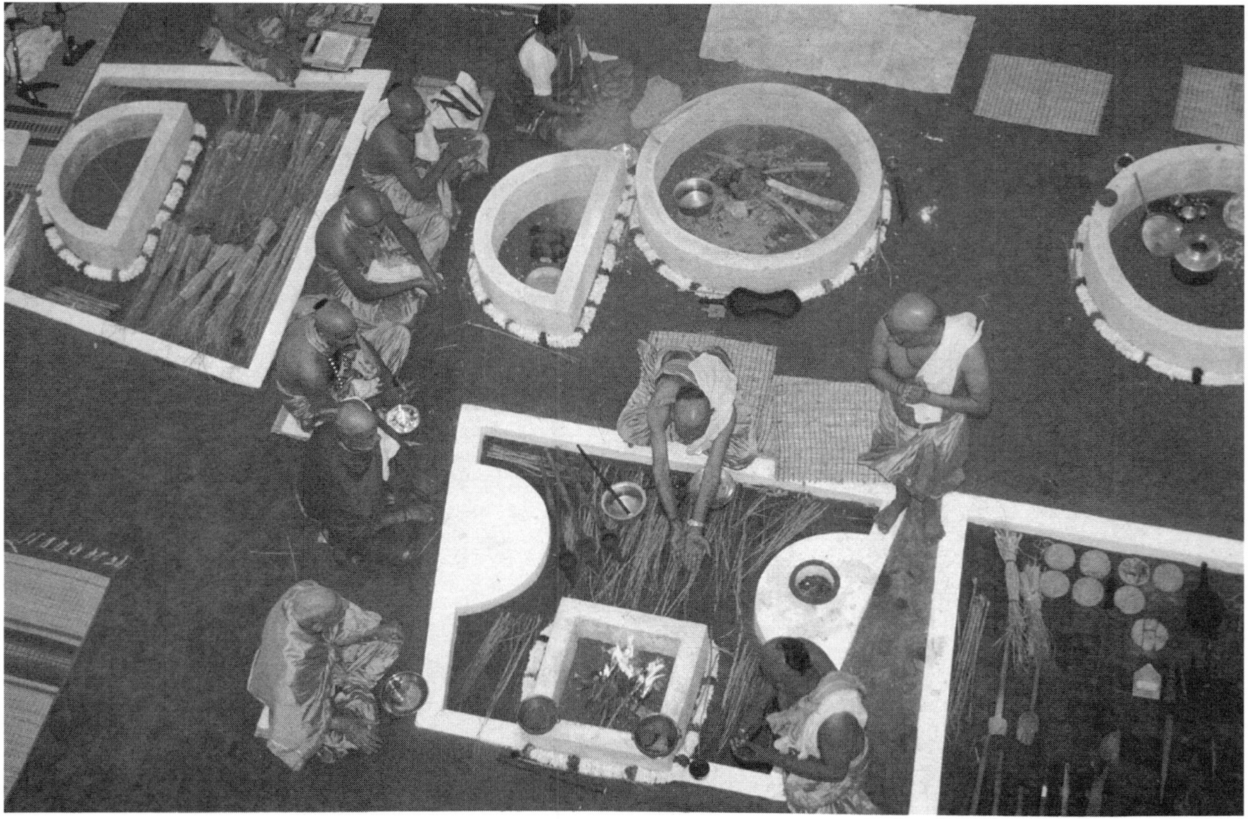

Fig. 17. A Caturmāsya Śrauta *yajña,* a 3,500-year-old Vedic ritual, held in Gurudev Siddha Peeth in 1990

West with the intention of giving shaktipat to many people and creating institutions that could carry the message of Siddha Yoga. Now, the institutions were in place. The original recipients of shaktipat had been practicing Siddha Yoga for upward of twenty years. Gurumayi had inherited Swami Muktananda's accomplishments, and she was in a position not only to refine and expand the existing teachings and organization but to guide her more experienced students to a far deeper experience of their spiritual potential. That she was aware of this is evident from a statement she made in 1985 to an interviewer who asked for a "message." "Meditate on your Self," she said. "God dwells within you as you." The interviewer protested, "But that's Muktananda's message." "I know," said Gurumayi. "My message is '*do it!*'"[270]

"These are beautiful teachings. And the only way they'll help you is if you put them into practice," said Swami Anantananda. "I see so much of Gurumayi's work is showing her students how to make these teachings a practical reality."[271]

For example, there was Swami Muktananda's statement, "See God in each other," which many students had treated more as an ideal than a practice. "There's a natural tendency among spiritual seekers, especially when the teaching is about personal liberation, to focus on staying in a lofty state and try to ignore everything that tends to bring you down to earth," said a student. "From early in her tenure, Gurumayi has made it clear that this wasn't enough, that seeing God in each other doesn't just mean having a lofty vision, it also means being kind, helpful, and above all, respectful of the people around you."[272] Her published writings reflect this concern. One of her books, *My Lord Loves a Pure Heart,* is a guide to developing qualities like compassion and freedom from anger; another, *Inner Treasures,* offers practical lessons about how to develop feelings of joy and peace:

> Now allow me to tell you what perfect joy is not. It is not the same as laughing at other people's mistakes. It never secretly gloats over another person's shortcomings or makes a joke at someone else's expense. It doesn't sit in a corner and fret. . . . It simply cannot stay where the people and things of this world are not rightly respected. . . . It isn't half-happy and half-doubtful. It isn't a quick smile arising from a sense of duty or courtesy.[273]

Many students maintain that Gurumayi has a particular genius for bringing her message into the day-to-day lives of individuals—often making use of small incidents to demonstrate a deeper point. A woman with a tendency to ignore others was once startled when Gurumayi interrupted a chant to ask her to move over so that a little girl could sit on the carpeted area rather than on the bare floor. "How do you expect to feel joy in your heart when you don't notice other people?" Gurumayi asked her.[274]

Swami Ishwarananda recalled how after one of his public talks

Gurumayi sent him a note that read, "It's one thing to love to talk. It's something else to love the people you're talking to." He commented, "I thought about that for a long time. What I came to see is that she was pushing me to see my teaching not as an act of personal expression, which is fundamentally self-seeking, but as service—as a way of serving people. She insists that we totally embody the teaching of Siddha Yoga. That teaching is about love, service, and sacrifice. As a spiritual organization, as a spiritual path, we have to be living what we teach. And when you become her student, she works on every single part of you that is out of line with the teachings until you learn how to live the teachings not just in public but also in every aspect of your private life."[275]

In support of this principle, Siddha Yoga courses often emphasize self-examination and learning to recognize and deal with negative personal tendencies—the "inner enemies" as they are called. Periodically in her Intensives and even public talks, Gurumayi will guide students in self-examination exercises, often culminating in an invocation to the power of grace, which Siddha Yoga students understand as the source of personal transformation as well as spiritual experience. Gurumayi's willingness to bring the teachings to a practical level, coupled with the historical fact that she is leading a group of people who have many more years of spiritual practice behind them than did most the people around Muktananda, has had several effects. Most notable has been the gradual development of a global community that is increasingly able to put the teachings into practice in mundane life in the world. Said a student from Germany, "When I was going through hard times a couple of years ago, it was quite routine for people from the Siddha Yoga center to call up to chat, to give me support. People here are unusually willing to go out of their way for each other."[276] Penny Clyne, who has practiced Siddha Yoga since 1974, said, "Recently, I looked at my life and I realized that I am surrounded by love. There is so much closeness in my family—and this is especially amazing since for years I felt that my family was the biggest obstacle to my spiritual practice. Somehow, just through the process of sadhana, we've learned to become treasures to each other."[277]

Clyne said that when a large group of people simultaneously act with the intent to see God in other people, the result is pleasant to behold. "What impresses me about Siddha Yoga in the 1980s and 1990s," agreed a journalist who regularly attends Siddha Yoga gatherings, "is that you can get into a wonderful state not only by being around the teacher, but by being around the students."[278]

It has not been an overnight process. Some students speak ruefully of the effort it took for them to learn Gurumayi's lessons of civility or service. A woman with a tendency toward chronic busy-ness recalled that several times over the course of a six-month period she heard Gurumayi say in her presence, "In Siddha Yoga, we don't just care about getting things done, we care about getting them done with love." Only later, the woman said, did she begin to apply this statement to herself.[279] One particularly feisty engineer reported that it took him five years of receiving hints and direct instruction from Gurumayi. "But it didn't seem to matter to her how long it took," he said. "She had a vision of me as a person who could manifest kindness, and she kept at it until I got it too."[280]

For many students, the process of spiritual maturation starts when they begin to internalize this vision, along with its subtler corollary: the point of balance between self-surrender and taking responsibility. "One of the misunderstandings that Westerners seem to have about a guru-centered path," said Martin Brost, a German businessman who is also a director of the Board of Trustees of the SYDA Foundation, "is that surrender to the guru means giving up responsibility for your own life. Actually, surrender is a much deeper and more difficult process—it's not about following rules or giving up your power to another person. It means learning to identify with your own higher Self—letting go of your feeling of being different from God, so that you can realize your own greatness and also your kinship with others. When individuals operate from that kind of understanding, it affects the group as a whole. As the individuals grow, the community also becomes more compassionate, more skillful, more self-aware."[281]

Gurumayi's 1995–96 tour to California, Mexico, and Europe provided for many observers a case in point. "Gurumayi had spent nearly five years working with the American and European communities to help them become more supportive of each other, to create a kind of culture of kindness," said Renato Rezende, a Brazilian who helped with the organization of the European segment of that tour. "For instance, the Germans and Italians were encouraged to see themselves not just as a part of their local community, but as Europeans working together. The northern and southern Californians were encouraged to work together."[282] The effects of the training were reflected in the experience of fellowship reported by many who encountered the Siddha Yoga community on that tour. Said a young Mexican man after a retreat with Gurumayi in Cuernavaca, "These two weeks were the happiest weeks of my whole life. They gave me a new vision of myself and the world we live in. Never in my life had I experienced so much love, nor did I know that so much love was possible. We just sat down to talk about the day and it was pure ecstasy. Or sometimes we just sat in silence looking at each other and we cried out of love."[283]

The Challenge of Growth

Siddha Yoga as a movement is expansive. The South Fallsburg ashram more than tripled in size during the late 1980s; the ashrams and centers see a steady influx of newcomers, spurred by Gurumayi's tours. Since the bestowal of shaktipat remains at the core of the movement, touring has been a constant. Throughout most of the 1980s, Gurumayi typically spent six months of the year in Gurudev Siddha Peeth, two months in South Fallsburg, and the rest of the year on tour. Siddha Yoga swamis and students traveled as well, sometimes alone, more often in groups, and wherever they went, new students were drawn to the path.

Expansion poses physical challenges—halls are periodically outgrown as the population swells, and accommodations during peak seasons can be crowded. Yet in a spiritual path based on the guru-disciple relationship, the most poignant issue raised by population growth is the potential effect on the very relationship that is the heart of the yoga. How, in a movement where as many as two thousand people regularly sit with the guru during a morning program, does a disciple maintain his or her connection to the guru?

It is not, of course, a new dilemma. Even in the late sixties, students accustomed to the intimacy of the tiny original circle around Swami Muktananda felt that the ashram was crowded when there were thirty people present instead of ten. A long-time student recalls a conversation with one of Muktananda's tour staff in 1974, during which she complained about the distance between Swami Muktananda's seat and her seat in the back of the hall. Then she added in a tone of amusement, "Of course, if he wants to say something to you, he can do that in a crowd of a thousand, and if he wants to ignore you, he'll do it even if you're alone in an elevator with him!"[284] She might have taken her insight a step further: Whether the movement is large or small, discipleship in Siddha Yoga must ultimately base itself on an inner connection with the guru, far more than on any external interaction. "There is no way you can see this as just an ordinary face-to-face relationship," said Mexican poet Elsa Cross. "Ultimately each devotee must learn to meet the guru at a very subtle level."[285] Without that inner connection, Gurumayi Chidvilasananda sometimes says, you miss the point of the relationship with the guru. "Everyone worries about getting attention from the guru," she said. "What you have to understand is that even if I go on talking to you forever, it will never be enough unless you find the guru inside."[286] In 1996, it was announced that the practice known as the "darshan line," where students had the opportunity to spend an individual moment with Gurumayi, would no longer be a regular part of programs with her. Students met in Siddha Yoga ashrams and centers to contemplate the impact of this shift on their personal relationship with Gurumayi, and as they discussed their experiences, many shared their realization that the deepest moments of communion with the guru had been internal, not based on physical or verbal interchanges.

Nonetheless, Gurumayi continues to create channels for making the physical connection, ranging from her teaching programs and Intensives—

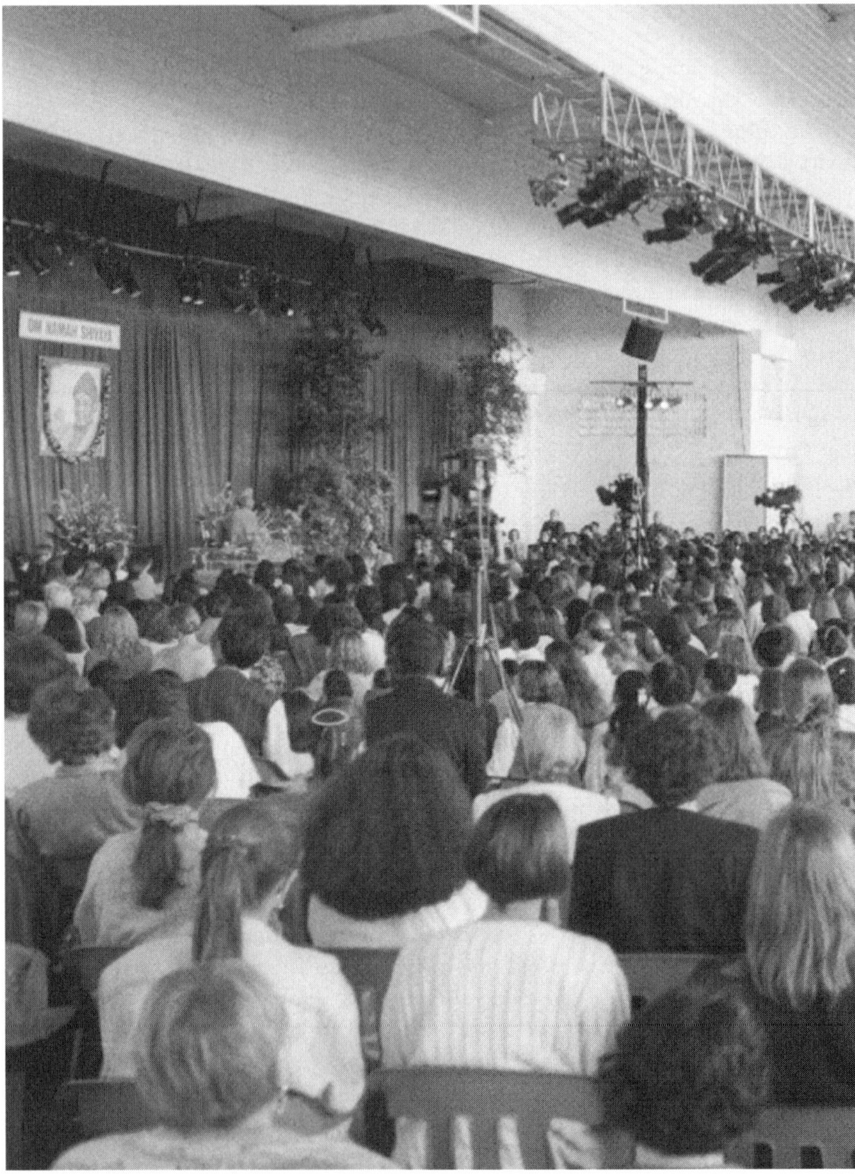

Fig. 18. Swami Chidvilasananda giving a talk in Mexico City in February 1996

some of which are transmitted internationally via satellite television—to the weekly gatherings at Siddha Yoga centers.

Making the Connection: How Siddha Yoga Works

In the world of Siddha Yoga in the 1990s, a strong thread of common practice connects most students, and for many the connection point is a Siddha Yoga meditation center. A student who lives near one of some three hundred centers in Europe, India, Australia, or North and South America usually attends weekly satsang programs, where students chant together, listen to readings or brief talks, and meditate. If the center is large enough, *haṭhayoga* exercise sessions might be offered. Courses on video are sent out from SYDA Foundation headquarters in South Fallsburg. Since the early nineties, all programs in centers and ashrams across the globe have been built around monthly themes like "Meditate on your Self" or "Make the Mind Your Friend," chosen from the teachings of Siddha Yoga. These create a unity of focus among practitioners otherwise separated by geography and language.

A student who wants to become more deeply involved can also support the center through offering service, a practice that Siddha Yoga, in common with spiritual traditions from Christianity to Zen, values as a primary avenue to spiritual progress. Siddha yogis' enthusiasm for such service—students regularly volunteer to chop vegetables for three or four hours at a clip, chanting all the while—is not always easy for outsiders to understand. Even some Siddha Yoga students are slow to grasp what *gurusevā* is about. "Work? I come here to meditate!" is not an uncommon remark. However, many consider *gurusevā* to be the most immediately transformative of Siddha Yoga practices. As a dishwasher in the South Fallsburg ashram wrote, in a rollickingly ingenuous paean to the suds:

> O my mind,
> how can you be blue?
> When there are heavenly dishes to do?
> My spirit becomes
> a shining light
> as each dish becomes
> so bright, clean and white.
> We all seek that
> which purifies and cleans.
> To know God is the goal
> and
> the dishes
> are
> THE MEANS![287]

These ingenuous lines express a truth that is as central to the Siddha Yoga ethos as it is to other spiritual traditions: that unselfish action purifies the mind. Siddha Yoga institutions encourage the notion of living life unselfishly—not simply because it is "nicer" but because acting unselfishly is one of the traditional ways to free oneself of the bondage of ego and come closer to the ultimate goal of realizing one's identity with God and the universe. Offering service as it is needed, without thought of reward, is valued as the most immediate means to cultivate unselfishness. *Gurusevā* also helps to bond students to the community and to the overall "mission" of Siddha Yoga; it gives them arenas for shared experiences, and according to many, attracts grace into their lives.

"When people offer service in one of the centers, that very act of offering their effort becomes the means by which they put the teachings into practice. It's easy to feel great in meditation, but a lot harder when you're working or interacting with people," said Alexandra Gonzalez, who helps coordinate the work of Siddha Yoga in Mexico. "*Gurusevā* offers a laboratory, so to speak, for developing yogic qualities, like detachment and skill in action. And once you've learned in the Guru's environment, it's a lot easier to apply these principles in your daily work."[288] In many ways, Siddha Yoga is a collective path; other students provide both the social support and the social friction that appears to be necessary for effective personal transformation. Swami Muktananda, asked how he personally worked on the egos of so many disciples, once said, "I don't have to work on them. I just put them together and they work on each other."[289] *Gurusevā* offers the arena where that process of ego-work can take place.

However, its primary purpose for Siddha Yoga students is to deepen their experience of the awakened *kuṇḍalinī*. *Gurusevā*, at its core, is a mystical practice like meditation, in which students who offer their service are "rewarded" by interior experiences, intuitive realizations, feelings of love, calm, and energy. *Gurusevā* is, for Siddha Yoga students, a primary means to attract grace into your life. A man who spent time doing *gurusevā* in one of the Siddha Yoga ashrams in the late 1980s wrote:

> There was no way I could have predicted that cleaning my room could make me feel grateful. That is the great thing about the Guru's Shakti: you can't ever predict the outcome of a certain linear act—cleaning a room, making a videotape, performing in a play, fixing flowers . . . sweeping the path—because while you are doing it, on some other level, the Guru is withdrawing some karma, some dirt, some obstruction in your life. Then you find that miracles happen . . . all because you helped build the Mandap. . . . You're more patient, or you're not as angry, or you love your wife more, or you had the most beautiful day with your children you can ever imagine, walking by the lake with the wind blowing, smelling the jasmine. Or you're just happy.

> You get to these subtle states where life is about as beautiful as it can be, where it seems to be the highest state of civilization, where God and man are in some kind of unity.[290]

A student who lives where there is no Siddha Yoga center at all can do "home seva"; tasks range from making meditation cushions or altar cloths for the Siddha Yoga bookstore, to graphic design, text editing, and typesetting. Another source of connection is the Siddha Yoga Correspondence Course, whose bimonthly lessons offer several thousand subscribers ongoing instructions for integrating Siddha Yoga teachings into daily life. Some students periodically take time off from work to spend a few months in one of the Siddha Yoga ashrams, and most students who have the means usually travel at least once a year to be with Gurumayi for a few days or weeks. She makes this easier by touring and by creating opportunities for personal contact through visits to centers. Students in northern California still talk about the day in 1989 when she walked through the neighborhood around the Oakland ashram. Devotee households put up orange flags to mark their houses, and Gurumayi visited every one—almost 150 homes in all—where she chatted, inspected personal treasures, and met family members. At centers, her manner is personal and intimate. "We have met one another in so many different ways, in so many different forms," she told a group in southern California in 1996. "Finally we meet in this form because it has been our wish. This is the promise we have kept. It is a promise being fulfilled."[291] Visiting holy shrines in Europe with local Siddha Yoga students—the Basilica of St. Francis in Assisi, the Shrine to the Black Virgin in Montserrat, the Church of the Black Madonna in Poland—she led her students, and anyone else who happened by, in informal chanting or impromptu meditation.*

Although moments in the physical presence of the guru are prized and often become the source of cherished lessons and instruction, even those who have no opportunity of ever being in Gurumayi's physical presence seem quite capable of experiencing the connection. Devotees introduced to the guru through the Siddha Yoga Prison Project, many of them serving long prison sentences, have reported experiences in which Gurumayi appeared in their meditation or their dreams, or guided them inwardly, and many say that they feel her support at crucial moments in their prison experience. And there is no lack of anecdotes from students thousands of miles away who "see" Gurumayi sitting before them, or "hear"

---

*Both Swami Muktananda and Gurumayi Chidvilasananda are strongly ecumenical. Not only are nuns, priests, and rabbis regular visitors to Siddha Yoga's ashrams, but Native American religious ceremonies have been held on the grounds of Shree Muktananda Ashram, performed by devotees who are Native Americans as well as by visiting tribal elders.

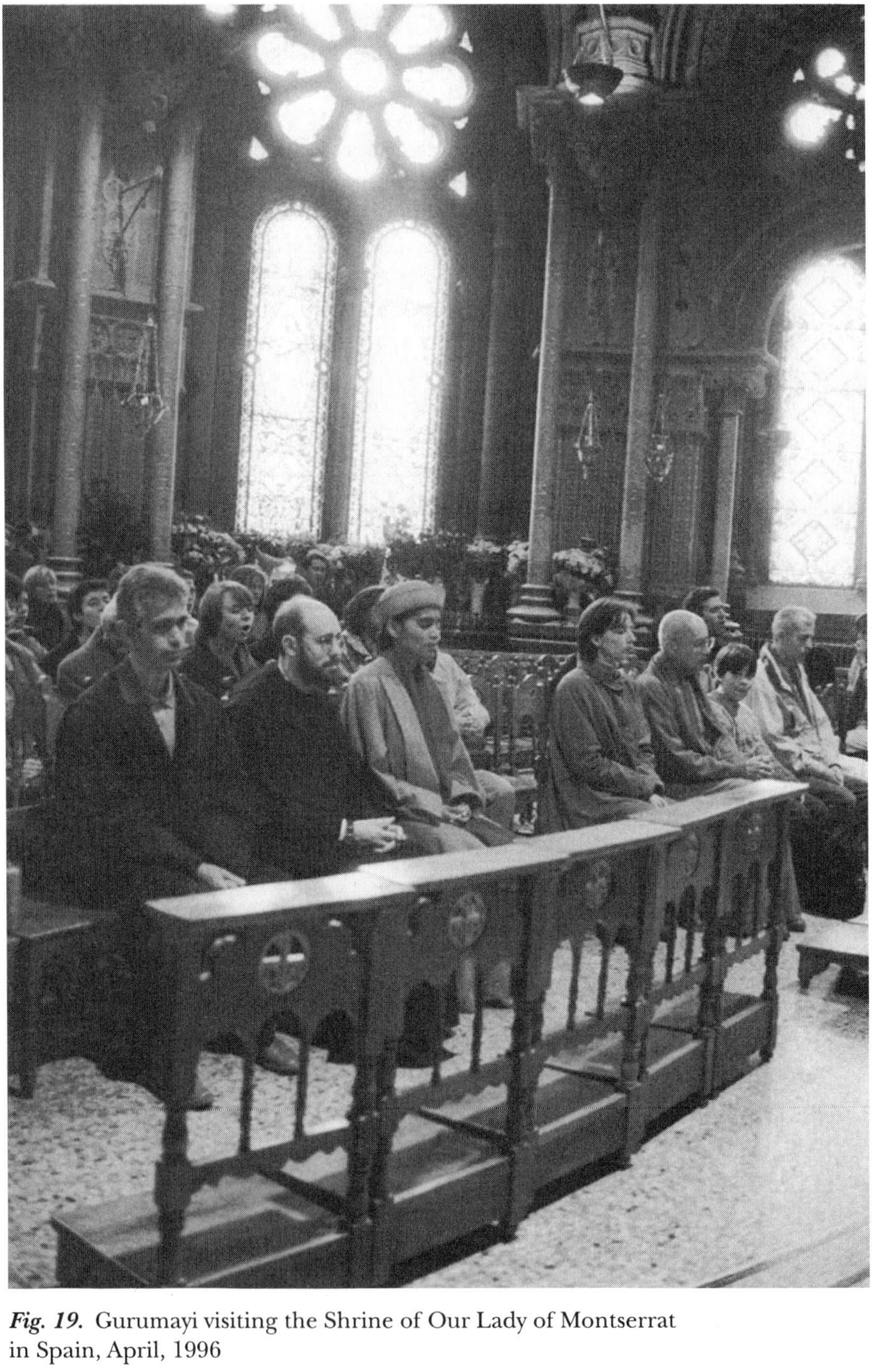

Fig. 19. Gurumayi visiting the Shrine of Our Lady of Montserrat in Spain, April, 1996

her guidance. That inner guidance occasionally turns out to echo an actual external message given by Gurumayi. Shubhada Vora of Bombay had just such an experience when her clothing factory burned down. As she described it, while she was watching her business go up in smoke, she heard an inner voice saying, "Don't worry. What was burned wasn't yours, and what's left isn't yours either." She said that she knew this was a message from her higher Self, and it led her into a deep contemplation through which she realized nothing external really belonged to her. The next day, she received a telephone call from one of the swamis with a message from Gurumayi, to whom she had sent word of the fire, though not of the inner voice. The message was, "Don't worry. What was burned wasn't really yours, and what's been saved isn't yours either."[292]

This mystical feeling of connection, where students experience Gurumayi's subtle presence at critical moments, is so widespread and so intrinsic to Siddha Yoga that in 1996, Catherine Parrish, the executive vice president of SYDA Foundation, described a series of such incidents reported by devotees during a single month:

> They tell us that Gurumayi was physically in Cuernavaca, Mexico. . . .
>
> But at the same time, the daughter of a devotee having an operation in Fresno, California, swears that she felt Gurumayi's presence in the hospital room with her family. She said that she not only felt Gurumayi's presence and the warmth of her blessings and support, but she also could smell her sweet fragrance.
>
> In Perth, Australia, a schoolteacher, who had been struggling with the angry behavior of a young student, saw Gurumayi come into her classroom and smile lovingly and approvingly at the boy. The schoolteacher did the same, feeling a rush of compassion for him. His behavior shifted and he can now do no wrong.
>
> In Canada, the niece of a devotee was about to play her first solo part in the symphony orchestra. She was so nervous that she thought that she might fail to even be able to play her violin at all. To her surprise and delight, her uncle's guru showed up in the front row smiling and silently cheering her on. She played beautifully.
>
> In a home in New York City, a house guest picked up *Darshan* magazine and became mesmerized by the love in the face of Gurumayi's picture, and had the life-altering realization that her own mother had indeed always loved her in spite of how it had seemed throughout her lonely childhood.
>
> An executive faced a difficult and intense situation in his company. From all evidence it seemed that some of his jealous colleagues were conniving to have him fired. He was pacing back and forth in his office when Gurumayi suddenly appeared sitting behind his desk. She smiled and said, "Remember the play of consciousness." He meditated on her words and found himself

> feeling playful, ready for anything, and confident that "everything happens for the best."
>
> Later that day he was called to a meeting where the chief executive laid out the accusations of incompetency that had been fabricated by the others. Our executive calmly spoke his perspective on the matters. He retained his position and gained the respect of everyone there.[293]

As these reports indicate, the guru in Siddha Yoga is experienced not only as a finite physical being, but as a subtle yet very real presence who guides the students wherever they happen to be. Swami Muktananda and Gurumayi identify the subtle aspect of the guru with the awakened *kuṇḍalinī.* They point out that once the guru has transmitted spiritual energy to a disciple, then the energy itself can teach the student from within.*

For this reason the responsibility for spiritual progress, satisfaction, and connection in Siddha Yoga ultimately belongs to the student. Siddha Yoga is, above all, a movement based on home practice—the time devoted to daily meditation, repetition of the mantra, reading the guru's books, chanting (which many students do in their cars, to the accompaniment of taped chants sold by the SYDA bookstore), applying the lessons of the Correspondence Course. "It's the internal work that matters," said Martin Brost, "and it's the internal work that bears fruit."[294]

New Forms for the Teachings

Growth creates another challenge: In a movement where shaktipat continually draws new students into the community, the content of programs and courses is often driven by the newcomers' need for basic instruction in the teachings and culture of Siddha Yoga. At the same time, students who have been practicing the yoga for fifteen or twenty years need a level of teaching that reflects their experience and concerns. Through the years, as teachers worked to reconcile the need to integrate new students with the demand of advanced students for increasing depth, Siddha Yoga courses, publications, and programs have gone through a continual process of refinement.

At the heart of the process has been the formal and informal teaching of Gurumayi Chidvilasananda herself. Her formal lectures at programs and Intensives often begin from a seed of scripture—a verse from the *Bhagavadgītā* or an Upaniṣad, interpreted for its relevance to a person per-

---

*In *Where Are You Going?* Swami Muktananda says, "Because I exist within my disciples in the form of the awakened Shakti, they can experience my presence everywhere and at all times, no matter where they live. I do not have to guide them, because they receive guidance from the inner Shakti. If I had to guide my disciples personally, then this would not be divine work. It would not be spontaneous yoga." (p. 137)

forming spiritual practice in New York, Paris, or Sydney, and enlivened with tales, anecdotes, and quotations from ancient and modern authors. At the same time, she has been known to teach spontaneously wherever a gathering occurs. When she is in residence at Shree Muktananda Ashram in South Fallsburg, informal satsangs have sometimes occurred weekly, and here her emphasis is on dialogue, discussion, and a kind of Socratic questioning. She might throw out a question to invite opinions and discussion, or have someone read a parable and then ask people what it means.

Typical of such impromptu teaching situations was a Sunday in March 1995, which found Gurumayi sitting in the big, sky-lit lobby of one of the buildings with nearly five-hundred students gathered around her. A swami announced the topic of discussion: What does it mean to leave the ego behind? Then he asked the question, "What does it mean to be free of ego?" Some hands were raised, and a New York woman volunteered, "To me it means being able to do everything with an empty mind." Another hand went up. "Does that mean you don't think?" someone asked. "Does losing your ego mean you stop using your mind?" "Aha," said the swami. "Let's look at this question. Is that the teaching? That you don't use your mind?" Hands went up all over the room. "The idea is that the mind should be still, so that when you use it, it can be sharp and clear. Not that you don't use your mind," a man offered. Gurumayi, from her seat at the front of the room, asked, "What is the role of the mind in sadhana?" and a visiting professor of Vedānta stood up to explain the philosophical perspective on the mind. "What we are doing here is self-inquiry," the swami said, "*ātmavicāra.* We are trying to climb the ladder to attain the higher Truth."

The discussion became more animated, with more and more people raising their hands to have their say. At the end of an hour, Gurumayi pulled the microphone toward her and began to comment—pointing out areas of confusion, clarifying questions that had not been completely answered. She said:

> Baba used to say, "Ego is not bad. You just need to know how to use it." He used to say, "Have *śuddhāham.*" *Aham* means "ego," and *śuddhāham* means the "pure ego." So have this consciousness, the pure "I am"—"I am that I am." Baba said, relate yourself to the higher "I am," to the greater you. You must understand that your greatness does not shift according to place, person, or time. Your greatness constantly remains as great as it is. When you compare yourself with your own great Self, you become greater and greater and greater. There is continuous expansion. There is no moment that is dull when you compare yourself with your own greatness.[295]

"For a while, we had these dialogues every week," said Swami Gitananda, who served as one of the facilitators. "It became a kind of group exercise in Vedāntic self-inquiry, a modern recreation of the Upaniṣadic dialogues between gurus and disciples. In the process, Gurumayi actually trained a large group of people in how to look beneath the surface of the teachings, to see what they really understood and what they were merely accepting without examining it."[296]

Said John Grimes, the scholar of Vedānta who participated in this discussion, "What I perceive here is that Gurumayi aims to preserve the most basic, classic experience of the guru-disciple relationship, where the Guru gives the disciple spiritual knowledge and then tests that knowledge. She is a genius at finding forms for that dialogue in a community where the group of disciples sitting with the guru is likely to be anywhere from fifty to two thousand people at a time."[297]

The dialogue-discussion model of scriptural study also prevails in the Gurudev Siddha Peeth program of scriptural study, required for all residents, which combines lectures by visiting professors with ongoing study groups in such texts as the *Kaṭha Upaniṣad* or the *Śiva Sūtras*. It is especially evident in the courses taught in South Fallsburg each summer by Siddha Yoga swamis and lay teachers as well as visiting university professors. These courses have ranged from explorations of scriptures like the *Śiva Sūtras* and Patañjali's *Yoga Sūtras*, to concentrated workshops in meditation and practical sadhana-oriented courses with titles like "Yoga of Daily Life," to *haṭhayoga* courses, courses for teenagers and children, and workshops that explore the symbolism behind major Hindu deities like Lakṣmī or Gaṇeśa. (For a complete list of Siddha Yoga courses and Intensives offered during one calendar year, see appendix 3.)

Outside the ashrams, courses in Siddha Yoga meditation are offered in centers, while ongoing training programs prepare new teachers, help speakers develop communication skills, and provide study programs for guided scriptural study.

The Intensive and Global Shaktipat

Yet the central vehicle for Siddha Yoga teaching remains the Intensive; since Swami Muktananda's time, this weekend program has functioned both as a vehicle for shaktipat and as a means for long-time students to reconnect to the purposeful transmission of their guru's spiritual energy. It is also the arena for the subtlest level of teachings. Gurumayi's students describe how, during her talks and meditation instructions, she often uses sacred sounds and visual imagery to guide students through subtle shifts of consciousness, to open inner spiritual centers, or to help students release inner blocks or obstacles.[298] Moreover, from 1989, when the first "satellite" Intensives were broadcast around the world, the term "global shaktipat" began to take on a literal meaning. A case in point: In 1994, an Intensive was broadcast by audio hookup to the tiny Siddha Yoga center in St. Petersburg,

Russia. The next year, a French student took a trip to Russia and, toward the end of his trip, spent some time in a Russian Orthodox monastery there. The abbott there noticed the student's photograph of Gurumayi. "Oh, you're with Gurumayi," the abbott said. Surprised, the student asked, "How do you know Gurumayi?" "Everyone knows Gurumayi," replied the abbott, explaining that her name and photograph were widely circulated in the Russian spiritual community[299]—no doubt by students who had taken that Intensive. One result was that when Gurumayi visited Poland in 1996, hundreds of people came from all over Eastern Europe to attend the Intensive. A similar story was told by students who visited the town of Shian in northern China, in 1992. They fell into conversation with a taxi driver, and when he heard that Gurumayi was their guru, he beamed and said, "She's my Guru, too."[300] Siddha Yoga meditation centers in Brazil sometimes have more than a hundred students taking satellite Intensives—many of whom have never met Gurumayi in person.

Such incidents epitomize what to many students looks like a shift in Siddha Yoga's relationship to the surrounding culture. Whereas non-Indian Siddha Yoga students of the seventies often experienced their involvement in yogic practices as a choice that took them out of the mainstream of their culture, Siddha Yoga under Gurumayi has tended to be increasingly mainstream in character. Her style as a teacher—her ability to blend tradition and modernity, keeping alive classical forms while recognizing the contemporary issues that color the spiritual lives of her students—makes her accessible to many who would have been uncomfortable in Bhagawan Nityananda's environs, or had difficulty in relating to the Hindi-speaking Muktananda. This accessibility, which draws people of a wide range of backgrounds and ages, has been of immense significance in the ongoing "meditation revolution" that Siddha Yoga sees as its primary mission. Though Siddha Yoga doesn't proselytize, Muktananda's legacy includes an ongoing commitment to helping people achieve knowledge and experience of the inner Self. "This work is for liberation, and not liberation just for one person," Gurumayi told a group of Siddha Yoga center leaders in 1986. "Baba's work is not only for individuals—it has a greater scope."[301] She has consistently emphasized the fact that meditation doesn't just benefit the individual who meditates. "When you meditate, it's not just for yourself," she often says. "As you become peaceful inside, your state also spreads to others."[302]

It is for this reason that the yoga emphasizes both turning inward—personal meditation practice—and a public accessibility that allows a constant expansion of the community.

These two polarities are exemplified by the relative situations of Gurudev Siddha Peeth in India and Shree Muktananda Ashram in the United States. Gurudev Siddha Peeth is run as an old-style *gurukula* with relatively few (between 150 and 500) students, each of whom is required to set aside time each day for scriptural study in addition to ashram service, personal practice, group chanting, and satsang, and where a prospective visitor must fill out an application form stating, among other things, his or her reasons for wanting to go to the ashram.

Though also run as a *gurukula,* Shree Muktananda Ashram is open throughout much of the year to students who might come for a weekend, a week, or several months to follow the daily schedule of chants and courses. Others may drive up for the day from nearby Manhattan or down from Boston to attend a morning program with Gurumayi, take a "Learn to Meditate" course, eat a vegetarian meal in the ashram's dining hall, and drive home.

The accessibility of the South Fallsburg ashram and the tours—where "closed" meditation retreats alternate with open public programs—is important to Siddha Yoga students, since interest in the yoga tends to spread among family members and friends. "Even when we don't have any personal interest in bringing people to the Siddha Yoga centers and programs," said Carmen Soria of Barcelona, "the people around us often ask us questions like, 'Why are you so happy?' And when they find that the answer is Siddha Yoga meditation, they want to know more, they want to try it too." She added that when a person experiences personal transformation, there seems to be a natural desire to share that experience: "Not only do we rejoice in our own experience, but we would like to see the whole world immersed in the experience of inner love."[303]

"With Siddha Yoga inner and outer transformation happen simultaneously," said Françoise Lexa. "When we change, our whole world changes."[304] One obvious manifestation of this is in the impulse to social service that activates many Siddha Yoga students.

SIDDHA YOGA IN THE ARENA OF SOCIAL SERVICE

Philanthropic work has always been a part of the Siddha Yoga movement, even though Swami Muktananda made it clear that social work was not his primary mission. He used to say that those who go out to help the world without having first come to know their own inner Self are like bankers who lend money they don't have. To really give to other people, he maintained, you have to have inner resources of love and understanding, otherwise your work doesn't truly nourish others. Nonetheless, social service—especially toward Gurudev Siddha Peeth's *ādivāsī* neighbors—was an ongoing concern from the earliest days of Bhagawan Nityananda's stay in the valley. Muktananda expanded Nityananda's philanthropic work. He had milk distributed daily to the protein-deprived schoolchildren in the region. He built a high school for *ādivāsī* children and had houses constructed for over five hundred homeless families near his ashram. Gurudev Siddha Peeth periodically donated money to famine and flood relief around India. It was Muktananda who first envisioned a mobile hospital that would travel to the villages in the region and give free medical care to the malnourished and sick of the valley. In 1978, he brought that vision to fulfillment when he inaugurated Shree Nityananda Mobile Hospital (now renamed Shree Muktananda Mobile Clinic), a modern dispensary created on a bus chassis donated by a devotee.

According to Swami Apoorvananda, an American doctor who headed the project for several years, the mobile clinic, with over 42,000 patient visits annually, has been instrumental in reducing the vitamin deficiencies and infectious diseases that are endemic among the tribal people. In the nineties, it became known locally as "Gurumayi's bus," offering prenatal care, immunizations, and minor surgery, as well as general medical diagnosis and treatment to people of all ages.

The PRASAD Project

In the mid-eighties, Swami Chidvilasananda began to expand the scope of Siddha Yoga's social service work beyond the borders of the Tansa Valley, and even beyond India itself.

The PRASAD Project, described in a 1993 newsletter as "a volunteer organization dedicated to improving the quality of life for people in need and to creating opportunities for their self-reliance," was incorporated in 1992 as an international not-for-profit corporation. Executive director Catherine Parrish, formerly the chief executive officer of an international nonprofit organization focused on ending world hunger, described PRASAD in 1996 as "an expression of the philosophy and teachings of Siddha Yoga in action." She added, "The 'action' we take in PRASAD is to work in partnership with people living in poverty to uplift the quality of their lives. It's a natural extension of people being kind and considerate, people being global citizens, people caring for their community and for each other."[305]

PRASAD (Hindi, *prasād*: "blessed gift") is also an acronym meaning Philanthropic Relief, Altruistic Service, And Development. True to the functions listed in its title, PRASAD carries out community development projects in the Tansa Valley, as well as in Sullivan County, New York (where Shree Muktananda Ashram is located), and in Mexico City. In India, it sponsors the Shree Muktananda Mobile Clinic and a free mobile dental clinic, and runs a large free eye-camp, Netraprakash ("light of the eyes"), where Indian and Western physician volunteers use state-of-the-art surgical techniques to remove cataracts and implant intraocular lenses.[306] By 1996, the eye-camps had restored sight to an estimated three thousand impoverished villagers.

The Prison Project

Siddha Yoga satsang programs have been going on in prisons since Swami Muktananda inaugurated the Prison Project in 1978 with a statement that has become something of a maxim for inmates on the program: "You can turn your prison cell into a paradise."[307] Since then, the Prison Project has regularly sent teams of Siddha Yoga volunteers into maximum security prisons, where they meet with groups of inmates to meditate, chant, and pass on some of the basic teachings of Siddha Yoga. In the early nineties, a survey showed that about fifteen hundred prison inmates were involved in the Prison Project programs, mostly through the Siddha Yoga Correspondence Course, whose bimonthly lessons are sent free to any inmate who requests them.

As elsewhere in Siddha Yoga, interest in the course spreads by word-of-mouth. Many inmates would hear about the course from cellmates or neighbors. Diego Santiago of New York City began receiving the Correspondence Course during a twenty-year sentence at Shawangunk Prison in Wallkill, New York. He wrote:

> The course started to take a lot of the hate and pain and bitterness from me. It was like the fetters came off.
>
> After I'd been taking the Correspondence Course for about eleven months, . . . I was reading some of Gurumayi's quotes in the back of the lessons, and I was feeling real good. Then the cell opened up and I walked out for chow, and I looked at the guys and I saw myself in all of them! And I said to myself, "This is what the lessons are talking about." I knew they were experiencing what I experienced, and I was experiencing what they experienced, and it was just remarkable. It was fantastic. A feeling of liberation.[308]

Santiago credited the Correspondence Course with a shift that has been significant for him as a prison inmate: He said that even though he still gets angry, he no longer holds onto his anger. During a recent cell-block confrontation, for instance, he was able to make peace with his opponent rather than allowing the confrontation to turn into a vendetta like many disagreements among prisoners.

Alan Gompers, who was released from prison in 1986 after serving six years of a fifteen-year drug sentence, wrote of a similar experience of being released from his anger and bitterness about his situation. Once, as a guard screamed at him for a minor infraction, he was able to feel compassion for the guard's anger. "I could really see that 'guard' and 'inmate' aren't different at all; what matters isn't the role, it's the feelings we carry. I kept feeling more love, more compassion."[309]

Tom Toomey, a former Catholic priest who began directing the program in 1979, has pointed out that the largest number of inmates enrolled in the program are in maximum security prisons, and some have even been on death row. "These are people who will do their entire sadhana in prison," he said. "The program is the difference for them between a state of despair and a meaningful life."[310]

FACE-TO-FACE WITH GURUMAYI

Over the years, despite changes in the forms and rhythms of Siddha Yoga culture, certain things remain constant. One of these is the Siddha Yoga satsang program—since the early 1970s, the setting where devotees and visitors can gather to hear the guru's teachings, to chant and meditate, and to experience the mystical transmission that occurs through *darshan,* the simple act of being in the presence of a God-realized person. Whether they are held in large conference centers or hotel ballrooms (as they often are during Gurumayi's tours), or in the open-air Shakti Mandap in South Fallsburg, these programs are usually the setting for Gurumayi's lectures—lectures that are carefully structured yet filled with improvisation, scriptural yet personal and anecdotal, and much cherished by her students.

A Morning Program with Gurumayi

During the 1990s, most programs have begun with a welcome delivered by a master of ceremonies, followed by a brief introductory talk by a Siddha Yoga teacher or devotee. Gurumayi might enter partway through the program, perhaps walking across the stage (if the program is held in a theater, as they generally are when she is on tour) or simply strolling in from the back of the hall in South Fallsburg, then bowing to the picture of her guru over her seat. Her entrance is sometimes greeted by emotional expressions of welcome, especially on the part of students who have not seen her for some time—during her 1996 visit to Mexico City, as she walked down the aisle of the Mexico City World Trade Center, observers say that so many happy, tearful people reached out to take her hand that it took her several minutes to reach her chair. In South Fallsburg, Gurumayi is likely to enter trailed by several of the ashram children. Her affection for children is famous, and so is her willingness to take them seriously as disciples. Children often accompany her on her walks, and those who are old enough to sit quietly occupy many of the seats closest to her chair.

On this summer morning, Gurumayi takes her seat as the introductory strains of a *nāmasaṃkīrtana,* a group chant, well up from the bank of musicians who occupy a spot to one side. Chanting is another area in which Gurumayi's refining power has been most apparent. Over the years, she has encouraged constant creative innovation in this core Siddha Yoga practice, holding chanting courses in which trained singers teach the basics of voice production and group singing, setting chants to traditional *rāgas*, Indian melodic patterns, and encouraging ashram musicians to experiment both with Western musical accompaniments and classical Indian instruments. Siddha Yoga students who are professional musicians often sit in on chanting sessions; along with the traditional harmonium, cymbals, and *mṛdaṅg*, synthesizers, electric keyboard, violin, cello, or flute may accompany the voices. By all accounts, the experience of these chants is relished, affecting not just the students but even those who drop in for the first time.

Writer Linda Johnsen described her first experience of chanting at such a program:

> The hall darkens and a harmonium begins to play. Gurumayi initiates the chant: "*Kali Durge Namo Namah!*" ("To the supreme Goddess I bow again and again!") I join in tentatively. Gradually, I note, with some satisfaction, that a few of the women sitting near me are just as approximate in following the melody as I.
>
> And then the chant swallows me. It is not coming from my mouth but from the root of my being. . . . Like a thousand other voices in that dark hall I am suddenly singing perfectly—and at the top of my lungs. I am a wave in an ocean of mantra as we cry out the Divine Mother's name over and over again. It is ecstatic: I am singing here, filled with bliss, and then I am gone. All that remains is the Inner Observer relishing the *nada*, the vibration of the . . . name.
>
> Abruptly, Gurumayi ends the chant and we are plunged into a silence so deep that not even thought disturbs it. The experience is awesome. Perhaps when the Siddha devotees claim their master can give one a glimpse of one's deepest self, this crystalline state of lucid serenity is what they mean.[311]

As the chant ends, Gurumayi sings out mantras, invoking her guru and the power of the lineage: her ritual prelude to beginning her talk. Part scriptural explication, part practical application, the talks are laden with illustrations and examples from her own life and the experiences of her students. They are also very much oriented toward practice—as in a talk on gentleness given during the summer of 1996:

> [Gentleness] is not a technique for making the mind or intellect numb so that you cannot think, or judge, or discriminate anymore. It is truly a means for extracting the perfection from each moment. God is perfect, this universe is perfect; therefore, perfection must be inherent in every particle of this universe. You may forget things, you may make mistakes, you may make blunders, you may do all kinds of things; yet, that doesn't mean there is no perfection in God, there is no perfection in God's universe. It is your sadhana to extract the perfection from each moment, from each particle of the universe. And how

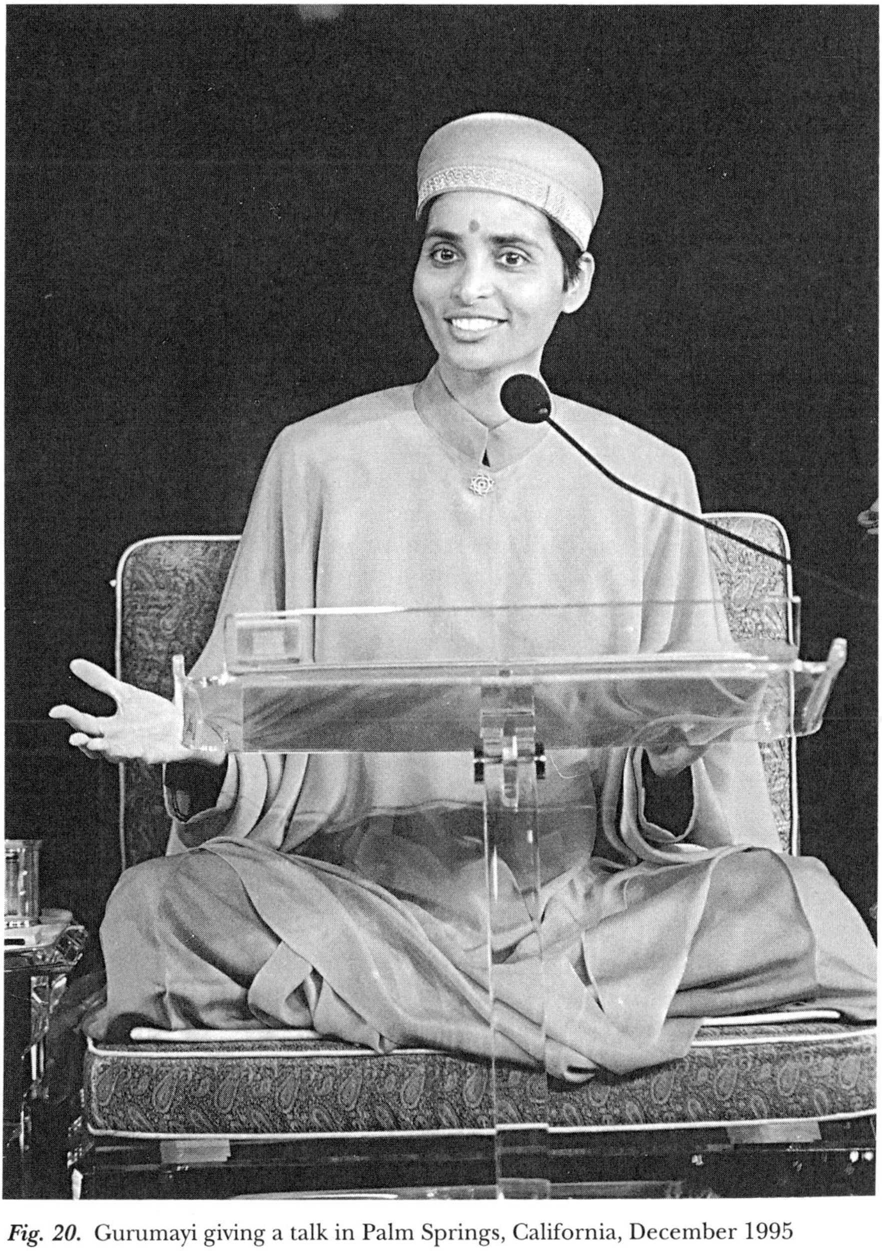

Fig. 20. Gurumayi giving a talk in Palm Springs, California, December 1995

> do you do that? In Siddha Yoga we do it through contemplation, continuous contemplation. Instead of allowing the mind to enter into a negative mode and prattle away until it devours the consciousness of the mind, or until it dries up the nectar of the mind, you fill the mind with the words of the siddhas, with the words of the scriptures, *Oṃ pūrṇamadaḥ, oṃ pūrṇamidaṃ*—"This is perfect. That is perfect." And as you do that, incredible understanding blossoms forth. You are able to receive wisdom from your own inner being, from the fountain of knowledge that is present within each person. When you are gentle, you are able to extract this perfection. And you must be truly gentle. You cannot force it. If you force it, you lose it. When you are gentle, you are able to extract perfection from every particle of this universe.[312]

Periodically, Gurumayi might break her discourse to lead the audience in a contemplative exercise or to direct them in a few moments of inner focus. When her talk is complete, and she begins instructing them in a visual meditation technique, most people in the hall already seem indrawn. The entire hall becomes deeply quiet during the fifteen minutes that follow. At the end of the meditation period, the master of ceremonies announces that on this occasion students will be able to come before Gurumayi one by one, to receive blessings through her long wand of peacock feathers, and ultimately, to experience a moment of inner communion. This practice, known as the "darshan line," was soon to disappear from Siddha Yoga programs, where the focus is increasingly on hearing the teachings and practicing in Gurumayi's company. So this afternoon's interactions are among the last examples of a practice that had once been a regular feature of Siddha Yoga life. "What do you receive when you have darshan of the Guru?" the emcee reminds the audience. "When we come before the Guru, she shows us our own Self. She shows us our own greatness. So stay focused in your heart."[313]

To observe Gurumayi meeting people is to note her apparently boundless capacity to connect to those who come before her. The line for this face-to-face darshan forms like a wide ribbon of humanity that stretches backward and out of the hall, snaking around the building. Friends and family are introduced. Gifts are given and received. Questions are asked. Yet communication is usually wordless; students say that a glance or simply a moment in her presence—even at a distance—can resolve questions without anything being said. Gurumayi greets many people by name, asking them simple questions such as "When did you come?" often attending to several things at once. "Did you get rest?" she asks the parents of a student who are visiting for the first time, then nods as the father says, "My son has a lot of faith in you." She hands the father a shawl, which he holds over his heart. "I feel so strange," the mother says as she walks away. "Why do I feel this way?" "She's a saint," the father tells her.[314]

"At times," wrote Marilyn Goldin in a newsletter from Gurumayi's 1996 tour where this form of darshan was held in most of the public programs, "these exchanges . . . are so simple that their dimension almost escapes you. For instance, seeing Gurumayi nodding and smiling at someone and saying, 'You were at the Flint Center.' It sounds like a simple, pleasant thing to say—until you remember that this was a brand-new devotee and that the Flint Center [in Cupertino, California] is an immense auditorium with several balconies that were filled to the rafters that day and darshan lines that went on around the block, and that the event was two weeks ago. . . . You find yourself thinking 'How can she remember everyone? What kind of knowledge is this?' and you start looking for answers beyond the limitations of the mind."[315]

Her interactions with the students run a wide gamut: they can be playful, confrontational, or instructive. In one program during the late eighties, someone gave Gurumayi a mirror. She spent the rest of the evening holding it up to the students' faces to show them their own expressions. "For some people, the surprise was how beautiful they looked," said an eyewitness of that event. "Other people were amazed at how much anxiety showed on their faces."[316] Many students relate that a simple exchange with Gurumayi—often during a moment when she passes them in a corridor and stops to speak a word or two—can provide food for long contemplation. A middle-aged Chicago woman described how, in 1991, she had brought her mother, with whom she had an angry, difficult relationship, to meet Gurumayi. The mother slipped as she was greeting Gurumayi, whereupon Gurumayi rose from her chair to catch the mother's arm. "Help your mother," she told the student. The student said later that as she contemplated these words, she decided that they weren't just for the moment, but contained an instruction for her life. So she began spending time with her mother, cooking for her, entertaining her—and in the process, she said, dissolving her lifelong resentment toward her parent.[317]

Yet for most of the students the impact of being in her presence has nothing to do with any outward exchange. It is the energy, the *śakti*, that surges up in her presence or in the environment around her that creates the inner shift. On this particular morning, as an Indian devotional song spills through the hall, a man tells the friend, who has brought him for his first visit to the ashram, "I don't understand what's happening to me!" Tears are streaming down his face. Nearby, an artist is describing to a friend her experience in meditation. "I felt myself going to a place of deep sadness," she says. "It felt as if it was the place of my most deeply held grief. Then I heard Gurumayi's voice saying, 'Go down, go down.' So what I did was I went into the sadness. Then all of a sudden it was like I went through the bottom of the sadness, and on the other side was love." A man from New York City sits against one of the windows, savoring a vision he has just

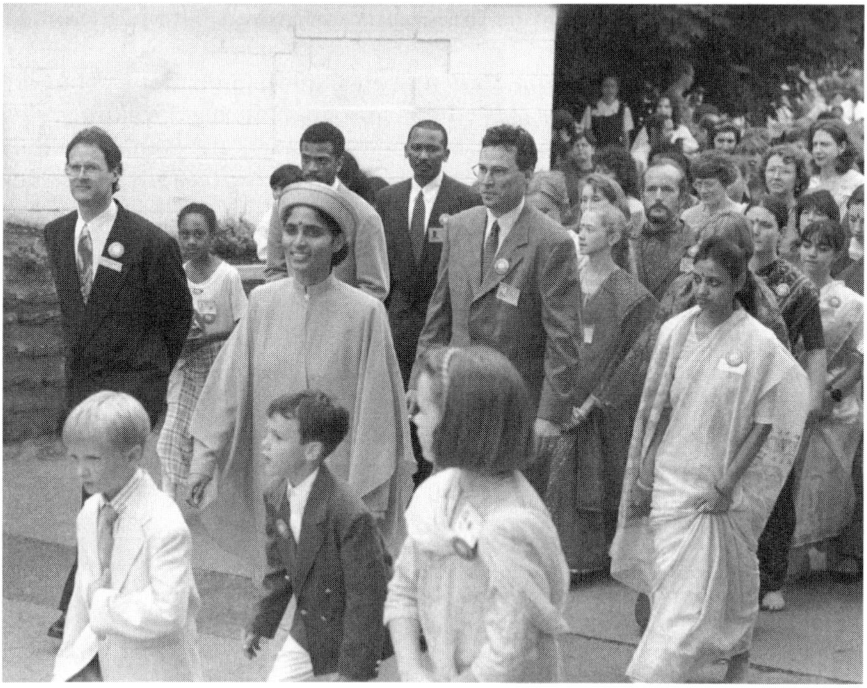

Fig. 21. Following a morning program in the Shakti Mandap, Gurumayi and some of her students on a walk on the grounds of Shree Muktananda Ashram; summer 1996

experienced in meditation—a vision he later described as a "vast field of blue light in my heart, out of which I heard this pulsating sound like "*Om, Om, Om.*"[318]

Each person's experience is profoundly subjective, many of them so ineffable that they can hardly be conveyed in words. Yet watching and listening to them, it is uncanny how their stories echo those told and written by previous generations of students—by Muktananda's and Nityananda's disciples. Despite differences of language, of culture, of time and place, certain fundamental experiences continue to characterize Siddha Yoga. The feeling of stillness, the awakening of tenderness, the bond of energy passing between guru and disciple, the tears that seem to come unbidden, signaling an inner opening or purification, the feeling of inner connection that remains despite physical distance—these are universal reactions to the reception of shaktipat at the hands of a siddha guru. In this sense, the history of Siddha Yoga is the history of millions of moments of connection between gurus and disciples, drawn together over miles and years and languages by the experience of the awakened *kuṇḍalinī,* and the inner bond of the heart.

Part 2
Theology

Chapter Two

The Siddha
Paradoxical Exemplar of Indian Spirituality

Paul E. Muller-Ortega

Samudre ca yathā toyaṃ
kṣīre kṣīraṃ ghṛte ghṛtam
bhinne kumbhe yathākāśas
tathātmā paramātmani

Just as water merges in the ocean,
milk in milk, ghee in ghee,
the space [inside the pot in the space outside] when a pot is broken,
so the individual soul [merges] in the universal soul

Gurugītā 162

UNDERSTANDING THE SIDDHA

The specific purpose of this essay is to inquire into what Swami Muktananda meant when he employed the term *siddha.* To one not familiar with the life and work of Swami Muktananda, it might not be immediately evident why one would inquire into such a topic. Muktananda gave the name "Siddha Yoga" to the spiritual teachings and practices that he brought to the world. He devoted his entire life to the discovery and revival of the specific practices and the deep, inner understandings of what may quite accurately be called the esoteric core of Indian spirituality. Such an esoteric core revolves around notions of human perfection and of possibilities of spiritual cultivation that are certainly ancient in India. Nevertheless, despite their ancient pedigree, by the early twentieth century such ideas and practices had fallen into obscurity and inaccessibility as far as the larger world was concerned. India has never been devoid of its enlightened saints and sages, but prior to Swami Muktananda, one would have been hard-pressed to discover living sources of shaktipat (Sanskrit, *śaktipāta*) initiation—and all that goes with it—who were willing to make this revelatory wisdom available in any widespread way. Swami Muktananda himself recounts his search throughout India for many years for the living spring of enlightened wisdom. This he finally found in the person of his teacher Bhagawan Nityananda, a twentieth-century exemplar of the figure of the siddha, the perfected human being.

It was the particular genius of Muktananda that even as he remained eminently faithful to the traditional spiritual teachings of India, he managed to make them accessible to modern practitioners by the sheer impact of his expressions. Such expressions revolved, in some large measure, around his unpacking of the notion of the siddha, the "perfected one." It is clear that if one wants to understand and delineate the particularities of Muktananda's contributions to modern spiritual practice, as well as to the history of religion and mysticism in the modern world, one must address oneself to his understandings of the notion of the siddha.

The following essay surveys and summarizes the essence of what Swami Muktananda had to say about this exemplar of Indian spirituality. This first section of the essay examines in a preliminary way the idea of the siddha and will propose the notion of enlightenment as crucial to Muktananda's understanding of the siddha. A second section will offer a specific example of the siddha in the figure of Bhagawan Nityananda. A third section offers a bird's-eye view of the historical traditions of the siddhas in India, especially highlighting those various siddha traditions with which Swami Muktananda was familiar. A next section offers a typology that argues for a spectrum of meanings in Muktananda's usage of the term *siddha*, as well as important variant meanings implicit in his usage of the expression *lineage of the siddhas*. This is followed by two final sections that attempt to lay bare the meanings of "perfection" and "spiritual enlightenment" that are implicit in the notion of the siddha. In these sections attention is given to the idea of the "path of the siddhas"; the ways of differentiating between the knowledge of the siddha and that of an ordinary person; and finally, interpretations of the various existential "gestures" of the siddha. In all, it is hoped that this essay will facilitate access by the reader to Swami Muktananda's clarification of the densely complex topic of Siddha Yoga.

It is well known that there have been many varieties of yoga taught in India. For example, one of the standard and venerable typologies found in the *Bhagavadgītā* divides the spiritual disciplines it teaches into the path of action (*karmayoga*), the path of devotion (*bhaktiyoga*), and the path of knowledge (*jñānayoga*). This early typology gives evidence of the varieties of yoga that were already present at the time of this early text. In addition, there are many other such typologies of yoga to be found in the texts and commentaries of the Indian tradition.[1]

It might be asked: What is the particular flavor or inflection inherent in the term *siddhayoga*? To inquire into the meaning of this term gives many clues as to the specific character of Swami Muktananda's understanding of yoga. The core of such a consideration must focus on the word *siddha*, which is clearly meant to indicate the particularity of spiritual discipline that is here at stake. In the term *siddhayoga*, the Sanskrit word *siddha* may be rendered in two different and equally significant ways. On one hand, *siddhayoga* means the yoga, the "spiritual discipline," of the siddhas, the "perfected ones." This rendering places the focus on the historical heritage from which the yoga has been received. On the other hand, it is just as correctly translated as the "perfected yoga." This rendering is intended to clarify the specific nature of such a form of spiritual practice. Though there are different inflections present in these two renderings, it is clear that by choosing "Siddha Yoga" as the name for the path of spirituality that he taught, Swami Muktananda meant to indicate its distinctive nature.

The idea of the siddha has a long and complex history in India that is only now beginning to be sorted out in very preliminary ways by historians of religion.[2] In order to understand the meaning of *siddha*, it is useful to explore some of this wider context. The term appears to have developed in specific environments in the Indian tradition that are predominantly Śaivite and Tantric in their orientation. What is particularly significant about the notion of the siddha is that it alludes to and draws together most—if not all!—of the major strands of Indian religion. Traces of these many strands of historical practice and belief are clearly present in Swami Muktananda's particular usage of the term *siddha*.

Thus, the primary focus of this essay will be to try to understand and describe what Muktananda meant by this term. In this sense, what follows is an attempt at sustained interpretation and reading of what Swami Muktananda put forward as the central value of Indian spirituality, the idea of human perfection. In such an enterprise, the Sanskrit meanings of the word *siddha* set the terms of inquiry. In Sanskrit, the word *siddha* means "perfected" or "that which has achieved an intrinsic perfection."[3] It implies a completion that culminates and terminates a long process of growth, development, or evolution; it is the successful fulfillment of a goal. Applied to a person, the term *siddha* denotes one who has achieved the highest perfection of which human life is capable, one who has completely unfolded the deepest or highest possibilities intrinsic to human existence. A siddha lives in a state of completion and perfection, of freedom and liberation experienced spontaneously, with ease, and total mastery. In response to a question, Swami Muktananda describes it in the following way:

> A Siddha's state is not something to just talk about, because it goes beyond words. A Siddha is one who has attained perfect freedom, who has become completely independent. One who has brought these inner senses and outer senses under his control is a Siddha. None of the senses can move him. His mind cannot be moved; it is always established in his own Self. He is completely absorbed in the bliss of the inner Self, and no one can separate him from that state. If someone has all these qualities, he is called a Siddha.[4]

At the outset, we can see that in this passage Muktananda is invoking the ineffability of what we seek to approach in this essay. His words echo the cautious provisos issued in so many traditions expressing the difficulties of capturing in words the subtle and mysterious flavor of the experience of the divine. Here, it is the experience of the one who has fully embodied perfection and freedom that proves similarly elusive and difficult to grasp. Moreover, Swami Muktananda seems to imply that the state of the siddha is not just a subject for idle discussion or intellectual conversation, for such discussion inevitably misses the point. Rather, he emphasizes that the siddha is the one who "is completely absorbed in the bliss of the inner Self."

Even more importantly, Muktananda's statement indicates that the state of being a siddha is not granted by outer circumstances of institutional allegiance or affiliation, or by the acquisition of institutional position or authority. Though there are siddhas in India who take this name by virtue of their adherence to a particular *sampradāya* or sect—members of the order of the Nātha siddhas constitute an important example—this is not what is meant here. What is being described is the experiential acquisition of a condition of perfection, an existential condition of freedom and perfection. *Therefore, for Swami Muktananda, an initial definition revolves around freedom, independence, autonomy, and total control over the senses. The siddha is established in the Self.*[5] When Muktananda speaks of the siddha, he is pointing at this inner accomplishment, this hard-won spiritual achievement that certainly cannot be granted by mere institutional decree. This is a crucial and primary distinction that must be kept in mind in all that follows. Swami Muktananda goes on to describe the state of mind of the siddha in the following terms:

> He lives in this body, but he is different from this body. He lives in this world, but he is different from this world. He lives among people, but even so he lives in a solitary way. Even though he performs actions, still he doesn't do anything. This is how a Siddha lives.[6]

Identified with the supreme consciousness, the siddha has a presence in the world that is both complex and profoundly paradoxical. The state of mind enjoyed by the siddha is conceived as the summit of human possibilities and, indeed, as the intersection of the human and the divine realms. Swami Muktananda continues his description, saying:

> The true Siddha has realized his own true nature through meditation and knowledge and has obliterated his ego and become one with the Universal Spirit. He unites with Shiva and becomes Shiva Himself. He is a true Siddha, a genuine Siddha. Such a Siddha was Ramakrishna, such a one was Sai Baba of Shirdi, and such a Siddha was Nityananda Baba; they all became one with Shiva and became Shiva.[7]

Here, knowledge that is acquired through meditation is indicated as central. Meditation can be broadly conceived and understood as the array of disciplines that lead beyond the limited ego to the knowledge of the absolute consciousness. This path of gnosis—which is also a path of devotion to God and of selfless service to God's creation—culminates in the obliteration of the limited sense of individuality or ego, and in union or merger with the universal Spirit. It is significant that Swami Muktananda—in referring to this absolute consciousness—here employs the name of the Hindu deity Śiva. This should not be misunderstood as a limited, sectarian connection, for Swami Muktananda's understanding of the notion of the siddha does not fit within such constricting religious boundaries. Evidence of this is his naming as siddhas in the same passage his guru, Bhagawan Nityananda; the nineteenth-century figure Ramakrishna;[8] and the early twentieth-century saint known as Shirdi Sai Baba,[9] all of whom confounded such sectarian identifications in their own lives and teachings. In addition, it must be noted that for Swami Muktananda, Śiva does not name one among many different Hindu deities but, rather, represents the supreme Deity or absolute consciousness to which, in his estimation, all the other names of Hindu deities equally refer. Nevertheless it must be noted that, from a historical vantage point, the various lineages that can be identified as siddha lineages seem to be preponderantly Śaivite in their orientation, vocabulary, and doctrines. We will later examine briefly some of the historical forebears of the mysterious and complex religious phenomena that comprise the traditions of the siddhas.

One of the most significant contributions of Swami Muktananda was his persistent attempt to clarify the figure of the siddha. It is by means of his teachings with regard to the siddha—teachings that might be said to pervade practically everything he ever said—that we gain an avenue of access and insight to a major phenomenon in Indian spirituality. It is true that the figure of the siddha has been little understood. Yet, by Swami Muktananda's own account, the siddha represents both one of the treasures and one of the deep mysteries of Indian thought and culture. We might begin by considering, for example, Muktananda's own depiction of one of the siddhas whom he met during his many travels in India. Muktananda says:

> Many are the ways of Siddhas. I knew a great Siddha, Zipruanna, who was always naked. He would lie on a heap of garbage. He ate whatever passersby gave him. Although he sat surrounded by filth, he was never affected by it. He saw only equality everywhere. He was always happy. Although he was in the body, he knew that he was totally different from it. He was an ecstatic Siddha.[10]

For one untutored in the images of Indian asceticism, this word-picture might prove a curious and, at first sight, even possibly alarming depiction of human perfection. What was it about this being that caused Swami Muktananda to call him a siddha? A naked person sitting on a garbage heap and surrounded by filth does not convey an initially appealing image. Yet it is clear that Muktananda was totally taken by this "ecstatic" being who "saw only equality everywhere." This fragment of narrative about a siddha whom Muktananda knew and loved allows us to see a siddha whose apparent eccentricity was based on the fact that he did not care about the world's ego-based and limited values. The siddha is an enlightened, ecstatic being for whom there has occurred a definitive overturning of the world's attachment and ignorance. Echoing the teachings of the *Bhagavadgītā*, Swami Muktananda would often emphasize that what is night for the ordinary person is day for the siddha who is awake in the Self, and that what is day for the ordinary person is considered the night of ignorance by the awakened yogi (Sanskrit, *yogī*). Herein we encounter a reversal of expectations that typifies the nature of the siddha. Zipruanna lived on a garbage heap, and yet Muktananda describes him as an ecstatic being. He says in another such description of Zipruanna:

> In the course of those wanderings, I ran into an unusual, naked saint named Zipruanna. He was very great. Although he appeared to be a fool to worldly minded fools, he was omniscient. He seemed a naked mendicant only to those who were spiritually naked, being without knowledge. However, he was the owner of a vast treasure of wisdom—a true millionaire. I loved him at first sight.[11]

This statement about Zipruanna is even more specific. It focuses on the wealth of knowledge that the saint possessed, calling him "omniscient," and "owner of a vast treasure of wisdom." Further, it hints that the ordinary person is not able to see the true reality of the saint by saying, "he appeared to be a fool to worldly minded fools." The siddha's virtue is obscured and concealed. It is not necessarily obvious at first sight, for it is the virtue of an absolute consciousness that is transcendent in its nature. Swami Muktananda continues his description of Zipruanna, saying:

> Zipruanna was omniscient. He had full knowledge of both past and future. He spoke in the Marāthi language, and his speech was simple and straightforward. In his village, he always roamed wherever and whenever he liked. If

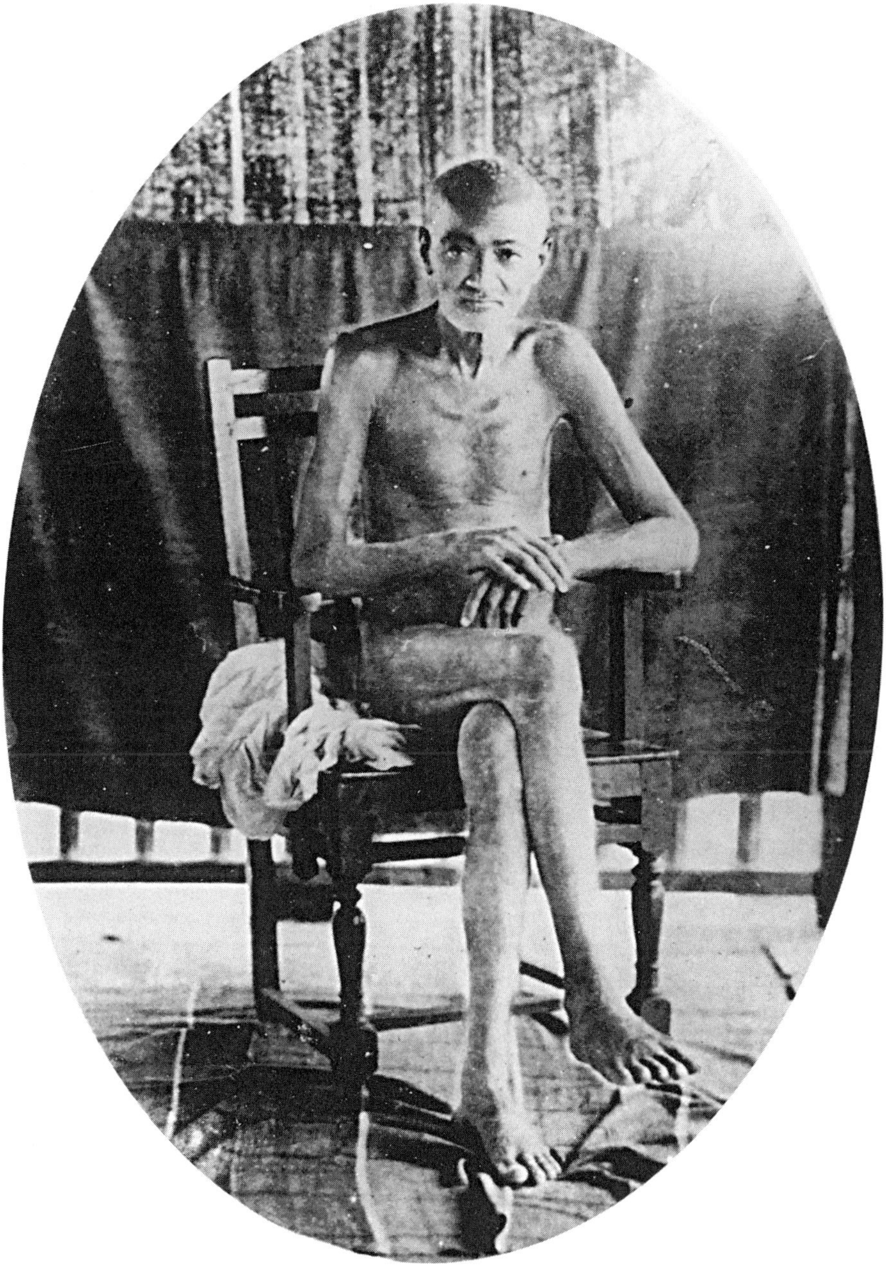

Fig. 22. Zipruanna in the village of Nasirabad in northern Maharashtra

anyone spoke to him, he would reply with only a few words. He was always ecstatic within himself. There were a large number of Hindus and Moslems in his village, and both groups respected him greatly. One has to be supremely fortunate to meet such a Siddha.[12]

One of the telling details in this passage is the statement that Zipruanna was respected by both Hindus and Muslims. We will return to this universality of appeal, which seems to be inherent to the siddha. In addition, he is praised again as an ecstatic siddha who knew the past and the future. It is abundantly evident that, despite the strange outer circumstances that this being lived in, what appealed to Swami Muktananda was derived from his understanding of the inner state of the siddha. It is also clear throughout this portrait that Muktananda loved this holy man greatly. From the first time he saw him, Muktananda recognized the perfection that was manifest in this naked saint, and he realized that he was "supremely fortunate" to be able to meet such a being. The descriptions of the siddhas that Swami Muktananda gives in his books, like these in *Secret of the Siddhas*, are compelling and challenging accounts. They present us with another face of wisdom, a guise for ultimate human perfection other than that which we might derive from most Western sources. It is by means of such statements that we are afforded a glimpse into a world that is very difficult to see, the world of the siddhas. Swami Muktananda describes many of these beings—Zipruanna, Sai Baba of Shirdi, Hari Giri Baba, Akalkot Swami, Siddharudha Swami, Ranchot Bapuji, Ranga Avadhut, and many others.[13] For example, in this brief narrative, he encapsulates the life of Hari Giri Baba, another eccentric and saintly being for whom he had great love:

There was another saint called Hari Giri Baba. I spent a good deal of time with him, too. He lived like a gentleman. He wore a turban of expensive silk with a gold border, an elegant coat, and costly shoes. He always roamed here and there, even at night. If anyone invited him for a meal, he would eat and then leave. His state was exceedingly strange. He talked to himself, and his speech was odd.

Most of the time, Hari Giri [Baba] wandered around a dry river bed. He would select tiny pebbles, talk to them, and stuff his pockets with them. Sometimes he would gaze off into the distance and scold. Occasionally he would talk to the wind. His was a curious state. Whenever I went through difficult times in my *sādhanā*, he would visit me. He would help me understand something and then leave immediately. He was a Siddha who knew the past, present and future.[14]

Again, we are faced with a portrait that is not, perhaps, immediately appealing. While this saint boasts a more elaborate sartorial presentation than the naked Zipruanna, we can still puzzle over the various forms of behavior that

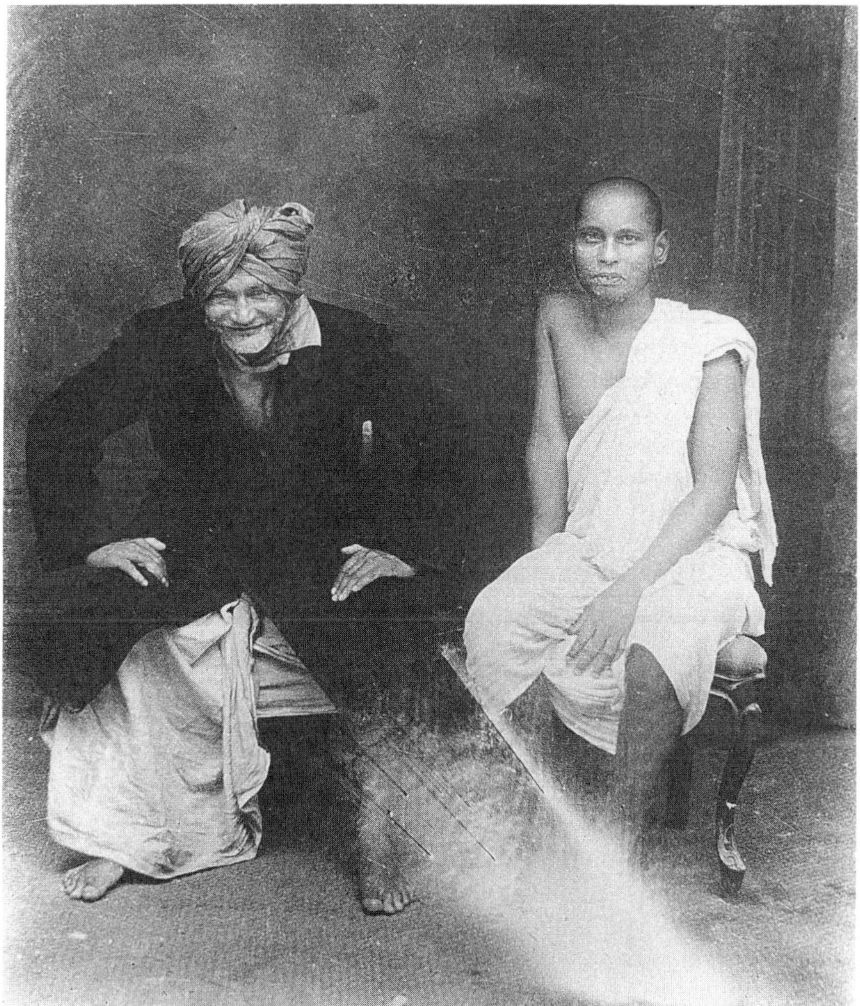

Fig. 23. Swami Muktananda with Hari Giri Baba in the village of Chalisgaon, 1953

are described: the pebbles, the talking to the wind, the strange demeanor that stares into the distance. Even Swami Muktananda allows that the speech of this saint was "odd" and that his state was "exceedingly strange" and "curious." Yet, this eccentric being would intercede at crucial moments in Swami Muktananda's spiritual journey, arriving unbidden to provide, in his own way, crucial secrets and potent clues that would serve to remove serious obstacles from Muktananda's path. Once again, it is abundantly clear that the rather level-headed Swami Muktananda loved and valued this being greatly.

Indian spirituality has long acknowledged that the dividing line between what the world would call madness, and what it might value as spiritual enlightenment, is thin indeed. The Sanskrit term *unmatta* can refer equally to those who are out of their minds because of some functional disorder or pathology and those who are "out of their minds" with the healing intoxication of spiritual bliss. It is not that these two domains are to be conflated or confused. In one case—that of madness—the individual is lost in pain and agitation. In the other case, the individuality of the person is lost in the bliss and wisdom of a transcendent merging. It is apparent that Swami Muktananda, a person of the most practical and orderly habits throughout his entire life, was not attracted by the pathologies of madness. Rather, in Zipruanna and Hari Giri Baba he recognized two siddhas—granted, of the more eccentric and exaggerated variety, but nonetheless siddhas—who were filled with love, wisdom, and an extraordinary and transforming power of spirituality.[15]

There is, consequently, a central question that must be addressed at this point: What is a siddha? What is it that makes a siddha a siddha? Clearly, in the above two cases, it was not the superficial eccentricity and convention-defying behavior that served as the true qualifications. If these expressions of individual personality have significance, it is only as symptoms of a deeper transformation. Moreover, not all siddhas fall into the category of those we have been terming eccentric in their outer demeanor. We find that there were many other beings whom Swami Muktananda called siddhas who were fairly conventional and apparently uneccentric in their behavior. Rather, it might be said that the true qualification of the siddha is that he dwells at the core of reality, at the very center of all being. The siddha is one who is stationed in the deepest point, at the center of the great *maṇḍala* of reality, merged with God, at one with the absolute. The siddha is the enlightened being who has reached the end of the path of liberation. Abiding as the living and embodied absolute consciousness, the siddha is the *jīvanmukta*, the "one who is liberated while still alive." The siddha has successfully carried out the ascent across the many "stages of yoga" (*yogabhūmikas*) to reach total enlightenment. The siddha has reached what is called *sahajasamādhi*, the "spontaneous, natural absorption" of total freedom. Here, the intrinsic "freedom" (*svātantrya*) of consciousness—which is the principal quality of the *śakti*, "divine power," according to Śaivism—has reached its supreme expression within human life.

Thus, the so-called "eccentricity" of the siddha can be understood quite differently. It is not merely the adoption of a particular mode of external behavior that makes one a siddha. The siddha abides and acts from a stance that is expressive of the viewpoint of the *jñānī*, the "one of knowledge," whose vision is profoundly nondual. In truth, one could reverse the argument and say that it is the ordinary person who might be seen as truly "eccentric," that is to say, absent from the center of things. The critique of the siddhas is that to live in the ordinary, unenlightened state is to be off center; it is to be in the superficial ego and so distort and filter everything from that limited and desire-filled perspective. It is for this reason that, from the uncentered perspective of the ordinary state, the actions and speech of the siddha, the one who swims in the all-pervasive consciousness of God, may seem to be eccentric or even mad. But as Swami Muktananda reminds us:

> You may call this state madness. O friend, correct your vision. Cure your own madness. Through the meditation and knowledge of the Siddhas, you will realize, "I was the one who was deluded."[16]

This powerful notion of a transformed vision will occupy our attention in what follows.

APPROACHING A SIDDHA: BHAGAWAN NITYANANDA

It seems appropriate at this juncture to present what is possibly the most important example of what Swami Muktananda meant by the word *siddha.* In his book *Secret of the Siddhas,* Muktananda gives a concise, inspired, and lovingly detailed portrait of his guru, Bhagawan Nityananda, as a siddha, a perfected being. It is evident that for him Bhagawan Nityananda was the preeminent siddha of Siddha Yoga. This portrait presents in a powerful way Swami Muktananda's own deepest understanding of who and what a *siddha* is. He writes:

> O Nityananda, you were perpetually bathed in bliss. Your name itself was bliss. When you laughed, joy and ecstasy burst forth from every pore of your body, as if your skin ripped open with the sudden onrush of your joy. You always spoke aphoristically. Although you might utter one brief word, it would contain as much meaning as a lengthy discourse. Sometimes you would remain silent for two or three days at a time. This is the extraordinary way of the Siddhas.[17]

This passage conveys the image of an amazing sage in the mode of the ancient traditions of India. In Swami Muktananda's description, we catch a glimpse of a being who dwells in perennial bliss. Like the descriptions of realized beings found in the religious literature of India, the first characteristic trait that Muktananda gives in this portrait is that of bliss. Nityananda is not described as a dour ascetic, though he was a very great renunciant. Rather, Muktananda chooses to place great emphasis on his guru's ecstasy: the state of perennial absorption in the bliss of consciousness that manifested as the "sudden onrush of joy." Commenting on the bliss of the siddhas, Muktananda says:

> Sometimes I used to come across great beings who kept laughing and laughing and laughing, and I would wonder, "Don't they get tired?" Now I understand why they are always laughing. They feel bliss and so they laugh, and then in the next moment they are in a new kind of bliss, so they have to laugh again. Because their bliss is ever-new, they have to keep laughing.[18]

In this portrait as well, we catch a glimpse of a *muni*, a "silent sage," absorbed in the contemplation of the bliss of the Self for days at a time, not needing to speak, but preferring to dwell in the inner fullness of bliss. Then, when the *muni* breaks his silence, it is not to pronounce long discourses: a single word is charged with the extraordinary weight of that fullness. Often, a single, aphoristic expression is sufficient to pierce the heart of the listener and to convey, in manifold ways, the message of the siddha. Swami Muktananda continues:

> O Nityananda, O Lord of *avadhūtas*, you had a dark body. Your belly was enlarged by the spontaneous retention of your breath. Although your eyes looked outward, your gaze was directed within. Your eyes were half-closed and shone like the morning sun. A smile always played upon your lips. Your hands were generous. When you walked, your gait was like that of an intoxicated elephant. You were a Siddha who stole everyone's mind.[19]

In the adoring gaze of the disciple—who had been completely transformed by his many years of contact with this siddha—the contemplation of the siddha guru presents a rich feast. We may rightly imagine that even as he penned this word-portrait, Swami Muktananda was inwardly gazing at his guru in memory, recalling the many such "sightings" or darshans (Sanskrit, *darśanas*) of the guru. Because the siddha is the embodiment of perfection, his body reveals the esoteric processes of yoga. As he gazed in this way, Muktananda found in his guru's physical form the signs and symptoms of his state of being an enlightened siddha. For Muktananda, the body of the siddha guru is like a book, and in this portrait he reads that text for us and transcribes its many yogic meanings.

In this passage, Swami Muktananda employs the term *avadhūta* to categorize his teacher. This term refers to the "shaking off" of all limitation, the "shaking off" of ignorance. Nityananda was not constrained or limited by an ordinary or conventional consciousness, and so in his physical appearance he had shaken off the constraining garments of clothing and was often dressed in a simple—and precariously loose—loincloth. However, it is not the outer garments that are particularly relevant here. The outer appearance of the siddha gives clues and signs to the inner state of such a being. Therefore, in Swami Muktananda's description of Nityananda as an *avadhūta*, the term resonates with the highest class of realized beings. It describes the siddha as one who has fully and completely shaken off the ties and limitations of ignorance, of karma, of the pull of the senses, of limited and false individuality, and of suffering. For Muktananda, the *avadhūta* Nityananda is the incarnation of freedom whose perfection radiates from his dark body.

Swami Muktananda sees much significance in the fact that Nityananda's body is dark: It is like the body of Kṛṣṇa or Śiva or, indeed, of Kālī. It is dark like the unfathomable void of the absolute, or like the spiritually illuminating darkness of the cave of the innermost heart. Such a darkness is, therefore, paradoxically illuminating. It shines with power. Moreover, Nityananda's body betrays the signs of his yogic state of perfection in another way: his enlarged belly. In traditional yoga, an enlarged belly has nothing to do with overindulgence in food, which in any event was not the case here, for Nityananda lived a spare and austere life. Rather, Nityananda's belly is swollen with the retained power of the breath. This is called *kumbhaka,* the spontaneous holding of the spiritual power that causes the body of a yogi to swell in this way.

The eyes, it is said, are the windows of the soul. Swami Muktananda lovingly describes his guru's eyes as shining "like the morning sun." Though the eyes of a siddha may be open, his gaze is always inwardly directed. He sees beyond both the world of physical forms and the subtle world of thoughts to the immense and deeply interior landscapes of the absolute consciousness. This is called the *śāmbhavīmudrā,* the "gesture of Śiva," in which the outer world and the inner world are both contemplated simultaneously. In such a gaze, it is the perception of *both* the inner and the outer world as absolute that predominates. Thus, the siddha is neither exclusively captivated by the limiting forms of the outer world nor is he exclusively given over to a state of meditative inwardness. Merging these two realms of being into one overarching perception of reality as the absolute consciousness, the siddha has transcended the polarity of inner and outer.

It is just such an enlightenment that causes a smile always to play upon the lips of the siddha. Such a smile is the genuine expression of freedom. It is neither socially manipulative nor the expression of a temporary levity or a

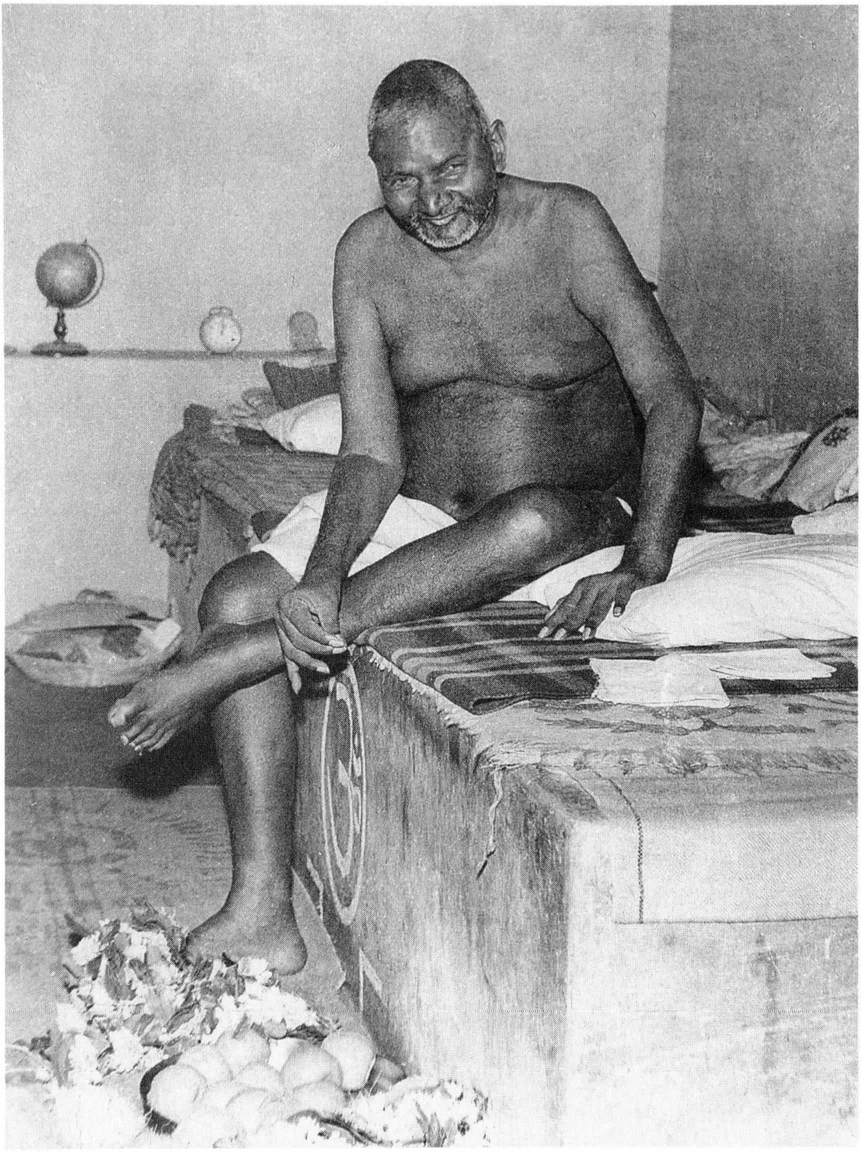

Fig. 24. Bhagawan Nityananda, in Kailas Bhavan, in Ganeshpuri village

passing state of pleasant good humor. Rather, it is the sign of the permanent bliss of the Self bubbling up continuously through the person of the siddha.

The siddha's hands are described as open wide—always ready to give, Swami Muktananda would always say. The generosity of the siddha is legendary for it is only such a being who can bestow what is considered to be the highest and most precious gift of all: enlightenment as the stabilized vision of the Self. Even in the gait of the siddha, there is manifested the intoxication of bliss, which is the result of continuously dwelling in the state of the Self. In his portrait, Muktananda confesses that the vision of the body of such a divine person, the body of an enlightened siddha, is captivating. It has a peculiar power to steal the minds of those who view it. What Swami Muktananda means here by "stealing the mind" is important to understand. He is not referring to some volitional act or cognitive control the siddha exerts on those who look at him. Rather, to gaze at the siddha is to have some of the siddha's inner state granted by a kind of divine contagion. This divine contagion enraptures the mind of the viewer and reveals a glimpse of the extraordinary bliss that is the siddha's constant state of experience. Swami Muktananda continues his portrait of his guru, saying:

> Sometimes when you closed your eyes, it would take you an hour or two to open them. Enjoying the natural state of a Siddha, at times you would sleep for hours on end, immersed in the ecstasy of your own Self. Although thousands of people came to see you, there was no noise; the atmosphere was hushed. You did not give lectures. Merely by seeing you, people would be consoled. You were the Lord of the Siddhas.[20]

Here is another fragment of the extraordinary picture of this rarest and most rarefied of beings, the siddha: not an orator or *paṇḍita* in the usual sense, not a ritualist or *brāhmaṇa* in the ordinary meaning of the word, the siddha is said to attract, teach, and uplift by the very fragrance of his being. Unconcerned with the world, immensely free, powerfully stabilized in the ultimate consciousness, the siddha abides in ecstasy. Immersed in the state of *samādhi,* he dwells in the eternal Self, even as his body continues to inhabit and illuminate this world.

It is interesting to imagine the scene alluded to here, a scene that was repeated again and again during the later years of Bhagawan Nityananda's life. For many years, thousands of people would make the pilgrimage to the small village of Ganeshpuri to have the darshan, the purifying and uplifting glimpse, of this rare being. In his presence, it is said, the perfumed and graceful breeze of spirituality wafted spontaneously into people's hearts, and their lives began to be transformed. The power of his presence was such that it evoked a spontaneous sensation of reverence, a sacredness, which was reflected in the hushed atmosphere that surrounded the siddha. Finally,

Swami Muktananda shares with us a few of the precious words that his siddha guru had spoken:

> O Nityananda, you used to say, "The Self is the Supreme Truth. There is nothing more sublime than the Self. Hey! The Self is within. Turn within." In this way, you taught with just a few words. For you, within and without were the same. You always dwelled within. What a great Siddha you were![21]

Here, finally, we receive the verbal message of the siddha. Condensed into a few brief words, the message announces the central themes of Indian spirituality. It points victoriously to the supremacy of the innermost consciousness. It urges the listener to taste the sublimity of the Self. It reveals the location of the Self as the deepest inwardness of being. And it gives the simplest yet most eloquent of commands, one that summarizes the path of the siddhas: "Turn within." In his comment on this phrase, Swami Muktananda elaborates, saying, "For you, within and without were the same." That is to say—and as we will see in detail later on—the Self, which was located at first in the deep inwardness of consciousness, later reveals to the siddha its paradoxical omnipresence. Because the siddha's experience is that of having become one with this inward and yet paradoxically omnipresent reality, Swami Muktananda is able to say, without fear of contradiction, "You always dwelled within." It is the perennial and conscious abiding in the Self that constitutes the greatness of the siddha.

In his spiritual autobiography, *Play of Consciousness*, Swami Muktananda adds to this portrait of Bhagawan Nityananda—a portrait he spent his life elaborating—saying:

> He was a perfect Siddha, one of the greatest Siddhas of Siddhaloka. The qualities of knowledge, yoga, devotion, and selfless action were perfectly blended in him. Though a yogi of great skill, he lived in a simple and ordinary way. He always lived in a thought-free state, as if his mind itself had become pure Consciousness. People knew Nityananda as a unique, ecstatic yogi. Although omniscient, he feigned ignorance. Everyone called him "Baba."[22]

For Swami Muktananda, this extraordinary exemplar completely embodied the true image and full understanding of what it meant to be a siddha. Though Muktananda had met many siddhas, it seems clear that for him none matched the illuminating power that he experienced in his guru. It is this power that he summarized in his statements about the nature and capacities of the guru, saying:

> On the Siddha Path, one needs a Guru who has been chosen by another Siddha of the true lineage of Siddhas. He must have complete knowledge and be proficient at transmitting energy and removing all obstacles. He should always be pure, simple, straightforward, capable of bestowing wisdom and making love flow. He must know that true Principle just as it is. He must have

> become one with That. He should be content with whatever comes to him and free of addictions. He must also be a master of diplomacy. One needs a Guru who can point out the path to attain the Self, but in addition one has to put forth self-effort.[23]

These words—like everything else Swami Muktananda ever said about the notion of the guru—are clearly born of his experience as a disciple of Bhagawan Nityananda. It is also interesting to note that it is probable that Bhagawan Nityananda did not apply the appellation "siddha" to himself. It seems to be a designation bestowed by his disciple as a retroactive identification of the true nature and condition of his guru. This is a curious and important fact because it matches historically the usage of this term in the Indian tradition. It seems to be the case that most often it has been the later tradition that has applied the nomenclature of "siddha" to earlier personages.[24] It tells us something about the nature of this term that it very often constituted a retroactive recognition, identification, and appropriation of an individual (or of a series of individuals) to this exalted status. In this process, we see Muktananda following established tradition by applying the name "siddha" not just to his guru but also to other historical personages within the Indian tradition for whom he deemed this appellation appropriate. Moreover, as we will see, the notion of the siddha became for Swami Muktananda a more universal category within which he also encompassed such figures as Moses, Jesus, and certain Western saints.

ON THE HISTORICAL BACKDROP OF THE SIDDHA TRADITIONS

As has already been mentioned, the historical backdrop of the siddha traditions in India is only now being sorted out in a preliminary way by historians of religion. The notion of the siddha appears to be a pan-Indian category that can be traced at least as far back as the fourth or fifth century. There are many traditions in India that have formulated notions of human perfection and developed them in the context of a terminology of the siddha. Certainly, one can look to the Śaivite traditions as they develop in many lineages in the north, particularly in Kashmir. Of particular interest here is the development of the Trika-Kaula synthesis, especially in the hands of the most famous exponent of Kashmiri Śaivism, Abhinavagupta.[25] In the south, especially in the Tamil region, there is the even earlier development of the tradition of the Sittars—also Śaivite in their orientation—associated particularly with a sage known as Tirumūlar, author of the classic work entitled the *Tirumandiram.*[26] There are also the important developments in the early traditions of the Maheśvara siddhas, devotional followers of Śiva who set the character of south Indian Śaivism.[27] In close association with the sacred mountain of Shri Shailam in Andhra Pradesh, there is the later evolution of the Vīraśaivas, founded by Basavaṇṇa.[28] The Nātha Yogīs, who elaborate esoteric teachings of *haṭhayoga*, develop in a widespread way in the north of India.[29] Central figures in this complex series of lineages are the teachers known as Matsyendranātha and Gorakhnātha. There are as well complex evolutions in the development of the alchemical siddhas of medieval India (Rasa or Raseśvara siddhas) who are very widespread but seem to be particularly strong in the western regions of India, especially Maharashtra.[30] There are also the lineages connected to the Paścimāmnāya ("Western Transmission"), Śāktas devoted to the goddess Kubjikā.[31] As well, there are numerous developments surrounding the later evolution of lineages of siddhas with a fervent devotional flavor in western India, particularly Maharashtra.[32] In addition, there are the important strains of Buddhist siddhas (especially as these develop in the region of Bengal), the Buddhist Tantrikas, Mahāsiddhas, and Siddhācāryas.[33] There are many other lineages.

This brief listing does no more than point to the complex and still very little studied chapters in the religious history of India that are the evolving traditions of the siddhas. What is most striking is that even if the historical complexities of these many disparate varieties of spiritual practice and teaching have not yet been fully sorted out from a historical point of view, it is still clear that the idea of the siddha—in various important inflections—is quite widespread. Seemingly, everywhere one looks in India from about the fifth century on, there are instances of a path leading to the condition of becoming a siddha. In all of these, the state of life enjoyed by the siddha is conceived—in a variety of different interpretations—as the summit of human perfection and as incarnating, in a paradoxical way, divinity in the human condition.

It is important to note, however, that while the ideology embodied in the term appears to be ancient, our capacity to trace the exact terminological usage of *siddha* from a historical vantage point in the Indian tradition is limited.[34] It appears to have developed, at the earliest, sometime in the fourth to seventh centuries, but the historically known traditions of the siddhas further evolve and take recognizable shape in the Tantric, Śaivite, alchemical, and *haṭha* yogic traditions during the seventh to thirteenth centuries. Moreover, it seems as if all of these traditions represent but one more "incarnation"—if that term can be used—of an ancient archetype in the Indian tradition: the enlightened being, the divinized being, the being who is the embodiment of a total wisdom, of a transcendent and supreme consciousness.

One of the earliest usages of the term *siddha* found in the religious literature of India points to a category of semi-divine beings who were givers of wisdom. Both in the *Yoga Sūtra* (usually dated to about the 4th century

C.E.), as well as in the commentary by Vyāsa, there occur references to siddhas of this sort.[35] By the evidence of this text, we can surmise that even at this period there was already a widespread cult of the worship of semi-divine beings known as siddhas[36] and that their worship was often associated with mountains. It might be noted that the connection of siddhas to mountains is important for the mountains often become places of pilgrimage, places where one may come into contact with the semi-divine siddhas and their transforming wisdom. It might be noted as well that the summits of mountains are associated with a mid-heaven or atmospheric domain, rather than with the highest possible heaven.[37] Gradually, this mountain-cult of semi-divine beings known as siddhas gave way to another concept: the notion that certain human beings may ascend to the state of a siddha by means of a series of religious practices differently elaborated in the various groups that compose the siddha traditions.

A reflection of the gradual evolution of various categories of siddhas, the classification encountered in the later tradition and used to distinguish between these two kinds of siddhas, is the notion of *ogha*, "stream." There are said to be three "streams" of siddhas.[38] The *divyaugha* refers to the "divine" siddhas who are at times identified as the supreme gods of Hinduism. Then there is the *siddhaugha*, the "perfected" stream, which corresponds to the early class of semi-divine beings associated with mountains. Finally, there is the *mānavaugha*, who are human beings who have ascended to the status of a siddha. As is often the case with many Indian typologies, this classification leaves room for ambiguity and uncertainty in its application. Nevertheless, its very existence indicates that there has occurred a shift in the meaning of the term *siddha* from naming a class of demigods to naming a class of human beings who have achieved the summit of spiritual liberation.[39]

One preliminary conclusion that might be drawn from all of this is that while there are numerous historical groups that appropriate the term *siddha* and employ it—each in its own distinctive way—it is also clear that even in these early environments the word *siddha* (and the ideologies and practices that cluster around the term) floated free of direct connection with any particular historical group. It began to function as a pervasive, descriptive category, often with quite varied meanings and connotations. This was certainly the case by the time Swami Muktananda appropriated and used the term *siddha.*

The important scholarly study of the traditions of the siddhas recently written by David White summarizes the array of historically known siddha traditions in the following way:

> As a proper noun, Siddha becomes a broad sectarian appellation, applying to devotees of Śiva in the Deccan (Maheśvara Siddhas), alchemists in Tamilnadu

> (Sittars), a group of early Buddhist tantrikas from Bengal (Mahāsiddhas, Siddhācāryas), the alchemists of medieval India (Rasa Siddhas) and most especially, a (generally) north Indian group known as the Nāth Siddhas. These latter two groups greatly overlapped one another, with many of the most important Nāth Siddhas—Gorakh, Matsyendra, Carpaṭī, Dattātreya, Nāgnāth, Ādināth and others—being the authors (if only by attribution) or transmitters of a wide array of revealed yogic and alchemical teachings. The medieval Nāth Siddhas and Rasa Siddhas further interacted with a third group. This was the Paścimāmnāya (Western Transmission), a Śākta sect devoted to the worship of the goddess Kubjikā which, based mainly in Nepal, also incorporated tantric, yogic, and alchemical elements into its doctrine and practice.[40]

From this survey, it is evident that the term *siddha* is applied in a historical sense to a wide array of geographically disparate and doctrinally differentiated groups. Commenting on this development of the siddha traditions, the distinguished historian of religions, Mircea Eliade, informs us:

> Hence we see that Sahajīyā tantrism (both Hindu and Buddhist), alchemy (Nāgārjuna, Carpaṭi), Haṭha Yoga (Gorakhnātha), and the Kāpālikas here coincide: their representatives are included in the lists both of the nine Nāthas and of the eighty-four Siddhas. This may perhaps give us the key to the symbolism of the Nāthas and Siddhas—at a certain point (probably between the seventh and eleventh century), a new "revelation" occurred, formulated by masters who no more claimed to be original than their predecessors had done (were they not "identified" with Śiva or with Vajrasattva?), but who had reinterpreted the timeless doctrines to conform to the needs of their day. One of the essential points of this new "revelation" was that it finally completed the synthesis among the elements of Vajrayāna and Śivaist tantrism, magic, alchemy, and Haṭha Yoga.[41]

Thus, what *is* known about the early groups of siddhas gives rise to the speculation that they have been a pervasive presence, a hidden and subtle presence, throughout Indian religious history, making important contributions to the philosophical, alchemical, and even medical traditions. Seen in this way, the siddhas constitute a presence that has revealed itself here and there, but that, it may be speculated, undoubtedly continued its existence many times far removed from the gaze of history. Moreover, the development of the historically identifiable lineages of the siddhas appears to take place in symbolic continuity with preexisting and more ancient formulations in India.

If we return to our initial point of departure—Swami Muktananda's usage of the term *siddha*—we find in it an important contrast. It is clear, at times, that Swami Muktananda is referring to the historical actions of actual siddhas, their teachings and writings, and so on. At other times, it is clear that he is employing the term *siddha* in ways that hearken back to its earliest usage and referring to what might be termed the transhistorical actions of siddhas inhabiting another realm called siddhaloka, the "world of the perfected ones." It is important to note that this contrastive usage is quite traditional and reflects ancient ambiguities and complexities, which, as we have seen, are present in the earliest usages of the term.

We have said that for Swami Muktananda, his guru, Bhagawan Nityananda, represented the preeminent example of the siddha. Nevertheless, if we scrutinize the published writings of Muktananda, we can see that there were many other siddhas whom he revered deeply. We encounter, for example, numerous references to the thirteenth-century Maharashtrian figure Jñāneśvar Mahārāj. Jñāneśvar was a Nātha siddha as is evidenced by the lineage of his gurus that he gives at the end of his masterly commentary on the *Bhagavadgītā,* the *Jñāneśvarī.* In one important passage, Jñāneśvar gives a narrative of the *paramparā,* the "inherited spiritual lineage," to which he belongs. He says:

> My Guru, Shri Nivrittinath, is so great that this writing is more the glory of his grace than my composition. I don't know when Lord Shiva communicated this wisdom to Parvati on the shore of the Milky Ocean, but it was found by Vishnu, who lay concealed within the womb of a fish in the waves of that ocean. On the Saptashringa mountain, Matsyendranath met the crippled Chaurangi, whose limbs at once became whole.
>
> Matsyendranath then conveyed this secret wisdom to Gorakshanath, who had a great desire to enjoy undisturbed contemplation. The great Matsyendranath enthroned Gorakshanath on the highest place of contemplation. Gorakshanath was like a lake of lotuses in the form of yoga and valiant in the destruction of sensual desires.
>
> Then Gorakshanath transmitted to Shri Gahininath the glory of the incomparable joy, with all its power, received from Shankara. When Gahininath saw that Kali was persecuting all creatures, he gave this command to Nivrittinath. This command has come down to us from Shankara, the great Guru, through the tradition of his disciples. You should take this and go quickly to relieve the distress of all those who are being vanquished by Kali.
>
> Now Shri Nivritti was compassionate by nature, and receiving this command from his Guru, he became like the clouds bursting with rain in the rainy season.[42]

In this passage, we can see the connection that the thirteenth-century Jñāneśvar claims to the famous founders of the Nātha siddha lineages. The names Matsyendranātha and Gorakṣanātha have accrued layers of legend that complicate their historical identification. Nevertheless, by mentioning these names of famous proponents of the *haṭhayoga* and Nātha siddhas, Jñāneśvar unmistakably situates himself as a member of an important and historically recognizable branch of the siddha lineage.[43] Swami Muktananda expresses his admiration for Jñāneśvar Mahārāj in very direct terms, saying:

> Jnaneshwar wrote his commentary not simply through the intellect but in the complete freedom of divine inspiration. Jnaneshwar's words seem to be the very words of the Lord. He has depicted the very heart of the Lord.
>
> Maharashtra has produced a large number of saints, both men and women, one more powerful than another, and these saints have come from all possible sections of society, from all classes. Though Jnaneshwar was the youngest of them all, yet he was the greatest. The oldest among them accepted Jnaneshwar as the king of knowledge. They all accepted his supremacy, and they sang his praises. Jnaneshwar's works are extremely fine. . . .
>
> During the period of my sadhana I was quite an avid reader. I had read so many works, and in none of them did I come across a satisfying description of the different stages of sadhana, the different spiritual experiences and visions that come to a seeker. It was only in the works of Jnaneshwar that I came across the perfect explanation of what had happened to me, a perfect description of all the visions. That was why I was so fascinated by him.[44]

By these words Swami Muktananda elaborated the primary reasons for his great admiration of Jñāneśvar: the recognition of a profound sympathy and affinity between his own experiences in sadhana (Sanskrit, *sādhana*) and that which is so carefully elaborated in the detailed expositions of this thirteenth-century text. It becomes evident that from a historical point of view, the figure of Jñāneśvar forms one of the most powerful links that Muktananda forges to the historical traditions of the siddhas, apart from his initiatory linkage through his own guru.

But Swami Muktananda revered many other siddhas in Maharashtra, including the figures of Tukārām Mahārāj, Eknāth, Nāmdev, and later, Shirdi Sai Baba. In addition, Muktananda was very fond of the sayings attributed to Kabīr[45] as well as being influenced by the traditions of Vīraśaivism originating with Basavaṇṇa, Allamaprabhu, and Akkamahādevī.[46] He was quite familiar with the connection of this tradition to the sacred mountain of Shri Shailam, a place he had visited where many siddhas are said to have carried out their practices, a place with ancient connections to the practice of alchemy.

Swami Muktananda was also well aware of the various traditions of Tamil Sittars, including such figures as Tirumūlar, Bhogar, and Agastya. He had visited, apparently more than once, the golden-domed temple of Palani in the south of India, which is located on top of a high hill and which also has ancient associations with many siddhas and with the practice of alchemy. In Maharashtra, Swami Muktananda knew about the cult of Dattātreya, a later synthetic deity who encompasses the traditional *trimūrti* of Hinduism and also has important links to siddha lineages.[47] It is also evident that in Muktananda's many travels around India, he had encountered the various lineages of the Nātha Yogīs and heard the many tales and legends associated with Gorakṣanātha and Matsyendranātha and the Nātha siddhas.

Beyond these many links to historical lineages of the siddhas, Muktananda retroactively attributed this term to many other figures of the Upaniṣadic tradition, from classical India and Purāṇic lore, as well as to figures in later Bhakti traditions. For example, in his spiritual autobiography, *Play of Consciousness,* he mentions many beings as belonging to the lineage of the siddhas:

> You do not know your ancestry, but when you visit Siddhaloka, you will gain a full knowledge of your lineage. In your family there is, first of all, the primordial Shiva, the wise, the blissful, the great Lord. Then there are Narada, the sage of the gods, and the great sage Vyasa. There are also Shesha, Shukadeva, Yajnavalkya, Kakabhushandi, Suta, Shaunaka, Shandilya, Bhishma, and King Janaka. There are the milkmaids of Vraja, who all attained perfection, and such kings as Prithu, Ambarisha, and Bharata.[48]

He continues, saying:

> Then there are countless other perfect beings, such as Prahlad, Dhruva, Sanaka, Hanuman, Akrura, Uddhava, Vidura, Sanjaya, Sudama, Kashyapa, Satapa, Prishni, Manu, Dasharatha, Kaushalya, and King Vibhishana. Belonging to our times are Sai Baba of Shirdi, my beloved Zipruanna of Nasirabad, and your Paramaguru, Bhagawan Shri Nityananda. In Siddhaloka there are millions and millions of Siddha yogis and yoginis to protect you. So do not falter or hesitate in any way, but stay firm and steadfast in the Siddhamarga, with absolute faith and devotion.[49]

In Swami Muktananda's understanding, the so-called "historical" siddhas exist in direct continuity with many other beings of the ancient Indian tradition for whom the term *siddha* might not have been employed in a strict historical sense but whom, nevertheless, he adjudged as fitting into the category of realized and perfected beings. As we survey this list of names, it seems clear that here Muktananda is employing the term *siddha* in a wider and more inclusive usage as a designation for practically all of the enlightened beings in the Indian religious and spiritual traditions. We will essay a typology of his usages of the term in what follows. We can conclude this section with a look at what one author has to say about the notion of the siddha. Keith Dowman, in his

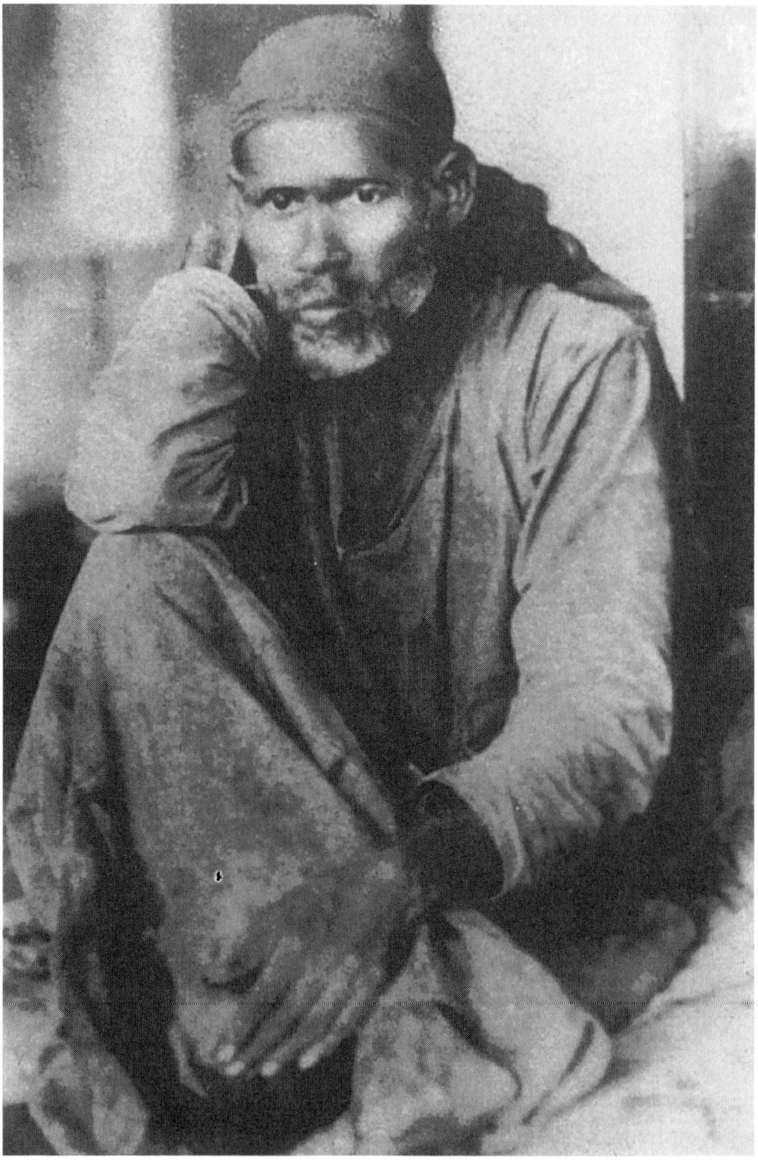

Fig. 25. Sai Baba of Shirdi

introduction to a book about the lives of the Mahāsiddhas in the Buddhist tradition, offers the following thoughts:

> Siddhas are practitioners of Tantra who are successful in attaining the goal of their meditation. This achievement is known as *siddhi*. It is twofold in that it confers both magical power (mundane) and enlightenment itself (supreme). The word "siddha" could be rendered "saint," "magus," "magician," or "adept." But even this is not sufficient, because "siddha" evokes an entire life style, a unique mode of being, and a very particular form of aspiration. For uninitiated Indians, the emphasis of their associations with siddhas is on magical power. If a yogin or yogini can walk through walls, fly in the sky, heal the sick, turn water into wine, levitate, read minds, they may gain the title "siddha." If those same practitioners have a crazy glint in their eyes, cover themselves in ashes, bring tears to the eyes with their songs, calm street mongrels by their very presence, induce faithful women to leave their families, wear vajras in the yard-long hair knots, eat out of a skull bowl, talk with birds, cry when they see spastic children, sleep with lepers, fearlessly upbraid powerful officials for moral laxity, or perform with conviction any act contrary to convention while demonstrating a "higher" reality, then they are doubly siddhas.
>
> However these are the popular notions of people who have no conception of the siddhas' spiritual and existential goal of mahamudra, which is Buddhahood. Of course, siddhas are also found working inconspicuously in offices, on farms, and in factories. A siddha may be a king, a monk, a servant, or a whore. The prefix "maha" means "great," "sublime," or "magnificent"; thus the mahasiddhas are the greatest of the most accomplished of the siddhas.[50]

These comments are illuminating and instructive as we attempt to understand what the notion of the siddha has meant in the wider ambit of Indian religion. It is true that from the perspective of the popular mind in Indian religious history, the siddha becomes identified with many forms of magic both benign and not so benign, with miracles and supernatural phenomena of all sorts, with healing and other types of divine interventions in human affairs, with alchemy and various other forms of esoteric arts, and perhaps most importantly with many categories of eccentric and unconventional speech and behavior. However, ultimately the reality of the siddha revolves around this most thoroughgoing and complete realization of freedom. This definition of freedom and enlightenment is so far distant from the usual presumptions and ordinary perspectives of human beings that it is considered to be quite difficult to grasp. Often, the traditions that taught these highest understandings of enlightenment did so in encoded, metaphorical, or veiled terms, and the understanding of the average person simply failed to penetrate to a proper assessment of the nature of the siddha.

SIDDHA: A TYPOLOGY OF MEANINGS

From this brief, initial survey of the notion of the siddha, we can discern initially three different if somewhat overlapping usages of the term *siddha.*

1) "Siddha" is a designation of affiliation to a particular and traceable historical lineage. In this sense, to be a siddha is to be a member of a particular initiatory lineage (or at least to claim to be a member of such a lineage). Here, the designation "siddha" does not denote a state of enlightenment and realization as much as it does an institutional connection granted by ritual entry and affiliation to a group. Certainly, the various groups called "siddhas" still recognized the achievement of enlightenment of some among their number and designated such beings as "siddhas," or indeed, "mahāsiddhas," that is to say, "great siddhas." As we have already mentioned, Swami Muktananda was not primarily interested in this purely institutional form of association, nor does he seem to have used the term *siddha* in this narrow, historical sense.

2) Connection to the siddha lineage is an initiatory affiliation, an inner and mystical linkage to a siddha guru. Here the term *siddha* denotes a much less institutional and much more inward and initiatory connection. To be called a "siddha" in this sense is to have asserted a claim of connection not just by virtue of institutional affiliation but by right of initiatory transmission and appropriation. It is a connection not just to a sociologically definable group but to a particular, individual siddha. It is also a connection that transmits not so much social identification of a quasi-familial sort but rather an ultimate identity of enlightenment.

There appear to be two elements in Swami Muktananda's use of the term *siddha* in this mode. One is clearly the designation of a particular state of completion of the spiritual journey: the abolition of the ego, the realization of oneness with Śiva, with the absolute consciousness. The other aspect of Muktananda's designation of the nature of the siddha is clearly initiatory and such an initiation must go beyond the merely superficial ritual of social integration into a group. The initiation in question must carry a profound existential and experiential impact.

For Swami Muktananda, it is impossible to become a siddha if one has not received the grace of a siddha master. One must belong to the "line" of the siddhas. Such a "belonging" is clearly established by an initiatory event that conveys the profound and powerful transmission of shaktipat. It is this which allows for the possibility of the completion of the spiritual journey. Says Muktananda:

> A true Siddha is he who receives the grace of a Siddha, who belongs to a line of Siddhas. As a result of that grace, he crosses all the stages of sadhana,

> mastering all the aspects of yoga which are described in the scriptures. He acquires full power. He has seen all that a yogi must see on the way to the highest perfection. He has experienced all that a yogi should experience during his spiritual journey.[51]

As Muktananda further emphasizes:

> What exactly is a Siddha? Is a Siddha a mere name, or does it denote a state of consciousness? Does Siddha denote a certain uniform, or does it refer to a certain state? You can never become a Siddha by yourself; you can become a Siddha only if another Siddha makes you a Siddha. Anyone who claims to be a Siddha can be tested with this question: "Who made you a Siddha?"[52]

It is this kind of initiatory impact of a profoundly transformative sort that transmits the core of what it means to be a siddha.

3) "Siddha" is a designation of affinity with a much larger group of enlightened beings as a result of having attained the state of the siddha, i.e., full enlightenment and realization. This final category most closely describes the deepest understanding of what Swami Muktananda means by the term *siddha.* In many ways, this does not constitute a separate category from the second one listed above. When Muktananda uses the term *siddha* in this sense, he does, however, extend the notion of the siddha to a wider ambit than that encompassed by any one particular, initiatory *paramparā.* A siddha is one who, having received the grace of a siddha guru, goes on to complete and perfect the highest state of enlightenment that is possible for a human being. Such a being may, in the final analysis, belong to *any* religious tradition—Eastern or Western. What is important to Muktananda in this regard is not the external or superficial details of cultural history but, finally, the state of consciousness.

The usage of the term *siddha* in this sense is coextensive with many of the other terms that have emerged in the course of the development of the Indian tradition to describe the one who abides in the state of enlightenment and perfection. The *jīvanmukta,* the "one who is liberated while still alive"; the *sādhu,* the "truly good person"; the disciplined *yogī*; the wise, all-seeing *ṛṣi*; the love-intoxicated *bhakta*; the knowledge-realizing *jñānī*; the awakened *buddha*; and many other such terms denote—each with their separate connotations—differing formulations and descriptions of one who lives in this most exalted of states of life.[53] We will further consider the meaning of this category in what follows.

A Typology of the Siddha Lineage

Before we do so, it might prove useful to attempt a similar analysis with regard to the notion of the lineage of the siddhas in terms of Swami

Muktananda's usages. Several different though interrelated meanings implicit in the notion of a lineage of siddhas appear in his usage. As we survey these meanings, it becomes apparent that this is a rather fluid category. Its differing levels of application function like a series of concentric circles, in which the most focused applications of the term expand continuously to give way to wider and wider usages. As we will see, there is a final sense in which the notion of the lineage of the siddhas seems to expand to encompass and appropriate all of the world's spiritual traditions and religious exemplars.

1) The siddha lineage is a "mystical" concept of connection to the primordial guru, Śiva. In this sense, the connection to the siddha lineage is one that occurs atemporally and even ahistorically. It is the assertion of a mystical and synchronic connection to Śiva as the fountainhead of all siddhas, a connection that occurs at every instant, both within and beyond time. In this sense, a true siddha experiences a direct linkage to the foundational source of the lineage, here understood or personified as the deity Śiva, symbolic of the absolute consciousness itself. Insofar as the absolute consciousness is present as the most intimate reality of a person's innermost being, that consciousness may manifest forms of connection directly to itself. This may occur by means of initiation in dreams, visions, the spontaneous evolution of spiritual experiences, and, in general, the autonomous evolution of consciousness unmediated by outer links of any sort. This direct and mystical link forms the most intimate meaning of the notion of "lineage." It is an inheritance of wisdom, power, and authority received directly from the ultimate source and unmediated by other, more usual forms of lineage. One of the famous accounts of initiation in a dream that Swami Muktananda used to tell involved the figure of Tukārām. He says:

> There was a great saint in Maharashtra named Tukaram; he received initiation in a dream from a being who had come from siddhaloka, the world of perfected beings. In one of his poems Tukaram says that though the supreme guru is master of the universe, he makes a tiny house, as tiny as a sesame seed, and lives in that. That tiny house is like a dot, like a *bindu*, and a meditator is able to see the forms of many gods and goddesses, many deities, appearing and disappearing within that dot, within that house. Tukaram says that though the bindu appears to be so tiny, it holds in its belly all the three worlds of the macrocosm and the three worlds of the microcosm—the worlds of waking, dream, and deep sleep. These, too, are held in the belly of that tiny bindu. All this exists in every person and that is why I say that a human being is very, very great.[54]

Beyond asserting the possibility of *authentic* initiation being received in a dream, that is to say from within one's own consciousness, this passage asserts the primacy of consciousness as symbolized in the image of the *bindu.*

The Sanskrit term *bindu,* which means something like a "drop" or a "point," is used to represent the inherent presence of the totality or the absolute consciousness within the individual. The *bindu* functions as an inherent inner source of revelatory wisdom, which may arise in many forms from within. The Kashmiri tradition talks of this possibility in terms of a person who is initiated directly by means of the *śakti* or inherent power of his or her very own consciousness. When such a being reaches the state of complete realization, he or she is termed in the tradition, *saṃsiddhika,* "self-perfected."[55]

On the other hand, the "outer" links may manifest because the siddhas who dwell in siddhaloka, the "world of the siddhas," may "descend" to initiate the individual at any time. The siddhas in siddhaloka are all around at all times. There is no limitation to the possibility of initiation by the siddhas in this sense. Therefore, it is considered to be the case that all the siddhas ultimately dwell in this direct and unmediated form of "lineage," whatever other sources of lineage connection might or might not apparently be there. This crucial notion "solves" the apparent contradiction between Swami Muktananda's statement that all siddhas are made to be siddhas by another siddha, and Bhagawan Nityananda's apparent lack of a physical guru figure. As we will see, Muktananda spoke of his own guru as a *janmasiddha,* that is to say, "one who is born enlightened," usually by virtue of practice performed in a previous life, and who therefore spontaneously regains or reassumes a state of embodied enlightenment in this life. While such figures are considered to be extremely rare, such a siddha enjoys this state of direct and apparently unmediated connection to the ultimate source of lineage, which is the absolute consciousness itself. Such figures are often instrumental in the revival of historical lineages, and such was certainly the case with Bhagawan Nityananda, whose life initiated a profound expression of the siddha lineage in the modern period.

2) The concept of the siddha lineage is a connection to the paramparā *of Bhagawan Nityananda: Nityananda as the preeminent siddha of Siddha Yoga.* It is clear that for Swami Muktananda the preeminent and most direct initiatory route present in his own life is that of his own connection to his teacher, Bhagawan Nityananda. Though seemingly not employing the *terminology* of siddhahood, Bhagawan Nityananda served as the direct and most proximate mediating source of both spiritual power and spiritual experience in Muktananda's life. Hence, the evolution of the *paramparā* of Siddha Yoga, from a recent and historical perspective, traces itself back to find its source in this extraordinary figure.

3) A wider context encompasses a series of lineages, present in different periods of time and in different geographical locales, all identifying themselves as siddhas. However, as we have seen, Swami Muktananda did not exclude other beings, either contemporary to himself or in the historical past, from belonging to the category of siddha, especially in the sense of perfectly enlightened beings. Muktananda seems to have been aware of a number of these, and to have come into contact with representatives or descendants of many of these individuals and the groups or organizations they may have brought into being. It is important that he gave a place of respect, honor, and recognition to such individuals even as he reserved the primary place of honor for his own teacher.

4) A yet wider context encompasses practically all of the traditions of Hindu spirituality and all of the venerated figures within these traditions and retroactively labels and attaches them to the siddha lineage. Often in his writings, it is clear that Swami Muktananda is bestowing the retroactive appellation of "siddha" (either in the sense of someone who belongs to a siddha lineage in the historical sense, or in the sense of someone who has reached the "state" of a siddha, or, in some cases, both meanings at once) to figures in Indian religious history who neither employed the designation for themselves or their teaching or who would not have accepted such a designation for a variety of reasons. The long passage from *Play of Consciousness* previously quoted gives many such examples.

5) The widest of the expanding circles moves out of Hinduism to assert that venerated figures in the spirituality of Islam, Buddhism, Jainism, Christianity, and, indeed, in practically every known historical spiritual tradition are in some way intrinsically connected or identified with the siddha lineage. This is a very important and also, perhaps, controversial level of identification. It essentially sets up the siddhas as a kind of meta-lineage. It then adduces the notion of an intrinsic and supreme current of spirituality and revelatory wisdom that has manifested in different ways in many different times and places. Such a current is conceived as preserving an unbroken connection with a single meta-tradition that then bears the appellation of the "siddhas." Here, the notion of lineage breaks down in any historical sense and implies, rather, that each of these traditions contains at its core an indefinable essence that connects and identifies it with the siddha "lineage." In some way, this last category thus reverts to the first category above. It propounds the notion that at the center of every authentic spiritual and religious tradition, there have existed individuals who might be termed "siddha," that is to say, "perfected, enlightened and complete." Such individuals—existing in a direct and unmediated "lineage," that is to say, existing in enlightened, conscious connection to the absolute consciousness—are able by virtue of such connection to have served as founders, impellers, revivers, and otherwise creators of historical lineages of spiritual teaching of various sorts. For example, Swami Muktananda would say:

> This is the new lotion which is applied to your eyes. No matter what religion a Siddha comes from—whether he has been a Sufi, a Muslim, or a Hindu—he is in the same state which transcends all man-made traditions and religions.[56]

In many ways, this is a recognizably "perennialist" and "universalist" move on the part of Swami Muktananda.[57] It seems apparent from his own internal logic that he finds himself both compelled and spontaneously moved to make this identification. In this way, Muktananda asserts his recognition of affinity and even identity with countless figures in the history of human spirituality. It must be noted that such a declaration of affinity and of recognition does not necessarily encompass the more exoteric religious traditions founded by such individuals or their followers. Rather, it asserts a "higher" order of congruence (and even of identity) with the intrinsic state of the individuals themselves as perceptible signs of their siddhahood appear in their writings or the narratives of their lives.

By the time of Swami Muktananda's early wanderings around India, it was evident that the concept of the siddha had become a pervasive classificatory category, not so much related to traceable lineages as it was to the declaration of someone belonging to this classificatory category by virtue of his or her having attained a certain state of being, a state of enlightenment. To assert that someone is a siddha becomes a transhistorical identification that need not be limited to its presence or expression in India alone. It therefore becomes a cross-cultural category of recognition of the state of the siddha, of the siddha's state of consciousness. For Swami Muktananda, such a recognition gives rise to a retroactive declaration of connection with a large array of beings. By universalizing the category to be highly inclusive of all enlightened beings both in the Indian tradition and elsewhere, it becomes a metacategory in the sense that we are describing here. At times, Swami Muktananda seems to indicate that if there is a relationship to "place," such a place is located on another plane of being; it includes all of the siddhas who dwell in siddhaloka.

It is only in this sense of the siddha as a transhistorical category that there is a universalizing and retroactive declaration of connection. The notion of the siddha thus becomes a highly inclusive descriptive category that embraces all beings who have been adjudged to have achieved enlightenment. Swami Muktananda seems to use it as a pervasive, classificatory category that is grounded in the transhistorical and mystical without in any way denying the reality of the historical lines of differentiation. He asserts the existence and the primacy of the category as a cosmic affinity group, a relationship of beings who are seen to have in common what could be called the "state" of the siddha—a particularly exalted conception of ultimate enlightenment and liberation—rather than any particular sectarian affiliation to an actual historical lineage. Further, this vision understands the variety of historical lineages of siddhas (in this widest sense) that have appeared as expressive of and supported by an invisible and larger cosmic connection or cosmic relationship: siddhas coming from siddhaloka and appearing at different historical moments to act and teach. Thus, it might be said that their wide-reaching affinity is not, in the first instance, one that is established by historically documentable and visible interactions. Rather, it is primarily undergirded by a cosmic connection to an original source, whether symbolized as a deity (Śiva), a place (siddhaloka), or a philosophical principle (Brahman, the absolute consciousness). Though Muktananda was aware of and respected historical siddha lineages—he himself had a hand in founding one—what was at stake for him was finally not a historical recognition or adjudication of connection to an historical lineage. It was about the siddha's own capacity to "recognize" other siddhas. Such a capacity is itself an expression and a function of the siddha's own state of enlightenment and expanded vision of reality. Indeed, it is finally *only* from such a state that a warrant of connection to the "siddha lineage" (in its deepest sense) has ultimate validity for Muktananda. Nevertheless, each such siddha can (at least potentially) be seen to establish with authenticity an historical "branch" of the siddha lineage, of this invisible and transhistorical lineage. For Swami Muktananda, both of these were crucially important.

A Typology of Siddhas Derived from Swami Muktananda's Interpretations

In one of his earliest statements about these matters, Swami Muktananda himself offered a classification or typology of the different kinds of siddhas. He tells us that there are essentially three kinds: *janmasiddhas*, *kṛpāsiddhas*, and *sādhanasiddhas*. Muktananda says:

> Siddhas are mainly of three types: (1) *janma* Siddhas are those who are born as Siddhas, (2) *kripa* Siddhas are those who obtain Siddhahood through grace, and (3) *sadhana* Siddhas are those who become Siddhas as a result of their own *sadhana*.[58]

About *janmasiddhas* he says:

> Those who have practiced *sadhana* in many previous lifetimes and complete it in this life without the help of a Guru are called *janma* Siddhas. In their former life, such individuals were not able to completely give up their identification with *jivahood* (individuality) and hence, could not entirely realize their Shivahood. In this life, they take up *sadhana* on their own without a Guru and become Siddhas. It is certain, however, that they must have had a Guru in their previous life. They resume *sadhana* in this life from whatever point they left it in their past life. They manifest *siddhis* at a very early age, for example, whatever they say comes true and they are able to foretell events. Sai Baba of

> Shirdi and Nityananda Baba were Siddhas of this type. *Siddhis* reside in such great beings right from their birth, but they are not even aware of them. Their *siddhis* work for them in a natural way without any effort on their part. In spite of having great powers, they act according to the will of God. Such *janma* Siddhas complete their *sadhana* without any effort on their part. Shakti Herself ensures that they complete it. Those saints who attained perfection after receiving mantra initiation in a dream also belong to the class of *janma* siddhas.[59]

At other times, Muktananda would include in this category Akalkot Swami, saying that Nityananda, Sai Baba, and Akalkot Swami, all *janmasiddhas*, were "the great Siddhas of the modern age."[60] It is evident that by elaborating this category, Swami Muktananda is accounting for those who would appear as perfected beings without seeming to have received initiation or made efforts at sadhana, spiritual practice, under the direction of a teacher. About *kṛpāsiddhas*, he says:

> Those who attain Siddhahood as a result of an inner awakening by the grace of a Siddha Guru are known as *kripa* Siddhas. . . .
>
> Later, they have the same powers as *janma* Siddhas including the ability to bestow grace on others. One who becomes a Siddha by receiving a mantra from a Guru also belongs to this class of Siddhas.[61]

About *sādhanasiddhas*, Muktananda says:

> Those who become Siddhas after practicing yoga and doing *sadhana* are known as *sadhana* Siddhas.[62]

Swami Muktananda concludes, saying:

> A *janma* Siddha has had a Guru in his past life and his *sadhana* proceeds automatically in this life. A *kripa* Siddha receives the Guru's grace and attains liberation without any strenuous effort.
>
> They are known as Siddha incarnations who come to this earth from Siddhaloka with a message from God or who come to fulfill a special mission. They may remain here till the end of the cycle. They are unaffected by pleasure or pain and they have infinite powers, but they cannot be called incarnations of God. [63]

This interesting classification not only goes toward solving several problems alluded to above, it also shows that Muktananda was attempting to grapple with the notion of the siddha in a creative and comprehensive fashion, drawing upon his own life experience in these matters—which was extensive—as well as from the traditional textual and scriptural sources.

For Swami Muktananda, the path of the siddhas is the *mahāyoga*, the "great" and spontaneous yoga, the extremely secret knowledge that allows entry into the innermost Self. It is this wisdom that, after so many years of searching all over India, he felt he had received from his preceptor and guide, Bhagawan Nityananda. Muktananda understood this path to be universal in its scope and all-encompassing in its outlook. For him, the path of the siddhas is the supremely subtle wisdom that reveals the most elusive and unique knowledge about the secrets of consciousness, the secrets of the most intimate being. The path of the siddhas reveals a sequence of insights that take place by a progressively deeper absorption into the great Heart, and so it progressively reveals the vision of nonduality.

This path has many elements as described by Swami Muktananda. Perhaps most centrally, it is understood to be a path of grace. It is by receiving *kṛpā*, the grace of his guru, that Muktananda experienced that the spontaneous and great yoga had been impelled within him. He defines it succinctly by saying:

> As I have already said many times, in Siddha Vidyā, *gurukripā hi kevalam gurorājñā hi kevalam,* "Only the Guru's grace, only the Guru's command."[64]

So the path of spontaneous *mahāyoga* is initiated by the reception of shaktipat initiation. Nevertheless, because this great yoga is considered to be the essential or root element of all such paths of yoga, it has many and various characteristics. First of all, it might be described as a path of reversion, of return. The individual soul returns to its own source in the Self. In this process, there occurs a spontaneous renunciation of the attachments and desires implicit in the mind and senses, as the Self is progressively discovered to be an arena of bliss, freedom, and fulfillment. Central on this path is the figure of the guru from whom the initiatory impulse is received. Because of this, the path described by Swami Muktananda can be termed a path of *gurubhakti,* a path of "devotion to the guru." In this context, there is a complex play between the figure of the outer, physical guru and the guru as the deepest impulse of liberating wisdom that is found in the innermost Self.

It might be said, then, that this path is one that discovers and uncovers the experience of the absolute consciousness, the great Self; it is a path of enlightenment and liberation, a path of transcendence of suffering, a path of the blissful dwelling in the absolute Self. In addition, it is very beautifully described by Swami Muktananda as a path of love, of supreme devotion (*parabhakti*)—a visionary, ecstatic path in which the deepest impulses of love, ecstasy, and devotion that are present in a human being are cultivated and brought forward into full manifestation in life. This path might also be described as a reversive path, one that reverses the flow of attention from the outer to the inner, that reverses the ordinary conceptions of this world; a topsy-turvy, against-the-grain path; an unexpected path that discovers a royal road where we would ordinarily not expect a path; a path of the extraordinary and astonishing. All of these elements are clearly present in

Muktananda's many descriptions of the spiritual discipline that he brought to the world. He says:

> Whatever anyone may say or think about me, I take great interest in my Guru. My love for him has become an addiction. That Siddha gave me one word which completely transformed me, but I had to spend such a long time with him to receive it. That word which I received after so many years spread through my body from head to toe like wildfire carried by the wind. It produced in me both inner heat and the coolness of joy.
>
> Before meeting my Guru, I had practiced many different kinds of yoga, but it was I who had practiced them. However, that word activated a spontaneous yoga within me. I was filled with amazement. What postures, *mudrās,* and breathing processes! Everything happened on its own. After attaining divine realization, I understood my compassionate Guru. [65]

For Swami Muktananda, the *siddhamārga,* the "pathway to perfection," is the supreme secret of existence. It is this path that, because of the impulse of grace of the guru, discloses and reveals the deepest secrets of human existence and puts a human being face to face with God, the consummate theophany, the vision of the Supreme. This highly secret path of the siddhas is considered to be eternal. For Swami Muktananda, there is the confidence that there has always existed this avenue of God's supernal compassion. For him, such a path exists eternally outside of time as the perfect and continuous expression of the grace of the siddhas. He always said it was an ancient path as well, though he recognized that we lose sight of it in the furthest reaches of recorded history. In a most consistent way, when asked to disclose the source of the *siddhamārga,* Swami Muktananda always named the figure of Śiva, or Paramaśiva, the supreme Śiva. In his mind, the path of the siddhas is allied with the command of the supreme deity Śiva. It is called the *Śiva-śāsana,* the "command of Śiva," the final and complete instruction that is given by Lord Śiva about the absolute consciousness. In a compelling passage, Muktananda says:

> Lord Shiva is the source of Guruhood. . . . [A]ll deities, sages, and seers have addressed Lord Shankara as the Guru of the entire world, the Lord of yogis, and the Guru of Gurus. The supreme knowledge of Siddha Yoga first manifested from the effulgence of Shiva and the form of Shakti, the supreme energy. It arose from the body of Uma Kumari, God's power of will. . . . For this reason, without the grace of yogini Kundalini, the great Shakti, the supreme state is difficult to attain. This Shakti of the *maha* yoga is the basis of everything. She is Consciousness.
>
> The *Maha Yoga Vijnana,* a great text of Siddha Yoga, explains how the Siddha Yoga lineage originates with Parashiva and was passed on to Lord Narayana, who assumed the form of a yogi and taught Siddha Yoga to all the sages.[66]

It is in this way that Swami Muktananda understood this path of the siddhas to be a supreme distillation of truth, fashioned by the fundamental intelligence of the absolute consciousness, and then arising in the insights and visions of the first sages. It was these original sages who then understood that what they unfolded within themselves as a vision of a path to the Supreme was revealed to them by the primordial Guru, by Śiva, the supreme teacher who fashioned the venerable, authentic, and potent path of enlightenment. In order to expound this understanding, Muktananda says:

> Siddha Yoga takes no interest in differences. It does not argue about bigotry or cults. In Siddha Yoga, there is no room for cultism. Siddha Yoga is the same as it was thousands of years ago at the creation of the universe. Then there were yogis and great sages who had transcended their minds, and Siddha Yoga was born from their arduous *sādhanā* and ultimate perfection. Siddha Yoga is the teaching of those great beings who had fully attained the Truth and who had become one with Paramashiva, the all-pervasive Consciousness and the Supreme Guru. This field of knowledge is beyond human ambition, beyond the mind and imagination. It is a venerable path to the realization of Truth. We follow it seeking the supreme love of our own inner Consciousness.[67]

It is this path which, in the estimation of Swami Muktananda, reveals that which is uncommon, paradoxical, and of difficult access. This is the reality of the Self, the absolute consciousness, the nature of which seems to run against the commonsense perspective of the ordinary world. Because it is a reality that is located beyond the limited mind and ego, its nature runs against the grain of what the ego wants, of what the senses and their desires continuously prompt the individual to do, of the consolations that the body-mind in its usual condition is always seeking. Such a path gives rise to a new mode of knowledge, a deep gnosis or insightful illumination of the nature of existence. It is to an examination of this notion of enlightenment that we now turn in some detail.

SIDDHA AND *SIDDHI*

It is precisely out of the paradoxical and seemingly contradictory nature of the absolute consciousness that the Indian philosophical tradition has always invoked, under a variety of names, what might be called a perspectival understanding of knowledge. In this context, it might be asked: What is the perspective of the siddhas, and how does it differ from that of the ordinary person? The contrast between these two perspectives is significant and instructive. In philosophical terms, this contrast stipulates an essential epistemological differential, which centers precisely on the achievement of the siddha: the state of enlightenment. How can this be understood? How does the siddha perceive reality and know things? What is the state of the knowledge and perception that the siddha has of himself, of others, and of the world?

It is in response to such queries of an epistemological sort that the Indian tradition invokes two different perspectives or conditions of knowledge, or what might be called epistemological perspectives.[68] On one hand, there is the ordinary perspective of the world, which considers differences, separation, and finiteness as the intrinsic realities of individual experience. This is called the "worldly" or "ordinary" (*laukika, vyavahārika, saṃvṛtti*) perspective. On the other hand, there is the perspective of the siddha who has seen through the surface differences and distinctions of existence and located the fundamental reality of consciousness as the true being of all things. This is called the "unworldly" (*alaukika*) viewpoint of the *jñānī*s, the "knowers of the truth." It might also be termed the "point of view of supreme truth" (*paramārthasatya*), or the *śivadṛṣṭi*, the "vision or viewpoint of Śiva." The tradition says that a person who has not made any efforts toward spirituality or the deeper understanding of reality is *laukika*, "worldly." Everything in such a person's awareness is filtered exclusively through his own limited ego, her sense of separateness, his desires. The understanding of such a person is narrowly focused on his or her sense of dilemma, of crisis, of suffering. For the *laukika* being, life is a problem that refuses to be solved. From the viewpoint of the *jñānī*, the "knower of reality," the *laukika*, "worldly," perspective is seen as ignorance.

What is the viewpoint of the *jñānī*? It might be said that the answer to this question is one of the wellsprings of Indian philosophy. For it is precisely in the attempt to transcribe the ineffable experience of the *jñānī* into words that the variety of philosophical positions in Indian thought arise. Hindu, Jaina, and Buddhist traditions each articulate a variety of different perspectives on the wisdom of the absolute. It is therefore important to note that strictly speaking there are various and competing answers to the question: What is the viewpoint of the *jñānī*? With this proviso in mind, it is possible to sketch in general terms what the Hindu nondual traditions have to say about the viewpoint of the *jñānī* in the following way. This world with all of its phenomena is the manifestation of a deeper, totally blissful, all-pervading and absolute consciousness. This ultimate consciousness dwells within everything and everyone as their inherent reality and perfection. The *jñānī* refuses to accept the ordinary viewpoint, which sees only the forms and shapes and limited experiences of this world as real. If the *laukika* being is focused on the ever-changing surface waves of the ocean, by contrast the *jñānī* cares only about the vast and eternal ocean itself. The shapes and forms of the waves come and go, but the ocean always remains the same.

Swami Muktananda elaborated on these two perspectives by telling a traditional story.

> The following story makes an important point: Once there lived a crow king and an owl king. Both had many companions. They lived with their friends in the same forest on their respective trees. One day they met, and the crow asked, "Why do you work at night?" The owl protested, "O Brother, it is you who works at night." This began a long, heated argument. As they argued, the day wore on and became night. The owl said, "O King of crows, now it is day." The crow replied, "No, brother it is night." Then they began to fight in earnest.
>
> At that point, a swan arrived and said, "Don't fight. You are both right. What is day for a crow is night for an owl. What is day for an owl is night for a crow."
>
> In the same way, an ignorant person's day of sense pleasures and possessions is night for a Siddha and is to be renounced. What is day for a Siddha—his awareness of the Self of all, the knowledge of "I am That," and the understanding of the all-pervasive light of bliss—is night for an ignorant person. Turn your night into day. Muktananda says, "Then Siddha Yoga is filled with ecstasy and joy."[69]

The *jñānīs*, the enlightened siddhas, teach nonduality (*advayavāda*) and refuse to accept as valid the distinctions and differences so valued from the worldly perspective. Rather, what is ultimately real is the unitary and unbreakable wholeness of divine consciousness, the domain of bliss beyond space and time, beyond limited individuality, beyond suffering. This is the *alaukika*, "non-worldly," nature of the path. For Muktananda, as we have seen, the core of this path revolves around the figure of the guru, the one who lives continuously ensconced in this enlightened perspective of the siddha. Using the metaphor of alchemy, such a being is likened to the philosopher's stone, which is capable of turning base metal into gold. That is to say, the guru is capable of bestowing his own state of enlightenment, his own perspective of knowledge of the absolute consciousness, to others. Says Muktananda:

> The Self, or *ātman*, of the Guru never changes in its perfection. Whoever merges with the Guru becomes one with his Self, and that Self does not become diminished, severed, warped, deteriorated, or even increased. Always remaining in the same changeless, irreversible state, the Guru transforms his disciples just as the philosopher's stone turns iron into gold. Like a magnet, he activates the divine Shakti lying inert in his disciples. And like the holy waters of the Ganges, he makes his disciples as pure as he is and thereby makes his disciples' disciples perfect like himself. Thus, one who is identical with Lord Shiva in every way, who has imparted to other spiritual aspirants the

> divine Shakti by which they can bring their disciples to perfection, and who is thoroughly capable of giving the divine authority of *gurupad* (mastership) to others, is alone Shri Guru. He is the transmitter of the *mantravīrya* (essence of mantra) to his disciples. There is not the slightest difference between the Guru and Lord Shiva.[70]

It is precisely because of the differential in perspectives of knowledge between the *laukika* and *alaukika* conditions of knowing that the tradition has always indicated its expectation that someone who is completely caught in a *laukika* perspective would not understand much about the reality of the great Self, the unbounded consciousness beyond space and time. The essence of the path elaborated by the siddhas is not really of interest to the world. It remains concealed and hidden because it is subtle and because the ordinary perspective of the *laukika* point of view cannot appreciate this subtlety.

To become a siddha, then, is to shift from one perspective to another by walking a path of great subtlety. Implicit within the notion of the siddha is the idea of a journey of mystical ascent, a movement from the ordinary state of waking consciousness—dominated by the limited perspective of the ego—toward the progressive reappropriation and expansive recognition of the divine Self. The siddha is one who has completed this most extraordinary of journeys and has thus relinquished forever the illusions and limitations of the ordinary and narrow ego-sense. Muktananda says:

> O friend, as waves are in water, fragrance in camphor, and brilliance in jewels, so a Siddha dwells in supreme unity. As warp and woof are inseparable from cloth, as clay is inseparable from pots, so a Siddha is entirely one with God. A Siddha yogi who has attained complete knowledge of That remains inseparably immersed in Consciousness; he is the Self of the universe. Perceiving only consciousness, he knows the seer as it is. Through his awareness of the Self in all objects, he knows the true nature of the seen.[71]

In this passage, Swami Muktananda articulates the core of the siddha's vision of reality: "Through his awareness of the Self in all objects, he knows the true nature of the seen." Traditionally, in India such perfected beings were considered to dwell in a paradoxical state of existence. To understand such a state, to understand the condition of the siddha, it is necessary to look into the state of perfection that the siddha is held to have achieved. Such perfection does not simply maximize the conceivable range of strictly *human* possibilities that might be imagined to exist within any given person. Rather, the perfection lived by the siddha grows out of discovering, unfolding, and stabilizing a condition of inner divinity. The siddha's perfection is grounded in the unfolding of the inherent autonomy and power of the ultimate consciousness. It is this divine and absolute consciousness that is thought to abide as the deepest reality beneath the relativities of human existence. The successful and complete unfolding of the total range of possibilities intrinsic to this ultimate and divine consciousness leads to the state of the siddha, the state of the perfected or enlightened one. Moreover, it leads to the achievement of a permanent state of identification with the ultimate reality, with the supreme creative potency from which the universe itself is said to have arisen. Describing this condition, Swami Muktananda says:

> A Siddha has this continual awareness: "That conscious Being is ancient. He is both unmanifest and manifest. I am controlled by the Supreme Power, and I am the controller as well. That Supreme Power is beginningless, indestructible, and fearless. It is both the support and that which is supported. I am self-born and exist in all forms as the inner Self. I am also beyond everything. I am new as well as old. I am the void as well as the whole. I am both large and small. I am every existing thing." This is the statement of the Siddhas.[72]

There is another, central meaning of the term *siddha.* A siddha is one who is possessed of *siddhis*, that is to say, one who has developed "supernatural capacities" of various sorts. In the traditional Yogic and Tantric literature of India, these *siddhis* are enumerated at great length. The practicing yogi in the *Yoga Sūtra,* for example, aspires—as one aspect of the practice put forward in this text—to achieve a variety of *vibhūtis*, "supernatural attainments": clairaudience, clairvoyance, telepathy, levitation, the ability to overcome hunger and thirst, the capacity to manipulate matter, to create a mind-made body, and many others.[73] In the later literature of the Tantric and *haṭha* yogic traditions, this list of *siddhis*—literally "attainments"—is expanded to include a variety of alchemical powers and capacities, focusing most centrally on the ability to transform the physical body from a state of mortality to a condition of physical immortality.[74]

In most of these traditions, however, it is simultaneously acknowledged that the development of such supernatural capacities, while forming a subordinate or secondary part of the yogic path, does not constitute the ultimate purpose or fulfillment of the mystical path of Yoga. There is, thus, a perceivable tension between the focus on the achievement of these supernatural capacities, which are generally thought of as epiphenomena or byproducts of the path of Yoga, and a higher focus on the ultimate goal. For this reason, there evolves in many of these traditions a distinction between these secondary *siddhis* and a supreme *siddhi,* supreme accomplishment. This is the so-called *parama-siddhi,* the "accomplishment of the intrinsic perfection" abiding as a perennial potentiality within all human beings.[75]

Swami Muktananda illustrates this focus on the supreme *siddhi* by telling a story of what happened to him when he dabbled in the lower or secondary *siddhis*:

When I was doing sadhana, I came across a person who was teaching *riddhis* and *siddhis*—how to attain supernatural power, so I studied under him for a while. He had the power to materialize a train or bus ticket. Of course, it was a fake ticket. He could also tear a piece of paper and it would become a five rupee bill—for five hours. Afterward, it changed back into plain paper. He could transport a piece of apple from one place to another. Or if someone had something in his pocket, he could transfer that object into somebody else's pocket. So I studied these things under him. It was all fake, it was phony. It wasn't God's grace, it was just a mediocre skill. It meant nothing.

Having learned all these tricks from this person, I went to see my Baba [Bhagawan Nityananda]. The moment I entered my Baba's place, he took out a long stick and began to scold me. He said, "You thief, you traitor, you rogue! What are you doing here? Get out of here!" I fled.

After I ran away, I began to think about it. He called me a thief? He called me a traitor? I never stole anything. I never betrayed anybody. Why did he say that? I just couldn't understand why he would say such a thing about me.

Again I peeked in because I really wanted to go inside to be with him. He got the stick out again, and he said, "You unworthy fool! Get out of here."

I went out and I began to think about it. I hadn't done anything like that. Why would he say such a thing about me? I was really upset; I felt that my heart was going to burst if he was going to be like that with me.

But my right understanding told me it did not matter what he did. The Guru's anger, the Guru's curse, the Guru's blessing—they are all the same, they are nothing but a bestowal of grace.

So I gathered myself and with great courage I went inside again. He had already thrown the long cane in my direction, so it wasn't close enough for him to reach. But he still had one more—a little one—and he hit me very hard with that, "Will you ever do that again?" He hit me so hard you can't even imagine.

With great humility, I said to him, "I don't understand what mistake I made."

"Didn't you learn those phony supernatural powers?" he said.

"Oh, yes." Then I promised, "Never again, never again."

He said, "In your entire life, will you ever use those supernatural powers? Will you ever try to fool others with those phony powers?"

And I said, "No."

Then he told me, "He is a sadhu, he is a holy being, who is totally absorbed in his own Self, totally immersed in his sadhana."[76]

This story is quite crucial in that it assists us in making the distinction between the kind of siddha who might be interested exclusively or primarily in the development of these secondary supernatural capacities, and the type of siddha who is focused exclusively or primarily on the highest spiritual goals.

The terms of discourse about this supreme *siddhi* are not couched in the language of power understood in any usual sense or even in a supernatural sense.[77] As Bhagawan Nityananda says in the above passage, "He is a sadhu, he is a holy being, who is totally absorbed in his own Self, totally immersed in his sadhana." The supreme *siddhi* does not revolve around the capacity to manipulate objects within space and time, or even around the capacity to deploy the body or the senses in a variety of extraordinary ways. The kind of power that is involved is the supreme and subtlest power of the ultimate consciousness itself. This supreme *siddhi* denotes the accomplishment of a truly extraordinary and even transcendent goal. It is the achievement, the unfoldment, the realization of the total range of the absolute consciousness. It is the achievement of that condition of consciousness that stands free beyond space and time; beyond the range of the senses; beyond the intellect, ego, or mind. The supreme *siddhi* is the discovery of the domain of perfection and totality, the domain of divinity, as the secret possibility of life that exists latently within all human beings. It is, as can be seen from what has previously been said, what makes a siddha a siddha.

This is a crucial point. So often the siddhas have been understood primarily or even exclusively in terms of their capacity to perform miracles and to display these secondary, albeit extraordinary, powers that are seemingly at their disposal. For example, it is well attested that the vast majority of persons who approached Bhagawan Nityananda during his lifetime did so seeking to witness this kind of extraordinary display or to receive this form of miraculous intercession of the siddha. They came seeking cures, solutions to worldly problems surrounding illness, work, marriage, the birth of children, money, politics, and so on. In the Indian tradition, the siddha is often seen as the living, wish-fulfilling tree, and many times these spiritually sensationalistic or outright worldly desires appear to have been in some way fulfilled. It is evident that such fulfillment only served to redouble the fame of the siddha as a saint; as a miracle worker; as an interceder with the divine; as a solver of karmic dilemmas; as a magician adept at the manipulation of nature, the elements, the senses, and more.

What is important in all of this is that because of the glamour and allure of the secondary *siddhis*, the primary and supreme "accomplishment" of the siddha remains obscured or at least partially veiled. The story narrated by Swami Muktananda shows that, at least in his case, his guru was completely intent both on preserving him from the distractions and perils inherent in the deployment of spiritual powers for worldly ends and was further intent on bestowing on him the full brunt and power of the revelatory, primary, and supreme *siddhi*.

In many places Swami Muktananda describes the profound experiential and revelatory impact that the reception of this primary *siddhi* had on him. Having received the initiatory force of this *siddhi* from his guru, a series of yogic repercussions began to occur. At one point, Muktananda comments on this, saying:

> After the awakening of the Shakti, this process of yogic movements began to take place within my entire body. What power the word had! I almost hesitate to write all of this. It revealed whatever was within me—in my heart and in my head. I saw my own double many times. In the *sahasrāra* at the crown of the head, I perceived the brilliance of a thousand suns. I also saw the Blue Being. Sometimes I would lose myself within; then I would regain consciousness. It was like a play, similar to that of the waking and dreaming states. Even now, I do not know where I lose my small self and from where it returns. It is so amusing—I lose myself, then find myself. I have seen the center of true joy; there I lose myself and from there I return. I am ecstatic! I have found the best place of all, right within myself.[78]

This description reveals in graphic detail the power of the supreme *siddhi.* Having received the initiatory stroke of his guru's enlightenment encapsulated in the form of the mantra, a series of yogic experiences of the highest sort begin spontaneously to unfold within him. Within the notion of the supreme *siddhi* there is implicit the discovery of the methods and mechanisms by which individual awareness is led to the supreme realization. The individual awareness is usually identified with the physical body and the limited range of a mind dominated almost entirely by the perceptions of the senses and by thoughts. The supreme *siddhi* is the mechanism that impels this ultimate realization that leads to the state of the siddha. It reveals the possibility of unfolding that individual consciousness so that its core reality is laid bare, so that its innermost essence is activated and made to live and breathe within a particular human being who is then called a siddha. In this sense, the supreme *siddhi* is both that which leads to such an enlightenment as well as the living state of enlightenment itself. Therefore, the mechanism of shaktipat[79] and its transformative consequences embody what is here being termed the supreme *siddhi.* Because of such an accomplished realization, the siddha stands triumphantly free of all limitation and is established in the domain of fullness, perfection, and the transcendent power of consciousness. This is described by Swami Muktananda in the following terms:

> "I am a Siddha and exist everywhere equally. I am filled with Consciousness." Through God's grace and his one-pointed devotion, a Siddha truly knows this. He is also aware that he is the knowledge of the experience of the Self. Just as an ignorant person naturally identifies himself with the body, a Siddha fully experiences himself as the embodiment of bliss. A Siddha lives in total freedom.[80]

Therefore, the siddha is not held by the pull of the senses, is not conditioned by the ever-changing states of the body, and is not identified with a limited and contracted ego. Rather, the siddha paradoxically incarnates within the human condition the freedom of the transcendent consciousness and the power of the realm of divine reality. Describing this condition Muktananda says:

> Such a blessed *sādhaka* loses his individuality. Initially, he perceived the world as full of misery and hardship and as a place of transient enjoyments. But when transformed by the practice of *japa yoga* [mantra repetition], he has the experience that, being one with the Guru, he is ageless and immortal. To him the universe now appears to be a paradise, and the world, the Sadguru, and all fellow beings look benign like Shiva. In the vast garden of the Universe, he proclaims, "I am Shiva," for, indeed, he has become Shiva. He neither loves nor hates, because for him all likes and dislikes have become Shiva, and the universe has become the form of Shiva. With the worshipful knowledge of the universe as Lord Shiva, he cheerfully fulfills his remaining *prārabdha* [karma]. . . . Just as one who is on the ocean sees nothing except water on all sides, similarly a *japa yogi*, devoid of the feeling of mine and yours, interior and exterior, higher and lower, sees only his own Self everywhere.[81]

It is precisely in this highest sense that Swami Muktananda employed and understood the notion of the siddha. His selection of the designation "Siddha Yoga" to denote the path of yogic practice and unfoldment that leads to the exalted goal of the state of the siddha was not arbitrary or casual. It was an intentional statement of the enormous—even limitless—possibilities that he considered to be inherent within all human beings and which could be made experientially and existentially available by means of the knowledge and path he was bringing to the world. It was as well a deliberate identification with one of the most esoteric and venerated as well as one of the least known and understood currents in the ambit of Indian spirituality.

THE ENLIGHTENMENT OF THE SIDDHA

It might be said that the ideology of the siddha we receive from Swami Muktananda's writings recapitulates and embodies each of the differing versions of liberation and enlightenment described in the various traditions of India. It is important to understand that each of these descriptions of what constitutes liberation or enlightenment—sometimes (though not exclusively) termed *mokṣa*—derives from a philosophical or doctrinal system that either explicitly or implicitly holds a view about the nature of the ultimate reality or purpose to be sought by that system.

For example, the early traditions of classical Yoga and Sāṃkhya define the fundamental reality in terms of a dyad of *puruṣa* and *prakṛti*. *Puruṣa* is the ultimate consciousness that resides within human beings as the possibility of freedom and as the silent witness of all actions. *Prakṛti* is the source of all material reality. These two principles, though essentially separate from one another, have somehow combined to give rise to the reality of human existence. For the traditions of classical Yoga and Sāṃkhya, the purpose of the system is to elaborate a pathway to the liberation of the *puruṣa* from its seeming entrapment in the folds of *prakṛti.* This goal is given the name *kaivalya,* which may be rendered both as "isolation" or "aloneness," as well as more interpretively, "unitive consciousness."[82]

Without entering into the complexities of this particular philosophical system, it is important to note that in this system the ultimate reality is realized as being completely separate from ordinary reality. Because these two early systems of Indian philosophy are quite influential, one of the fundamental notions about liberation that develops in the Indian tradition defines the ultimate goal as a progressive, systematic, and thoroughgoing *transcendence* of the ordinary reality. The path of yoga that develops out of these traditions emphasizes a radical meditational process of going beyond every form of identification with what is not the *puruṣa.*

This movement of transcendence is equally present in the early teachings of the Upaniṣads, which speak of the universal Self (Ātman) as dwelling beyond the individual self. This universal Self is regarded as identical with a cosmic, absolute Being (Brahman). The path that develops out of the Upaniṣads emphasizes both transcendence and renunciation. There grows out of this tradition the spiritual ideal of the *tyāgin* or *sannyāsin,* the "renunciant" who is liberated from any desires, attachments, or motives toward action.[83] In both of these examples, the one who has reached the ultimate goal functions as an embodiment of this absolute transcendence, impersonality, freedom, and separateness of that absolute as present *within* the conditions of relative existence—thus, the paradox of the siddha's existence.

In a parallel way, in traditions that focus on a theistic ideal of devotion to and union with a personally defined deity, the image of ultimate realization that develops is one in which the realized being takes on—quasi avatar-like—the qualities of that deity. For the followers of Kṛṣṇa, the supreme goal involves a merger in the deity Kṛṣṇa, and an identification with the roles, moods, attributes, and functions of Kṛṣṇa as theologically defined.[84]

There are, as well, the Buddhist traditions in which a *nirvāṇic* abolition of the illusion of a separate self is sought. From these there grows the very ancient concept of *nirvāṇa* as elaborated in early Buddhism, which presents a paradigmatic image of the liberated being who—though still dwelling in a body—has in fact transcended and shattered all forms of limitation and individuality.[85] Other formulations are found in early Jainism and its concept of the *kaivalya* or isolation of the spirit (*jīva*) from all traces of materiality.

The Jaina traditions teach that the physically binding power of karma must be dissolved through extreme acts of the repudiation of all forms of action.[86] All of these ideas form the core of the early Indian formulation of an "ultimate human goal or purpose" (*paramārtha*). In each case, what appears as the nature of the absolute—as philosophically or doctrinally described in each system—clearly *determines* the nature of the descriptions of liberation and enlightenment.

As the notion of the siddha evolved historically—as a potent and many times free-floating symbolism in the Indian tradition—it gathered up to itself all of these various definitions and prescriptions of the fully realized being. The siddha is the one who comes to embody and to fulfill each of these differing and already existent ideals that describe the nature of the realized being. The siddha becomes a paradoxical being: he embodies the conjunction of the absolute and relative; he is the master of space and time, free and possessionless yet the emperor of the universe. Swami Muktananda describes it in the following way:

> The state of the Siddha is beyond both knowing and not knowing. In that state, bliss is embraced with bliss. Joy is experienced through joy. Success is gained through success. Light dwells within light. Shaivism says that the stages of yoga are filled with amazing phenomena. [*Śiva Sūtras*, 1-12] In that state, astonishment drowns in astonishment. All dos and don'ts are silenced. Rest attains total rest. Experience delights in experience. The state of the Siddha is the attainment of total perfection. Siddhas are like this. O friend, read this very carefully.[87]

Even a brief survey of what many of these traditions teach demonstrates that there exist numerous variations in the details describing the exact nature of this ultimate goal and how it is to be achieved. For example, one argument that divided early forms of Śaivism centered on whether the ultimate liberation is achievable only at the time of death (*videhamukti*: "disembodied perfection") or can be achieved while still subject to the limitations of physical embodiment (*jīvanmukti*).[88]

Further discussions center on the nature of the afterlife state of liberation. The more austere traditions of the Vedānta, for example, describe it in terms of the impersonal Brahman, the qualityless, limitless, and indescribable objective absolute. Other traditions imagine the state of liberation in terms of some kind of transcendent heavenly realm: the Vaikuntha of the Vaiṣṇava traditions is a deliberate critique of the disembodied, "impersonalist" notions of ultimate liberation of the Vedānta. Similar to this (but with different inflections that seem to combine aspects of both) is Swami Muktananda's description of siddhaloka as a world of transcendent ecstasy and bliss where all liberated beings who have become siddhas are said to dwell. Other notions that developed in the later alchemical siddha traditions have to do with the achievement of an immortalized physical body (as taught by the Nātha siddha traditions attributed to Gorakṣanātha), as opposed to those traditions that seek the achievement of an ethereal spiritualized body of enlightenment (as represented by the Vīraśaiva saint Allamaprabhu). In all of these cases, the notions of *videhamukti* and *jīvanmukti* have varying meanings. It is very clear that for Swami Muktananda, the siddha represents an extremely important example of the *jīvanmukta*, the "one who is liberated while still alive."

At the same time, in his many teachings, Muktananda emphasizes the location that he calls siddhaloka, the world of the siddhas:

> There are many, many of your predecessors living in Siddhaloka. All Siddhas—from the supremely perfect primordial Lord Shiva and the Seven Sages, to the innumerable Siddha seers who have appeared since the earliest time—live in Siddhaloka possessing all their powers. They grant you Shakti, activate your yoga sadhana, and are always ready to protect you, to obtain what you need and preserve what you already have. You should not feel that you are the student of your Guru alone. You are a true descendant of the line of the inhabitants of Siddhaloka.[89]

Swami Muktananda describes his own meditational visits to this plane of siddhaloka in his spiritual autobiography. He says:

> One day [the blue pearl] took me far away, and set me down in the most beautiful world, the most entrancing of all those I had seen. I cannot describe its beauty, for words would be an insult to it. In this world I came upon a fascinating path, and, following it, I saw many woods, caves both large and small, flowing streams of pure water, white, blue, and green deer, and also some white peacocks. The atmosphere was very calm and peaceful, and there was a beautiful blue light everywhere, such as you would see if you looked at the early morning sun through a piece of blue glass. There was no sun or moon, only light spreading everywhere. When I arrived I felt such strong waves and impulses of Shakti that I knew intuitively that I was going to have the *darshan* of the ancient seers. I started to move around with the speed of thought. And then what? This was Siddhaloka, the world of the Siddhas! I saw many Siddhas, all of them deeply absorbed in meditation. Each one was in a different *mudrā*. None of them looked at me. Some had long, matted hair, some were clean-shaven, and some had pierced ears. Some were sitting under trees, some were sitting on stone, and some were inside caves. I also saw the great seers I had read about in the Puranas. I saw Sai Baba of Shirdi. Though Nityananda Baba was in Ganeshpuri, he was here, too. Each Siddha had his own hut or cave or house made in styles I had never seen. Some of the Siddhas were sitting quietly.
>
> The climate was very good and the light very pleasing. I found that I now

> knew everything. I recognized the seers and sages of ancient times and, moving on a little, saw many *yoginīs*, all sitting steadily in their various divine mudras. I spent a long time wandering around Siddhaloka looking at the yoginis and Siddha saints. I was very fascinated by Siddhaloka. No other world had seemed so good to me. I did not feel like leaving and thought it would be very nice if I could stay.[90]

This remarkable passage shows the vision of a cosmic destination, a location that is far away in some other, heavenly realm and yet available to be seen by the siddha. It is a destination where the true being of the siddha eternally resides even as the siddha takes physical residence in this world for a brief sojourn. As Swami Muktananda further describes it:

> Siddhas dwell in their own world, Siddhaloka, the world of Siddhas. That is situated very high above. There nature offers no resistance, no obstacle, no impediment. There is neither sun nor shade, day nor night in that world. Physical suffering is nonexistent. Siddhaloka is a vast realm, surging with bliss. It gets illumined without the sun or moon. In that world, everything is made of the light of pure Consciousness. All its trees, flowers and creepers, gardens and mountains are filled with conscious radiance. Only Consciousness glows and shimmers there. That world is fashioned by the great Kundalini from the material of Her own nature.[91]

The idea of siddhaloka as elaborated in these and other passages forms a central consideration in understanding Swami Muktananda's vision of the reality of the siddha. Whether we wish to interpret the idea of siddhaloka quite literally or to read it as a metaphoric transcription of the realm of enlightenment into a vocabulary of physical location, it is a crucial component of the idea of the siddha. The siddha has his true residence elsewhere. The presence of the siddha on earth is an extension or aspect of his total being, which is carefully protected and ensconced elsewhere. By means of the siddhaloka idea, Swami Muktananda elaborates an understanding of his own mystical experiences of his own guru's indwelling presence, experiences that go to the very core of his own entrance into the condition of being a siddha.

Nevertheless, there still remain interesting questions with regard to the elaboration of what the state of *jīvanmukti* represents. That is to say, how is this state of enlightenment described philosophically? With regard to the actual description of what constitutes the achievement of enlightenment, one of the classical early formulas is outlined in the *Yoga Sūtra* and its allied commentarial literature, which prescribe the attainment of the *asaṃprajñāta-samādhi* as the highest goal of the yogi. Here, the yogi enters into a state of meditative absorption in which all thoughts, all activities and movements of his awareness have ceased. This form of spiritual attainment is thought to conclude and culminate a program of interiorization, of eradicating or negating all the *vṛtti*s, the "activities," of the body-mind complex.

Thus, in addition to embodying already existing definitions of liberation, the evolving ideologies of the siddhas brought with them creative new definitions of the ultimate goal. The term *siddha* developed to describe a new and yet more encompassing and exalted formulation of the condition of enlightenment. *This is the gradual innovation of the siddhas: the redefinition of the condition of enlightenment as something that is no longer incompatible with bodily activity, and with sensory and intellectual functioning.*

While many prior traditions of Hindu religious and philosophical thought have emphasized the nature of enlightenment as a progressive transcendence of the material and manifested world, there now begin to develop explicit notions of a mysticism of immanence spelled out in great, technical detail. This form of mysticism was not seen to supplant or subvert the prior teachings of transcendence but, rather, to form a yet higher evolution that began where the other left off. It must be emphasized that, like everything else in Indian spirituality, these immanentist developments have long precedent in the earlier tradition, particularly in the Upaniṣads. The history of the evolution of this new goal is complex and has not really been adequately traced.

In contradistinction to earlier teachings, the traditions of the siddhas assert, for the most part, that such an interior, ascensional transcendence is an important *stage* in the path of mysticism that leads to perfection. But they also assert that such an exclusively interiorized path does *not* deliver the highest goal of yoga. Ultimately, they teach, the distinction between high and low, between interiority and exteriority, between subject and object must be overcome. Swami Chidvilasananda has described a vision of this goal in the following words:

> Do you want to know one of the most magical things about God? He is both transcendent and immanent. You cannot separate God from his own creation.
>
> The sages do not hesitate to say, Every form is the form of God, every form is the form of Truth. In every form is the eternal Witness.
>
> Baba used to say, This world, with all its objects and subjects, is nothing but an outfit for God, different clothes for the same Lord, for supreme Consciousness.
>
> The same supreme Consciousness has become an ant and also an elephant, a pebble as well as a mountain, a fool and also a scholar—all that is and all that is not. Having experienced the splendor in all things and all beings, all times and all places, the sages burst forth into songs of praise, attempting to capture the experience in syllables, which are themselves a form of the light of God.[92]

Describing how this happens, the Kashmiri siddha Abhinavagupta asserts in his writings that at the culmination of the ascensional, interiorized path of yoga, there arises a new and outwardly expansive movement in consciousness. This new movement descends or expands down from the highest consciousness itself and invades and overtakes all of the subtle structures of individuality, and then moving out from the senses, it sweeps down and out into the world to overtake all in an embrace of unity and nondifferentiation.[93] This extroversive "wave" of consciousness arises from the heart, from the depths of consciousness, and it establishes a very different state of enlightened perception. It is in this way that the so-called closed-eyed (*nimīlana*) or "enstatic" levels of *samādhi* so carefully mapped in the classic Pātañjala yoga are superseded in the traditions of the siddhas by states of truly "ecstatic" or open-eyed *samādhi.*[94] Describing this condition of natural *samādhi,* Swami Muktananda says:

> The yogi in this state understands God as the one who appears in an infinity of forms, who is the whole and indivisible support of the phenomenal universe, and who also pervades all physical objects and all living creatures. This [yogi] experiences the continual influence of God in all that he does. Just as the shape of a fruit, its juice, and its smell and all its various characteristics exist as a simple unity, so the yogi discovers that external objects, the knowledge of these objects, and the one who knows them are all one with the all-pervading God, the fundamental basis of all things. Thus, the yogi discovers this in everyone.[95]

Thus, the accomplished siddha has no need of closing the eyes or of shutting off the sensory functions in order to perceive the all-pervading consciousness. Because of the reversive, all-encompassing wave of unified consciousness that sweeps out to enfold everything—the activities of the mind, the apperceptional sensations of the body, the functioning of the limited senses, the experience of the objects of perception in the world—all of these are transformed. Whereas before these may have formed limiting structures needing to be excluded and transcended by the ascending and interiorizing yogi, they now stand awash in the ultimate consciousness. What was once apprehended as the world—filled only with diversity, shot through with multiple possibilities for suffering, a never-ending kaleidoscopic display of forms and experiences that succeed each other continuously in a seemingly chaotic and dynamic change—all of this now reveals a new dimension to the eye of the ecstatic yogi, the accomplished siddha. It is *all* consciousness. It is *all* divine. It is *all* perfect. In a great paradox, the great Self of consciousness—which the yogi was once capable of discovering only as the supreme and transcendent experience revealed in the depths of an interiorized *samādhi*—this great Self now begins to be discovered through and in each and every object of perception, through and in each moment of experience. For such a siddha, life becomes the successive revelation—moment by moment—of the pulsating presence and eternal reality of the ultimate consciousness. In his writings, Swami Muktananda eloquently and beautifully describes his own experiences of this state of revelation. For example, in his spiritual autobiography, *Play of Consciousness*, he writes:

> As I gazed at the tiny Blue Pearl, I saw it expand, spreading its radiance in all directions so that the whole sky and earth were illuminated by it. It was no longer a Pearl but had become a shining, blazing, infinite Light; the Light which the writers of the scriptures and those who have realized the Truth have called the divine Light of Chiti. The Light pervaded everywhere in the form of the universe. I saw the earth being born and expanding from the Light of Consciousness, just as one can see smoke rising from a fire. I could actually see the world within this conscious Light, and the Light within the world, like threads in a piece of cloth, and cloth in the threads. Just as a seed becomes a tree, with branches, leaves, flowers, and fruit, so within Her own being Chiti becomes animals, birds, germs, insects, gods, demons, men, and women. I could see this radiance of Consciousness, resplendent and utterly beautiful, silently pulsing as supreme ecstasy within me, outside me, above me, below me. I was meditating even though my eyes were open. Just as a man who is completely submerged in water can look around and say, "I am in the midst of water, I am surrounded on all sides by water; there is nothing else," so was I completely surrounded by the Light of Consciousness.[96]

To be completely surrounded by the light of consciousness is the intrinsic nature of the state of the siddha. It is for this reason that the siddha who dwells in such a condition no longer apprehends the world as different from himself or herself. This state has often been called *sahajasamādhi*, the "spontaneous" *samādhi*. The siddha who dwells there continuously abides as the cresting wave of the ultimate consciousness. Such a wave breaks continuously to express, in supreme ecstasy, the pulsation of life. Yet at the same time such a wave retains its wholeness, purity, and perfection. Therefore, the siddha does not get lost in the delusion that there is anything like a separateness or differentiation to be found in anything that appears in the field of awareness. It is not that the world or the body has disappeared. It is that these so-called external and objective structures are now evaluated completely differently. They are now seen to be encompassed seamlessly in the ocean of unity, in the field of nondifferentiation. Forms, differences, and diversity are encompassed and melded, held and irradiated, in the ocean of the formless, the nondifferentiated, and the unitive. There has surged into operation a mysterious alchemy of transmutation that reveals within the leaden world the glow of the golden light of consciousness.

Such is the condition of the overwhelming divine realization described and taught by the traditions of the siddhas. The objective world is no longer experienced as an opaque objectivity. Rather, the objective world is now seen to emit the light of consciousness itself from everywhere, to be, in effect, nothing more or less than that light of consciousness engaged in its boundless and delightful play. Bathed in the radiance of the Supreme, all forms of life reveal their intrinsic purity, perfection, and formlessness. The *sahajasamādhi* of the siddhas is so total, so radical, and so complete that it cannot be impeded or even diminished in any way by the ordinary conditions of life. If, as the philosophical teachings of many siddha lineages instruct, all existing things are but modifications of an intrinsic and supreme consciousness, and, if the siddha has completely realized and unfolded the deepest and most authentic reality of that all-pervasive consciousness, then nothing can impede or stand in the way of such a realization. What appears in the field of experience of such a being is stably and completely realized as the supreme consciousness. Reality and all experience has been melted into that which is of "one flavor" (*ekarasa*).[97] Swami Muktananda describes this state in his book *Play of Consciousness*, saying:

> When, through the yoga of meditation, the Siddha student attains this knowledge of Chiti [consciousness], he sees the entire world, inner and outer, as Her play, sees Her vibrating in every action, and finds supreme joy in all his work and activities. This is because, through his insight, the Siddha student is constantly and completely aware of the expansion of the Chiti. He knows that everything that happens in the world, because it is the flowering of Chiti, is Chiti.[98]

This redefinition of the nature of enlightenment is crucial to an understanding of the ideologies of the traditions of the siddhas. For example, such an understanding of enlightenment brings about a subtle but potently important redefinition, a further precision, in the definition of renunciation. Many of the historical siddha traditions will continue to implement existing and traditional ritual forms of renunciation. Nevertheless, their approach to the meaning and nature of such renunciatory practices is altered by this understanding of the nature of the state of siddhahood itself. Says Swami Muktananda:

> [Y]ou are conscious, all-pervasive, and perfect. The universe is not all different from you. What is it that you want to renounce? What are you running after to possess? There is nothing in the world but you. It is you who pervades the universe, who are the perfect and undying principle. There is no difference between you and the world. There is no duality. You fill the whole universe, without differentiation. You are the serene, imperishable, and pure Kundalini, the light of Consciousness.[99]

If the siddha dwells in the pervasive and fully stabilized realization that there exists only the ultimate consciousness and that all that appears in the mind, all that pulsates in the senses, all that stands in the world is now perceived as but a modification of this consciousness—a "modification" that does not in any way alter the intrinsic perfection and purity of that consciousness—then what need is there for renunciation as it is traditionally understood? The siddha does not seek to escape the world. The siddha does not pronounce the world to be an illusion, a nonentity, or even impure. Rather, if the siddha adopts the mode of life of a renunciant, it is because such a mode of life is appropriate and most reflective of the state of one who has fully realized that ultimate consciousness. What else could the siddha who dwells in this state of *sahajasamādhi* seek or desire to experience? The supreme secret, which reveals everything to be nothing but God, has opened before her eyes. What could be added to that? Seeking nothing because he has everything, desiring nothing because he dwells in the ecstatic, cresting wave of the bliss of the ultimate consciousness at every moment, owning nothing because he has become like an emperor of consciousness, having no set social role or function, because he has become the supreme friend and well-wisher to all the world, the siddha dwells and abides in his own bliss, freedom, and perfection. Says Muktananda:

> There never was and never will be any ignorance in you. You are the play of universal Consciousness. You are not *rajasic* or *tamasic*; you are not dominated by any particular element. You are *nirguna* and *saguna*, God without form and God with form. You are the untainted and unchangeable play of pure Chiti. Golden bangles, bracelets, anklets and necklaces are all gold; in the same way, the world born from the blossoming forth of the Shakti of Parashiva is nothing other than Chiti! The effect cannot run counter to the cause.[100]

The renunciant seeks to realize that fundamental consciousness in its most native and fundamental state, of which the world is but a conditional and temporary manifestation and modification. The siddha does not repudiate the world. The "world" in and of itself is not the enemy. Rather, it is the constriction and limitation of awareness that does not permit the world to be properly evaluated and understood which stands as the enemy to be overcome. *Siddhaḥ svatantrabhāvaḥ*, "Freedom is achieved," is the concise and aphoristic judgment of the *Śiva Sūtra*.[101] It is described by Swami Muktananda as follows:

> As long as "possession and renunciation" control you, you will still be bound to the world. While they exist the world will exist for you, but a man who forgets about "possession and renunciation" goes beyond worldly existence. Neither renounce "possession/renunciation" nor accept it. Become absorbed in your inner reality. Think of the world as the play of Chitshakti and find true peace. If you can always be aware of Chiti when you are hearing, seeing, touching, smelling, eating, drinking, waking, and sleeping, you will

> never be depressed or sad. Such a Siddha student is perpetually liberated. The wise man who is unattached like the sky and never at any time allows his mind to become agitated has perfected his meditation, for he has become one with Chiti. He is extremely fortunate.[102]

So the path of the siddhas projects the achievement of a condition of freedom in which that intrinsic constriction and limitation of awareness is forever undone. Then, all of the limiting and constraining misunderstandings and misperceptions will be forever undermined and abandoned. Then, the world will be revealed and seen for what it truly is, an unfolding display of that ultimate consciousness itself. Says Muktananda:

> Wherever you look, whatever you see, is all your own light. Nothing is different from you. You are present in everything. You should not think of such distinctions as "I am here, I am not there." Instead, your constant meditation should be the thought "I am everywhere, I am the Self of all." Nothing other than you exists in the world. The *Shiva Sūtras* [3:30] say, *svashakti-prachayo'sya vishvam,* "The universe is the expansion of one's own Shakti." The illusion called the universe has arisen in you solely through your own mental impurities. Worship goddess Chiti, and as you become free from impurities, the universe will appear as the resting place of Chiti. You are pure Consciousness; you are pure Reality.[103]

The siddha seeks to live in the state of *sahajasamādhi,* a spontaneous and natural *samādhi,* which is neither the same as the ordinary state of waking nor an exclusively introverted and ascended state of meditative absorption. Rather it is an even higher condition in which the directionality of inner and outer, the polarity of higher and lower, the distinction of pure and impure, the division between matter and mind, all of these divisive and polarizing constructs have been overcome and have melted into the all-encompassing and all-pervasive condition of the ocean of consciousness. Says Swami Muktananda:

> The whole world is simply an illusion. From the point of view of Ultimate Reality, it is the play of Chiti. The eternal and everlasting reality of Shiva pulsates throughout the entire universe. The Siddha student who knows that everything is the pure light of Consciousness, composed of the red, white, black, and blue lights, is himself the very image of Chiti. He has completed his *sādhanā.* He has achieved nonattachment to differentiation, renunciation, and forms. He has heard, reflected on, and contemplated Mother Chiti, and established Her in his heart. The enlightened man who knows directly the identity of the Self and the Absolute is a true Siddha student. He is blessed and worthy of being honored by the world. He has recognized his own Self in the many different forms. He is no longer concerned with the body or anything else. He considers everything as Chitshakti *vilās,* the play of divine Conscious-

> ness. He is established in wisdom, ever free; he has found the divine joy of the Absolute. Such a Siddha student is liberated while still in this body.[104]

These notions about freedom, about the expansion of human possibilities, about the nature of consciousness and of personal identity, and about the paradoxical figure known as the siddha form the core of the teachings that Swami Muktananda brought to the world. As we have seen, these ideas are ancient in Indian spirituality, and they express the deepest perceptions of the ancient wisdoms of that tradition. Cast in modern garb, expressed in ways that made them accessible to the twentieth century, these notions formed the explanatory backdrop for the extraordinary form of spiritual initiation known as shaktipat, which constituted the gift that Muktananda sought to give to all. In describing his own teacher from whom he had received this gift that he gave to others, Muktananda says:

> O Nityananda, your words were mantras; your speech was scripture. Your behavior embodied the teachings of yoga. The place where you lived was immaculate; it always looked freshly scrubbed no matter how many thousands of people came to see you.
>
> O Shrī Gurudev, in you one could see that the sublime *shaivī khecarī mudrā* of Shaivism had taken up residence. Lord Shiva described this *shaivī mudrā,* this pure *khecarī* which is the state of Shiva. He said that the eyes remain fixed and unblinking but see nothing. Although they appear to look outward, the gaze is directed within. The mind is quiet, not dwelling on any thought, and the vital force is still but not forcibly retained. O Nityananda, you lived in this sublime *mudrā* of the Siddhas.[105]

As a concluding consideration we might linger for a moment on this notion of the *mudrā* or what might be called in a wider sense the "gesture" of the siddhas. This specific gesture, as Swami Muktananda tells us, is called the *khecarīmudrā. Khecarī* means something like "moving in the void," in this case, the voidness or spaciousness of the ultimate consciousness. It is also called the *bhairavīmudrā,* or the "gesture of Bhairava" (who is a form of Śiva), in the traditions of Śaivism. It is the gesture that is expressive of the siddha's state of complete and total enlightenment. It is expressive of the perfection and freedom of the siddha, whose enlightenment encompasses both outer and inner in the embrace of an absolute consciousness.

In a wider sense, one could say that the gesture of the siddha is the totality of everything that the siddha says and does, the siddha's spontaneous perfection of speech and action. It derives from an attunement to the whole. It is omniscience in the sense that there is such purity and transparency of consciousness that anything the siddha desires to know can be known. But it is also omniscience in the sense that the siddha is unthinkingly and unhesitatingly expressive of perfection, of the wisdom of every moment. The absolute perfectly unfolds and explicates itself in every moment of the siddha's existence.

Because the siddha dwells at the core, at the center, at the deepest source point of reality, there is no ego, no barrier, no pretension, no limitation to the expression of the highest truth. It is for this reason that the siddha's speech, the siddha's word is mantra; it is revelation. The *Śiva Sūtra* says *kathā-japaḥ*, "His ordinary conversation has the power of the recitation of mantra."[106] The siddha's words are said to be able to pierce the mind and heart, to resonate powerfully in one's deepest being. The siddha's words magically speak to the deepest thoughts, the hidden desires and deepest aspirations, and the concealed faults and virtues of humankind. The siddha's speech is held to be the pulsation of the deepest Self, engendering in the human heart a profound and uncanny sense of recognition, intimacy, and love. The siddha's speech is experienced as the scripture of the heart. Even seemingly casual phrases are mysteriously charged with grace.

The *mudrā* or gesture of the siddha is the continuous gesture of revelation, of gracefulness, of pointing out the path that is so totally apparent to him, the pathless path, for the siddha's gesture is the gesture of immersion in the ocean of consciousness. It is a gesture of teaching, of compassion, of supreme freedom. It is a gesture that subverts the ordinary in this world, so that it may continuously reveal the extraordinary, a gesture that grants the experience of the ever-new bliss of consciousness. Swami Muktananda talks about the *śaivi-khecarīmudrā*, which is known by many names, the gesture that appears to look out into the world, and is yet ever attuned to the inner delight of the Self, a Self that is no longer inner or inward because it has become all-pervasive. This teaching gesture of the siddha expresses itself in so many and even seemingly contradictory ways. The siddha is the supporter of dharma, the clarifier of that which upholds life and the truth, the reviver of dharma, the one who breathes the living breath of God into the law that becomes stale in the rigid and uninsightful hands of the unenlightened. The teaching gesture of the siddha is the transmission of the sacred tradition, of the supreme and eternal path that leads to God. But in this gesture that is supportive of the true and deepest sacred traditions, the siddha often brings a revolution. Not a revolution of violence, nor even a revolution that accuses or separates—a revolution of nonduality. As Swami Muktananda said, a meditation revolution was his mission. And while this revolution welcomes all, it contains an implicit inspiration toward change. Muktananda minced no words to describe the ignorance he was doing battle against: the limitations and faults of the ego.

Just so, some of the siddhas come as cosmic revolutionaries, inspiring reform, great change, evolution, and using the tool of criticism when it is necessary to point out the defects of the current situation. The siddha loves the world as the very divine consciousness, but the siddha criticizes the world inasmuch as the world fails to express and live the possibility of divinity.

The teaching gesture of the siddha is expressed in the writings, the spoken word, the instructions, the continuous inspirational words, the admonishments, in short, all of the manifold forms of *upadeśa*, "instruction," that he or she brings. But this is also expressed in the actions of the siddha, the *līlā*, "play," of the siddha, the divine actions and gestures of love, the gestures of ecstasy, the gestures of revelation, the gestures of the great vision of God that seem magically to emanate from the siddha's person. As Swami Muktananda said of his own guru, "O Nityananda, you lived in this sublime mudra of the Siddhas."[107] There is so much more to say about the state of the siddha. We might conclude by mentioning again the central import of this essay: The siddha lives in enlightenment. The siddha's state is one of dwelling in *sahajasamādhi*, the eternal and astonished recognition of God in every moment, the cresting wave of the ecstasy of the *śakti*, the breaking wave of the ever-unfolding, infinite, and absolute consciousness. This is the open-eyed *samādhi* that has recognized the Self both deep inside as well as dwelling in and as all things. Speaking about this state, Swami Chidvilasananda has said:

> Baba said, joy is constantly bubbling up in your heart. Not only was this Baba's experience, he also unlocked this experience in thousands of hearts. Perfect joy. Joy without dependency. Joy that is whole. Joy that is everlasting. Joy that never decays. Joy that is free from likes and dislikes. Joy that places itself in the service of God, that never leaves His presence for a second. Joy that is contagious, that is giving. Such perfect joy does exist in everyone's heart.[108]

Chapter Three

The Guru-Disciple Relationship
The Context for Transformation

William K. Mahony

THE LIBERATING PROMISE OF THE "WAY OF THE GURU"

In the love, honor, and reverence its devotees afford the guru and in the importance it sees in the guru-disciple relationship as an indispensable element of spiritual life, Siddha Yoga gives contemporary texture and shape to some of the most pervasive and certainly some of the oldest of all Indian religious sensibilities. Those contours give form to a set of values, perspectives, and disciplines centered on what would be known in Indian spirituality by such terms as *gurubhakti*, "devotion to the guru"; *gurūpāsana*, "reverence for the guru"; *gurūpāsti*, "adoration of the guru"; and perhaps the most inclusive, the *gurumārga*, "the path of the guru" or "the spiritual way of the guru."

A hymn from the *Atharvaveda*, extolling what it presents as the fundamentally significant spiritual dimensions of the relationship between a student and a teacher, suggests that such an idea dates in India to at least 1000 B.C.E.[1] That this particular type of relationship has been regarded with such value is suggested by the fact that many of India's most highly honored religious texts take the form of dialogues between a teacher and a student. The Upaniṣads (ca. eighth to third century B.C.E.), for example, typically present their insights in the form of lessons given by wise teachers to a variety of spiritual seekers. The *Bṛhadāraṇyaka Upaniṣad* (ca. eighth century B.C.E.) recounts lessons given by such teachers as Yājñavalkya to a number of seekers, including a number of wise philosophers, his wife Maitreyī, and Janaka, the king of Videha. So, too, the *Chāndogya Upaniṣad* (also eighth century B.C.E) includes teachings given not only by Prajāpati to Indra, the king of the gods, but also, among others, by the sage Uddālaka Āruṇeya to a number of students (including his son Śvetaketu), Sanatkumāra to the philosopher Nārada, Gautama to Satyakāma, and Satyakāma to Upakosala. The *Bhagavadgītā* (ca. fourth to first centuries B.C.E.), perhaps the most influential and well known of all Indian religious texts, revolves around teachings given to Arjuna by Lord Kṛṣṇa, and virtually all of the many Tantras codified in the seventh to twelfth centuries C.E. take the form of pedagogical lessons given by God as Śiva to one or another of the forms of the universal Goddess, usually Pārvatī.

So important to spiritual life is the function of the teacher that even Indra, the king of the gods, is said to have approached Prajāpati as a student in order to learn from the Lord of Creatures the nature of ultimate reality.[2] According to the *Rāmāyaṇa*, many gods and goddesses and other divine spirits turn to Bṛhaspati for guidance and counsel,[3] and Lord Rāma himself, who is said in that highly influential devotional epic to be the very incarnation of God as Viṣṇu, bowed down to the wise teacher Viśvāmitra. The story told in the *Yogavāsiṣṭha*, a sixth- or seventh-century Kashmiri text to which Swami Muktananda and Swami Chidvilasananda have frequently referred, revolves around the lessons given to Lord Rāma by his teacher, Vasiṣṭha.

In his characteristically straightforward way, Swami Muktananda noted the necessity of a teacher:

> It is universally true that in all fields, if there is a student, then there must also be a teacher. In this world, there is a teacher for every subject. This is nothing new. If there is a music student, there is also a music teacher. . . . Similarly, if there is a spiritual seeker, there must also be a guide to point out the right path. In Siddha Yoga, the Siddha Guru guides the seeker unerringly.[4]

Recounting his own spiritual search, Swami Muktananda said:

> I had earlier visited sixty great saints, including Shri Siddharudha Swami, Shri Zipruanna, Shri Hari Giri Baba, Shri Madivala Swami, Athani Shivayogi, and Shri Narsingh Swami and Shri Bapu Mai of Pandharpur, and I had heard the same thing from all of them: "There is no higher path than that of meditation on, obedience and service to, the Guru!"[5]

After having found his own guru in Bhagawan Nityananda, Muktananda noted:

> When I was pursuing my sadhana [spiritual discipline], I followed many teachers and many paths. I read a great deal about saints and came to the conclusion that I could know my own inner Self only with the help of a Guru. And that was true: I received everything from my Guru, and even now I receive blessings from him. That is why I always say that there is nothing greater or more valuable than the Guru.[6]

Muktananda's weighty reference here to the importance of the guru in his coming to know the "inner Self" does not reflect a narcissistic preoccupation on his part. By "inner Self" (*antarātman*) he is referring to the soul itself, which—following Indian spiritual thought in general and Vedāntic Hindu thought in particular[7]—he regarded as the sublime presence deep within the human heart of the divine power that fashions and supports all things in this universe. The inner Self Muktananda sought is identical, he taught, to the ultimate source and ground of all things in the world, that is, to God himself. From this perspective, to know God inwardly is to experience the deep significance and unwavering value of existence itself. According to the *Brahma Upaniṣad:*

> There is one divine power that lives hidden within all creatures.
> All-pervasive, he is the inward soul of all beings.
> He is the controller of all actions, resides within all beings.
> He is the inner witness, autonomous, conscious, and free of all attributes.
> He is the sole controller, the inward soul of all beings.
> He has one form, but makes it many.
> Those who realize Him as the Self within
> have eternal happiness, they and no others.[8]

In looking to his guru for help in knowing the inner Self, Muktananda therefore sought knowledge of the very foundation not only of his own being but of Being itself. Indian thought has long held that a seeker of such knowledge needs the help of a teacher, for the absolute is inconceivable to the mind that has not made the shift in awareness necessary to comprehend its own source, namely, ultimate reality itself. The *Kena Upaniṣad* (ca. seventh century B.C.E), for example, asserts, "There the eye goes not; language cannot go there, nor the mind. Indeed [the absolute] is other than the known and even above the unknown."[9] Since it cannot be fully grasped through one's own mental effort, one who wishes to know the absolute must rely on the favor of a teacher who already abides in that knowledge. As the *Kaṭha Upaniṣad* holds:

> Unless taught by a teacher [who truly understands], there is no access there,
> for—being more subtle than the subtle—
> [ultimate reality] is inconceivable.
> Dearest one! This knowledge is not attained through reasoning.
> Truly, for ease of understanding
> it must be taught by another.[10]

Indian tradition holds that a student without a teacher is like a person who has been blindfolded and led into the wilderness without being given directions out of those wilds. But the person who has such a teacher "becomes conscious" and finds the way revealed.[11] A passage from the *Ṛgveda* (ca. 1200 B.C.E.) states:

> The one who does not know the way asks of him who knows it:
> taught by that knowing guide, one travels forward.
> Truly, this is the splendid blessing of instruction:
> one finds the path that leads onward.[12]

If, according to the perspective of the *gurumārga*, the way to reach union with God is by means of the guru-disciple relationship, then we must ask this: Who (or what) is the guru?

WHO IS THE GURU?

It is important to know at the outset that according to the teachings of Siddha Yoga, as well as those of the long spiritual traditions in India from which they are drawn, there are different forms or aspects of the guru. We will return at some length to this idea in a subsequent section of this chapter. For now, we might simply say that the physical person is only one of those forms. This is the outer guru, or physical guru, the human teacher for whom devotees have expressed deep love and reverence. One cannot overstate the intensity and the depth of affection and appreciation devotees seem to have felt for Bhagawan Nityananda, Swami Muktananda, and now Swami Chidvilasananda—just as countless devotees have felt for their teachers in centuries past. Each person's relationship with the guru is unique. But in Siddha Yoga, as in the Indian devotional tradition as a whole, there appears to be one essential quality that marks all of those unique relationships: each is grounded on a powerful love shared by guru and disciple. Not infrequently one will hear a person say that he or she has "fallen in love" with the guru, not in the ordinary way that two people fall in love but rather in the sense that, having met the guru, he or she has discovered or uncovered a boundless fountain of love within his or her own heart and that the guru-disciple relationship allows him or her to express that love unconditionally. Many devotees report that meeting Bhagawan Nityananda, Swami Muktananda, or Swami Chidvilasananda has completely changed their lives and that they continue to find guidance in their relationship with the guru.

Muktananda's own words reflect his experience of such love gained through his devotion to Bhagawan Nityananda. To him Nityananda was the embodiment of that incomprehensible and majestic divine love that sustains and holds this whole world together. Loving Nityananda, Swami Muktananda thereby loved the entire universe. Loving the universe,

Muktananda became one with that divine force itself, for—as he put it—there "is only love, love, nothing but love."

> When two sticks are rubbed together, an exquisite flame arises. By the churning of milk, butter is produced. Similarly, joy arises from the love of [the mantra] *Guru Om* [which gives voice to the presence of the Guru] and from the churning of the love between the Guru and the disciple. Only the Guru can know that delight and taste the elixir which arises in every pore of the body. This love cannot be attained through practicing yoga, through indulging in sense pleasures, or through prattling about knowledge.
>
> Only when a river merges into the ocean can it fully know the splendor of the ocean. Only when I lost myself in the ecstasy of Nityananda did I realize who he was. He is the nectar of love which arises when everything, sentient and insentient, becomes one. He is the beauty of the world. He pervades all forms, conscious and inert. He is the luminous sun, the moon, and the stars in the heavens. He frolics and sways with love in the blowing of the wind. His consciousness glimmers in men and women. There is only Nityananda, nothing but Nityananda. He is the bliss of the Absolute, the bliss of the Self, the bliss of freedom, and the bliss of love. There is only love, love, nothing but love.[13]

The guru, for Swami Muktananda, was the unfathomable reality and power of transcendent love itself. The guru is therefore not bound by any one physical body or another. The guru is "the luminous sun, the moon, and the stars in the heavens." Coming to know the abiding Self which is the source of this love,[14] "one is flooded with the awareness of inner contentment. A fountain of joy wells up in one's heart when one's awareness becomes stable."[15] For such a seeker, everything in the world of multiplicity reflects and becomes one with this universal power of love. As Muktananda put it:

> When the sun rises, all the stars fade away in its brilliance. Similarly, when the sun of knowledge rises in the heart and a person experiences the essence of the Self, the universe of diversity with its countless beings and objects is dissolved for him. Duality perishes. The radiant sun of the Self blazes in his eyes. Its flame radiates through every pore of his body. As it flashes, his entire body is filled with the nectar of love. Drops of nectar from the stream of love flow from his eyes. His words shower love.[16]

Muktananda referred to the guru as "Gurudev," which we may translate as "divine teacher." He traced his very being to the grounding and compassionate love of Gurudev. "My attainment is Gurudev," he proclaimed. "My *sādhanā* is Gurudev. My realization is Gurudev. My mantra is Gurudev. What is the formless or the attributeless? What is realization of the form? It is all delusion created by words."[17] But, although he understood the guru in this most cosmic of ways, Muktananda also found that this universal love was perfectly and fully embodied in the person of Bhagawan Nityananda, and it was to this, his physical guru, that Muktananda directed his devotion.

According to tradition, there are various kinds of physical gurus. The *Kulārṇava Tantra* (eleventh century) identifies six: "one who sets [the disciple] in motion, one who shows [the way], one who explains [the teachings], one who reveals [the truth], one who possesses effective knowledge, and one who awakens [the disciple's spirit]."[18] Of those listed here, the sixth—*bodhaka*, "one who awakens"—is, according to the *Kulārṇava Tantra*, the most important, for "the first five are the result, as it were, of the last, [which serves as their] cause."[19] By this the Tantra means that the guru as *bodhaka* awakens the disciple into all other forms of spiritual learning and development. Such a guru blesses and directs the whole of the disciple's spiritual life. Such a guru is one "who performs the full initiation [*purṇābhiṣekakartṛ*]."[20] For many of those who practice Siddha Yoga, Bhagawan Nityananda, Swami Muktananda, and Swami Chidvilasananda seem to have subsumed in their persons all six types of gurus at once. They have "awakened" the love already residing within these disciples and, having done so, set their spiritual lives in motion and directed their continuing spiritual growth through effective guidance and teaching.

Yet, as we have just seen, there is more to the guru than the physical teacher. According to Siddha Yoga teachings, the guru exists not only in the form of the outward teacher but also within one's own being. This is the inner guru who abides within as the individual seeker's innermost spirit and who is approached through meditation, contemplation, dreams, and the other means by which one is said to gain access to subtler dimensions of one's own being. The physical guru may be understood to be a manifestation or outer expression of the inner guru. The latter itself may be envisioned as having a subtle form; some Indian contemplative traditions, for example, describe various "seats" of the guru in the subtle system, the most powerful being in the *sahasrāra*, the thousand-petaled divine lotus blooming at the top of the head.[21] The guru is also inwardly heard in the form of subtle inner sounds, replicated by the various mantras the outer guru gives the disciple. The inner guru may also be experienced as without form, in which case it may be experienced as the plethoral silence and infinite spaciousness of the expansive heart.

According to Siddha Yoga teachings, all physical forms have subtle, inner aspects that are in some ways equally or even more real—that is, more lasting—than their external expressions. In some Indian traditions, the world-creation itself is seen as a simultaneous and continuous event in which the "stages" of manifestation are actually levels of subtlety, each being contained within and superseded by the level of greater subtlety that precedes it. These levels—from the supreme being all the way down to the many manifold objects of the physical world—are known as *tattvas*, "universal principles" of creation, which demonstrate a pertinent concept of Indian philosophy: that which is more subtle is closer to God.

The guru is the *tattva* at the most subtle level of creation—that is, the guru is said to be the vital force that creates and sustains and, therefore, infuses the whole of the outer and inner universes. For Swami Muktananda, this universal principle is equivalent to the unconditional, unending love that holds and nourishes all things. The fact that the cosmos exists in all its wondrous complexity is said in the teachings of Siddha Yoga to be due to the continuing presence of this guru-principle (*gurutattva*). One's heart would not beat, one's mind would not think, without the presence of this enlivening, sustaining, and incomprehensibly intelligent force that guides all of creation. The guru as *gurutattva* is therefore equivalent to the universal power of consciousness that is said to give rise to and support to the universe and all things in it.

Siddha Yoga teachings hold that the guru-principle is also the power of redemptive transformation. It is through this power that anything has the ability to turn toward the divine. This is what Kṣemarāja, an eleventh-century Śaiva theologian from Kashmir, seems to have meant when he said, "The Guru is the grace-bestowing power of God."[22] Swami Muktananda expressed essentially the same sentiment when he taught, "Infinite grace from God is always showering; we call it the grace of the Guru."[23]

In the context of Siddha Yoga, the word *God* represents a galaxy of epithets for what is held to be the supreme Deity, which the tradition generally, but not always, recognizes by the name Śiva, the "Benevolent One" or the "Auspicious One." According to Śaivism in general—Śaivism being that immensely rich, varied, and yet systematic set of beliefs and practices centered on the worship of God as Śiva—not only is Śiva the creator and sustainer of the universe but also he is its guru. Śiva is said to be the "original guru" (Ādiguru) and the "supreme teacher" (Paramaguru) because God is said not only to form all objects in the universe and to direct all of the universe's myriad movements, but also to illuminate the meaning and significance of that creation, thereby bringing light and clarity and joy to the human spirit where otherwise there may be darkness and confusion and despair. One of Śiva's main forms for his devotees is that of Dakṣināmūrti, that is, "sublime teacher." Śiva's guiding and illuminating presence in the world is thus one of compassion and love, and therefore an expression of the divine power of grace (*anugraha-śakti*).

Swami Muktananda once said, "God's power of grace dwells in the Guru," a statement that is theologically consistent with the classical Tantric and Śaiva concept that the human guru reveals on the physical plane of existence the universal but otherwise formless guru-principle. Noting that "Śiva is, in truth, all-pervading, subtle, beyond the [power of] the mind [to grasp], without features, imperishable, ethereal in nature, eternal, and infinite," a passage from the *Kulārṇava Tantra* asks, "Then how can such a [sublime, ultimate reality] be worshiped?" The text then answers: "That is why Śiva takes the physical form of the Guru and, when worshiped with loving devotion, gives fulfillment and liberation."[24] Similarly, the *Yoginī Tantra* speaks of Ādinātha Mahākāla, the transcendent Lord who lives outside of the structure of time on the heights of Kailasa, the sacred mountain that supports the universe and around which the universe turns; that supreme Lord is said to enter into and speak through the human guru when that physical guru gives a disciple a mantra.[25]

According to Siddha Yoga teachings, the physical guru is assumed to have become one with God through his or her own diligent spiritual discipline and through the grace of his or her own guru. Like their predecessors in the siddha lineage, Bhagawan Nityananda, Swami Muktananda, and Swami Chidvilasananda are described as *brahmaniṣṭha*, that is, they abide in a state of firm and constant awareness of the absolute. It is precisely this—the unwavering vision of the divine in all things—that makes the physical guru not a human being in the ordinary manner, for ordinary human beings tend, more or less frequently, to forget God's constant presence and then to act accordingly. The guru is understood to have no mundane human motivations as such—the desire for power or prestige or control over others, for example. That the guru is firmly established in the awareness of God is one of the primary assumptions of the *gurumārga* in general. If he or she were an ordinary person with the various motivations and inclinations that so often drive human actions, then there would be the dangerous likelihood that the guru would exploit his or her disciples for selfish purposes.

Indian tradition in general holds that a true devotee similarly works to become free from egoism. Since the time the *Bhagavadgītā* was first sung—before the first century B.C.E.—an influential strand of religious thought in India has held that a sign of spiritual maturity is the lack of self-centered motivation. The same view is held in those traditions based on the *gurumārga*. Commenting on Kṛṣṇa's lesson to Arjuna—"He who is free from wants, pure, capable, disinterested, free from anxiety, who has abandoned all [self-centered] undertakings and is devoted to Me, is dear to Me"—the great thirteenth-century poet-saint from Maharashtra, Jñāneśvar, said, "Such a person, O Arjuna, is free from ambition, and his very existence causes joy to increase."[26] Jñāneśvar held that the experience of God's presence in one's life is a cleansing and powerful one, but that a seeker must be willing to become absorbed in that divine presence if such grace is to take effect. "The Ganges [River] is pure, and all sin and passion are purified in its waters," he taught, "but one must sink in them."[27]

We will return in a subsequent section of this chapter to a discussion of various forms of the guru. For the moment, however, it is important to understand that, according to Siddha Yoga, to be in a guru-disciple relationship is to be in relationship with any or all of the different forms and aspects of the guru. The disciple of Bhagawan Nityananda, Swami Muktananda, or Swami Chidvilasananda follows the guru's teachings and loves these great siddhas in their outer manifestation for the power of grace they embody. In following the guru's command, the disciple also enters into relationship with, and thereby aligns himself or herself with, the graceful inner power and wisdom that fashions, supports, and directs the movements of the universe as a whole. From the perspective of Siddha Yoga, to listen to and follow the guru's command is to be receptive to God's grace and to act in consonance with that grace. It is to hear and be true to God's will (*īśvarasaṃkalpa*), and to be true to God's will is to be true to the inherent integrity and dignity of the soul itself.

THE GURU-DISCIPLE RELATIONSHIP AND THE REVELATION OF THE DIVINE

Swami Muktananda often would invite his devotees to bring their spiritual concerns to him in the context of question-and-answer sessions. On one such occasion, he was asked a question regarding the nature of spiritual discipleship. He responded:

> He is a disciple who has lost himself in the Guru. He is the Guru who has entered into the disciple. Jnaneshwar Maharaj said, "When the Guru and the disciple come together, when the Guru and the disciple become one, God reveals Himself." In Siddha Yoga, we say that he is the Guru who can awaken the energy of a disciple. He is the disciple who becomes the Guru's. So, the oneness of the Guru and the disciple is called Siddha Yoga.[28]

In his reply, Swami Muktananda presents a number of the central teachings of Siddha Yoga. We see, for instance, the idea that a disciple is one who has "lost himself in the Guru," that is, who has given or surrendered himself completely to the guru. We see also that the guru is one who can "awaken" the transformative spiritual energy that resides deep within the disciple's own being. Using language consistent with ideas from the classical Tantric tradition, Muktananda frequently described this energy as the inward presence of divine consciousness, the transformative and substantive power that gives rise to and moves within all things.[29] Here Muktananda's response implies that, at least at one level, the guru and the disciple are separate entities. This must, in part, be so. Otherwise, how could the disciple surrender completely to the guru, and how could the guru awaken the disciple? Yet in this response, Muktananda also teaches that the two—guru and disciple—can become "one." In fact, in this statement Swami

Muktananda defines Siddha Yoga itself as that very unity of guru and disciple.

Following an important Indian custom in general and Siddha Yoga tradition in particular, in which a teacher acknowledges the lessons of an earlier teacher from the same tradition, Swami Muktananda in the lesson above quotes Jñāneśvar, for whom he held great affection and reverence. The teaching Muktananda gives in this way is precise and unequivocal: It is when this union of guru and disciple takes place that "God reveals Himself." Thus Muktananda says that God's presence can indeed be revealed in one's life and that it is precisely in the relationship between guru and disciple that such a revelation takes place.

Elsewhere, Muktananda said, "Realization of God is possible only through a Guru . . . . By his grace alone, the inner Shakti [divine power] is unfolded. The glory of the Guru is full of mystery and is supremely divine. He gives a new birth to man, he gives him the experience of knowledge, he shows him sadhana and makes him a lover of God."[30]

Swami Chidvilasananda, Muktananda's spiritual heir, has said, "Of all the relationships in the world, the relationship between the Guru and disciple is considered to be the most sublime."[31] She has also noted, "It is through this relationship where the Guru teaches and the disciple learns, that all progress takes place."[32] And, "If the disciple is able to imbibe the teachings the Guru gives, this beautiful relationship becomes invincible."[33] Chidvilasananda holds that such a relationship allows the seeker to experience and share in what she describes as a "divine presence," and that the guru and disciple enter into that relationship only through divine grace. God's grace is thus the origin and fulfillment of this sublime and momentous relationship. As Chidvilasananda has said, "The relationship between Guru and disciple is based solely on the experience of God."[34]

Like her predecessors in the siddha lineage, Swami Chidvilasananda also teaches that it is in the relationship between guru and disciple that God reveals himself. In a poem she dedicated to her guru, Swami Muktananda, she writes:

> Baba, I give thanks to God
> For having your form incarnate on this earth.
> Through your form, I have come to love
> The most elusive nature of God. . . .
>
> As your sweet, enchanting form became my goal,
> An incredible thing happened—I disappeared.
> As I went still deeper into you, form itself dissolved;
> Nothing remained but light—boundless, radiant light!
> No color, no sound, no touch, no smell, no taste survived.

> Beyond the grasp of the senses, nothing was left to describe;
> The sole reality was the experience of God. . . .
>
> No wonder, no wonder that I love you![35]

This poem expresses the disciple's experience of self-transcendence and complete absorption into the guru's "sweet, enchanting form," and of the ineffable unity of the divine, a formless and resplendent "sole reality" that lies beyond or within all form. The disciple has entered the guru's realm of "boundless, radiant light."

FULFILLING DISCIPLINE AND LIBERATING DISCIPLESHIP

According to Indian spiritual traditions, the truth that wise teachers share with their students is not bound by the constraints of time, space, and causality. Existing of its own autonomous and independent nature, this "One without a second," as Indian texts have called it, cannot be said to have been created. Ancient sages are said to have heard the uncreated truth resonating from the depths of eternity itself. In fact, in those religious traditions of India that align themselves in some way or another with Vedic thought—and this includes most of them—revelation of the divine is regarded as *śruti,* "that which has been heard."

In other words, truth is not fashioned by the human mind; truth is revealed to the mind. Hence the importance in Indian tradition of the practice of learning the truth by listening to one who speaks it. This is known as *śravaṇa,* "hearing." But hearing the truth is not enough. The student must internalize it, mull it over, imbibe it. There must therefore be a process of reflecting or "meditating" on it (*manana*), and there must also be a process of "contemplating" (*nididhyāsana*) the insights thus gained so that that student is better able to apply that truth in his or her own life.

The teacher's own understanding must necessarily have involved the process of *śravaṇa,* as well. A true teacher listened to his or her own teacher, who was in turn taught by a previous teacher. Since the earliest years of Indian religious history, the teacher has therefore been regarded as the heir of a long lineage (*vaṃsa, paramparā),* a line of teachers that is believed to stretch back to the eternal moment "before" the beginning of time itself. The *Bṛhadāraṇyaka Upaniṣad* notes that its lessons have been taught by a lineage of sixty teachers. According to that text, the original teacher was the god Brahmā, the divine personification of the absolute.[36] The great philosopher and systematizer of yoga, Patañjali, who lived somewhere between the fifth century B.C.E. and the second century C.E., taught that God "was also the guru of the ancient [sages] because [in him] there is no limitation brought about by [the flow of] time."[37]

Siddha Yoga holds a similar view: One truly learns when one is taught by a true teacher who shares the knowledge he has gained from a long line of previous teachers.[38] Both Swami Muktananda and Swami Chidvilasananda have stated over and over again that they owe all of their accomplishment not to themselves but rather to the grace of the guru. "Only through the grace of another Guru can you become a Guru," Swami Muktananda firmly maintained. "You cannot become a Guru according to your own whim."[39] He dedicated his book *The Perfect Relationship: The Guru and Disciple* with these words: "I dedicate this book to the lotus feet of my supreme father, Sadguru Nityananda, to whom I owe my existence."

Indian tradition holds that the revelation given to the student by the teacher is itself derived from the transformative power of the same divine grace through which one is born into this world and through which one comes to freedom from cycles of disappointment and confusion. This idea is succinctly presented by the *Vivekacūḍāmaṇi*—an eighth-century C.E. text from the Advaita Vedānta tradition attributed to the great philosopher Śaṅkarācārya—which asserts:

> These three things are rare indeed and are due to the grace of God—namely a human birth, the longing for liberation, and the protecting care of a perfected sage.[40]

Swami Muktananda taught that the guru-disciple relationship is the key to religious fulfillment. He has said in this regard:

> The ancient sages expounded various means—such as austerity, penance, repetition of the divine name, charity, religious vows, fasting, pilgrimages, image worship, and meditation on the Formless—for acquiring fame and fortune and becoming pure and noble. They are, no doubt, true and rewarding. Even so, for a genuine *sādhaka*, a seeker of the highest Truth, Shishya Yoga—that is, accepting discipleship under a Sadguru and proceeding on the spiritual path according to his teachings, instructions, and guidance—is the best. Shishya Yoga, the path of discipleship, is great in every respect.[41]

Although Swami Muktananda himself is regarded by thousands of people as a *sadguru*, a "true guru," he thought of himself first and foremost as Bhagawan Nityananda's disciple. He once said, "If someone were to ask me what gives meaning to my life, I would say, 'The name of my Guru.' I discovered everything within me by my Guru's grace."[42]

In a collection of poems in which he addresses the reader as himself, a style used for centuries by the devotional poet-saints of India, Muktananda wrote:

Discipleship is the key to yoga.
It is the sadhana of knowledge
and the perfect path to liberation.
Muktananda,
become a perfect disciple.

All sadhanas are fulfilled in discipleship.
The true disciple gets the fruit of all austerities.
God becomes his support.
Muktananda,
become a perfect disciple.[43]

According to the precepts of Siddha Yoga, to enter into and sustain a relationship with the guru is the most beneficial activity one can pursue. This relationship is said to be indispensable for a disciple's sadhana, for his or her spiritual discipline, and sadhana is literally "that which leads to completion or wholeness." In Siddha Yoga, the disciple must necessarily be a *sādhaka*, one who practices such a sadhana. The contemporary disciple who gives his or her whole being to that spiritual discipline is a modern version of the traditional Indian *sādhu*, "one who goes straight toward the goal."

To enter into this relationship with the guru is thus to become a disciplined disciple of the guru; for a "disciple" is one who practices a "discipline." If the Sanskrit words *sādhaka* and *sādhana* both connote an ongoing process of completion, the English words *disciple* and *discipline* suggest the process of giving one's trust completely to a teacher and of aligning one's life in a way that is true to the vision that guide presents.[44] In classical Indian traditions, a disciple was known by such terms as *chāttra*, "one who is sheltered" by the guru's enveloping care; *adhikārin* (nominative: *adhikārī*), "one who is qualified" to study with the guru because he or she has demonstrated the willingness to live a necessarily disciplined spiritual life; *śaikṣa*, one who has just begun formal studies; *vidyārthin* (nominative, *vidyārthī*), one who is an already accomplished student who wishes more advanced scholarly training. The most important and encompassing of the terms referring to the student is *śiṣya*, "one to be taught" by the wisdom the guru holds. The *śiṣya* is more than one who simply wants knowledge, although that is, of course, extremely important. A *śiṣya* realizes that true knowledge can be gained only through the grace of God and through the compassionate teaching of the guru. A *śiṣya* is, therefore, one who becomes a disciple of that guru, practicing spiritual discipline.

Such spiritual discipline—the diligent practice of meditation, mantra repetition, chanting sacred texts, scriptural study, selfless service to the guru and thus to others, in addition to leading a healthful life, performing one's moral responsibilities, and so on—may at times be quite difficult for the disciple. Such discipline is said necessarily to involve a challenge to what are long-established yet limited ways of understanding oneself as inadequate, as irreconcilably separated from others and from God. Following Kashmiri Śaiva thought, Siddha Yoga interprets this misunderstanding to be an expression of the three rings of impurity (the three *malas*) that wrap the soul, keeping it trapped in bondage: the *āṇavamala*, which is the sense of smallness and inadequacy; the *māyīyamala*, the misguided sense of reality caused by illusion; and the *kārmamala*, the false sense that one's actions are one's own rather than God's.[45] Imprisoned by the effect of the three *malas*, one feels alienated from God and isolated from others and leads one's life while under the sway of the sum total of these misunderstandings. Siddha Yoga holds that the challenge of spiritual discipline, if properly monitored by a loving and compassionate guide, ultimately frees the disciple from the constraints of a life lived in the confusion that necessarily arises from a mistaken sense of alienation from the divine. One who is thus liberated is said to experience union and profound love.

THE GRACE OF GOD AND THE GRACE OF THE SIDDHA GURU

Informed by and drawing on the ideas presented by Vedāntic, Tantric, Yogic, and especially Hindu devotional (*bhakti*) sensibilities, the Siddha Yoga gurus hold that the power of that graceful love resides and finds expression within each and every human being as the vital force of life itself, but that in most people this divine inner presence remains only imperfectly realized and is said, therefore, to lie dormant. Swami Muktananda identified this vital force of being as the goddess Kuṇḍalinī, the inner presence of the creative, substantive, and transformative power of universal consciousness, the latter of which he revered as the goddess Citi Śaktī.[46] Siddha Yoga gurus teach that throughout history there have been people who have "fulfilled" or "completed" or "perfected" (Sanskrit, *siddha*) that inherent, divinely given love in their own lives. Such a "perfected" human being is known, therefore, as a siddha.

Since a full presentation on the topic has appeared elsewhere in this collection, there is no need here to describe the nature and function of the siddha.[47] For our present discussion, however, we should note two pertinent ideas. First, the primary qualification of a spiritual master is that he or she be a siddha. Second, a siddha who has the power to awaken the *kuṇḍalinī* lying dormant in another person through the process of shaktipat (Sanskrit, *śaktipāta*: the grace-filled "descent of divine power")[48] and then to guide that person in the spiritual discipline that is necessary to maintain, purify, and perfect that newly found love, is known as a siddha guru. Siddha

Yoga holds that there have been many siddha gurus throughout history and that, in fact, the world has never been without at least one such compassionate being; for it is through the siddha guru that God's fulfilling grace is said to flow to the human world in a perfect and complete way. Swami Chidvilasananda has said:

> *Shaktipat* initiation, the awakening of Kundalini Shakti, is the supreme act of the Master's grace. It is the lightning bolt that reveals the greatest treasure within. It is the ultimate gesture of compassion, the breath of the Absolute that breaks the chains of endless death and rebirth and sets you free once and for all.[49]

Each siddha guru is said to have been trained and guided and tested by another in the long lineage of such gurus, and each is said to owe his or her authority and power to the legitimating installation by his or her predecessor. Each siddha guru is, first and foremost, a perfect disciple of his or her guru. Siddha Yoga as a spiritual tradition maintains that Bhagawan Nityananda, Nityananda's disciple Swami Muktananda, and now Muktananda's disciple Swami Chidvilasananda are such siddha gurus and, accordingly, holds them in the highest possible esteem.[50]

To be in relationship with a siddha guru is, in Swami Muktananda's own words, to be in the *satyasambandha*, that is, in "the true relationship" or what has been translated as "the perfect relationship."[51] Why might he say this? It is the true relationship because it is aligned with and enveloped by the truth that stands at the foundation of all life, namely, by God's encompassing and selfless love. Furthermore, such a relationship is perfect because it is through this relationship that the inherent dignity of the human spirit is understood to become "perfected." This does not mean that the disciple in this relationship no longer has any faults. Far from it: the continual cleansing and purifying of one's thoughts and actions as well as one's diligent attention to one's responsibility to others constitute some of the central elements of spiritual discipline in response to this awakening. To become "perfected" means that, through his or her relationship with the guru, the disciple fulfills—completes, makes whole, "perfects"—what Siddha Yoga maintains are his or her otherwise divinely ordained but often hidden human virtues: confidence and yet deep humility, both of which are born from the surrender of one's self-centered will to the will of God; unpretentiousness and the ability to celebrate others' as well as one's own unique contribution to the world; benevolence and compassion; patience, forgiveness, steadfastness, straightforwardness, self-control. Siddha Yoga holds that such a relationship allows the disciple to realize his or her inherent dignity and to recognize that same dignity in others. For Siddha Yoga devotees, such a powerful realization is experienced as nothing less than a result of the grace of God.

Following a long tradition in India, Siddha Yoga holds that the realization of this divine presence, mediated through shaktipat and spiritual practice, is made possible through the guru's compassion for the disciple and his or her skill in bringing the disciple past all inner impediments. Said differently, it is through the siddha guru's grace-filled gift of shaktipat that the religious seeker's heart is opened and softened so that it may experience and imbibe the presence of the divine already residing therein.

Swami Muktananda was careful to locate the ultimate source of this graceful power not in a human teacher, but in God: "Through the means of Shri Guru, *shaktipat* is bestowed. This process does not originate from a human being, but from God. Therefore, to approach the Guru is to approach God."[52] Swami Chidvilasananda similarly has said, "The Guru is not the body; the Guru is the universal Consciousness, it is the Shakti, it is the divine force."[53] Again: "The grace of the Guru is the supreme power, which itself is not different from the divine Self."[54] Like the various *bhakti-* and guru-oriented Indian religious traditions on which they draw, Siddha Yoga gurus teach that to receive the grace of the guru is therefore to receive the grace of God. According to Swami Muktananda:

> The Guru's grace is the inner awakening. It is called Guru's grace when you attain the love of God. As man continuously revels in the external world, his inner path is blocked. When that path is prevented, he can neither understand himself nor others, nor can he experience any peace. Through the Guru's grace, the inner path is opened. Then man enters within and finds the abode of peace. When this happens, he understands himself and others, and his life is filled with bliss. . . .
>
> To attain that you have to have an earnest desire within you. That is called *mumukshutva.* The scriptures call it a longing for liberation. You have to have this longing, this fire of love burning within yourself. You must wonder, "When will I meet Him? When will I attain Him? When you have a true longing to attain Him, at that very minute you do attain Him.[55]

Muktananda has also said:

> The Guru is the one who bestows the grace of God; he is the bestower of God's Shakti—he is not an individual being. Through grace, the Guru transmits God's energy into you. After transmitting that energy into you, he awakens your own inner energy and then spontaneous yoga begins to happen. That is the Guru's grace. The Guru applies the lotion of his grace to your eyes. Then the veil of ignorance is destroyed. Afterward, there is great delight in watching the world—you see the world as it is.[56]

THE GURU AS COMPASSIONATE TEACHER, THE DISCIPLE AS WILLING STUDENT

At its most basic level the relationship between guru and disciple is that of one between a teacher and a student. The Sanskrit word *guru* is, in fact, usually translated as "teacher." This is perfectly appropriate, if perhaps somewhat limiting. Actually, its earliest attestations show that the word functioned as an adjective meaning, literally, "heavy" in the sense of "extraordinarily powerful" or "unusually influential," a connotation that does not always apply to a teacher. The *Ṛgveda* (ca. 1200 B.C.E.) includes a passage in which the term *guru* modifies the word *mantra,* possibly because such a powerful sacred word or phrase is "weighty" in its influence.[57] But by around the eighth century B.C.E., the word *guru* had also become a noun referring to a teacher, probably due to the fact that, in ancient Indian culture, the function of teaching was held in high esteem because teachers were said to understand and, therefore, to possess powerful truths. For this reason the teacher was afforded in ancient India certain "weighty" prestige. One of the earliest uses of the term *guru* in reference to a vitally important spiritual teacher appears in a text dating to about the fourth century B.C.E. "For the sake of this knowledge [of the absolute]," the *Muṇḍaka Upaniṣad* teaches, "let him take fuel [for the sacred fire] in hand and approach a guru who is learned in the scriptures and firmly established in the Absolute."[58]

But *guru* must generally refer to a special kind of teacher, for since the most ancient of times in India there have been many other words besides *guru* to describe one who instructs another. A *śāstṛ,* for example, is one who has mastered a particular field of knowledge and presents that knowledge to the student in a disciplined and ordered fashion. An *upadeṣṭṛ* or *upadeśika* teaches by pointing out the content of what is to be learned and by guiding the student as he or she pursues that knowledge; a *śikṣika* is one who wishes to be of assistance to another by instructing that person in various fields of knowledge; a *prādhyāpaka* is a seasoned teacher who instructs advanced students and other teachers; a *bodhaka,* as we have already noted, awakens or rouses a student's mind and spirit.

Perhaps the oldest term in India referring to a teacher is *ācārya,* "one who knows and teaches the proper mode of conduct," a meaning that suggests an ancient notion that true teaching involves more than simply conveying information. The *ācārya* was not primarily concerned with his student's acquisition of factual knowledge but rather with his spiritual development, for in classical India, as represented by texts drawn from a variety of sources, formal education was directed to what is known as *brahmavarcasa,* to the understanding and experience of the "splendor of Brahman," the "brilliance of the absolute." The *ācārya* taught not only through formal instruction but also, more importantly, by example.

As one who "moves along the universal Way," the *ācārya* brought his students to an increasingly fuller understanding of what it is to live in harmony with the forces of the universe. A story from the *Chāndogya Upaniṣad* has the various divine forces of nature teach the student Upakosala the ways in which they reveal the universal Self (Ātman),[59] but then they tell him that only the *ācārya* can give to him the fullness and meaning of that truth. "You now have this knowledge of ourselves and of the Self," the fire says to Upakosala, "but only the *ācārya* can tell you the Way."[60]

The fact that the *ācārya* can show the student the "Way" [*gati*] that encompasses all of life is due to the fact that he himself lives in harmony with what are experienced as universal and eternal truths. Traditional means of gaining wisdom regarding Brahman—the absolute, the timeless and boundless ground of being from which all things emerge and on which all things find their foundation—centered on the proper understanding of the function and performance of sacred rituals and other forms of hallowed action (such ceremonies were understood to link the human and the divine worlds), the diligent study of sacred texts, and the disciplined practice of meditation and contemplation.

The student who sought such wisdom from an *ācārya* was known in Sanskrit as a *brahmacārin* (nominative, *brahmacārī*: "one who moves in Brahman"), that is, as one who dedicates him or herself to the understanding of the absolute. Conducting himself in a way that is in harmony with the absolute, a *brahmacārī* practiced *brahmacarya*, "holy living," which enabled, supported, and encouraged spiritual growth and the understanding of sacred truths.

In the sixth or fifth century B.C.E., the great Sanskrit grammarian and linguist Pāṇini referred to the teacher of sacred knowledge by using a variety of terms: a *pravacanīya*, for example, spoke forth sacred lessons,[61] while an *anūcāna* recited sacred texts perfectly.[62] Pāṇini also distinguished three classes of teachers besides the *ācārya*:[63] a *pravaktṛ* taught students sacred texts, but did so always under the general guidance of an *ācārya*; a *śrotriya* was one who, having memorized them syllable-by-syllable, recited the metrical songs of the Veda to his pupils;[64] and an *adhyāpaka* taught students practical lessons and recited treatises pertaining to the secular life.[65]

But, for Pāṇini, the most important of all teachers remained the *ācārya*. He noted that a student who had been initiated by an *ācārya* into the study of holy texts was known as an *antevāsin*[66] (nominative: *antevāsī*, literally, "one who lives at the boundary"), that is, as one who lived with a teacher in a quiet retreat in the forest far from the distracting bustle of everyday village life.[67] He described the student as *śuśrūṣu*, "one who intently listens" to the teacher's lessons,[68] and noted that the teacher and student were always "close to each other" (*upasthānīya*).[69] According to Pāṇini, the relationship between a *brahmacārī* and an *ācārya* was a spiritual bond (*vidyāsambandha*)[70] based on the sacred knowledge they studied together, and was just as real as the relationship one has with the very womb from which one has been born (*yonisambandha*).

In saying this, Pāṇini echoed an ancient Indian understanding that the teacher and student share with each other an exceptionally close inner connection. The inward effect on the student of the teacher's knowledge is said to be remarkably transformative. A song from the *Atharvaveda* (ca. 1000 B.C.E.) in praise of the *brahmacārī* speaks of the teacher's effect on the inward life of the student in the language of rebirth: "Taking [him] in charge," a verse reads, "the teacher makes the student an embryo within."[71] This internal transformation brought about by the student's contact with the teacher is said in ancient texts to link the two so intimately that it seems in some way they become one. As one text from roughly the ninth century B.C.E. notes, "When he does what his teacher asks [him to do], and when he performs any work for the teacher, he redeems that part of himself that is in the teacher; and having purified it he takes it into himself. It enters him."[72]

QUALITIES OF THE GURU AND DISCIPLE

Because of the extraordinarily close and vital relationship between a master and a disciple, Indian spiritual tradition has long held that the guru and the *śiṣya* must treat each other properly and, accordingly, both be of sound character—or, at least in the case of the student, *trying* to be of sound character. There is a certain amount of austerity (*tapas, tapasya*) involved, for spiritual education directed toward *brahmavarcasa* depends on the continued purification of the body, mind, and spirit.

The whole guru-disciple relationship itself is said to be built around the guru's compassion for the disciple and the trust the disciple must have in the guru. In a poem to her guru, Swami Chidvilasananda has written:

> The essence of the Guru-disciple relationship
> Is the Guru's compassion.
> It is limitless and unfathomable.
> So subtle yet infinitely powerful,
> It takes a disciple across
> The ocean of birth and death.[73]

A disciple's experience of the guru's compassion allows him or her to trust the guru's instructions, and thus to gain fuller understanding of the blissful nature of the divine truth said to dwell within the human heart. Swami Chidvilasananda has said, "The best way to reach the highest dharma, the knowledge of the Self, is to follow the teachings of your Guru. This is what all the Indian scriptures have advocated down through the centuries. By following the teachings of the master, you reach the pinnacle of joy without a doubt."[74] Similarly, she said, "The Guru is a benevolent force. The Guru's entire being vibrates with love. The Guru's sole purpose is to elevate the disciple to a higher state of consciousness. Little by little, the Guru transforms the disciple until he becomes the embodiment of perfection."[75] This understanding is consistent with teachings presented by devotional texts from various Indian religious traditions, which maintain that the guru offers guidance out of his or her deep compassion. Śaṅkarācārya is thought to have written this description of such teachers:

> There are pure souls who have attained peace and magnanimity. Like the coming of springtime [after winter], they bring goodness to others; for they themselves have crossed the dreadful ocean of this world and, without any [selfish] motives whatsoever, help others to cross [it, too]. It is the very nature of these magnanimous ones to endeavor, of their own choice, to remove the troubles of others, like the moon of its own cools the earth parched by the burning rays of the sun.[76]

That the guru is compassionate is a keystone of the *gurumārga* in general. Even the goddess Pārvatī is said to have recognized this potential compassion in her teacher, Śiva. According to the *Gurugītā*, the "Song of the Guru," sung every morning in Siddha Yoga ashrams, "On the beautiful summit of Mount Kailasa, Pārvatī, having bowed with reverence to Lord Śiva, who is the master of uniting one with devotion," offered her salutations to her beloved, the "teacher of the universe" (*jagadguru*). There, she asked him to initiate her into the knowledge of the guru. She said, "O Lord, by which path can an embodied soul become one with Brahman? Have compassion on me, O Lord! I bow to your feet."[77]

From the perspective of Hindu theological devotionalism, a person's misery and suffering (*duḥkha)* in the repeated cycles of life are due to his or her own distance from God. Traditions aligned with the *gurumārga* hold that it is the work of the guru that allows the disciple to bridge that distance and return to God. This point is made in a story told by Kabīr, a fifteenth-century north Indian devotional poet who described going to a marketplace one night to play devotional music and contemplate the splendid nature of God. Seeing a woman there grinding grain with a mortar and pestle, Kabīr began to weep, suddenly overcome with despair. A holy man, Nipāt Nirañjan, asked him why he was crying. "O good guru," Kabīr replied:

> As I saw the mill being turned, I saw the grains of wheat turn to flour. Just such is my condition. I have fallen between the millstones of this earthly existence. I was therefore seized with fear, and have manifested this violent grief.

"Why do you mourn in vain?" Nipāt gently asked Kabīr. "I will remove your doubts on this question." The wise man then showed Kabīr that adhering to the axle of the grinding wheel were grains of wheat that were untouched by the stones. He said:

> It is when you discard the central prop and wander about that you become as it were, flour in the mill of *kal* (death). Just as grain in the mill adhering to the central prop is not turned to flour, so those who are devoted to the worship of Shri Ram are not caught in the cycle of death.

The narrative then proclaims, "Hearing him say this, Kabīr was awakened to the truth, and the two embraced one another with feelings of love."[78]

A north Indian devotional song attributed to Kabīr also tells of this incident:

> Seeing the grinding mill turning made Kabīr begin to weep;
> Between the two grinding stones, nothing at all is saved.
> The stones keep grinding, but the axle reaches far beyond the sky.
> Sadhus and saints were saved by this, by sticking close to the axle.[79]

Swami Muktananda often told this story, saying that the axle was a metaphor for the guru, and that by adhering to the teachings of his spiritual master a disciple would be saved.[80]

If the guru teaches the student out of deep compassion, the student must also give his or her trust to the guru. Without this trust, the student is consumed by doubts and insecurities. Swami Chidvilasananda has said:

> As much as the Guru's grace is abundant, the disciple's grace must be very generous too; then the eternal bond between the Guru and disciple can flourish. Baba called the Guru-disciple relationship "the perfect relationship." Unless you trust the Guru fully and in every way, you are eaten up by your own shortcomings. A true Guru wishes only the best for his disciple, only the disciple's upliftment. The Guru totally sacrifices himself to redeem his beloved disciple. The Guru bears every pain to purify the disciple and have him experience the vision of God.[81]

Indian tradition has recognized a number of ways in which such trust is established. The *Laws of Manu*, an influential second-century text on dharma, outlines in some detail the way a disciple is to behave when with the teacher; he is, for example, to refrain from sensual indulgence, to cultivate humility and industriousness, and to act always in a respectful and dignified manner toward his teacher.[82] For his part, the teacher is to honor his student by teaching him with compassion and gentility.[83]

The Vedāntic perspective of the true guru-disciple relationship revolves, in part, around the idea that the disciple must be genuine in his or her longing to know the eternal Self and must act in a way that is consistent with this aspiration. The Vedānta also stipulates that the guru truly and lovingly lead such a seeker toward the liberating experience of the Self. Such a relationship is suggested by these lines from the *Muṇḍaka Upaniṣad*:

> To [a seeker] who has approached him in a proper manner—
> whose mind is calm and who has gained peace—
> may the wise [teacher] teach the knowledge of the Absolute
> [*brahmavidyā*]
> in its very truth, [the knowledge] by which
> one knows the true, imperishable Self.[84]

According to the Vedāntic tradition, the guru's compassionate work with the disciple (*śiṣya*) is based on the teacher's firm commitment to the disciple's liberation from spiritual bondage. The *Upadeśasāhasrī* ("A Thousand Teachings"), a work attributed to Śaṅkarācārya (eighth to ninth century), presents the Vedāntic idea that the teacher removes the impurities from the student's karmic situation, the residue of which is preventing the disciple from true understanding. "When he discovers from [various] signs that the disciple has not properly understood," Śaṅkarācārya is reported to have said, "the teacher should remove those causes of noncomprehension, which are [the result] of improper and profane acts [*adharmalaukika*] in the past and present. . . . He should also impress upon the disciple [the importance of] qualities, such as humility, that lead to knowledge."[85]

Several verses toward the beginning of the *Vivekacūḍāmaṇi* ("The Crest-Jewel of Discrimination"), another work traditionally attributed to Śaṅkarācārya, present in concise form a Vedāntic perspective regarding the qualifications of a true seeker of liberation and the qualities such a disciple is to cultivate. It is worth quoting these lines at some length, for they give us much to consider regarding the Vedāntic understanding of spiritual discipline in the context of discipleship. We note, initially, the importance of one's spiritual yearning and openness to the guiding wisdom of a teacher. We see, too, that one is to cultivate tranquillity and other contemplative virtues. But we are also to note that, in giving his or her trust to the teacher, the true disciple is *not* thereby to abandon the power of reason and judgment. In fact, the text holds that it is one's diligent practice of reasoned examination or discerning reflection (*vicāra*) that, finally, allows one to discriminate between truth and unreality.

> Having given up his craving for pleasure from external objects, the wise person should strive diligently for freedom. He should approach a great and generous teacher and imbibe deeply the truth that is given to him.
>
> Having become absorbed in the nature of contemplative discipline, one should rescue one's soul, which lies drowned in the ocean of birth and death, by means of one's devotion to proper discrimination. . . .

> Firm knowledge of the truth is gained only through discerning examination of the great teachings of the wise. . . . Therefore, let one who would know the reality that is the Self [*ātman*] turn to reasoned examination. But first one should approach a Guru who is a perfect knower of Brahman and who is an ocean of compassion.[86]

The teacher welcomes the disciple because the student has demonstrated his or her genuine yearning to learn. Śaṅkara described the true spiritual seeker in this way:

> One who discriminates [between the real and the unreal] and who is disenchanted [with the unreal], who possesses tranquillity and related virtues, and who longs for liberation: only that one may be considered qualified to study Brahman.[87]

The text states that wise teachers have recognized four requirements for genuine spiritual discipline:

> In this connection, the sages have spoken of four means of attainment. If they are present, one's devotion to truth becomes fulfilled. If they are absent, it fails.[88]

> The first mentioned is discrimination between the eternal and the noneternal. The next is renunciation of the fruits [of one's actions], both here [in this world] and in the hereafter. Next come the group of six attainments, beginning with tranquillity. The [fourth], certainly, is the yearning for liberation.[89]

The text then expands on the nature of these four basic requirements. It begins by explaining what is meant by discrimination (*viveka*).

> Brahman is real; the world is unreal. The firm conviction that this is so is said to be discrimination between the eternal and the transitory.[90]

It defines renunciation or "dispassion" (*vairāgya*, elsewhere in the text also *virāga*) as the turning away from ephemeral means of gratification, which it regards as the sensual pleasures not only of the physical body but also those enjoyed by a sublime or heavenly body:

> Renunciation is the giving up of pleasures ranging from those beginning with seeing and hearing and the rest all the way to the highest kind of divine body.[91]

The text then turns to the group of six "attainments" (*ṣaṭkasampatti*), which it identifies as tranquillity, self-control, mental equanimity, patient forbearance, trust, and a certain settledness or deep contentment within one's heart.

> To detach the mind from sense objects by continuously noting their defects and to direct it firmly toward its goal [of liberation]: this is called "tranquillity" [*śama*].
>
> To detach both kinds of sense-organs [that is, the organs of perception and the organs of action] from objective things and to place them in their proper centers: this is called "self-control" [*dama*].
>
> The best mental equanimity [*uparati*] consists in the mind's ceasing to be affected by external events.
>
> To endure all kinds of afflictions without resentment, anxiety, or complaint: this is called "forbearance" [*titikṣa*].
>
> A firm conviction, based on reasoned understanding, that what the scriptures and the guru say is true: this is called "trust" [*śraddhā*] by which reality is known.
>
> To concentrate the intellect constantly and steadfastly on the pure Brahman: this is called "settledness" [of one's spirit or "contemplative composure," *samādhāna*]. This does not mean merely indulging one's mind [in pleasant or soothing thoughts].[92]

The passage then defines what it means by the fourth of the four basic qualities of the true seeker, namely, the yearning for liberation:

> The yearning for freedom [*mumukṣutva*] is the longing to be free from all bondages created through ignorance—ranging from [the bondage] due to egoism to [the bondage to] the body—through the realization of one's true nature.[93]

Having outlined the qualities that it regards to be necessary for genuine discipleship, the *Vivekacūḍāmaṇi* implies rather directly that the most important are first, *mumukṣutva* and second, *vairāgya*; for, when combined with the compassionate grace of the guru, the seeker's true yearning for liberation from the cycles of worldly existence and the renunciation of the fleeting pleasures that bind him or her to that world eventually lead to the practice of the other components of sadhana. When these two are strong, the other attainments come readily. Without them, there can be no true discipleship. We read that—

> Even though it may be slight or mediocre, this longing for freedom will increase through the grace of the guru and through the practice of renunciation and of the attainments such as tranquillity. It will bear fruit.

> For one whose renunciation and yearning for freedom are intense, then the practice of tranquillity and the other attainments are genuinely meaningful and are fruitful.
>
> [However,] when this renunciation and longing for freedom are weak, then tranquillity and the other attainments are an illusion, like a mirage in the desert.[94]

The *Vivekacūḍāmaṇi* concludes this particular set of verses on the qualifications of the disciple by returning to the supreme importance of the disciple's loving devotion (*bhakti*) in the process of liberation. The text does not say to whom this love is to be directed. Perhaps it is to the universal Self (Ātman), or perhaps it is to the guru. (As we will see later, Siddha Yoga holds that in fact, at a very deep level, the Self and the guru are one and the same.)

> Among all means of liberation, loving devotion alone is supreme. Loving devotion is understood to be the seeking after one's own true nature.
>
> Another way [to say it] is that loving devotion is defined as the inquiry into the truth of one's own Self. The seeker of the truth of the Self, one who possesses the qualifications mentioned [in the verses] above, should approach a wise guru, who gives liberation from bondage.[95]

Having noted the important qualities of the disciple, the text then describes the guru and encourages the disciple to entrust the guru with any questions he or she may have regarding the nature of the Self.

> [The guru] is deeply versed in the sacred scriptures, pure, untouched by [selfish] desire, the highest knower of Brahman. [The guru] abides firmly in Brahman and is calm like a flame that has consumed all of its fuel. [The guru] is an ocean of unconditional love, a friend to all good people who humbly present themselves before him.
>
> Let the seeker approach the guru with loving devotion. Having pleased him with humility, love, and service, let one ask whatever he wishes to know of the Self.[96]

In a way, the Vedāntic vision of the guru-disciple relationship is summarized in a subsequent verse from the *Vivekacūḍāmaṇi*. Here, we see the idea that the student must be a true seeker and that the guru teaches such a disciple out of graceful compassion:

> To one who has sought his protection, to one who yearns for liberation, to one who has properly performed [his or her responsibilities according] to the scriptures, to one whose mind has become tranquil and who has become

calm, [to such a one] the teacher, out of grace, proceeds to teach the truth.[97]

The Tantric tradition of Hindu spirituality presents a similar image of the guru-disciple relationship. A section of the *Kulārṇava Tantra* presents a number of characteristics of the guru and the *śiṣya*. It is too long to present in its entirety here, but it is worth looking at an abridged version. The *śiṣya* is described as follows:

> . . . steady in the practice of spiritual disciplines that lead to wholeness, pure in nature, clean in body and dress, intent on wisdom, dedicated to ethical responsibility, pure of mind, steady in the observance of religious obligations, abiding in the practice of the truth, infused with both faith and devotion, diligent, thoughtful, engaged in service to others without selfish motive, free of the poverty of the mind, skillful in action, clean, grateful, wary of misconduct, dedicated to the welfare of all beings. [The disciple is to be] one who has trust and modesty [and] does not deceive others in regards to wealth and physical appearance, achieves [what otherwise may seem] impossible. [The disciple] is courageous, enthusiastic, and strong, and engages in beneficial work; he avoids intoxication; is capable, helpful to others, and truthful. [The disciple] is not obsequious and is reserved in speech; he refuses to blame others, understands [what is taught] after it is said just one time. [The disciple] prefers not to hear others praise him and does not turn from their criticism. He is the master of his senses, intelligent, sexually responsible. [The disciple] is free from worry, malaise, fickleness, delusion and doubt.[98]

In a subsequent description of the guru, the *Kulārṇava Tantra* emphasizes, among other points, the guru's reverence for his own guru.

> The guru must be skilled in meditation. He must praise his guru and speak well of him. He must worship and bow to God, be devoted to the divine guru. He should remain in the company of the guru, please the guru, and be engaged at all times in serving the guru by means of his mind, speech, and body. He should obey the guru's command, spread the glory of the guru, and know the authority of the guru's word. He should be a servant to the guru, free from arrogant pride due to his social class, prestige, or wealth. [The guru] knows the truth of the scriptures and knows how to apply all of the mantras. He rids [the disciple] of delusion and doubt. [The guru's] attention is directed inward, although he may be looking outward. [The guru] conquers the six enemies: desire, anger, greed, delusion, jealousy, pride. He contains the power of the mantra. Constant and merciful, the guru feels at one with all [and] is supremely dedicated to the performance of moral responsibility.[99]

The Yogic tradition holds similar perspectives regarding the guru and the disciple, and the nature of the proper attitude of the disciple (*adhikārin*). A classic text from that tradition, the *Śiva Saṃhitā*, holds:

> The first condition of success [for the *adhikārin*] is the firm belief that [the knowledge his guru gives him] will come to fulfillment and be fruitful. The second is to have trust in [that knowledge]. The third is to honor the guru. The fourth is to have equanimity. The fifth to have controlled the senses. The sixth is to eat in moderation. . . . Having received instructions in [the practice of] yoga, and having met a guru who knows yoga, he should practice [yoga] with diligence and insight, according to the method taught by the guru.[100]

Like their Vedāntic, Tantric, and Yogic counterparts, so too the Bhakti spiritual traditions in India teach that the disciple is to cultivate important virtues with the help of his or her guru's guidance. The *Jñāneśvarī*, for example—the thirteenth-century saint Jñāneśvar's magnificent commentary in Marathi verse on the *Bhagavadgītā*—presents a number of extended passages on various virtues a disciple is to cultivate.[101] Jñāneśvar stresses the importance of humility and unpretentiousness; of maintaining a nonviolent attitude; of patience and straightforwardness; of purity, steadfastness, self-control, dispassion, and selflessness.

In our own time, Swami Chidvilasananda has directed her devotees' attention to the importance of cultivating virtues. She has spoken at length, for example, about the importance in spiritual life of practicing fearlessness, purity of being, steadfastness, freedom from anger, compassion, humility, respect, and selfless service.[102]

THE TRANSFORMATIVE FUNCTION OF *GURUSEVĀ*

According to Swami Chidvilasananda, the last virtue just mentioned—selfless service—is one of the most important practices of a disciple. Siddha Yoga gurus are, of course, not unique in this view. Traditional thought in India holds that to contribute to the ongoing welfare of one's community and to perform one's responsibilities without selfish motivations are the key components of a meaningful and moral life. One might justly say that the fundamental lesson of the *Bhagavadgītā* is this one point: To act selflessly in the world is to serve God.[103] Swami Chidvilasananda has quoted Kṛṣṇa's description of such activity as "pure" in nature because it is not tainted by any self-centeredness:

> That action, which is prescribed by the scriptures,
> which is free from all attachments,
> performed without passion and without hate,
> by one who has no desire for any reward,
> is said to be sattvic or pure.[104]

In a set of teachings regarding such selfless activity, Chidvilasananda has also referred to Jñāneśvar's comment on this verse:

> This daily duty, supported by periodic rites, is good and is like
> fragrance added to gold.
> Just as a mother will devote all the strength of her body and life to
> caring for a child without thinking of her own weariness,
> In the same way, a good person will perform his duty wholeheartedly, without a thought for its fruit, and by offering it to God.[105]

In the context of religious sensibilities centered around the *gurumārga*, such service to the world, and thus to God, is often described as "selfless service to the guru," a phrase which translates the Sanskrit *gurusevā* as well as the more classical *ācāryopāsana*, "attendance on the teacher." In one of her talks, Swami Chidvilasananda called *ācāryopāsana* "one of the best qualities." She added, "The whole of Siddha Yoga is built on seva, service," and she quoted this passage from Jñāneśvar:

> The service of a true disciple has no limitations
> of time and space.
> When he is serving, he does not think
> about day or night,
> Nor does he regard any service
> as either greater or lesser.
> The harder the work the Guru gives,
> the fresher and stronger he becomes.[106]

Chidvilasananda teaches, "When there is this longing, when there is this desire for service, discipleship comes automatically." She has recounted some of the many things her guru, Swami Muktananda, did in establishing the many ashrams and spiritual as well as social programs around the world. "He gave and kept on giving. There was absolute, total service. There was complete one-pointedness. He always said, 'My Guru asked me to do it, and that is why I do it.'"[107] Ideas and values associated with the practice of selfless service to the guru are closely connected with the notion that in a perfect guru-disciple relationship, the disciple is to "follow the guru's command."

There is in India a long history of such sentiments. We have already noted that, as early as the fourth century B.C.E., a disciple was instructed to gather wood to burn in his teacher's sacred fires,[108] which suggests that the disciple was to help the teacher maintain the guru's household (*gurukula*) in an appropriate manner. Similar teachings and perspectives appear, for example, in Vedāntic, Yogic, and Bhakti traditions. Writing from the perspective of the Advaita Vedānta, Śaṅkara says:

> Let [the seeker] approach the guru with reverence and devotion [*bhakti*]. Then, when he has pleased him with humility, love and service, let him ask whatever is to be known of the Self. [He should say], "O Master, O friend of all devotees, the ocean of compassion, I honor you. I have fallen into the [turbulent] sea of the world. Save me with [your] steadfast look which sheds supreme grace, like ambrosia.[109]

The Yogic perspective, given in the *Śiva Saṃhitā,* is this:

> One who is dedicated to [gaining] knowledge readily gains the fruit of that knowledge if he or she serves the guru in every way. There is no doubt that the guru is the father. The guru is the mother. The guru is even God. As such, he should be served by all [disciples] in their thought, word, and act. It is through the guru's blessing that everything good pertaining to one's self is gained. Therefore, the guru should be served daily. Otherwise, no goodness can come to be.[110]

Writing from the *bhakti* perspective, Jñāneśvar said this:

> I will become the Guru's house. I will be his servant and do all his work. I will be the threshold of the door over which my Guru passes when entering or leaving his house. I will both be the door and his doorkeeper. I will become his shoes and will also put them on his feet. I will become his umbrella as well as the one who holds it. I will be his herald and the one who holds his fly whisk. I will be his forerunner. I will prepare his betel nut and serve his personal needs. I will make the preparations for his bath. I will become the seat on which he rests, his garments, his ornaments, sandalwood paste, and all other articles for his use. . . . I will become his throne. Thus I will serve him in every way.[111]

The idea that a disciple is to undertake selfless service to the guru may make people who are unfamiliar with the *gurumārga* in Indian tradition somewhat uncomfortable. There is some good reason for this, for the late twentieth century has seen a number of unfortunate incidents of gullible people surrendering their judgment and integrity to follow so-called religious leaders, sometimes bringing great harm to themselves and others.

Swami Muktananda himself was well aware of Westerners' unfamiliarity with the role of the guru in the religious traditions of India. He also seems to have understood that many people legitimately distrust religious teachers whose followers express inordinate deference, and he often spoke about the danger of surrendering oneself to a false guru. "The Guru-disciple relationship has a long tradition," he once said in a conversation with a devotee. "It exists in the East, but the West takes hardly any interest in the subject. Some people become very unhappy when they even hear about this relationship. It gives them a headache, but that's understandable because there are some bad gurus around. So choose a good Guru."[112] Another time he warned, "With all the Gurus that are coming, the disciple should stay alert. He should look and see how much of what the guru is saying is really in the guru."[113]

Muktananda appears to have been equally firm in maintaining that "the disciple . . . must choose his Guru after a great deal of thought and deliberation,"[114] and that "if there is a command from the Guru which seems to go against the scriptures, which would alienate you from your own Self, you have to pause and think very deeply whether you should obey or not."[115] He seems to have been especially concerned that some false gurus demand that their followers surrender to them in an unhealthy way. In response to a statement that "many people think that by following a Guru, they will be allowing their lives to fall under someone else's control," he said:

> A Guru doesn't make a person weak and keep him under his control. Instead, he frees him from dependency. The job of a Guru is not to bind a disciple, but to give him the freedom of the Self. People think that if they accept the authority of a Guru, they will lose their individual freedom and become slaves. . . . When I took refuge in my Guru, I became completely free of dependence.[116]

Muktananda explored this apparent paradox—that by taking refuge in the guru one becomes independent—saying that the goal of discipleship is not to remain a mere disciple. "The relationship between a Guru and a disciple is divine," he said. "It is so great that as time passes by, the disciple becomes the Guru."[117] By saying this Muktananda did not mean that a disciple necessarily becomes a spiritual teacher, but rather that the disciple in some way turns from his or her former way of looking at the world and shares the guru's state of awareness. The guru is the "finished" or "complete" form of the disciple, as it were. The guru is also a disciple himself; the guru has been over the same terrain, and therefore guides from experience. The *Taittirīya Upaniṣad* (ca. fifth century B.C.E.) says, "The teacher is the older form; the student is the younger form. Knowledge is their meeting point; instruction is the connection."[118]

According to Muktananda, a person who "becomes a disciple like this does not remain stuck in discipleship. He does not become small and weak; he does not become a mere slave. Instead, he becomes established in the state the Guru has attained. By surrendering to the Guru, he himself becomes the Guru."[119] Similarly: "A true Guru is not one who makes everybody his disciple and keeps them in that condition. . . . Only he is a true Guru who . . . takes discipleship away from his disciples and turns them into beings like himself."[120] Muktananda also said, "The disciple loses himself in the teachings of the Guru. The Guru-disciple relationship is this: The Guru commands and the disciple obeys. Then the disciple becomes the Guru yet does not lose his discipleship. This is the perfect Guru-disciple relationship. It is based on the disciple's constant remembrance of his identity with the Guru."[121]

This is yet another essential paradox inherent in the disciple's relationship with the guru: By following the guru's command the disciple becomes "empty" and, in a sense, "disappears"; at the same time, the disciple becomes "whole" and finds fulfillment, completion. The key to resolving this paradox is found in the understanding that it is the sense of alienation from God due to the three *malas* discussed earlier that keeps the disciple trapped in various cycles of confusion, discouragement, and even despair. Swamis Muktananda and Chidvilasananda locate the source of this misunderstanding in what they call the "ego." Here the term *ego* is not being used as Sigmund Freud would have used it, in reference to the beneficial capacity of the mind that balances various conflicting internal and cultural imperatives. In the context of Indian philosophy, the word *ego* translates such Sanskrit terms as *ahaṃkāra*, which literally means "I-maker." Spiritual teachers in India have long regarded *ahaṃkāra* to be that function of the mind which leads one to think of oneself as separate from the world; it is this perspective that leads one to identify one's emotions, thoughts, problems, and even physical body as one's "own," when in reality they are all part of the larger universe as a whole, inseparable from the interwoven fabric of Being. The extent to which this sense of alienation is dissolved is the degree to which the disciple returns to the already-intimate reality of God's constant presence.

To lose the false ego is, therefore, to open oneself to experience the fullness of God. The guru helps the disciple do precisely this. The guru can do so because he has become free of the ego himself. According to the *Haṃsabheda Tantra*:

> Many are those Masters who are honored and served, resplendent with consciousness and discrimination. But . . . it is hard to find that Master who [himself free of ego] can destroy the egos of others. It is through him that revelation is communicated, through him that all things are accomplished, through him that, freed of ego, one recognizes oneself in one's essential purity (*kevala*).[122]

Because he has no ego, the guru sees no distinction between guru and disciple or between guru and God. To the guru, all things emerge from, return to, and embody in their various ways a single Self, which is the Self of the universe. This perspective is similar to that presented by Advaita Vedānta, the nondualist philosophy that holds that there is only one true "Self" in the universe and that this Self is the singular reality of Being. It is also similar to important strands of Hindu theism, which hold that this universal Self is none other than God, variously regarded as Śiva, Viṣṇu, or one of the forms of the Goddess. Finally, it is closely aligned with the long tradition of Hindu devotionalism, which experiences this divine Self as of the nature of supreme love. Hindu thought in general maintains that one comes to taste the nectarean essence of this universal divine Self when one unlocks the debilitating and delimiting mental structures that separate one from that vital, fundamental, and independent reality.[123]

The guru is understood as the one who helps the disciple taste this nectar by dissolving the disciple's false sense of separation from God, that is, by taking power away from the disciple's identification with the mundane world. Sometimes this takes the form of testing the disciple. This "testing" is not to be understood in a negative sense. The purpose of the guru's test is to break down the self-centered and spiritually counterproductive pride that often accompanies *ahaṃkāra.* In describing this aspect of the guru's work with the disciple, Kabīr used the metaphor of a potter forming a pot:

> Guru is potter, disciple is pot. He [the potter] removes the faults one by one. Giving a supporting hand inside, he beats hard outside.[124]

Swami Muktananda has recounted one of the ways that his Guru worked with him in this regard:

> Bhagawan Nityananda helped me a great deal in my sadhana. He was especially helpful in crushing my ego. I was kind of a half-scholar. I had read some books and had some knowledge of the scriptures. So I had the pride of that knowledge. Above all, I wore the clothes of a *sannyāsi* [a monk], and I was always playing that role. My Guru must have undergone a lot of trouble trying to straighten me out. But he did it.
>
> He had his own ways of testing me. Sometimes he would allow me to come close to him, and sometimes he would not. Devotees would bring him piles of sweets and fruits, which he would then distribute as *prasād* [blessed food]. I would get into the line of people waiting for prasad, but sometimes when he saw me he would hold the fruit aside and say, "No, not for you." . . .
>
> Even when the Guru teases a disciple, he is really praising him.[125]

According to Muktananda, this "testing" is an act of supreme beneficence, for it frees the disciple from the constraints of a limited sense of who he or she truly is. "The more my Guru tested me," Muktananda said, "the more I advanced in my sadhana. . . . To live for a long time with the Guru, a disciple must have great endurance."[126] The disciple opens his or her being to receive such a gift by performing the spiritual disciplines that help weaken the ego's grip. Among such disciplines is that of *ācāryopāsana* or *gurusevā.* This service is undertaken not for the guru's benefit but rather for the disciple's. Furthermore, it is to be performed selflessly, for the less identification there is in such discipline, the more the ego dissolves. To use a term from the parlance of Siddha Yoga, the less one has a sense of "doership" in one's service to the guru, the closer one comes to union with the guru.

Service to the guru allows one to be free of the forces of *ahaṃkāra* and thus to come closer to an experience of the Self. As one Siddha Yoga teacher has said, "When we go beyond ego we go beyond the limitations of time and space; we enter into eternity. We experience the sensation of the Self, which is unconditional love. It is like coming home. Free from the ego, we begin to enjoy the life which all the sages and saints have known. When the ego is transcended all that is left is the pure Self; then we abide in our true nature—peaceful, content, and fulfilled. Such is the gift of the Guru."[127]

Swami Chidvilasananda has quoted the poet-saint Kabīr in this regard:

As long as I existed,
I had not met my true Master.
Now that I no longer exist,
There is no more ego,
There is only the Guru.[128]

It is by means of the dissolution of the ego, therefore, that the disciple becomes one with the guru. This is important for, as we have mentioned before and will explore further, the essential being of the guru is indistinguishable from the essence of God; the ultimate guru is God himself. Serving the guru, the disciple offers his or her otherwise ego-driven self to the encompassing wisdom of God. The disciple then sees everything from the perspective of a joyful and liberating humility, free from the burden of self-centeredness.

Siddha Yoga and the traditions on which it draws hold that when one has surrendered one's ego to the wisdom of God, one finds complete fulfillment in following the will of God. Jñāneśvar quotes Arjuna saying this to his guru, whom he had come to recognize as the very incarnation of God:

> O Lord Krishna, You are my great Guru, whom I must serve in simple devotion. Shouldn't I consider this to be Your blessing of oneness with God? The door of separation which stood between You and me has been transformed into the happiness of joyful service. Now, O Lord of all the gods, I will obey Your commands, whatever you may demand of me.[129]

The "guru's command" impels the disciple to continue further on the path to spontaneity, joy, and a deep affirmation of life; and to "follow the guru's command" is to direct one's life according to the loving and liberating vision the guru holds for one's self. Inspired by the guru, such discipline leads finally to ultimate freedom and to the pervasive celebration of the fullness of being. It was such discipline that led to Jñāneśvar's ability to proclaim this of his guru, Nivṛttināth:

Now I offer salutations to Him
Who is the well-spring to the garden of sadhana,
The auspicious thread of divine Will . . . .

I offer salutations to Him
Who comes to the aid of the Self
Which is suffering limitation
In the wilderness of ignorance. . . .

By his mere glance,
Bondage becomes liberation,
And the Knower becomes the known.

He distributes the gold of liberation to all,
Both the great and the small;
It is He who gives the vision of the Self.[130]

In Siddha Yoga the guru gives this command in a number of ways: through public lectures and published books; through outward lessons on how to perform various spiritual practices that discipline the body, mind, and spirit; and also by means of the quiet inner voice in which the disciple inwardly hears words of support and guidance. The disciple follows the guru's command by meditating on and diligently putting into effect in his or her life the teachings and practices the guru gives.

With genuine and healthy humility, the true disciple offers his or her entire life, not to the ego, but rather to God. Swami Chidvilasananda has said:

> When you have true humility and God becomes your whole life, you offer everything to Him. Everything is offered to one place, to one Principle, to one God. This is the sadhana of discipleship. . . .
>
> [Discipleship] does not involve becoming someone else's slave or servant. It involves the way we conduct ourselves in every situation, in every circumstance, at every moment, with everyone. The sadhana of discipleship is the sadhana of life itself.[131]

SOTERIOLOGICAL ASPECTS OF THE GURU-DISCIPLE RELATIONSHIP

In traditional Indian thought, as represented by the Upaniṣads, the *ācārya* was generally regarded as a *brāhmaṇa*, "one who knows Brahman." In these classical texts we see suggestions that because he possessed full knowledge of God, the teacher was considered an embodiment of God. Therefore, the Upaniṣadic student yearning to know Brahman demonstrated devotion to his teacher, for the reality of the former was revealed in and by the person of the latter. This is particularly apparent in the more theistic Upaniṣads,[132] which depict the absolute in such personal terms as *bhagavān*, "the Beloved One"; *īśa*, the "Lord"; and *deva*, "God." The epilogue to the *Śvetāśvatara Upaniṣad*, for example, states, "One who [has] the highest devotion to God and for his guru as God: to that great-souled one these teachings will shine forth."[133]

Drawing on Upaniṣadic perspectives, the Advaita Vedāntic tradition regards the purpose of spiritual study to be the attainment of a liberating freedom from the pernicious ignorance which is said to trap the human spirit in cycles of confusion and its resulting suffering. The *Vivekacūḍāmaṇi*, for example, identifies three forces that lead to liberation:

> Faith, devotion, and the yoga of meditation—these are mentioned by the revealed scriptures as the immediate factors of liberation in the case of the seeker; whoever abides in these gets liberation from the bondage of the body, which is the conjuring of ignorance.[134]

The text characterizes faith (*śraddhā*) as the "acceptance by firm judgment as true of what the scriptures and the guru instruct . . . by means of which the Real is perceived."[135] It defines devotion (*bhakti*) as "the seeking after one's real nature" and asserts that one who has such devotion should study with a guru who can lead him to knowledge of that true nature and, thus, to freedom from ignorance.

> Among things conducive to liberation, devotion alone holds the supreme place. The seeking after one's real nature is designated as devotion. Others maintain that the inquiry into the truth of one's own Self is devotion. The inquirer about the truth of the Atman who is possessed of the above-mentioned means of attainment should approach a wise preceptor [*guru*], who confers emancipation from bondage."[136]

These Vedic and Vedāntic texts suggest that the absolute can be revealed through the person of the guru, and that this revelation can bring about the disciple's spiritual fulfillment. This notion is consonant with the one that emerged in India in the later centuries of the first millennium B.C.E. and that found full expression in the rise of the Bhakti movements beginning in the seventh century C.E., namely, an otherwise eternal and transcendent deity can and does enter the world of time and space in a process described as a "crossing over" (*avatāraṇa*) of the distance between the two realms.

Tradition describes such an "incarnation" of God as an *avatāra*. The most influential of early texts holding such a view must undoubtedly be the

Bhagavadgītā, the "Song of the Beloved One," in which the *avatāra* Kṛṣṇa acts as divine guru and teaches the confused and distraught Arjuna of the nature of ultimate reality and of the importance of following one's dharma in support of that reality.

"Explain to me further in detail your power and manifestation," Arjuna pleads of Kṛṣṇa; "I am never satiated with hearing your nectar-like words."[137]

Kṛṣṇa replies, "To you I shall explain in full this knowledge, along with [its] realization; [it] having been understood, nothing remains to be known here in this world." (Jñāneśvar, in his commentary, has the Lord add, "Now I will impart to you knowledge and direct experience, so you will know me fully, like a jewel that is lying on the palm of your hand.")[138]

Arjuna's despair disappears when he comes to see that Kṛṣṇa is indeed God himself, and he surrenders his misdirected ego in accepting the moral guidance his divine guru has given him. The song ends with Arjuna's affirmation to Kṛṣṇa: "Through your grace my delusion is gone and wisdom gained, O Constant One! I stand now with doubt dispelled." Seeing now that God is the ultimate agent of all activity and that dharmic behavior is that which is aligned with the divine will, Arjuna tells the beloved One, *kariṣye vacanaṃ tava*: "I will follow your teaching."[139]

Expanding on this verse, Jñāneśvar has Arjuna add:

> You are that visible form which destroys all other visible things, which though separate swallows up all separateness, which is one and yet dwells eternally in all. Bondage to You brings liberation from all bonds, desire for You destroys all desires, and in meeting You one is revealed to oneself. You are my supreme Guru, who comes to the aid of the lonely and for whose sake one must pass over into the realization of union.[140]

Jñāneśvar has Kṛṣṇa be so delighted with his disciple that he "began to dance with joy" and proclaimed that "Arjuna has become the fruit of the tree of the universe, which is I Myself."[141]

According to this line of thought, the guru-disciple relationship revolves around the guru's compassionate concern for the disciple, and the disciple's willingness to conduct his life in accordance with the divine will, as revealed by the guru's teachings. God as guru frees the disciple from ignorance and brings that disciple back into conscious unity with the divine. In this kind of theological setting, the ideal relationship between the guru and a disciple is therefore that of God and his faithful devotee.

Selfless devotion to God thus allows one to open oneself to and in a sense merge with the divine presence. The *Bhagavadgītā* notes that Kṛṣṇa—according to that text, God himself—told Arjuna, "By devotion to Me, he comes to know who I am in truth; then having known Me in truth, he enters Me immediately."[142] The Indian devotional tradition holds that such a union takes place, not in some distant realm, but rather deep within the human spirit, for God already lives within the devotee's heart. The seeker's task is to uncover this already-present divine love. Jñāneśvar expands on this verse by adding the teaching that "treasures lie concealed within the earth, fire is latent in wood, and milk is contained in the udder of a cow. But to obtain these things, one must use the right methods. I must also be reached by certain means."[143] And what, according to Jñāneśvar are the "right methods"? The poet-saint has Kṛṣṇa tell Arjuna, "The established way to reach union with Me is through each disciple's relationship with his Guru."[144]

It is precisely in this type of soteriological relationship—one that links God and guru and devotee—that Indian religious traditions based on *īśvarabhakti*, "devotion to God," and *gurubhakti*, "devotion to the guru," most overlap; the attainment comes when the worshiper offers his or her full love and devotion.

Key components of devotional thought appear in the *Nārada Bhakti Sūtras*, a set of short aphorisms on loving devotion attributed to the sage Nārada. In this work Nārada uses the word *bhakti* in two ways. On one hand, it refers to ultimate reality, which according to Nārada takes the form of the transcendent love one tastes as divine nectar (*amṛta*).[145] Gaining that state, a person becomes complete (*siddha*) and fully contented. "Immersed in the bliss of the universal Self," one "becomes intoxicated, by this [love]."[146] Nārada calls this bliss of the universal Self *parābhakti*, a term we might translate as "supreme love." To abide in *parābhakti* is to be freed from self-centeredness and absorbed in God's perfect and perfecting love.

The other way Nārada uses the term *bhakti* is in reference to the process or discipline that leads to the experience of ultimate reality as supreme love. This he calls *aparābhakti*, "secondary devotional love." By "secondary" or "less than supreme," he does not mean that this is in some way less valuable than supreme love. Rather, he refers to a set of spiritual attitudes, perspectives, and practices that support and thus lead the devotee to the final state. In other words, supreme love is the goal, and secondary devotional love is a form of spiritual discipline by which the spiritual seeker reaches that goal.

Such discipline includes the devotee's performing acts of devotional worship, speaking lovingly about sacred subjects, and cultivating an inner equanimity so that the delight of the Self is not disturbed.[147] For Nārada, the disciple who best expresses this love is one who "lives constantly in the state of consecrating all activities [to God], in self-surrender, and in deep anguish if [God] is forgotten."[148] He holds that such divine love alone "should be grasped [as the goal] for those who yearn for freedom."[149]

Nārada further distinguishes secondary devotional love into two levels. The more advanced he describes as "love with one purpose" and as "higher love" (*ekāntabhakti* and *mukhyabhakti*, respectively). This form of loving devotion is practiced by those who "have one-pointed [love for God]":[150]

> Conversing with each other, their voices choking [from love], with tears in their eyes [and] their bodies thrilled [by the excitement of divine love], they purify [not only their] families but the land [they live on]. They sanctify places of pilgrimage [with their presence], render holy all beneficial actions, and authenticate the scriptures [by the way they live].[151]

Nārada encourages those who do not yet have such a one-pointed *gurubhakti* to practice a more preliminary form of secondary devotional love: *gauṇabhakti*, loving devotion to a physical object. Nārada teaches that "this form of devotion is more readily attained"[152] and thus more easily practiced than are the others. *Gauṇabhakti* is of three different types according to the quality of the devotee's mind. In this context, Nārada refers to the three *guṇas*, the three fundamental qualities of the psychological and physical world. He thus implies that, depending on the devotee's own proclivities, loving devotion can be directed toward that which is unmanifest, pure, or sublime (in other words, that which is *sāttvika*); or toward that which is energetic (*rājasa*); or to that which is physically manifest (*tāmasa*). In any case, offering his or her love, the devotee moves closer and closer to the experience of what Nārada calls "the good" (*śreyas*). He writes:

> Devotion directed to an object with characteristics is of three kinds, according to the quality of its physical nature. . . . [But] each preceding one leads to a better succeeding one for the sake of the good.[153]

How does one come to begin one's spiritual discipline at the secondary level of devotional love and thus to experience supreme love? Nārada says that this all comes through the grace of the physical guru. That grace may be very subtle and mysterious in its effect, Nārada says, yet it is undeniably fruitful. He says that the grace of the guru is more immediate than that of God, perhaps because the grace of God is mediated through the grace of the guru. Nārada is careful to add that, ultimately, there is no difference between the grace of the guru and the grace of God:

> [Divine Love experienced at the level of *parābhakti*] is gained primarily through the grace of great souls [*mahatkṛpa*] or in a small part through the grace of the Lord. Yet it is extremely difficult to come into the presence of a great soul [thus] and to benefit [from his teachings. The influence such a guru has on the seeker] is incomprehensible and unfailing. Nevertheless, [divine love] is indeed attainable through his grace alone, because between him [God] and his creatures there is no difference![154]

In his *Bhakti Sūtras*, Nārada presents the idea that intoxicating divine love can indeed be experienced, for God is of the nature of love itself. Because it is said to lead to liberation from the constraints of selfishness and all the pain this selfishness brings, such ecstasy serves a truly soteriological or redemptive function. Nārada also points out that the way to experience this divine love is through the practice of loving devotion. He notes that such devotion can be directed to the pure, unmanifest essence at the *sāttvika* level of *mukhyabhakti,* but he also teaches that this devotion can be expressed to manifest forms, as well.

The perfect physical form toward which one could express one's inherent love would be, of course, the perfectly loving person, the physical guru, called by Nārada the "great soul." Then, advancing into more subtle forms of *bhakti,* the seeker's devotion moves from the material to the energetic, from the energetic to the sublime, and from the sublime to the divine formlessness experienced at the "one-pointed" or "higher" level of secondary devotional love. The seeker ultimately reaches the state of supreme love in which he or she "lives constantly in the state of consecrating all activities [to God], in self-surrender."[155]

Supreme love is thus a state of renunciation. But Nārada holds that his renunciation leads to what he calls *ananyatā* ("not-otherness"), by which he means the "abandonment of all other [forms of] support."[156] The state of supreme love is therefore one in which there is love without an object.

Thus for Nārada the final submergence into the formless bliss of *parābhakti* begins with *gauṇabhakti,* the devotion to a being with physical characteristics. This is the physical guru. In linking the seeker's devotion to the guru with his or her devotion to God, Nārada states lessons presented by the devotional strand in Indian spirituality in general. The *Bhagavadgītā* has Kṛṣṇa, who is both God and guru, say to Arjuna:

> Know this! Through humble submission, through inquiry, through service (on your own part), the knowing ones, the perceivers of Truth, will be led to teach you knowledge.[157]

To this verse, Jñāneśvar adds:

> They [the knowing ones] are the dwelling place of all knowledge, and service to them is the threshold by which you can enter. Take hold of it, O Arjuna. Therefore, prostrate yourself at their feet with your body, mind, and soul, and serve them in all humility. Then, whatever you ask, they will explain it to you. Your heart will be enlightened, and all your desires will vanish.[158]

"Your heart will be enlightened," Jñāneśvar says here. The poet-saint was fond of describing the guru in language denoting the brilliance of a darkness-rending light:

> Hail to the Guru, that resplendent sun which has risen, dispelling the illusion of the universe and causing the lotus of nonduality to unfold its petals! He

swallows up the night of ignorance . . . and brings in the day of enlightenment for the wise.[159]

Other traditions on which Siddha Yoga draws regard the guru not only as God or (said differently) God as guru, but also see him or her as that soteriologically transformative force which brings illumination and clarity to a life otherwise characterized by darkness and confusion. Following a Tantric pedagogical and interpretative tradition in which a pertinent word—here, *guru*—is afforded a number of etymologies, the *Kulārṇava Tantra*, a Śaivite Kaula text, says:

The syllable *gu* signifies darkness; *ru* what restrains it.
He who restrains darkness of ignorance is the guru.[160]
Ga signifies giver of fulfillment; *r* server of sin, *u* Viṣṇu.
He who contains all the three in himself is the supreme guru.
Ga signifies wealth of knowledge; *r* illuminator; *u* identity with Śiva.
He who contains these in himself is the guru.[161]

Siddha Yoga theology and practice reflect similar devotional and soteriological ideas as those found in Vedāntic, Tantric, and Bhakti traditions. For instance the *Āratī*, a hymn of worship swamis Muktananda and Chidvilasananda have taught devotees to sing in their ashrams' temples each morning and evening, describes the worship of God as Śiva, who is revealed through the guru's compassionate love:

Oṃ. Salutations to the Guru, who is Śiva!
His form is being, consciousness, and bliss.
He is transcendent, calm, free from all support, and luminous.

Salutations to Nityananda, the Guru,
who rescues his disciples from the cycle of birth and death,
who has assumed a body to meet the needs of his devotees,
and whose nature is consciousness and being.[162]

Similar teachings find expression in the *Gurugītā*, the "Song of the Guru," a text that is apparently drawn from many sources and which Swami Muktananda regarded as "the one indispensable text" for Siddha Yoga.[163] Here, the guru is defined as a transformative power:

He by whose light (true knowledge) arises is known by the word Guru. . . . The syllable *gu* is darkness, and the syllable *ru* is said to be light. There is no doubt that the Guru is indeed the supreme knowledge that swallows (the darkness) of ignorance. The first syllable *gu* represents the principles such as *māyā*, and the second syllable *ru* the supreme knowledge that destroys the illusion of *māyā*.[164]

The rise of classical Vedāntic, Yogic, and especially Tantric and Bhakti movements in Hindu spirituality thus brought with them a shift in perspective in which the guru served not only pedagogical but genuinely soteriological functions. The latter idea revolves in part around the assumption that the human soul can in some way come to know or experience its own fulfillment in the context of a divine reality. Put into more explicitly theological terms, these various spiritual traditions maintain that the soul can, indeed, abide in God.

GURURĀTMĀ ĪŚVARETI: "THE GURU IS THE SELF AS WELL AS GOD"

As we have seen, Indian religious traditions based on the *gurumārga* hold that such experience or knowledge of God takes place by means of the guru-disciple relationship. It is understood that God can be revealed, experienced, and known through such a special relationship due to the ultimate identity of the guru, God, and the seeker's highest Self. Swami Muktananda wrote, "The great beings say, *gururātmā īśvareti*—'The Guru is the Self as well as God.'"[165] This is not to be understood as a hubristic statement on Muktananda's part (because of the nature of Sanskrit syntax, the phrase could also be translated as "God is the Self as well as the guru"), but one in which he affirmed a number of the ideas that have a long history in the religions of India. The phrase *gururātmā īśvareti* echoes the Vedāntic notion that there is finally only one Self in the universe, an idea that finds expression in Indian spirituality as early as the Upaniṣads. The *Śvetāśvatara Upaniṣad* (ca. fourth century B.C.E.), for example, describes this single Self of the universe as a sublime essence shared by all beings:

> As oil in sesame seeds, as butter in cream,
> as water in river beds, as fire in friction sticks,
> so is the Self held within one's own soul [*ātman*],
> if one looks for it with truthfulness and austerity.
> The Self which pervades all things,
> as butter lies within milk,
> which is the root of self-knowledge and austerity:
> that is the supreme secret teaching of the knower of Brahman![166]

The idea that the essence of one's own innermost Self is identical to the essence of all things in the world is developed at great length and in intricate detail in the seventh to eighth centuries C.E. by such proponents of Advaita Vedānta as Gauḍapāda, Śaṅkara, Maṇḍana Miśra, Sureśvara, Padmapāda, and others.

In teaching that "the Guru is the Self as well as God," Swami Muktananda rephrased a line from the *Āratī*: *īśvaro gururātmeti*, "The Lord is [the same as] the Guru and the Self."[167] He made a similar point when he translated a verse of the *Gurugītā* for a devotee—*mannāthaḥ śrījagannātho madgurus trijagadguruḥ*—saying, "My Lord, or my Master, the Master of my inner Self, is the Master of the entire universe. My Guru is the Guru of the whole world, and he is my inner Self."[168]

Muktananda's lesson that the guru is the Self as well as God further implies not only that there is only one true Self in the universe but also that this Self is God, a point made by most theistic traditions of Hinduism,[169] the textual sources of which can be traced to the Upaniṣads. One of those ancient texts opens, for example, with the proclamation, "All of this [universe], whatever moves in the moving world: [all of this] is enveloped by God."[170]

When people would ask him "Do you see yourself as God?" Swami Muktananda would say, "Yes, and if I am God, you are God, too!"[171] Similarly, when once asked, "What is the Self?" Swami Muktananda replied, "The Self is the light of God. The Self is God." His inquirer continued: "When you say 'Self,' I think of the body or the ego or the mind—but you are not talking about any of those?" Muktananda said, "No. The body, the mind, the ego, and so on are just instruments which allow the Self to be in this body." His student asked, "But the Self is God?" Muktananda replied, "Absolutely." [172]

We should note, then, the Siddha Yoga teaching that for a disciple to be in a proper relationship with the guru is, therefore, to be in relationship not only with God but also with his or her deepest and truest Self, which is understood to share in the essence of God.

"GOD-GURU-SELF" FROM THE PERSPECTIVE OF THE *GURUMĀRGA*

If God, guru, and Self are the same, then we can also say that, from the perspective of the *gurumārga*, to be in relationship with the true Self is not only to be in relationship with God but also to be in relationship with the guru. Furthermore, when one experiences this identity, the otherwise apparent division between worshipful subject and divine object collapses. Swami Muktananda has said:

> The moment a disciple merges into the Guru, neither the disciple nor the Guru exists as a separate entity any longer. The moment a devotee merges into the Lord, he is no longer a devotee and the Lord is no longer a separate entity. Names and forms disappear. Guru and disciple, Lord and devotee are

relative terms, one depending on the other; if one in these pairs vanishes, the other vanishes by itself.[173]

Drawing on this idea that the Self, the guru, and God dissolve into a transcendent unity of being, we might say that, in the guru-disciple relationship, God is in relationship with God. On the other hand, we could say that the Self is in relationship with the Self. Of course, then, we could also say that the guru is in relationship with the guru. This nondualist perspective finds delightful expression in the following verses from chapter 2 of Jñāneśvar's long poetic work, the *Amṛtānubhāv* ("The Nectar of Self-Awareness") in which this poet-saint describes how it is that the guru, who is one with the highest, can be in what looks like a relationship with a disciple. For Jñāneśvar, that apparent relationship is in fact the guru's playful game he enjoys with himself:

> By these verses I have made a finish of duality,
> And also honored my beloved Shri Guru.
>
> How wonderful is his friendship!
> He has manifested duality
> In the form of Guru and disciple
> Where there is not even a place for one!
>
> How does he have a close relationship with himself
> When there is no one other than himself?
> He can never become anything other than himself! . . .
>
> The words, "Guru" and "disciple"
> Refer to but one;
> The Guru alone exists as both these forms. . . .
>
> If a person awakes in a solitary place
> When no one else is about,
> Then one may be sure that he is both
> The awakened and the awakener as well.
>
> Just as the awakened and awakener are the same,
> The Guru is both the receiver of knowledge
> And the one who imparts it as well.
> In this way he upholds the relationship
> Between the Master and the disciple.
>
> If one could see his own eye without a mirror,
> There would be no need of this sport of the Guru.[174]

In this song Jñāneśvar gives poetic voice to the experience in which all separation between guru and disciple has disappeared. The guru is none other than the disciple, who is none other than the guru, for the "Guru alone exists as both these forms." All is one in the game in which the guru fashions, enters into, and enlivens the apparent relationship between a master and a seeker for the purpose of play. The guru lives in and enjoys all realms of being simultaneously. This divine play is not to be understood as frivolous. As we have seen in an earlier section of this chapter, the guru's presence in the world serves fully salvific purposes.

THE DISCIPLE'S RELATIONSHIP WITH THE MULTILAYERED UNITY OF THE GURU

According to Siddha Yoga as well as to the long spiritual traditions in India with which it is aligned, not only are God, guru, and Self ultimately one and the same but also there are different forms or aspects of the guru. As we noted earlier, the physical person is only one of them. This is the outer guru, for whom those who practice Siddha Yoga express deep love, appreciation, affection, and reverence. But the guru also takes other, inner forms and has other aspects, as well.

The physical manifestation of the guru's presence to his or her disciples is necessarily constrained by the structures of time and space. This is not so for other forms of the guru, which in their own various ways are immediately accessible to the disciple despite the fact that the physical guru may be quite distant. Swami Chidvilasananda has reported, "Many people ask, 'How can I learn anything if I don't have a Master physically right in front of me?'" a question to which she has responded by saying, "It is your bhava [attitude], it is your devotion, that determines what you attain."[175] Siddha Yoga holds that one need not be in the presence of the physical guru in order to benefit from the guru's grace. As Swami Muktananda taught:

> The greater your reverence, the greater your devotion, the higher you consider him to be, the more you will gain from him. If you have full devotion, reverence, and love for him, there is not the least doubt that you will receive all that the Guru has within him to give. But you must be free from affectation, hypocrisy, and pretense. Your devotion must be genuine.[176]

Elsewhere, Muktananda noted, "To maintain that contact [with the Guru] you should sustain a pure inner love for the Guru, a pure inner affection, and follow his teachings. Then you will be continually in contact with him."[177]

The Practice of "Absorption in the Guru"

In teaching the importance of such devotion despite the absence of the physical guru, swamis Muktananda and Chidvilasananda have often told a story of Ekalavya (or Eklavya, the modern spelling), a poor, uneducated boy who lived in the wilds of the forest and was shunned by others because of his low social standing.[178] Ekalavya yearned to become a great archer. He admired the great Droṇa, the best teacher of archery in all the land, but Droṇa was not able to accept him as a student because he already was teaching a number of young men from the upper reaches of the social order. Ekalavya would come to Droṇa's ashram every day. Sitting unnoticed in a distant corner, he would watch Droṇa intently. Having gazed in this manner on Droṇa's form, Ekalavya returned to his forest home, where with fine precision he sculpted a clay statue of the teacher that was true in every detail to Droṇa's own body. Ekalavya sat in meditation in front of the image, contemplating Droṇa's very being, internalizing his form. As Swami Muktananda tells the story:

> [Eklavya] identified his eyes with the Guru's eyes, his ears with the Guru's ears, his mouth with the Guru's mouth, and so on. He was submerged in the Guru. . . . Just as one becomes possessed by anger or attachment or greed by the force of his thoughts, likewise Eklavya became possessed by his Guru, Dronacharya, by thinking of him continually. As Eklavya was possessed entirely by the Guru's spirit all the Guru's knowledge passed into him.[179]

Infused in this way with the teacher's inward presence, Ekalavya received all of Droṇa's knowledge. As a result of his devotion to Droṇa, Ekalavya came to be the greatest archer in the kingdom, despite the fact that his teacher was physically absent. Muktananda concluded his teaching regarding this story by saying, "Such is the power of devotion to the Guru."[180]

Once when asked about the nature of the guru-disciple relationship, Swami Muktananda noted:

> [M]y Guru's picture has been placed here and incense sticks have been burned in front of it. This is not going to do any good to him. By installing his picture and doing *pūjā* to it, I am not doing a favor to him, I am doing a favor to myself. In this way I am hoping to receive his grace.
>
> So worship the Guru within your inner being for your own sake, for your own welfare, for your own good, and don't think you are doing a favor to the Guru. If your devotion to him is genuine, you will receive all his knowledge.[181]

This devoted absorption in the guru is known as *gurubhāva,* a term also translated as "meditation on the guru's form." The technique has similarities to some of the visualization practices used by Tantric forms of Hindu and Buddhist meditation. Muktananda made fruitful use of this technique in his own spiritual discipline. In his spiritual autobiography, he recalls how he would "look at him [Nityananda] with my eyes wide open, sometimes with them closed. What I saw looking outward I would bring inward in meditation. . . . And as I meditated on him, I began to get a feeling of complete oneness with him." As Muktananda did so, he would repeat the mantra, *dhyānamūlaṃ gurormūrtiḥ*, "The root of meditation is the Guru's form."[182] He reports how helpful the text *Jñāna Sindhu* was for him in this regard. This text teaches a spiritual seeker to perform this contemplation:

> [M]editate on the Guru, imagining him to be in every part of you. . . . Let your body become filled with him. Remember that just as a cloth is composed of threads, with cloth present in every thread, so are you in the Guru, and he in you. With this kind of vision, see the Guru and yourself as one. A pitcher is no different from the clay it is made of, and your Guru is no different from you. . . . [S]it down, become perfectly peaceful, and adopt a meditative posture. . . . Keep repeating in your mind *Guru Om, Guru Om, Guru Om*. . . . Implant the Guru in every part of your body, . . . saying *Guru Om*, so that you, yourself, are the Guru, you are the mantra, you are everything, you are in the Guru and the Guru is in you.[183]

The *Jñāna Sindhu*, apparently one of Muktananda's favorite texts, calls this contemplative technique the meditation on the guru "with form" (*saguṇa*). "[I]n solitude, with secret feeling," it says, "meditate in your heart on the supreme Guru, becoming the Guru." Such *gurubhāva* is said to be an effective way of strengthening the guru-disciple relationship. As the *Jñāna Sindhu* notes, the "*saguṇa* discipline of meditating on the Guru, worshipping him, remembering the Guru mantra, and installing him in every hair of the body, quickly brings a great change in the heart of the disciple."[184]

The Disciple's Relationship with the Inner Guru

In Siddha Yoga, great emphasis is given to the powerful presence of what it calls the "inner" guru. In fact, in some ways the inner guru is more powerful because he or she is more accessible than the physical or "outer" guru. Swami Muktananda has said, "We should honor such a Guru with the greatest devotion and reverence because he works within us, transforming us. . . . The Guru within is much closer than any outer teacher. After receiving a Guru's Shakti, you will see him in meditation, in visions, and in dreams."[185] For Swami Muktananda, the inner guru was none other than the inner Self, which as we have seen, he regarded as identical to the universal Self and thus to God. In response to a question, "Is my inner Self my own Guru?" he replied:

> The inner Self is your Guru if you have access to your inner Self. A Guru is one who can show you the way. If your inner Self can show you the way, very good.

In meditation you should look for the inner Self and see if you can receive guidance from it.[186]

A disciple approaches the inner guru not only through dreams and visions but also through meditation, contemplation, devotional worship (*pūjā*) and other means by which one gains access to subtler dimensions of one's being. Like just about everything else in Siddha Yoga, this idea has a long history. In the thirteenth century Jñāneśvar wrote of performing a mental *pūjā* by envisioning and then honoring the guru's feet within his own heart (the feet being understood in Indian tradition to hold the most intensely focused power of the guru's *śakti*):

> Now on the altar of my heart I will place my Guru's feet. Pouring my senses as flowers into the cupped hands of the experience of union with the Supreme, I offer a handful of these flowers at his feet. My desire, washed clean by the pure water of devotion, will be the sandalwood paste. Making anklets of the pure gold of my love for him, I will adorn his beautiful feet. My strong, pure, and one-pointed devotion to him will be a pair of rings for his toes. I will place on them the bud of pure emotions with the fragrance of bliss, and the full-blown eight-petalled lotus. Then I will burn before him the incense of egoism, I will wave before him the lamp of union with the Self, and I will embrace him with the experience of oneness with the Absolute. I will put on his feet the sandals of my body and my vital force, and I will wave around them the neem leaves of experience and liberation.[187]

If he or she may be approached through inward *pūjā*, the inner guru may also be envisioned in the process of contemplation as dwelling in the light-filled *sahasrāra*, the spiritual center in the crown of one's head. Swami Muktananda has noted, "The Guru lives in the sahasrara as much as he lives outside."[188] Drawing on Yogic and Tantric teachings and practices, the *Gurugītā* states:

> The (Guru's) lotus feet, which extinguish the raging fires of all mundane existence, are situated in the center of the white lotus in the region of the moon in the Brahmarandhra (the hollow space of the head).
>
> In the round space of the thousand-petaled lotus, there is a triangular lotus, which is formed by the three lines beginning with *a*, *ka*, and *tha* and which has *ham* and *sah* on two sides. One should remember the Guru, who is seated in its center.[189]

Muktananda once told a student that the important Siddha Yoga mantra, *So 'ham* ("I am That") arises in that inner space. "Right in the center of this triangle the Guru dwells," he said, "For this reason, you don't have to continue to search for a Guru," for "The Guru neither leaves nor comes. He always stays inside constantly." Accordingly, he taught, "If you experience this relationship between a Guru and a disciple, even for a moment, it is more than enough."[190]

The Disciple's Relationship to the Guru as the Mantra

Swami Muktananda thus taught that the inner guru who lives in the *sahasrāra* is associated with, and accessible by the disciple's use of, the mantra. We will remember that the siddha guru infuses powerfully transformative spiritual energy (*śakti*) into the disciple when he or she initiates that disciple into the use of the mantra. We will remember, too, that according to traditions represented by texts such as the *Kulārṇava Tantra,* the most important kind of guru is the *bodhaka* who serves as the *pūrṇābhiṣekakartṛ,* that is, as the one who "awakens" the disciple by acting as the agent who "gives the full initiation." Once when asked, "Is it necessary to meditate on a mantra?" Muktananda replied, "Yes it's very necessary. . . . [The] mantra is shakti. It is very powerful. It's difficult to understand it at the beginning. The Guru transmits his shakti through the mantra and the shakti enters the disciple through the mantra. It is essential."[191]

For Swami Muktananda, the guru is therefore closely associated with the mantra with which he or she initiates the disciple. His teaching is consistent in this regard with Tantric thought; the *Kulārṇava Tantra,* for example, notes that *mantramūlaṃ guror vākyaṃ*: "The root of mantra is the guru's word," a teaching presented also in the *Gurugītā.*[192] Muktananda regarded this association to be so close that he used to tell his students that the mantra is a form of the guru himself. He once said:

> If the Guru has planted the seed of yoga within you, and if by that means he has activated the inner yoga in you, he will always be working within you in the form of Shakti. The Guru always lives in your heart in the form of the mantra. See him right there—that is the best way of maintaining contact with him. A true Guru is one who can activate a mantra within the heart of his disciple and fill a disciple's heart with love and peace.[193]

Consistent with teachings presented by some Tantric traditions, Siddha Yoga holds that the inner guru's "sandals" or "feet" themselves contain the liberating power of the mantra. The inner sandals and feet are not physical objects, but rather manifestations of the guru's energy in the subtle body. Two of the verses of the *Śrī Guru Pādukā-Pañcakam* ("Five Stanzas on the Sandals of Śrī Guru"), an invocatory chant sung in Siddha Yoga ashrams each day before the *Gurugītā,* read:

> Salutations again and again to Śrī Guru's sandals, which are endowed with the mystery of (the seed letters) *aim* and *hrīm* and with the great glory of the profound meaning of (the seed letter) *śrīm* and which expound the secret of *Oṃ.*

> Salutations again and again to Śrī Guru's sandals, which are a boat (with which) to cross the endless ocean of the world, which bestow steadfast devotion, and which are a raging fire to dry the ocean of spiritual insensitivity.[194]

When asked once about the presence of the inner guru, Swami Muktananda replied in a manner that is consistent with the teachings of the *Kulārṇava Tantra,* saying that in the *sahasrāra,* at the crown of the head, "are two feet, *ham* and *sa,* and these are the feet of the Guru."[195]

Since the inner guru is so closely associated and even identified with the mantra, the disciple can enter into relationship with the guru by turning his or her attention to the mantra, just as the guru has become one with the mantra. Swami Muktananda said once that "Being a disciple is not a matter of being close to me or giving me wealth or doing a lot of *sevā.* The true disciple is the one who has become like the Guru. The Guru is always immersed in [the mantra] *So'ham.* When the disciple becomes that *So'ham,* he is a true disciple."[196]

*The Guru as the Guru Principle (*Gurutattva*) and as Universal Śakti*

As the essence and power of the mantra *So'ham,* "That, I am"—a universal mantra invoking a universe in which all multiplicity veils an underlying unity of being—the guru is understood to be identical to the essence and power of that unity. From this perspective, the guru is regarded as the *gurutattva,* which, as was mentioned earlier, means the "guru principle." The *gurutattva* is the force that creates and sustains all life and that therefore girds and directs the whole of the outer and inner universes; as the *Gurugītā* proclaims, it "moves and moves not. It is far as well as near. It is inside everything as well as outside everything."[197] The *gurutattva* necessarily transcends the limitations of time and space, for time and space are products of this creative principle and vital power. Siddha Yoga holds that this universal principle of being is identical with the universal being, consciousness, and bliss that is the nature of God. Swami Muktananda has said:

> The Guru principle has not come into existence recently. It existed even before the universe was created, and just like water, earth, air, fire, and ether, it has been a part of creation ever since it began. The Guru principle is within everyone as the inner Self, so when we pay our respects to the Guru, we are paying respects to our own Self. The Guru is the Self; he is nothing but supreme consciousness and supreme bliss.[198]

The guru as *gurutattva* is therefore equivalent to *citi-śakti,* the supreme consciousness that fashions, supports and transforms the entire universe itself and all things in it. The *Kulārṇava Tantra* refers to this idea when it says that all "activities in the world are based on the Guru."[199] Like other Indian spiritual traditions, Siddha Yoga holds that the *citi-śakti* is reflected or embodied most fully in the person of the physical guru who awakens a disciple to the reality of this universal power through the graceful gift of shaktipat.

This idea also seems to lie behind Swami Muktananda's statement, "An individual is not the Guru; Shakti is the Guru, and that Shakti resides in one who is a Guru."[200] In this, Muktananda is theologically consistent with the classical Tantric teaching that the human guru is a physical embodiment of the universal but otherwise formless ground of being that gives rise to and supports all things. We can recall the *Kulārṇava Tantra*'s assertion that, out of compassion for those who are seeking him, the eternal god, Śiva, becomes visible in the form of the physical guru who, when "worshiped with devotion, brings fulfillment and liberation."[201] Accordingly, that text states, "Fulfillment [*siddhi*] is close at hand for one who remembers with devotion, 'My Guru is Śiva himself, who grants liberation and enjoyment.'"[202]

The Guru as the Power of Divine Grace

The guru as *gurutattva* is not only the power of universal creation and sustenance but also of effective and redemptive transformation. It is through this power that anything—including the human heart—has the ability to turn toward the divine. The *Śiva Sūtra* succinctly states that *gururupāyaḥ*, "The Guru is the means." Commenting on this *sūtra*, the eleventh-century sage Kṣemarāja wrote that the guru "is the way by which one attains the potency" of sacred mantras and other powerful forces.[203] As was mentioned earlier, Kṣemarāja also said that *gururvā pārameśvarī anugrāhikā śaktiḥ*, "The Guru is the grace-bestowing power of God."[204] From his own more devotionally oriented perspective the poet-saint Jñāneśvar sang out to his guru, "Hail to you, O grace-bestowing power, who are pure, famous for your generosity, and always pouring out showers of joy!"[205]

Swami Muktananda made a similar point in saying, "It is important to understand that the Guru is not merely a human being but an eternal principle, the power of grace."[206] Similarly he taught:

> Guru, Self, and God are one and the same, and therefore love for the Guru is love for the Self. To repeat the Guru's name is to repeat the name of the Self; love for the Guru becomes love for God. God's power of grace dwells in the Guru. An individual is not the Guru; Shakti is the Guru, and that Shakti resides in one who is a Guru.[207]

As the divine power of grace itself, the guru may be known and approached both outwardly and inwardly. Nevertheless, Swami Muktananda held that the closest connection with the power of divine grace is through the disciple's relationship with the inner guru. Responding to the question, "What is the difference between the outer form of the guru and the inner guru?" he replied:

> That is the true Guru who dwells inside. The true Guru has no form. The scriptures say that the Guru is the Self, so the inner Self is the true Guru.
>
> As long as you do not receive the grace of the inner Self, outer wisdom is not going to work for you. The outer Guru dwells inside too. Remember that the Guru is not this body; the Guru is the grace-bestowing power of God. Lord Shiva said, "O Goddess, understand that I am the Guru who makes the mantra active and who makes the Shakti work inside." So the inner Shakti is the Guru.[208]

The Guru as Ultimate Reality

From the perspective of Siddha Yoga, which holds that "guru, Self, and God are one and the same," the guru is ultimately understood to be equivalent to supreme reality. This is, of course, not to say that the extent of the physical guru is identical to the extent of supreme reality, for the physical guru exists within certain limitations of time and space. It is to say that the foundational essence of the physical guru—pure existence, pure consciousness, and pure bliss—is identical to that of the absolute. It is also to say that the absolute is of the nature of compassionate teacher and that the guru is the form the absolute takes in order to bestow grace. As was mentioned earlier, God himself is described in many Indian texts as the supreme guru, who frees struggling seekers of the truth from the pain of confusion, doubt, and fear. It is from this latter perspective that Jñāneśvar declared:

> Hail to you, O Guru, greatest of all the gods, rising sun of pure intellect, and dawn of happiness. O refuge of all, delight of the realization of union with God, you are the ocean on which the waves of the various worlds arise.[209]

We see similar sentiments in the following verses from the *Gurugītā*, which hold not only that the gods themselves are forms of the guru but also that the guru is greater than any of the gods.

> The Guru is Brahmā. The Guru is Viṣṇu. The Guru is Lord Śiva. The Guru is indeed Parabrahman. Salutations to Śrī Guru.[210]

> Indeed, the Guru is the whole universe, consisting of Brahmā, Viṣṇu, and Śiva. There is nothing higher than the Guru. Therefore, worship the Guru.[211]

> Nothing exists which is higher than he. . . . It is by the grace of the Guru and only through service to the Guru that Brahmā, Viṣṇu, and Śiva become capable of creation (sustenance, and destruction.)[212]

Accordingly, the guru is none other than the absolute itself. Transcendent of time and form, the guru is the supreme existence, consciousness, and bliss on which the universe rests:

> Salutations to Shrī Guru. The Guru is the beginning (of all, but) he is without a beginning. The Guru is the supreme deity. There is nothing higher than the Guru. I bow to the Guru, who is Brahman, eternal and pure. He is beyond perception, formless, and without taint. He is eternal knowledge, consciousness, and bliss.[213]

The Unity of the Guru

In the context of the guru as the absolute, the guru-disciple relationship comes to its completion when the disciple realizes the final unity of guru, Self, and God. Swami Chidvilasananda has said:

> The last step is samadhi. Samadhi is the conscious awareness "God and I are not different from each other; there is no difference between God and me." Everything merges. There is no Guru, there is no disciple; there is no God, there is no devotee; there is no universe, there is no you. There is absolute oneness. This is called *purno aham vimarsha,* pure I-consciousness. Because of this experience of samadhi, you understand the Pure Being, the One without a second.[214]

The disciple of Bhagawan Nityananda, Swami Muktananda, or Swami Chidvilasananda follows the siddha guru's teachings and reveres the guru, in part for the power of grace he or she is believed to embody. But, because the guru—broadly defined—is also the guru principle and ultimate ground of being, in following the guru's teachings the disciple is also understood to enter into relationship with and align himself with the fundamental forces that fashion and sustain life and that, therefore, direct the movements of the cosmos as a whole. According to Siddha Yoga teachings, to listen to and to follow the guru's command is to hear and to be true to God, and to be true to God is to be true to what God has created, not only in putting the universe together but in becoming the human soul with all of its inherent dignity. Once again, there is the fundamental teaching: God, guru, and Self are one.

Just as God, guru, and Self are one, so too all of the forms of the guru function as one, for they are, themselves, a unity. And just as there is only one Self in the universe, there is, according to Siddha Yoga teachings, only one guru. Perhaps this is why the siddhas teach their disciples that they become one with the guru when they follow the guru's teachings. It may also be why they teach that a disciple enters into relationship with the guru by chanting the mantra, for the guru lives in the disciple in the form of the mantra. And perhaps it is why, too, they encourage the disciple to meditate, for it is in the quiet attention to one's own divinely ordained soul that one discovers the presence of the guru and the Self residing within one's own being. This is, in Swami Muktananda's restatement of the *Jñāneśvarī*, to find that the timeless presence within one's own being is "God Himself."

THE MOMENT OF DARSHAN

Of the various moments in the spiritual life of a student of Siddha Yoga, the most cherished by virtually all accounts is that which takes place when the disciple and physical guru see each other face to face. It is a moment of unmatched intensity and focus and can be an experience of what is described by many disciples as unbounded love. This is a time of darshan, that is, of being in the presence of the guru. The word comes from the Sanskrit *darśana,* which literally means "seeing." In the context of the spiritual life this is more than the ordinary experience of having someone in one's sight, or being seen by another. It is to make oneself available to the guru at all levels of one's being; it is to present oneself to the guru unadorned and uncloaked, as it were, by the many ways in which people both hide themselves and hide from themselves. It is an act of utter openness and honesty and, accordingly, of deep trust born of what disciples describe as the experience of the guru's understanding, concern, and unfathomed compassion. It is a time in which the disciple can put aside all enervating pretense and return to the inner but often veiled integrity of his or her own being. It is to just such a return to this inward integrity that all other practices of Siddha Yoga are said to lead: meditation, the inward repetition of mantra, the study of sacred texts, the singing of devotional songs, service to the community; and to be in the guru's "vision" is to experience the integrity of the Self in the passing yet somehow timeless depths of the moment at hand. It is a moment filled with *śakti.*

Darshan may occur at any time. It may take place in a large lecture hall or in a quiet room. It might take place as the guru walks through the ashram kitchen or along a path winding through a garden. Fifty years ago, people would walk miles along muddy jungle paths, sometimes for days, to sit for only a moment or two in the presence of Bhagawan Nityananda. Often he would say nothing to them or would utter just a few words. Nevertheless, reports indicate that his devotees were extraordinarily moved by the experience.[215]

Swami Muktananda allowed for a more structured, outward opportunity for darshan by sitting in a chair on a regular basis and after public programs so that devotees could come to meet him. Swami Chidvilasananda continued this same practice for many years, but in late 1996 she discontinued it. Siddha Yoga students still had opportunity to be with her physically in programs, during Intensives, and so on, but Chidvilasananda stressed to her followers the importance of seeing the guru within their own hearts.

That the disciple is to cultivate this inner contact with the guru is consistent with the values and practices of the *gurumārga* as a whole, which teaches that the guru need not physically be present for darshan to take place. Siddha Yoga maintains that the guru in some way continues to hold the devotee in his or her vision even when physically separated by long distance or across long stretches of time. Some devotees of the Siddha Yoga gurus report that they have had the guru's darshan when looking at a photograph of the guru or while singing a song or chanting a mantra. The experience of inner darshan can be quite powerful and transformative, and its effects can be long-lasting. Disciples note that they feel that in some way the guru lives deep within themselves as their very being and that they meet the guru's constant and unmediated presence through meditation, prayer, and other means of inward and quiet attentiveness. The guru sometimes speaks most clearly in the silence of the heart.

To hear the voice of the guru is to hear the voice of the divine Self abiding within one's own timeless soul, and to listen to the voice of the soul is in a very real sense to hear the word of God. Following a long spiritual tradition in India, Bhagawan Nityananda, Swami Muktananda, and Swami Chidvilasananda have taught that to keep one's inner vision on the guru, and thus to open oneself completely to the divine and loving presence of God, is to enter into a life of wholeness and integrity. To dwell in the guru-disciple relationship is to remember God's grace-filled and wondrous gift of life, a gift that God is said in Siddha Yoga to bestow out of the sheer and expansive joy of his own being.

Chapter Four

The Canons of Siddha Yoga

The Body of Scripture and the Form of the Guru

Douglas Renfrew Brooks

INTRODUCTION: THE CANON AND THE TEACHERS OF SIDDHA YOGA

Canons as Lineage Traditions

Swami Muktananda and his successor, Gurumayi Chidvilasananda, have drawn upon a vast array of oral and written sources from the legacy of Indian spirituality. Occasionally, they have also drawn parallels with ideas and practices of spiritual and literary traditions that are not of Indian origin. The "canon of Siddha Yoga" means that authoritative body of lineage teachings and practices presented by the gurus for the purpose of instructing disciples. This includes both the oral and written selections specially infused with the gurus' intentionality (*saṅkalpa*) and, more particularly, their own words, teachings, and interpretations. However, in the case of Siddha Yoga as well as in other spiritual traditions, a *canon* can also refer to much more than scriptural resources. In this sense, we can speak of more than one canon in Siddha Yoga, that is, authoritative resources other than texts and teachings. We should begin, however, with a note of explanation to the reader about what lies ahead in this investigation. The entire issue of mapping and comprehending the meaning of a canon in guru-centered mystical traditions, such as Siddha Yoga, is largely uncharted scholarly territory. We will need multiple perspectives to appreciate the complex materials and nuanced situations under consideration; and we will need methods and models for understanding that have not before been applied. It is in this more theoretical realm of creating methods and models for understanding that the reader will be particularly challenged. We are looking into a subject for which there are few direct antecedents in scholarship. First, however, we should clarify what we mean by the term *canon* in the most general sense.

By definition a canon is that authoritative body of texts and teachings decided upon by a given community's leadership. A canon represents both continuity and innovation, since the *content* as well as the interpretation of the canon can (and often does) change over the history of a religious community. Canons are never truly "fixed" in this sense but rather are themselves processes by which sacred teachings are set apart from those less authoritative or those ideas that lie beyond the scope of the tradition. Canons help create a register and catalog of sources that speak to the meaning of a tradition. The first meaning of *canon* is a list of authoritative sources. In this sense, canons help create "tradition," literally "that which is carried down or continued," but like traditions they too must be understood as more complex and subtle than simply a set of unchanging texts. Rather, like traditions, canons are living representations of the sacred as it unfolds in the hearts and minds of the spiritual community. They can change, be added to and amended, and most importantly, be interpreted differently over the course of time.

Another, second meaning of *canon* is that it is the ideal, the norm, and the authoritative voice of tradition. This meaning of *canon* is not restricted to written or oral sources. A canon's authoritative voice can be a living master, whose choices and interpretations guide tradition forward.[1]

In the spiritual traditions of siddhas, rooted as they are in the ultimate authority and empowerment of the guru, the guru is a living canon. This subtle notion will be crucial for developing our understanding of the notions of power and authority that are vested in the guru as well as for delving more deeply into the guru's relationship to scripture and tradition. The guru is a living canon in that the guru's own experiences and instructive interpretations are what make texts and teachings sacred and therefore scriptural. Texts, however instructive or edifying, are not fully canonical unless and until they "come alive" through the guru's teachings and intentions. "Scripture" refers precisely to those sources that the guru has empowered through teaching (*upadeśa*) or intention (*saṅkalpa*) to reveal the truths of tradition. Put in terms familiar to Hindu-inspired mystical yoga, texts become sacred and enter into the canon when they are infused with the divine *śakti*, the empowering force that pervades the universe. Only then, with the *śakti* awakened because of the presence of the siddha guru, can scriptures impart the grace-bestowing power (*anugraha-śakti*) of the divine.

We should distinguish, then, three typologies of texts that determine their relationship to the sacred in Siddha Yoga:

1) texts the guru treats as sacred either by declaring them to be or by explicitly endorsing their use;

2) texts, written or oral, that are taught, recited, or used by the guru to impart a given teaching; and

3) texts the guru uses to teach or make a particular point. Texts in this latter group may or may not achieve a canonical status, depending upon whether they fall into one of the other two categories.

It is with these three types of texts in mind, marked as they are by their usage, that we can begin to probe what makes them sacred or authoritative.

At the most fundamental level we should note that the guru's choices and uses of texts make them scriptural; it is not that a given text is simply sacred apart from the place the guru assigns to it. This is a crucial distinction. In some religious traditions, including in some facets of Hinduism, a text or body of texts is authoritative as such. We see in some forms of Christianity, for example, that the Bible is canonical teaching quite apart from any other authoritative voice. That is, the Bible is authoritative "apart from its interpreter" or without an empowering voice to enunciate its teaching. However in Siddha Yoga, as in certain other mystical yoga traditions, there is another facet to gaining canonical status: the guru who presides over texts and tradition as arbiter of authority. In Siddha Yoga a text is authoritative only when the guru's intention (*saṅkalpa*), that is, the guru's innate power (*śakti*) determines its content, meaning, and usage. Understanding how a canon is chosen and interpreted requires a thorough examination of the role of the guru as both the arbiter of scriptural teachings and as the embodiment of spiritual ideals.

Historically there is no preordained body of texts that defines *the* siddha tradition's canon at large. Siddha traditions have not organized themselves around a given or fixed body of texts, concepts, or values. Instead, they have created bodies of thought from which lineage gurus draw and to which they contribute. There are many texts from the larger body of siddha works that can be identified as expressing Siddha Yoga teachings and many more from which the siddha gurus draw more selectively. However, it is difficult even to speak of "the siddha tradition" as if it were a unified body of ideas and practices. Rather, there are siddhas and siddha traditions in which there are many common sources and familiar strategies for understanding and interpreting scriptures. It is the siddha guru who decides a lineage's canon both as its interpreter and as a vital contributor. More significantly, it is the siddha guru's values that define the boundaries of the scriptural canon; siddha gurus undoubtedly allow their ethics, their understanding of truth, and their method for teaching to be reflected in the scriptures they choose to regard as canonical. While the siddha stands for perfect freedom, the scriptures of a lineage speak to the ways that freedom expresses itself.

Each siddha guru contributes to the process of developing his or her own lineage's canon, though not necessarily by writing or even speaking.

The guru's presence and the lore that surrounds him or her may suffice as a canonical contribution. Some gurus write, others do not; some teach with words, others only by example. In any case the siddha is at the heart of the canon by defining what *is* true, authoritative, and appropriate within the lineage or for a disciple.

Each siddha lineage has its own canon of gurus, scriptures, and oral bodies of knowledge that make it unique. These distinct lineages are like members of an extended family who often bear close resemblances. One lineage's canon may be very similar, or nearly indistinguishable from another's. Sharing a canon of scriptures across lineages is not the same as sharing gurus. Since the guru is a canon as well, it is clear then that *each lineage* has a distinctive canon composed of texts and gurus. However, no two lineages will likely have exactly the same scriptural canon.[2] Many may have very different teachings and values. Even when lineages claim the same gurus or canonical links, they are likely to differ over interpretation or even content. The *intention* of the gurus may also be understood differently.

To use a different image, siddha gurus are like artists who paint from a palette of many colors that represent the long history of siddha traditions. Each guru contributes to a great collage that represents the collective effort of their lineage. The paints themselves are the truths of traditional texts and teachings; but the task of mixing colors, creating hues, textures, and tones, and ultimately creating the work of art falls to the siddha guru. Each generation of the lineage adds to the collage and each lineage defines its own canon by drawing from the palette of traditional resources. Thus, while there are many yogas and lineages of the siddhas, properly speaking there is only one Siddha Yoga as defined by swamis Muktananda and Chidvilasananda.[3] The Siddha Yoga gurus have created their own distinctive collage of canonical sources *and* they have put their own spiritual intentions into it to empower the teachings for their devotees. It is this combination of factors that distinguishes Siddha Yoga as a canonical body of teaching, practices, and experiences. The canons of Siddha Yoga are both the scriptural choices of the lineage gurus *and* their infusion into those scriptures of their own spiritual power (*śakti*).

Throughout this discussion, we should be aware of the concepts and values that apply to siddha traditions in general, those that apply to other siddha lineages, and those that pertain to Siddha Yoga.

The Scriptural Sources of Siddha Yoga

We can imagine Siddha Yoga's canon of texts in a number of ways. One can sometimes picture them like nesting Russian dolls, so that one teaching presumes a larger body of ideas into which it "fits." One teaching may presume or depend on another. At other times the canonical selections are like intersecting circles, which have areas of inclusion and exclusion. Ideas may be connected or related partially so that unwanted ideas and practices are left outside the canon.

Given the oceanic body of potential resources from which the Siddha Yoga gurus might choose, we can make two preliminary observations. *First, the Siddha Yoga gurus will reiterate certain crucial teachings, with subtle variations and elaborations. Interpretations are consistent inasmuch as there are very specific values and aims in mind.* These teachings may have diverse historical, cultural, or textual origins. The vast majority of resources come from Hindu-inspired yoga and mysticism. These traditions are assimilative and cumulative; in other words, they absorb virtually every tradition with which they have contact and they add teachings and concepts as they progress through time and across space.

What connects texts and teachings is that the gurus have established a relationship with a certain goal or understanding. For example, to teach the essential unity of all reality the Siddha Yoga gurus might draw from the oral poetry of north Indian mystics known as Sants (such as Kabīr or Nānak) and the highly crafted, technical commentaries of nondualist Vedānta philosophers (such as Śaṅkara or Sureśvara). Historically speaking, these sources have quite different origins and, culturally and socially, few connections within them. The Sants and Vedānta philosophers each produce "separate" traditions as such. *Yet these texts become part of a broader tradition because they are brought together by the guru.* To put this matter slightly differently, guru traditions *create* tradition *from* traditions. In the case we just noted, the Sants and Vedāntins are brought together around a single important concept—the unity of Being. In other instances, these same traditions might be called upon separately for the sake of developing another teaching or practice that they do not share. However they may be invoked, it is the guru who decides to what purpose they might be put.

In Siddha Yoga, a wide variety of texts support a core of teachings and practices that disciples recognize as familiar. There are texts, teachings, and practices that virtually any experienced Siddha Yoga student could identify as canonical—for example, any of the texts included in the Siddha Yoga collection of scriptures entitled *The Nectar of Chanting.* This is not to say that these are the only texts or that they are considered necessarily *more* important than others. On the contrary, the variety of forms the teachings take permit the Siddha Yoga gurus to add nuance and subtlety. When reading a text or listening to a guru, we must also consider to whom the instruction is directed: some teachings are meant for individuals, others for larger groups, and still others for everyone.

Second, as the core of teachings and practices expands and develops along with the textual canon, we notice consistent values and beliefs that guide interpretation. These values and beliefs are the guideposts to understanding the direction and the tone of the lineage's teaching. Behind the selections of texts and the teachings themselves are the gurus' principles that guide the choices and interpretations. These principles reflect their deepest ethical values and spiritual knowledge. For example, the Siddha Yoga gurus reject outright any teachings that suggest moral lassitude or prejudice based on gender, caste, or ethnicity. Such value-centered decisions are vital to understanding *potential* canonical choices. A particular passage of text that violates these values would not be considered a candidate for the canon.

By first organizing the basic scriptural canon of the Siddha Yoga gurus, we will be able to consider the more complex issues that connect these diverse resources to one another and the values that guide their selection. A careful review of the teachings of swamis Muktananda and Chidvilasananda reveal their keenest interest in sources from the Indian tradition that we can organize under five general headings. We will explore these five types of sources, but first we need simply to list them:

1) the traditionalist canon of Revelation and Recollection;

2) the esoteric canon of the Tantras and the "in-between" texts;

3) the tradition of treatises and aphorisms;

4) the tradition of songs and oral teachings;

5) the teachings of the Siddha Yoga gurus.

The Traditionalist Canon of Revelation and Recollection

At Siddha Yoga's textual core are the most basic resources of the Vedic and Hindu tradition, classified as Revelation (*śruti*) and Recollection (*smṛti*). The Siddha Yoga gurus recognize this traditional classification but are not particularly interested in using it as an important principle of choice. Revelation generally refers to the texts of the so-called Vedic corpus: the hymns (*saṃhitā*), the ritual instructions (*brāhmaṇa*), the "forest-texts" of reflection on ritual (*āraṇyaka*), and the mystic instructions of the Upaniṣads. Recollection refers to anything else in the corpus of Hindu texts written in the Sanskrit language, but particularly the great epics (i.e., *Mahābhārata* and *Rāmāyaṇa*), the mythic lore (*purāṇa*), and all the bodies of traditional learning from law (*dharmaśāstra*) to philosophy (*darśana*) and grammar (*vyākaraṇa*). As far as Revelation texts are concerned, the Siddha Yoga gurus refer to the hymns from the four Vedas frequently but center their attention on the Upaniṣads, a vast body of teachings and a wide variety of different texts that include metaphysics, yoga, and practical instruction.

Within the body of Recollection, the mythic lore and the epics are important and frequently cited. The *Bhagavadgītā*, which stands within the *Mahābhārata*, deserves special mention since it is such an important teaching resource. When discussing the *Bhagavadgītā*, the Siddha Yoga gurus draw from a wide variety of commentarial sources, which span many regions, languages, historical periods, and even philosophical schools and traditions. Their primary interest, however, is in the works of the philosophical nondualists and particularly the poet-saint Jñāneśvar who wrote in the Marathi language in the thirteenth century, the nondualist or Advaita Vedāntin Śaṅkara (c. 750 C.E.), and the Kashmiri Śaivite Abhinavagupta (c. 1000 C.E.) More needs to be said about these specific resources. The point to emphasize here is that the Siddha Yoga gurus are fully aware of the traditional division employed in Hinduism between Revelation and Recollection and invoke it occasionally as part of their teaching. However, as is clear from the range of texts and traditions from which they draw, they also feel no limitation from assuming this categorical distinction. In other words, while the body of texts that make up the Revelation and Recollection is important to the Siddha Yoga gurus, the distinction itself between these classes of texts is not as significant as the teachings.

The Siddha Yoga gurus choose from these sources primarily on the grounds of relevance and importance to their understanding of spiritual discipline or sadhana (Sanskrit, *sādhana*). There is little interest expressed in historical or polemical differences. This process of choice creates a canon in two tiers.

The first tier consists of the enormous *inclusive canon* made up of the entire body of traditional genres and literatures. The inclusive canon simply means the entire body of texts that Hindu tradition classifies as Revelation and Recollection written in Sanskrit as well as in other languages, such as Hindi, Marathi, and Tamil. There is no agreement among Hindus as to the precise content of this inclusive canon, that is, which texts or teachings are "in" or "out." In fact, the important point is that the inclusive canon is *not a list* of sources as such but *a concept*. That concept is meant to create the belief that there exists a body of sacred texts and traditions from which one can select. The inclusive canon has for its content oral and written sources; it is composed in many languages; and it comes from across the expanse of India's complex landscape of traditions.

Selecting sources and defining a lineage canon from Revelation and Recollection is the common work of all gurus. In other words, from the *concept* of the inclusive canon comes an actual body of texts and teachings that is selected by a lineage guru. The guru thus creates from his or her concept of the inclusive canon the lineage canon, that is, those particular texts and teachings that one locates within the larger body of tradition. Siddha Yoga, like other guru-centered traditions, leaves it to the gurus to select the sources that make up the Siddha Yoga lineage canon. The point here is simply that the first resource from which the Siddha Yoga gurus draw is the inclusive canon, the entire body of Hindu-inspired literature and lore as such.

Gurus may not mention all the sources that they would include in their concept of the inclusive canon. Rather, the inclusive canon acts as a conceptual backdrop that is made up of thousands of resources from which they *might* draw. We can only judge what a guru *might* have in mind by looking carefully at texts he does mention and then those texts that we can assume he presupposes from the ones he mentions. For example, the nondualist philosophies of Advaita Vedānta and Kashmiri Śaivism, which are central to Siddha Yoga, presuppose the inclusive canon's concern with grammar, logic, and ritual. These sorts of topics are rarely mentioned by Siddha Yoga gurus who have little interest in expounding on Sanskrit grammar, the methods of Indian logic, or the formalities of ritual. And yet these texts form a deep background and contain the foundation for understanding the philosophical systems that the gurus are deeply interested in explaining. The traditional study of Vedānta and Kashmiri Śaivism *presupposes* some understanding of these other arts and sciences. In some sense, these background sources are an invisible floor on which Siddha Yoga builds its scriptural house.

So beyond the first tier of the inclusive canon of *potential resources* is the second tier of tradition, which we can call the *lineage canon.* The lineage canon consists of the precise scriptural selections, interpretations, and works of the gurus. The lineage canon is, in part, drawn from the inclusive canon which stands as the body of all possible resources. The Siddha Yoga gurus draw from the vast array of Hindu-inspired sources, and thus they make selections that are canonical, that is, that are authoritative for the purposes of understanding spiritual practice and thought. In addition to the common sources of the Hindu tradition from which the Siddha Yoga gurus might draw, there are sources that are exclusive to the lineage since they are the lineage gurus' own words and teachings.[4] The lineage canon grows as the gurus come forward with their teachings. Everything mentioned as the lineage canon is sacred teaching, that is, canonical or authoritative. The inclusive canon, however, is treated somewhat differently.

The inclusive canon treats the *whole body* of revelatory and recollected texts as greater than the sum of its parts. Thus whole texts or genres of texts can be "affirmed" as canonical. For example, the Siddha Yoga gurus affirm the entirety of the so-called Vedic corpus of Revelation, which Hindu traditionalists regard with the highest canonical authority. *But this affirmation is made without endorsing or prescribing every idea or practice that appears within it.* This creates a notion of the Siddha Yoga lineage canon that does not include every word or teaching of the texts that may be cited in part. The actual lineage canon must go beyond the words of the texts to reflect the intention of the guru. Thus, it is possible to hear the Siddha Yoga gurus affirm that "the Vedas are sacred truth"—this being the sense of inclusive canon—and yet this statement does not mean that every word or idea in the Vedic corpus provides an authoritative teaching for Siddha Yoga. This latter selective process whereby portions of the Vedic corpus, for example, are commented upon is what creates the lineage canon. This same process of inclusion and selection is repeated again and again, no matter which texts are involved.

According to Hindu tradition, the Vedas as Revelation are held in higher regard than such Recollected texts as the epics (*Mahābhārata* and *Rāmāyaṇa*) or mythologies (i.e., the Purāṇas). The Siddha Yoga gurus, following the general line of tradition, will concur with this principle and distinguish these levels of authority in scripture. However, the important point is that the Siddha Yoga gurus will treat both types of texts in essentially the same way. That is, they will select what is of interest to them as teachings appropriate for their disciples and so create a lineage canon of selections. This process of selecting teachings from the whole body of traditional sources may involve mentioning some explicitly while suggesting others implicitly. It would take a rather encyclopedic knowledge of the entire body of potential sources and citations to know which texts or teachings are being implied as others are mentioned explicitly. At times, however, we will see the Siddha Yoga gurus speak in more general terms. This allows them to endorse the Vedas or the Purāṇas or some other part of the scriptural tradition *carte blanche* without stating which teachings or practices are to be followed or studied by disciples.

It is important then to distinguish the lineage canon—the sources and specific selections cited by the gurus—to understand the strict scriptural boundaries of Siddha Yoga teaching. Since their focus is on lineage teachings, practices, and interpretations rather than on the texts per se, guru-centered siddha traditions are under no burden to account for everything contained in the traditional body of teachings, the inclusive canon. In other words, there may be sources, teachings, or practices within the inclusive canon that gurus do not advocate even while they endorse the whole. To make a simple comparison, the Bible includes mention of slavery and even appears in certain instances to condone it. This does not mean, however, that a person who believes the Bible to be scripture endorses or condones slavery. Similarly, there are teachings in the inclusive canon of Hindu-inspired scripture that gurus would not claim as their own views. We might simply say that the canonical baby is not thrown out with the scriptural bathwater!

In guru-centered traditions like Siddha Yoga, the guru is free to affirm, reject, or even ignore specifics on the grounds that such teachings are not appropriate or skillful means (*upāya*) either to the lineage, in the current times, or even on an individual basis. Siddha lineages almost without exception (and including Siddha Yoga) endorse some notion of the inclusive canon of Hindu-based resources—the body of texts that as a whole plays the important symbolic role of representing tradition and confirming historical identity. However, gurus who begin from this common body of resources will create their own different lineage canons based on their selections, omissions, and interpretations.

Swamis Muktananda and Chidvilasananda are no exception to this general practice we observe in guru-centered traditions.[5] For example, the Siddha Yoga gurus' interest in the nondualist Vedānta of Śaṅkara should be understood in light of their understanding of Kashmiri Śaivism. Not all proponents of Vedānta or Kashmiri Śaivism understand them as complementary teachings, the way we see them portrayed in Siddha Yoga. Traditionally speaking, Vedānta and Kashmiri Śaivism are distinctive and even separate theological traditions that divide over many issues. This is not how the Siddha Yoga gurus treat them, however—the Siddha Yoga gurus are no more strict Advaita Vedāntins than they are exclusively Kashmiri Śaivites and the gurus do not engage in the polemics that divide these theological traditions. The Siddha Yoga gurus' connection with Kashmiri Śaivism, which deeply influences their interpretation of Vedānta, clearly distinguishes them from other modern gurus. There are well-known traditions of gurus who teach Śāṅkara Vedānta without this Kashmiri Śaivite influence, such as Swami Vivekananda or Ramana Maharshi. The point is that guru-based traditions do not necessarily follow established traditions of sectarian philosophy or worship—gurus may cross doctrinal, historical, regional, linguistic, and social boundaries to make their points. This is precisely what the Siddha Yoga gurus do in creating their own body of authoritative teachings.

Siddha Yoga's canon also reserves a place for the resources of ethics and law (*dharma*), sacrificial ritual (*yajña*), and worship (*pūjā*) common to the Hindu traditions that are called *smārta* traditions. Literally "based on the Recollections" (*smṛti*), *smārta* sources reinterpret the Vedic legacy and center worship on an expanding pantheon of deities and concepts. *Smārta* traditions were originally created by the priestly class of brahmins (Sanskrit, *brāhmaṇa*) as classical Hinduism crystallized from its ancient Vedic past. However, *smārta* resources have not stayed within any caste or regional boundaries; instead they have become common sources for many traditionalists, including the Siddha Yoga gurus.

Smārta sources particularly emphasize the five principal deities or *pañcāyatanadevatā*: Sūrya (the Sun), Viṣṇu, Śiva, Devī (the Goddess), and Gaṇeśa. Surrounding these deities are traditions of worship, mythology, ethics, and social custom. Historically, *smārta* traditions define themselves in contrast to traditions that make use of the texts known as Tantras and

Āgamas; formally speaking, what is *smārta* is not Tantric. However, this formal distinction is not always upheld even within *smārta* traditions. Many *smārta* followers are deeply interested in the Tantras and draw from them extensively. In other words, the formal distinction between *smārta* sources and the Tantras is anything but hard and fast. We need instead to look carefully at who is using the texts and for what reasons. Certainly some caste-conscious brahmins affirm a kind of sectarian distinction that allows them to refer to themselves as exclusively *smārta*. Others who use *smārta* texts and appropriate *smārta* traditions of worship or ritual are not the least bit interested in making the *smārta* canon a boundary for community identity. The Siddha Yoga gurus, for example, use many *smārta* texts and traditions with none of the sectarian interest that marks them elsewhere. Thus, while *smārta* traditions also have community and caste identities, these are entirely foreign to Siddha Yoga. One can speak of *smārta* traditions both in terms of social communities and textual resources.

The Siddha Yoga gurus draw freely from both *smārta* and Tantric literatures without imposing the formal *smārta* distinction based on different canons.[6] Further, Siddha Yoga evinces little interest in *smārta* sectarianism as a cultural and social reality that defines certain communities by their identification with a canon of texts and teachings. In fact, the same must be said of the Tantras and Āgamas that produce an alternative social and cultural vision that is non-*smārta* or even anti-*smārta*. The Siddha Yoga gurus do not identify with the social and cultural roles of the Tantras and Āgamas either but, rather, draw upon certain teachings contained in them. In sum, Siddha Yoga has shown a remarkable ability to keep itself apart from the different sorts of social, cultural, and political identifications that often accompany scriptures and canonical bodies of teaching. Instead, the Siddha Yoga gurus draw freely upon resources that suit their spiritual agenda and meet their ethical standards.

Historically, written and oral canons often represent the communities whose history is tied to their composition and use. Siddha Yoga, like some other guru-based traditions, identifies with scriptural teachings but not with their traditional social and cultural counterparts. We can, for example, contrast Siddha Yoga to certain forms of the Viṣṇu tradition. Many Viṣṇu-based or Vaiṣṇava traditions are not *smārta* and reject *smārta* values. Siddha Yoga clearly finds little affinity with these orthodox Viṣṇu-worshipers or with their non-*smārta* texts and customs. However, neither does Siddha Yoga identify with those segments of the brahmin *smārta* tradition that are exclusive in theological dogmas, deeply caste-conscious, or doctrinally anti-Tantric. Siddha Yoga gurus may cite many sources from Viṣṇu-centered traditions (*smārta* or not) and include important elements of the brahmin tradition, but they do not identify with any sort of Hindu sectarianism, communalism, or caste identity.

Rather than distinguish Siddha Yoga by the exclusion of others or by an identification with historical institutions, texts, or communities' interests, swamis Muktananda and Chidvilasananda take a different strategy. Their approach is rooted in the claim that the unity of being renders all dogmatism ineffective. The canon of texts and teachings, like all forms of Siddha Yoga teaching and practice, is defined in terms of its positive contribution to realizing this deeper truth. Swami Muktananda makes this point rhetorically when he says, "When there is nothing different from Shiva, what can be accepted or rejected? Siddha Yoga upholds equality."[7] This is a crucial and even defining feature of Siddha Yoga: Siddha Yoga is not a "religion" in the sense of a social, intellectual, or spiritual tradition that defines itself in opposition or in contrast with others. It identifies with no caste or communal interest. Neither is Siddha Yoga a Hindu cult within a given sectarianism, that is, it is not a "type" of *smārta* or Tantric tradition, or any other philosophical or doctrinal (*siddhānta*) group. Swami Muktananda states, "In Siddha Yoga there is no room for cultism. . . . Siddha Yoga considers all castes, religions, and sects to be its own and loves everyone with an open heart."[8] Further, since "the Supreme Being dwells in the space of the inner heart," Siddha Yoga seeks to put an end "to arguments and disputes, to the race-track competition among people, and to the futile rushing toward a dream of progress."[9] Thus Swami Muktananda states unequivocally, "Siddha Yoga . . . [does] not oppose any religion, sect, or code of ethics. . . . Siddha Yoga takes no interest in differences. It does not argue about bigotry or cults."[10] Swami Chidvilasananda reiterates the point by emphasizing the deeper truth behind the appearance of differences:

> As we perform our duties and become the duty, we become the Way. Then this separation between the Lord and the devotee vanishes. The Master and the disciple and all people become one. As all rivers merge into the ocean, we all merge into the ocean of the Truth.[11]

The Siddha Yoga gurus' tolerance for others' religions is not a blanket endorsement of all religious beliefs or practices; neither does it dismiss the fact that different texts or strata of tradition have differing views. Rather, the point is that one should not confuse the sometimes competing, conflicting, or antagonistic relations among texts and communities with teachings that lead to the highest realization.

While there are sound historical reasons to see many of the texts and genres in the Siddha Yoga canon as distinct in origin and even in conflict with one another, the Siddha Yoga gurus treat these differences as opportunities for developing a higher and deeper understanding. Their question is not whether a text is "ours" or "theirs" but whether it makes a contribution to understanding the unity of ultimate truth. What others believe to be dogmatic or communal statements, swamis Muktananda and Chidvilasananda treat as ideas and practices that either lead to harmony and insight or do not. There are other values at work as well, such as ethics, but these deserve their own discussion. Working within the largest scope of Hindu-based textuality and lore, the Siddha Yoga gurus are both traditionalists by their "acceptance" of the inclusive canon, and they are reformers who adapt, adopt, and reshape these sources beyond "original" boundaries.

The Esoteric Canon of the Tantras and the "In-Between" Texts

In addition to the resources common to virtually all Hindus and the *smārta* sources, the Siddha Yoga gurus have taken a special interest in the "Post-Vedic" or "Extra-Vedic" resources known as Tantras and Āgamas. The Tantras are a vast body of literature and teachings, nearly all of which presuppose oral commentary and secretive levels of initiate learning. While the earliest Hindu Tantras do not reach a written form until about the ninth century, they contain concepts (and indeed whole systems of practice) that speak to very ancient origins.[12] In many cases *tantra* is a term interchangeable with *āgama*, though the latter eventually takes on a more specialized meaning with regard to ritual texts and other sectarian divisions.

Defined in more conceptual terms, the Tantras are self-restricting and elitist. Most Tantras say their texts and teachings are not meant for those without highly specialized qualifications (*adhikāra*) and initiations (*dīkṣā*). By any standard, the Tantras are not within the sphere of the "ordinary" inclusive canon of Hindu sources. Their claim is that they are the exoteric canon's higher, esoteric extension meant only for the few. The Siddha Yoga gurus share no such elitist vision and use the Tantras as they would any other texts, though more selectively since they avoid both their sectarianism and their social boundary-defying attitudes.

Despite their claims, the Tantras are not nearly so secretive or remote from the mainstreams of Indian spirituality. Tantric influences have been pervasive in India since at least the sixth century and permeate the entire fabric of Hindu spirituality, especially yogic practices and ritual.[13] It is from Tantric literature, for example, that we gain the most insight into the role of the guru as the transmitter of spiritual power and the dispenser of grace; and it is the Tantras that outline the mysteries of the inner yogic journey as well as the theory and practice of *kuṇḍalinīyoga*. While the Siddha Yoga gurus reject much of their content on moral, ideological, and practical grounds, Tantric texts elaborate some of the Siddha Yoga lineage's most important teachings, including the guru's ability to infuse a divine awakening of spiritual energy (*śaktipāta*) and the internalization of divinity as the form of the yogi's own subtle body.

Unconcerned with Tantric claims to elitist teaching, the Siddha Yoga gurus utilize the Tantras to describe and refine these and other seminal ideas. Tantras are referred to explicitly by name, but perhaps more significant is their implicit role as background sources for key Siddha Yoga ideas. However, in contrast to the exoteric canon of Hindu Revelations and Recollections, the Siddha Yoga gurus are careful not to offer the same sort of traditional blanket approval to the Tantras. There is simply too much in the Tantras that gives rise to ethical abuse or is considered inappropriate or unnecessary to Siddha Yoga. For example, Tantric ritual initiations and extremely elaborate forms of deity worship involving mantras and *yantras* is not of much interest to the Siddha Yoga gurus. Occasionally important theoretical or practical teachings which are, properly speaking, most likely Tantric in origin and articulation make their way into Siddha Yoga, but these are treated as part of the larger tradition of mystical yoga. Siddha Yoga does not imagine or call itself a "Tantric tradition" though in many ways its mystical yoga and emphasis on the *guruvāda*, or "guru's way," is quintessentially Tantric.

In this sense we might, for scholarly purposes, place Siddha Yoga among the "Right-Current Path" (*dakṣiṇamārga/dakṣiṇācāra*) Tantric traditions. Put most simply, these traditions preserve the doctrine of the siddha's absolute freedom (*svātantryavāda*) but do not encourage or advocate boundary-defying modes of behavior on the part of gurus or disciples. This is not to say that the guru who follows this path sacrifices his or her freedom or any of the prerogatives of freedom that come with the perfection (*siddha*) of consciousness. Rather, the idea is that the guru *is* free to choose whatever conventions or boundaries are deemed useful and supportive of spiritual practice. Put differently, the guru is so free that there is no necessity to engage in any *deliberate* efforts to defy or violate social, cultural, or religious boundaries. There is, as it were, no point to be made by enacting freedom through boundary-defiance. The Right-Current understands freedom as boundless rather than as boundary-breaking. In this way, the Right-Current Tantric guru offers his own implicit criticism of the "Left-Current" (*vāmamārga/vāmācāra*) in which the violation of norms is part and parcel of affirming a libertarian state. In this *conceptual sense*, the Siddha Yoga gurus appear as part of the Right-Current though there is no formal "affiliation" with this terminology or the sectarian traditions that use it. As a conceptual model, it is quite important for understanding the *potential resources* (as well as the actual texts) selected by the Siddha Yoga gurus. Any selection of a text that makes a deliberate effort to subvert or undermine the most fundamental ethical codes of human conduct in order to assert freedom as beyond any boundary is *not* likely to be cited by the Siddha Yoga gurus. In other words, the Siddha Yoga canons are Right-Current in their notion of absolute freedom, not Left-Current.

Some important Siddha Yoga scriptures curiously stand between the exoteric sources of Revelation and Recollection and esoteric Tantric categories. The most important of these is the *Gurugītā*, which Swami

Muktananda calls "the one indispensable text of Siddha Yoga."[14] Said to be within either the *Skanda Purāṇa* or, more rarely, the *Padma Purāṇa*—which would identify the *Gurugītā* as part of the exoteric canon's Recollections (*smṛti*)—certain verses appear also in the *Kulārṇava Tantra* and other Tantric sources.[15] Much of the content of the *Gurugītā* resonates deeply with Tantric teachings and ideas: the esoteric qualities of the divinities, the interest in mantra and ritual yogic arts, and, of course, the mystical qualities of the guru. There are even ascriptions of the *Gurugītā* to the Tantras, such as the *Viśvasāra Tantra*. But the *Gurugītā* itself has a less than certain origin whether it be as a portion of the *Skanda Purāṇa*, as a section of another text known as the *Gurucaritra*, or as an independent quasi-Tantric text. This status is similarly not unusual for sources belonging to traditions of mystical yoga; they may have multiple "stations" in the larger canon, sometimes belonging to the exoteric Recollections and sometimes associating with the esoteric Tantras. This is due largely to the fact that Tantric sources seek frequently to *include* themselves as esoteric forms of exoteric works, in other words, as secrets concealed or appearing within more public resources.

The same sort of multiple appearances in different scriptures and categories of scriptures is true of many of the hymns (*stava, stotra*) chanted in Siddha Yoga ashrams. These hymns often have "Tantric" content but exoteric forms of attribution. For example, the *Śivamānasapūjā*, which extols the god Śiva's inner "mental" reality, is thoroughly Tantric in the ways it internalizes and esotericizes the yogi's identification with Śiva. Yet this text is part of the exoteric tradition associated with the Advaita Vedāntin Śaṅkarācārya. Whether it is a "Śaṅkara text" is irrelevant to the fact that Śāṅkara-based traditions have a stake in it and that its Tantric conceptual framework is as "mainstream" as it is esoteric. Furthermore, there is nothing particularly unusual about this example; many sources have these multiple or ambiguous origins and many have a share in more than one strand of Hindu tradition. From a vast array of materials in this "in-between" category of exoteric and esoteric texts, the Siddha Yoga gurus select certain individual texts and passages.

Since the Siddha Yoga gurus are not proponents of any one form of doctrinal worship (*siddhānta*), they are not committed to traditionalist "schools" of thought or particular philosophical identities. For example, while Siddha Yoga draws from both Śāṅkara Advaita Vedānta and the larger movement scholars called Kashmiri Śaivism, it does not identify with either (or any particular school within these traditions) in any formal sense. This has created an even greater opportunity for the gurus to draw upon the wealth of scriptural resources without drawing sectarian or denominational lines. As we shall see, this strategy is not unique to Siddha Yoga among the various forms of Indian spirituality.

The Tradition of Treatises and Aphorisms

Next, there are the learned traditions of aphorisms (*sūtra*), treatises, and commentaries called Śāstras composed by India's sages and philosophers. *The distinctive feature of all Śāstra texts is their attributed authorship and their espousal of specific viewpoints and teachings from within intellectual traditions.* In contrast, the works of Revelation and Recollection belong to so-called "great sage" traditions or have divine (or quasi-divine) authorship. Tantras similarly are attributed to divinities, particularly Śiva, or to quasi-divine beings. Śāstra texts not only have an attributed author, who may gain the status of a sage, but they are also usually grounded in some particular tradition or sect. While Siddha Yoga has little interest in the sectarian features surrounding these sources, the gurus are not reluctant to consider their content.

These Śāstra works range the entire historical spectrum from ancient to late medieval India. While some of these texts belong to the larger traditionalist canon, others are more clearly associated with *smārta* traditions, and still others are Tantric. Such texts as the *Yoga Sūtra* of Patañjali as well as selections from the philosopher sages Bhartṛhari, Manu, and others are part of this category. All the basic sources of the so-called six philosophical schools (*ṣaḍdarśana*) from Logic (*nyāya*) to Ritualism (*mīmāṃsā*) and Vedānta, should be considered here as well, at least in the sense of providing a background against which more important sources are considered.[16] In addition to the first layer of these traditions, such as Patañjali's *Yoga Sūtra*, we would include as well the entire corpus of yoga scriptures growing out of the larger Vedic and Hindu legacy, including the Tantric influenced texts of *haṭha*, *rāja*, *laya*, and *kuṇḍalinī* yoga. These texts are all part of the sagely tradition of treatises and teaching. Not every word is of interest to the Siddha Yoga gurus and certainly not the historical and polemical positions of the authors. The purpose of scholarship is to contribute to the guru's work of Self-realization. Gurumayi Chidvilasananda makes this point clearly when speaking about study in her main Western ashram, Shree Muktananda Ashram in South Fallsburg, New York:

> During the summer in South Fallsburg, we offer many different courses. Almost every course is designed for the same purpose: coming to know one's own Self. It isn't just intellectual wisdom that is being dispensed. What you are being offered is the experience of the supreme Self, which dwells within you. In fact, the professors, the scholars, the swamis who give these courses all speak from their own experience. They don't teach these classes to shock your brains, or to impress you intellectually, or to find glory for themselves. They speak from the depth of their own being. When you hear a teaching that is being given from someone's experience, it has the power to affect you, to purify your mind, your heart, and your body.[17]

The same principle is applied to the study of canonical scriptures. Formal study, even when it includes much that is technical or complex, is commended when it serves the purpose of transforming a person's experience and leads to purification and Self-awakening.

Like others within Indian spirituality, the Siddha Yoga gurus may take note of particular schools of thought or periods of intellectual development in order to distinguish their own teaching, but they apparently have no interest in the polemics or argumentation that are so pervasive in these texts. It is common, for example, for one of the Siddha Yoga gurus to mention a part of the history of a text or its attribution. However, this is only to locate it in the larger realm of scripture-as-that-which-aids-realization, as Swami Chidvilasananda notes above. In general, the Siddha Yoga gurus draw from the entire "mature" tradition of Indian spirituality in order to interpret the whole through the lens of their lineage experience. Since it is their experiential claim of nondual insight that governs the choice and interpretation of the texts, principles lead scriptures, not vice versa. From their standpoint as siddhas, any dispute or doctrinal difference dissolves with the vision of the nondual absolute.

More should be said about the two philosophical/worship traditions (*siddhāntas*) upon which the Siddha Yoga gurus have drawn most directly: the Advaita Vedānta of Śaṅkara and his disciples and the traditions of ecstatic Śaiva yoga known as Kashmiri Śaivism and its related Goddess-centered or Śākta offshoots, including the Spanda, Krama, and Śrīvidyā schools.[18] Though these traditions originate historically in rather different social and intellectual climates, their intersections become more frequent and important after the ninth century. In keeping with other South Indian traditionalists, including the practitioners of the goddess-centered Śrīvidyā, the Siddha Yoga gurus show little interest in the disputes that divide Vedānta and Kashmiri Śaivism from one another and within themselves.[19] This is not to say that swamis Muktananda and Chidvilasananda are unaware of these differences but rather that they see no need to "take sides."[20] In Siddha Yoga it is a matter of theological principle to engage texts and viewpoints in this fashion; it is the command of the guru to see scriptures only in terms of their role in Self-realization. There is, as such, *no* doctrinal stance in the formal sense. Swami Muktananda quotes his own guru, Nityananda, admonishing him to see beyond all such disputes:

> God has created the play of the world for His own pleasure. . . .
>
> Change your outlook. Correct your understanding. Then see that the world is just a play, an entertaining movie. It is neither true nor false. Know this secret. . . .
>
> All religions belong to the One. All sects are formed for Him alone. Nevertheless, through their own inspiration, the people who found sects give many

forms to that One. No matter how many ornaments one makes, they all come from the same gold.[21]

Precisely which texts and teachings are chosen by the Siddha Yoga gurus and how the traditions of Advaita Vedānta and Kashmiri Śaivism are synthesized is a matter we should address separately. For now suffice to say that these are as much distinct historical traditions of texts as they are different spiritual, social, and cultural practices.

In Advaita Vedānta the primary sources are the Upaniṣads, the *Bhagavadgītā,* and the *Brahma Sūtra.* These are augmented by the treatises of the philosopher-yogis Gauḍapāda, Śaṅkara, Sureśvara, and others. The Kashmiri Śaiva focus on the Tantras, Āgamas, and related Śākta scriptures includes the *Śiva Sūtra* of Vasugupta, the *Pratyabhijñāhṛdayam* of Kṣemarāja, and much of the work of the great eleventh-century intellectual mystic, Abhinavagupta.[22] All of these texts, like those of the traditionalist canon of Revelation and Recollection, are written in the Sanskrit language.

Another distinctive feature of the Treatise (*śāstra*) traditions is their reliance on interpretive commentaries. These are used by their saintly exponents to put divinely revealed or inspired recollections within specific intellectual and doctrinal contexts. Just as the inclusive canon concept allows the "acceptance" or "endorsement" of whole texts or traditions of texts without affirming every teaching within them, similarly the Siddha Yoga gurus recognize many of the great philosophers and theologians as siddhas without endorsing their every word. This is true not only of Advaita Vedāntins and Kashmiri Śaivas, but of other philosopher-sages of the Indian tradition. Swamis Muktananda and Chidvilasananda will occasionally cite traditional Indian philosophical qualified nondualists such as the eleventh-century Rāmānuja or the fifteenth-century Caitanya if their aims are suited by some aspect of these philosophers' teachings or lives. At the same time, the Siddha Yoga gurus do not endorse their philosophical positions.

This inclusive view of the philosopher-saints is itself a part of Siddha Yoga's own canonical belief that the nondual absolute is beyond any disputation. In this way even traditional "opponents" or "qualifiers" of nondualist thinking in India are made part of Siddha Yoga when it suits the aims of the gurus. To put this simply, any teaching that is useful in gaining insight into the truth of nondualism—the perfect identity of one's own consciousness with the divine—is a potential candidate for the Siddha Yoga gurus' selection. The authority of these sources rests on their theological interpretation *and* the intentionality (*saṅkalpa*) of the Siddha Yoga gurus to make them authoritative resources for contemplation. Thus the Siddha Yoga gurus can remain interested in ideas and even in theological doctrines without having any interest in social, religious, political, or cultural sectarianism. Siddha Yoga does indeed have theological principles, such as the ultimate unity of being and the non-competitive nature of truth, though these ideas themselves might be drawn out of virtually any resource. Those resources that particularly espouse the nondualist vision quite naturally gain a canonical authority when accompanied by the gurus' own intention to lead others to this experience.

The Tradition of Songs and Oral Teachings

The works of the saints known as perfected ones (*siddha*), saints (*sant*), and devotees (*bhakta*) are particularly important in the formulation of Siddha Yoga.[23] In contrast to most of the texts to which we have alluded, these sources are not usually composed in Sanskrit but in vernacular Indian languages like Hindi, Marathi, Tamil, Kannada, or Punjabi.

Bhagawan Nityananda and Swami Muktananda were both South Indians by birth; their travels eventually brought them to the area near Ganeshpuri, Maharashtra. It comes as little surprise, given their eventual central western Indian location, that these natives of the south became deeply immersed in the works of poet-sages of West and North India. The same is true of Swami Chidvilasananda. Again, we see an interest in the lives and teachings of these saints with little attachment to the sectarian traditions that have followed after them.

The location of the Siddha Yoga mother ashram in western India also has not diminished the Siddha Yoga gurus' interest in South Indian siddha traditions. Swami Chidvilasananda, for example, frequently quotes the saints of the Kannada-speaking Vīraśaiva tradition, particularly Akkamahādevī and Allamaprabhu. Occasionally we hear reference to Tamil siddhas including Tirumūlar, who happens to be associated with the beginning of the dualistic Śaiva Siddhānta movement. However, the Siddha Yoga gurus focus on the great medieval and modern saints who composed in Marathi, Hindi, and Punjabi.[24] While we hear frequently of Tukārām, Eknāth, Kabīr, and Mīrābāī, we also are told stories of lesser known figures such as Sundardās and Banārsidās.

Among these medieval siddhas, swamis Muktananda and Chidvilasananda hold a special place for the Maratha *sant* Jñāneśvar, author of the beautiful and richly complex *Jñāneśvarī*, a commentary on the *Bhagavadgītā*. The gurus do not, however, identify with the institutions and traditions of worship that surround the cult of Jñāneśvar in Pandharpur. This sectarian group, known as the Vārkarīs, practices Viṣṇu-centered worship and possesses a strong sense of communal and social identity.

The *Jñāneśvarī* may be the most frequently cited scriptural resource in Siddha Yoga, though it is not a devotional focus nor the canonical centerpiece for spiritual practices; that distinction belongs to the *Gurugītā*. The *Jñāneśvarī*, however, epitomizes Siddha Yoga's understanding that the paths of knowledge (*jñāna*), action (*karma*), and devotion (*bhakti*) primary to the

Bhagavadgītā are each necessary as well as inclusive and complementary of each other. This philosophical stance whereby all three paths (*mārga*) of the *Bhagavadgītā* are given equal stature and importance is both Jñāneśvar's view and that of the Siddha Yoga gurus. It stands in contrast, for example, to the strict doctrinal interpretation of Śaṅkara, the Advaita Vedāntin, though the Siddha Yoga gurus are just as likely to cite Śaṅkara as they are Jñāneśvar. Thus Jñāneśvar's standpoint contrasts vividly with other commentators who either see the paths successively (e.g., devotion as preliminary to knowledge), or as separate and unequal (e.g., devotion is superior to knowledge or vice versa.)[25] Like the Siddha Yoga gurus and unlike most *Bhagavadgītā* commentators, Jñāneśvar does not presume a doctrinal position (*siddhānta*) which he defends; neither does he engage in polemics to discredit less "desirable" views. Further, Jñāneśvar integrates the most esoteric teachings of *kuṇḍalinīyoga* into devotion to the guru by seeing both as forms of knowledge and embodiments of the divine play of consciousness. (This level or understanding of yoga is, for example, entirely absent in Śaṅkara's commentary on the *Bhagavadgītā* but is clearly in evidence in the Kashmiri Śaivite view of Abhinavagupta's commentary.)

The Siddha Yoga gurus teach that every practice—from selfless service (*sevā*) to silent meditation or scriptural study—is efficacious to Self-realization because knowledge, devotion, and action are ultimately identical. All originate from the same source and all are forms of a higher knowledge. As Swami Chidvilasananda notes, "When your knowledge is pure, you are functioning from the deepest part of your being, from the great heart where the truth abides."[26] Thus we see in their treatment of the *Bhagavadgītā* a crucial theological stance, one that would seem formally to align the Siddha Yoga gurus more with the theology of Jñāneśvar than any other commentator on this text. However, the important point is that the Siddha Yoga gurus are *not* particularly interested in choosing a doctrinal line of commentarial discourse or at least one over another. Rather, they feel free to choose from among these sources to make their own position clear. The *Jñāneśvarī* nonetheless stands as a constant resource of Siddha Yoga and one that devotees can look to nearly without exception as holding "the Siddha Yoga viewpoint."

The Siddha Yoga gurus also make occasional reference to the Sikh gurus, especially Guru Nānak whose vision centers on the qualityless (*nirguṇa*) absolute and the liberating force of the name of God given by the guru. Both of these are core Siddha Yoga teachings. Much of the so-called *Nām* or Name theology of the Sikhs, along with their mystical understanding of mantras and belief in the divine's nondualist nature, is in consonance with the Siddha Yoga gurus' teachings. And, as is ever the case, the Siddha Yoga gurus evince little interest in Sikh customs or traditions that don't bear directly on either their mystical theology or their core human ethics. There is no political or cultural alignment that follows from their interest in Sikh spirituality or the *kinds of spirituality* we see in evidence in the Sikh gurus.

Swamis Muktananda and Chidvilasananda seem as well to be versed in the lore of other religious traditions and quote liberally from the scriptural sources and saintly traditions of Christianity, Buddhism, Taoism, and mystical Islam. Swami Chidvilasananda in particular draws from an especially wide range of religious and philosophical works across Western and Eastern traditions. Inasmuch as they cite these sources specifically and contextually, they might be counted as part of the larger Siddha Yoga canon. Worthy of particular mention is the use of Sufi lore often in the form of stories. Many of the so-called Sheikh Nasruddin episodes and parables that frequently appear in the teachings of the Siddha Yoga gurus are likely Sufi in origin. This liberal use of materials originating in non-Hindu and even non-Indian spiritual traditions is part of the Siddha Yoga gurus' effort to place teachings ahead of dogmas or religious communal identity.

However, the Siddha Yoga gurus are not interested in creating either a new theosophical (or now, "New Age") religion, or a "new" Siddha Yoga vocabulary divorced from the sources of Indian tradition. Rather, there is an openness to the voices of others and a willingness to consider their insights in light of Siddha Yoga's understanding of reality. It is their own experience that Siddha Yoga gurus are interested in teaching and to which they refer when citing textual resources. There is clearly conveyed, however, the idea that this experience is "ancient" in the diachronic sense of being part of the tradition of the siddhas and that it is "eternal" in the synchronic sense of being forever and always true. This notion of an experiential core of meaning permits the Siddha Yoga gurus to refer to texts beyond the usual core of "siddha" or Indian traditions as works of "siddhas." It is not, however, a means of expanding or diluting traditions as such.

Swamis Muktananda and Chidvilasananda treat the "siddha" not as a category of texts or even of persons but rather as a state of divine consciousness that one can see reflected across all religious differences and historical traditions. It is with this understanding in mind that texts and teachings may be cited by the gurus regardless of their original source or context.

In addition, swamis Muktananda and Chidvilasananda draw from the lore of other modern saints treated as siddhas, many of whom were either Muktananda's contemporaries or were well-known to him. While much of this is oral lore passed through Muktananda's own writings, there is also the mention of other nineteenth- and twentieth-century saints, including Ramakrishna Paramahamsa, and Sai Baba of Shirdi. We may even hear of so-called "great souls" such as Mohandas Gandhi if it suits the gurus' effort to convey the meaning and the content of their experience.[27] To this type of saintly lore we should add Swami Muktananda's interest in "scholarly literature." These works, written largely in Hindi or Marathi as compilations and recapitulations of siddha and yoga lore, offered Muktananda a lens through which to view his own experiences and provided him at least some of the vocabulary he used to teach disciples. Several of these works he mentions by name in his spiritual autobiography, *Play of Consciousness,* as resources that aided his own understanding, particular the *Mahāyoga Vijñāna, Yoga Vāṇi,* and the *Gurucaritra.* While these texts are important in tracing Swami Muktananda's own interest in scriptural concepts, they are not part of the Siddha Yoga canon in any formal sense: They are not authoritative teachings nor are they prescribed (ritually or as study aids) for disciples except as sources of enrichment. To put this differently, while the content of these sources may speak to the siddha's experience, the sources themselves are not canonical in the sense of being either authoritative resources or scriptures that deserve study and contemplation.

In addition to these works mentioned by the Siddha Yoga gurus that speak more generally to their experience, we might also mention a handful of hymns and stanzas written by devotees for Swami Muktananda that have become part of Siddha Yoga lore *and* part of its canon, particularly *Jyota se Jyota* and *Āratī Karūṅ,* which appear in the book of chants and meditations called *The Nectar of Chanting.* These texts are not scriptural in the sense that they are important resources of teachings, though they are sometimes used for formal contemplation. Rather, they are canonical inasmuch as they provide *means for the enactment of devotion* or because they are *evocative of the inner experience* that the gurus extend to devotees.

Though the Siddha Yoga gurus may occasionally direct disciples to read or study a given text, this instruction itself does not *necessarily* make the source canonical. Rather, other factors establish authority; the guru's own interest or selective reference is only an indication of the importance of a text. A selection or source can even become "temporarily scriptural" in the sense that for a certain person or at a certain moment that resource is infused with the guru's intentionality (*saṅkalpa*) and power (*śakti*). The point is that it is the guru who is "the canon behind the canon," and that without which a text remains "inert" or "unawakened" (*jaḍa*).

The secondary scholarly texts in Indian vernacular languages, like other books or persons mentioned by the gurus, warrant discussion because they seem to offer resources for the Siddha Yoga gurus' interpretations of meditative experience as well as siddha and yogic traditions.

The Teachings of the Siddha Yoga Gurus

The final canonical resource for Siddha Yoga is also the most important: the words of the three lineage gurus and the texts they set specifically aside. *The Nectar of Chanting,* first published by Shree Gurudev Ashram in 1972, is a compilation of texts that is the primary example of Siddha Yoga scriptural canon-making. Its sources are drawn from across the spectrum of the exoteric and esoteric canon of Hindu-based spirituality. Sometimes works are taken in their entirety, like the *Viṣṇu Sahasranāma*, or in part, like the so-called "Introductory Mantras," the "Āratī," and the "Upanishad Mantras," which come from a variety of sources and oral lore. *The Nectar of Chanting* includes as well those texts specifically composed for Siddha Yoga like *Jyota se Jyota* and *Āratī Karūṅ*. In keeping with the spirit of their own inclusivism, *The Nectar of Chanting* does nothing to indicate the differences between these sources either historically or doctrinally. While the *Gurugītā* is singled out, we gain very little from the text of *The Nectar of Chanting* to indicate the importance of other texts included either for their teachings or their practical use. These sorts of instructions are gained from within Siddha Yoga by experience, instruction, custom, and practice. Just to make a simple comparison, one learns very little about the importance of teachings or practices from looking at a church prayerbook. To understand those dimensions of the text requires participation and involvement.

Beyond this resource of texts, we must also consider the Siddha Yoga gurus' teachings as canonical. From the standpoint of Siddha Yoga, Bhagawan Nityananda's words and teachings are viewed primarily through Swami Muktananda's recollections, experiences, and interpretations. The crucial canonical fact is that Nityananda left no written records from his own hand and only a few instances of his recorded voice. The record then is a small number of laconic sayings, stories *about* Nityananda, and other lore passed by longtime devotees.[28] Texts attributed to Bhagawan Nityananda, especially the so-called *Nitya Sutras*, are not regarded by the Siddha Yoga gurus as either particularly authoritative or even authentic. Though much in this text resonates with Siddha Yoga teaching and Swami Muktananda's understanding of his guru's teaching, it is not part of the Siddha Yoga canon.[29] What follows from the lore of Bhagawan Nityananda is not at all uncommon to that which follows other charismatic siddhas who leave no formal record or teaching but who do have traditions of discipleship. For example, in Ram Dass's collection entitled *Miracle of Love: Stories About Neem Karoli Baba*, we see disciples gathering hundreds of tales and stories by and about their guru. This is not, however, anything like an "authorized" record or account of the guru's teachings, but one that "surrounds" him. A similar, if less systematic, body of lore "surrounds" Bhagawan Nityananda. From the standpoint of Siddha Yoga, however, it is the portrayal of Bhagawan Nityananda by the Siddha Yoga gurus that defines his lore and teachings.

In contrast to the largely oral corpus of his guru, Swami Muktananda's teachings were kept first as notes and later as recordings and on videotape, often with his eventual successor Gurumayi Chidvilasananda by his side as his interpreter. Many of Swami Muktananda's and Swami Chidvilasananda's published writings originated as transcriptions of oral discourses—as is often the case in India, even many formal teachings that reach written form are discourses, dictations, or combinations of written and dictated work. These written compilations admit an editorial hand in the process of canon-making. This does not mean that they are not the guru's words since the talks included in such collections were in fact written by the guru. Moreover, their transformation into printed formats comes precisely with the guru's intentionality (*saṅkalpa*). Thus it is the guru's *saṅkalpa* as much as the guru's words that defines what is authoritative and therefore "canonical."

In the case of the Siddha Yoga gurus, some works are composed originally as written texts. In Swami Muktananda's case this includes his spiritual autobiography *Play of Consciousness*, the essays in *Light on the Path*, the poetry entitled *Mukteshwari* and *Reflections of the Self*, his rendering of the Kashmiri poetess saint Lalleshwari, *The Perfect Relationship*, *Secret of the Siddhas*, and the textual commentaries that make up *Siddha Meditation*.[30] Much of Swami Chidvilasananda's *Ashes at My Guru's Feet* was likewise written as a text rather than compiled from orations. While we may note important distinctions between works the gurus have dictated or spoken and those written, these will not prove crucial to understanding what is distinctive to Siddha Yoga teachings. What is canonical as such is that which comes with the Siddha Yoga gurus intentionality, their *saṅkalpa*; the format is secondary.

Since, however, only a fraction of the Siddha Yoga gurus' recorded words are to date publicly available and since more continue to be recorded, the canon of Siddha Yoga will in all likelihood continue to grow as Swami Chidvilasananda sees fit to expand the legacy of her guru and to publish more of her own discourses. Presumably future lineage gurus will make contributions to the canon or draw upon the archives of swamis Muktananda and Chidvilasananda.

My own access to the archives of Siddha Yoga has confirmed, as Swami Chidvilasananda has often said publicly, that all the essential teachings of Siddha Yoga are before the devotees. There are no "hidden" doctrines or practices yet to be revealed nor is there a principle in place, such as the Tibetan Buddhist concept of *gter ma*, or "treasure," that makes it possible for new texts to appear in the future that will alter or shift the core of Siddha Yoga teachings. However, with the presence of the living guru, there is a dynamic and organic quality to the dissemination and elaboration of Siddha Yoga that will invariably bring refinement and nuance to the unfolding understanding of practitioners. In other words, there will continue to be growth and development of Siddha Yoga teachings, just as Siddha Yoga culture will continue to evolve with the living gurus. Our point is that Siddha Yoga does not have a body of concealed teaching that stands behind its public presentation nor is there a "layering" of teachings that creates a hierarchy of initiation. (Though Siddha Yoga teachers have developed a graduated curriculum, so that advanced scriptural and oral teachings are given only after students have completed the necessary background studies.) All Siddha Yoga devotees, in effect, receive the "same" essential body of teachings, practices, and initiations; devotees have no "rank" or "spiritual status" as is the case in many Tantric lineages or in institutional traditions such as the Roman Catholic Church.

Particularly interesting to the development of Siddha Yoga teachings is the increasing role technology plays in developing canonical authority. Swami Chidvilasananda, taking advantage of other media, has utilized spoken tapes and video as means of communicating teachings. These media are deliberately utilized rather than simply films or recordings of the guru. In this way she has introduced "new" technologies as formats of canon-making. Unlike Swami Muktananda, who spoke mostly in Hindi, English is her primary medium. However, how she might appear—on video, in satellite broadcasts, in recordings, in print, or in person—is part of the canon-making process.

The Principle of the Gurutattva: Achieving Canonical Status

That the words of one's own guru have a canonical status is not the least bit unusual in the Indian tradition: we may consider the entire tradition of Śāstras written by sage-philosophers to be just that—the words of lineage gurus who are, in the eyes of their disciples, no less authoritative than any other scriptural resource. This means only the words of the living guru who embodies the guru principle (*gurutattva*) can be considered potentially canonical. The guru may appoint or sanction at a particular moment many different persons to speak on behalf of the lineage teachings but this is not to say that they bear canonical authority, any more than a representative of the Roman Catholic Church can be said to be as authoritative as the Pope or stand for scriptures of the canon. To put the matter succinctly, only the words of the guru have canonical status and then only when the guru indicates or implies as much by the context and form of their presentation.

It is a relatively simple task to list the sources the Siddha Yoga gurus have chosen and then to classify them by genres, languages, and currents of tradition. This would prove an efficient way to define the scriptural body of Siddha Yoga, *if* such a list, or more properly such a collection of lists, were truly all we needed to create the boundaries of the lineage tradition. Were this true we could say that when texts or even selections from texts were not on the list then they would be beyond the boundaries of Siddha Yoga.

However, the teachings of siddha lineages are not defined solely by their textual selections. In other words, no matter how carefully one constructs lists of sources from which the gurus choose, there are literally thousands of others which they *might* choose. Since siddha gurus are not bound to any one body of texts nor confined to fixed lists of scriptures which they must accept and interpret, their choices reflect their particular *experiences* from within an enormous spectrum of potential resources. In siddha traditions, there is nothing like the Bible or the Qur'an that defines *the* essential canonical resource even though there appear to be groups of texts or teachings, such as the Vedas or the *Bhagavadgītā*, which nearly all gurus "admit" into their canons. Though siddha gurus begin with the canon of texts chosen by their own gurus and treat their guru's words as canonical, this does not mean that they are limited only to texts *already* chosen by the previous lineage gurus.

To define Siddha Yoga we will need to understand the guiding principles of choice that point to the *potential canon*—those sources that the gurus might well choose. The notion of a potential canon is first an acknowledgment of the dynamic presence of the guru. Perhaps more importantly, the potential canon points beyond the scriptural choices themselves and toward the guiding forces that inform the siddha guru's experience. In addition, we will need to think about the organization and content of teachings themselves.

The siddha guru is considered absolutely free (*svatantrya*) in every respect; yet, at the same time, the authority of the guru is understood as a result of continued discipleship. The simultaneous role the siddha guru plays as guru and as disciple are the keys to understanding their prerogatives as innovators and conservators of tradition. It is in these roles that we gain a deeper understanding of the notion of canon as a body of texts and teachings and as the intentionality of the guru to convey the experience of the siddha. This dual role of guru and disciple demands our further consideration. We should begin by considering why spiritual traditions invest in canons, that is, in authoritative bodies of teaching and practice.

WHO SPEAKS FOR SPIRITUAL TRADITIONS: MAKING CANONS AND BECOMING HUMAN

One of the defining features of being human is our truly remarkable ability to acquire empowering knowledge that we pass down from one generation to another. We might even go so far as to say that a society keeps its promise to be human when it bequeaths to its children its important traditions, whether these are religious, social, or scientific. In part, fulfilling the promise of tradition involves recognizing and enshrining ideas, beliefs, memories, and skills in the form of texts and teachings that become canons. *Canons formulate and preserve basic truths essential to personal development and collective identity because they are continually authenticated by experience.*

Spiritual or religious canons are meant to withstand the malleability of evolving human knowledge and so address our condition across the divides of history, culture, or circumstance. This, in part, is what makes canons *sacred*: For in the face of our mortal condition, humans entrust their deepest convictions to a language of the immortal, setting apart the sacred from the profane. Canons are one way by which human beings create the notion of the sacred and they are an important way by which we can tell the difference between sacred and profane, transcendent and ordinary.

Canons are more than the written or oral resources for tradition. They are also sources of authority that remain when individuals pass away. In this way, canons help create a tradition's structure and content. Just as the frame of a house creates structure and the furnishings provide content, so a canon stands on its own, built by tradition. Canons endure after those who built them have gone. However, we must not forget that houses are built by experts whose continued involvement means they will tear down what is no longer useful, or make additions, and in this way insure worth. In addition, those "owners" of tradition must live in the canonical house; their role in maintaining it is crucial. Without the "owners," the house is empty, lifeless, and liable to deterioration. A canon requires a living presence just as a house needs a family to become a home.

Spiritual canons usually take the form of words, actions, gestures, or examples that are remembered and reaffirmed. A canon is not simply words that once spoken become sacred; rather it is the process by which they are recalled and the situations that prompt their remembrance. Above all canons are resources that speak to the experiences of people; they provide a means by which future generations can receive guidance and probe the meaning of tradition. The Bible, the Qur'an, the *Bhagavadgītā*, and other scriptures all fulfill this same human need. Though all canons have a history, undergo change, and demand interpretation, they are significant because their sense of authority creates boundary: They allow people to say, "This is truth," "These are our beliefs and our stories," or "What is said here speaks to all human beings." Such canonical boundaries do not necessarily exclude other persons nor do they always distinguish "us" from "them," though they are sometimes used this way. Canons may be unconcerned with those outside the community or have other aims; they may seek to distinguish truth from falsehood or the perennial and timeless from that which is merely relevant or timely.

In this way, canon-making is an important part of how we learn who we have been, who we are, and what we want to become. Canons help to describe what we know and want to know, and how we should go about fulfilling hopes and expectations. From whom we learn and how we pass along our lessons, whether in memories, in words, or by examples, is as significant as the knowledge itself, for this helps us to decide if the knowledge is valuable enough to remember and if the tradition is worthy of being continued. In this sense, traditional knowledge and those who know traditions are vital to everything we think, say, or do. When we are able to take things for granted, we are reaping one of the benefits of tradition in the form of things we think we already know. When we gain a new or deeper understanding, it is because others have fulfilled their promise and created a basis from which to grow.

Traditions succeed when human beings invest both in the knowledge that is transmitted and in the people who transmit it. In these ways, canons of spiritual teachings form the reservoir of knowledge from which people drink to refresh their minds and hearts. Importantly, the process of refreshment is recurrent rather than once and for all. By imbibing the knowledge of the canon, a person gains a sense of identity, belonging, and continuity with the wisdom and the people who have gone before. In addition, one learns and relearns the lessons that speak to an individual's personal experience as a human being. Canons are places to which people can return to reestablish their place in the world as well as within themselves.

Understanding the different ways knowledge is transmitted helps also to reveal the subtle and distinctive ways in which traditions differ from one another. While it may seem obvious that there are many different traditions and types of knowledge, it might not be apparent that traditions transmit their knowledge in different ways as well. In other words, canons of different traditions distinguish themselves not only in content but in formation and transmission. These ways of transmitting knowledge are as much "traditions" as the knowledge itself. When we investigate the structure of a spiritual canon, we gain a deeper understanding of a tradition's ideas and practices. We also gain a perspective on the choices people make to keep traditions alive. *Behind every tradition's canon is the story of how that canon came about and who is responsible for its creation, development, and transmission.* How people transfer and confer their knowledge may shape their understanding of tradition as profoundly as the knowledge received.

Messages and Their Media: Transmitting Tradition in Canons

Looking at traditions other than one's own, one will find there are not only different messages but also different media and different ways of establishing tradition. Canons contain more than a tradition's messages and instructions. They are also an important medium through which traditional knowledge is transmitted. One's opinion of people and of traditions is influenced by both the messages they send *and* the various media they use.

Those of us educated by contemporary Western methods, for example, have likely spent little time memorizing texts and have mixed feelings about this kind of learning. We admire but may also be suspicious or even disdainful of such learning. Knowing things "by heart" can be dismissed as mere memorization without understanding. As the body of knowledge becomes increasingly more voluminous and beyond our memories, we increase our investment in technologies that encourage us to consider other activities implicitly more valuable. The use of computers, for example, can suggest to us that knowing things by heart is unnecessary or a waste of time. We may place more value on our abilities to retrieve information than actually to know it. In this way, the value of the technology that delivers access to knowledge might for us outweigh the value of the knowledge itself.

In contrast, traditional Indian society has been ambivalent about learning that is not by heart. It is especially wary of the authority of words written and read over those spoken and heard. Extraordinary, even superhuman, efforts have been made to secure the power and insure the integrity of knowledge passed orally: The sacred texts of the Vedas, called *śruti* because they reveal the divine reality heard resonating in the universe, have been memorized and transmitted scrupulously syllable by syllable for at least three thousand years. Other sacred texts, by contrast, are afforded a lesser status because they are merely "remembered" (*smṛti*). *Writing* a text or studying one is yet another sort of activity, one whose value is not only dependent on oral revelation and remembrance but is derived from it. In this way written knowledge presumes a mastery of oral teachings and, importantly, the relationship of teacher and disciple.

In Hindu spirituality, the relationship between oral and written knowledge implies that spiritual teachings *must* flow through living reservoirs of learning, that is, through sages, gurus, or divine beings who speak either directly or indirectly. In this sense, the power of a text and its authority does not depend on its being written down so that it can become an autonomous "being" whose life stands apart from its transmission. Rather, the underlying assumption is quite the opposite. Hindu spiritual texts are powerful *when* they come through teachers believed to have embodied and experienced for themselves the very essence of their meaning.[31] Though Hindus believe that the Vedas resonate the eternal truth and so do not rely on humans to be true, every hymn and verse is attributed to a sage (or a divine being) who is named and credited with the transmission. Practically speaking, Vedic traditions sanctified not only the text but the relationship of guru and disciple through which the eternal was understood to flow.

Not all spiritual traditions, even those from India, place the authority or the power of living gurus ahead of canonical texts. But in guru-centered traditions, gurus are more than simply indispensable: They become embodiments of the canon in order to represent the truths that tradition sustains. In this way, gurus are not the same as priests, renunciants, yogis, or scholars, though they may be all of these as well.

The Tradition of Guruvāda, or the Doctrine of the Guru

In the case of Hindu spirituality rooted in *guruvāda*, or the "doctrine of the guru," it is difficult to imagine what purpose a canon would serve in the absence of a "living" master.[32] This is quite different than in certain other segments of Indian religion or in other religious traditions where the opposite seems to be true. For example, within certain Buddhist and Christian traditions, canons serve as forms of truth *in the absence of the living teacher.* Here the essence of the teaching is made to stand apart, "untainted" by those who might corrupt its meaning and available to everyone as that form of truth not dependent on the traditions of transmission.

In this sense, Buddhists deem their canon a form of the highest truth (*dharma*) and so a "refuge" (*śaraṇam*) whose authority, power, and importance is considered equal to the Buddha and the community.[33] Certain Buddhists therefore suggest that canonical truths should not be confused with canonical interpretations.[34] One might say that the Buddha's legendary refusal to appoint a successor was a step in the formation of a canon meant to represent him in his absence. As the story goes, the community (*saṅgha*) gathered for their first council upon the Buddha's passing. At least part of the reason for their gathering was to compile and authorize a canon that would help to take his place. In the absence of a single authoritative spiritual lineage, Buddhists have often canonized traditions and relocated authority in these canons. Similarly, Islam and certain strands of Christianity have conceptualized their Qur'anic and biblical canons as means for reinforcing the principle that scriptural truths should not be confused with or linked too intimately to those who transmit them. The goal in these cases is to create an authority that is not the individual who teaches the canon. The "preacher" is therefore not identified with the "preached," but rather the scripture is autonomous and an inviolate expression of truth. In such traditions, ultimate authority is not human authority and so the sacred is represented in canonical teachings rather than in persons.

In contrast to guru-centered canonical traditions, some Buddhists and Christians identify scriptural truths through the authority they vest in their communities—monks, priests, churches, and other institutional spiritual authorities gathered in great councils or congregations have been charged to define the boundaries of the canon.[35] In this way, the power to decide tradition is decentralized and the tradition's meanings, purposes, and forms are made institutional knowledge. The institutions become the arbiters of authority, and canonical texts become an important resource by which to sustain that authority. Of course, individuals may sometimes be given or assume powerful and significant decision- and meaning-making roles. The Pope, for example, sometimes serves in roles that are comparable to those of the siddha guru when he declares the meaning of scriptures, doctrines, practices, or declares new dogmas. However, certain Buddhists and Christians have created and used their canons of scriptures in part to represent and to complement their institutions, their founders, and their sacred truths *rather than their leaders.* This distinction is important because it means that some Buddhist or Christian leaders inherit a canon of teachings whose authority is deliberately separated from the human beings who interpret or exemplify it. This role for canon is quite different in those particular guru-centered traditions in which scriptural sources gain their authority because gurus embody and represent them.

Whether the canon is thought to exist *autonomously* apart from spiritual leaders or whether the canon is *embodied* in a spiritual leader, in every tradition there is the implicit acknowledgment that humans *must* take responsibility for the interpretation of the canon. Precisely where authority for interpretation *should* lie is a matter upon which traditions have differed significantly. All spiritual traditions grapple with the issue of maintaining sacred teachings while affirming a presence in the profane world. Just as certain Buddhists and Christians have conceptualized a canon to protect the sacred from human foibles and abuse, so the advocates of the guru-centered approach understood the dangers of investing so much authority in human beings. Guru traditions, however, deem the possible benefits fully worth the risks involved.[36]

To understand how human beings might confer such power and responsibility to gurus, one must see the *guruvāda* tradition as more than submission and surrender to a human treated as a divine being. Rather, one must affirm the possibility of perfection embodied both in the guru and, potentially, within oneself. Disciples *must* become gurus if guru traditions are to continue. From Siddha Yoga's standpoint, the guru is both a human being who stands for the power and authority of the tradition *and* a spiritual principle that can be identified as one's own inner nature or Self (*ātman*).

One must also consider the scope of the guru's authority and her or his own deference to traditions of discipleship, teaching, and practice. While guru-centered traditions are vulnerable to becoming cults of personality, the canons of these traditions explicitly denounce self-appointed authority and insist upon the vigilance of disciples. *The guru's power is ideally not so much the commanding exercise of authority but the restraining discipline of discipleship.* It is not that disciples "decide" who is the guru, rather it is the guru who gains authority *by virtue of enacting the principle of the* gurutattva, *the ideal of the embodied truth.*

Disciples of siddhas who become individual authorities are to do so by their achievements of spiritual discipline (*sādhana*) and the grace-bestowing power (*anugraha-śakti*) of their gurus. Gurumayi Chidvilasananda was appointed and ritually bequeathed the power and authority to assume the leadership of the Siddha Yoga lineage by Swami Muktananda. Her continuing empowerment, however, is understood in terms of the relationship between spiritual discipline rooted in her devotion and yogic commitment and the transformative effects of her guru's grace. Put simply, her vows to discipleship continue to express the will and intentionality (*saṅkalpa*) of her guru. It is this continuous, uninterrupted commitment that Siddha Yoga understands as a mark of the true guru (*sadguru*).

As spiritual leaders, Siddha Yoga gurus are neither elected nor self-appointed. Instead their power and authority originates in and is sustained by their relationship with their own guru and appears in the form of their self-discipline, relationship with tradition, and ability to lead disciples to Self-realization. Though siddhas have composed texts that become canonical for their disciples, in Siddha Yoga and other *guruvāda* traditions even these texts cannot substitute or serve as an authority *apart from the siddha guru*. In other words, texts do not stand apart from living gurus who embody the experience or state of the siddha that the texts describe. A siddha guru's authority is not dependent on or derived from a relationship to canons of texts or teachings per se. This is true even when siddha lineages express clear allegiances to the principles that link them to certain texts or selections from texts. In some cases, such as in the Śāṅkara traditions, there is an institutional framework within which the guru resides and from which he derives authority. In Siddha Yoga, however, the essence of the *guruvāda* is that the power and authority of the siddha guru is ultimately based on the siddha's own inner experiential state rather than on an institutional authority. This inner experiential state is marked by the unremitting commitment to discipleship as it is defined by lineage gurus. Textual sources then go on to confirm and offer measures by which persons can examine the qualities of both guru and disciple.

In Sanskrit, the word *siddha* means "proven" as well as "accomplished" and "perfected." In every case it suggests a continuing condition that is "final" and from which one does not regress or "take a break." When the spiritual state of siddha is disavowed or an individual fails to continue in some substantial way to exemplify its claims, then that person's power and authority naturally become suspect. In other words, when a person is not *siddha*, or is "disproved" by the canonical norms that define and describe *siddha*, then the power to act as the guru is not present. What is lost is the alignment of the disciple with his or her guru's *saṅkalpa*. Muktananda adds a moral dimension to the commitment of the siddha and infuses this ethical standard with his own *saṅkalpa*. His remarks are as much a description as a command to disciples:

> A person may claim to be a great being, a Siddha, or a leader. He may be a performer of miracles. He may claim to hold the degree of God. But if he does not behave properly, he will lead people astray. The behavior of a great being

is the greatest example for others, and they follow it. Become true, sublime, perfect, and pure.[37]

To give another example, in the traditions of Indian argumentation an assumption is *siddha* when it is "proven" and "accepted" as a ground for further discussion. Without this common point of departure there is no means by which to reach a correct conclusion. In siddha traditions the guru is both the point of departure for further understanding and the evidence that there is, in fact, conclusive knowledge. When something or someone is *not siddha* or is bereft-of-being-*siddha* (*asiddha*) then they (or it) will simply fail. What will be conspicuously absent are the qualities of the siddha. Scriptures as well as gurus offer means by which to measure the standards that create proven (*siddha*) knowledge. However, demonstrating what is *siddha* cannot be reduced to a show of hands, that is, it is not a mere majority opinion. An individual or group's assertion does not make something true, any more than the assertion that the world is flat is true if someone we admire says so or we all simply agree. Rather, there must be means by which to measure the truth of a claim. These means make clear the extent of truth present in any given case. In the Indian intellectual tradition there are methods for establishing truth known as *pramāṇam* that in their basic forms are beyond dispute. This clarity in understanding and measurement of truth is precisely what the traditions of the siddha gurus seek through their investment in the guru and the scriptures.[38]

To appreciate more fully how the concept that the guru is both a sustaining and a transformative source of tradition and how the guru acts as the arbiter of sacred knowledge kept in oral and written sources, we must investigate more deeply the concept of *gurutattva*, the guru principle discussed in Chapter 3.

THE PRINCIPLE OF THE GURU AND THE BASIS OF CANONICAL TEACHING

Gurureva jagatsarvaṃ
brahmaviṣṇuśivātmakam
guroḥ parataraṃ nāsti
tasmāt sampūjayed gurum

The Guru alone is the entire universe,
the nature of Brahma, Viṣṇu, and Śiva;
There is nothing beyond the Guru.
Therefore one ought to worship the Guru.

Gurugītā 80

Gurutattva, *the Guru Principle as the Foundation for Empowerment*

Nowhere is the guru principle more clearly established as the mystical and practical foundation of spiritual empowerment and worldly authority than in the Śiva-centered yoga traditions of philosophical nondualism. In these traditions, the fundamental principle is that the unity of being, its singularity in essence, is entirely uncompromised by its manifestation into a plurality of forms. To put this differently, the One reality becomes many and yet remains One; the many are nothing but facets and forms of the One. In the language of this yoga the One is portrayed as the male divinity Śiva, and the many as the female Śakti. From the philosophical point of view, this vision is rooted in nondualism (Sanskrit, *advaya* or *advaita*), the notion that the experience of the world through the lens of subject and object relationships is rooted in the singularity of reality. It is not the rejection of subject/object duality, as such, but rather the affirmation that this duality exists as the result of their complementary presence. Subject and object arise out of that single reality, which continues and sustains them as they exist, and into which they ultimately dissolve. From the theological point of view, this nondualism is theistic not only in the sense that it "uses" the deities Śiva and Śakti to express this philosophical truth as such. It is theistic in that this entire process of creation, perseverance, and dissolution are the willful, intelligent play of the divine consciousness assuming the forms of consciousness.

To elaborate this vision we need to understand as well that Śiva, the eternal One, is inert and amorphous when he is without Śakti; Śakti never exists apart from Śiva from whom she derives her essential being. Thus Śiva always appears in the form of Śakti, and Śakti is always nothing other than Śiva. The singular essence who is Śiva, appearing as the manifest forms of Śakti, is nothing other than one's deepest Self, which appears in the form of an embodied person (*jīva*). By this logic, the same Self resides in the heart of all beings and in all things; the appearance of the Self as a being or a thing is the manifestation of Śiva as Śakti, and the Self as the embodied personality (*jīva*), which appears as multiple and different in each case. The Self, like all things, manifests in and through the nearly infinite embodiments it assumes as creation; these embodiments, while they are nothing other than the Self, appear not as One but as many. Thus the forms of experience are manifold (as is Śakti) while the true experiencer is a single being (Śiva).

The goal of nondualist Śaiva yoga is to reunite the forms of experience with the source of these experiences, that is, to join all of the forms of self that appear to one's consciousness with the Self who is their source. To restate this in the language of Śaiva yoga, the goal is to reunite Śakti with Śiva and so experience the ecstasy of seeing the One in many and the many as only One. The divine has assumed this guise of Śiva and Śakti, of Self and embodiment, and engages in this play of the One and the many purely for the sake of its own enjoyment. Creation, as such, exists for the purpose of experiencing the joyful ecstasy of the divine at play. This is the divine's own willful intention (*saṅkalpa*); it is what the divine has chosen to do of its own free will (*svatantra*), solely for the purpose of experiencing its own blissful nature (*ānanda*).

The guru is nothing other than that essential Self within a person and so is none other than Śiva. The guru is also that form that Śiva takes to guide the seeker to this experience and so is the intelligent, willful Śakti whose intention is to reunite with Śiva. The guru's intention is that of the intelligent Śakti (*citi-śakti*): to bring the disciple to the experiential realization of being liberated while yet still embodied (*jīvanmukta*), having Śakti as embodied energy and Śiva as eternal Self. As a being who has realized his own nature is both Śiva and Śakti, the guru is the key to liberation (*mukti*) and to the recognition of joy (*bhukti*) as the divine's own state of being. The *gurutattva* is this subtle notion of the guru as the divine's own form and as the form of the divine play of Śiva and Śakti. The goal of Siddha Yoga is to join the seeker's deepest, liberative awareness with the experience of it as his or her own embodied manifestation. That is, the goal is to realize and so become the *gurutattva*, the principle of the guru, as the highest form of one's own Self and the very nature of the manifold universe.

This theological vision means that the canon of any siddha tradition depends not only on the guru as an interpretive presence but on the very concept of the guru principle (*gurutattva*). The Siddha Yoga gurus' interpretation of the *gurutattva* not only takes us to the heart of Siddha Yoga's scriptural sources but to the ideological and practical foundation upon which they base their scriptural choices. The Siddha Yoga gurus' standards of ethics and understanding of the usefulness and importance of tradition, as well as their basic ideological stance as theists and nondualists, are rooted in their interpretation of the guru principle. While undoubtedly highly personalized, the innovations of the Siddha Yoga gurus are more correctly understood as characteristic of Śaivite gurus rather than as idiosyncracies. *As swamis Muktananda and Chidvilasananda engage teachings and practices, they put principles ahead of texts and the reality of their own experiences before doctrines or dogmas.* This concept is at the very core of understanding how the *gurutattva* appears in the form of the canon. How then does the *gurutattva* become a canon, a resource that embodies the sacred?

While Hindu thinkers might agree that the Vedas are the ultimate source of knowledge, they differ significantly over their origin and interpretation. Are the Vedas origin-less (*apauruṣeya*) as the Ritualist Mīmāṃsākas would have it? Or did they come from the divine godhead Śiva as the yogic philosophers of Kashmir and South India say? Importantly, both sides would agree that all knowledge, Vedic or otherwise, becomes empowered, useful, and beneficial when it is taught by a realized guru. For the Śaiva yogis the guru is more than a mere instrument of knowledge. Rather, knowledge is embodied in the form of a guru, and more specifically one's *own* guru. In this sense the guru not only chooses which sources are authoritative but is regarded as the very form (*svarūpa*) of the truth expressed in them. Though it is appropriate to honor and take instruction from all of one's gurus, including one's father and mother, Śaiva and goddess-centered Śākta yoga traditions emphasize devotion (*bhakti*) and service (*sevā*) to the *one* guru who embodies ultimacy and teaches the path to its realization. As the *Gurugītā* states:

> The supreme austerity is to have one god, one religion (*ekadharma*), and one foundation (*ekaniṣṭhā*). There is no other more supreme than the Guru. There is no principle (*tattva*) more supreme than the Guru.[39]

Thus, while everyone has many teachers, there is a special place and a special type of power and authority associated with the siddha guru. Ultimately, the guru's authority is rooted in the continuity of discipleship within a lineage that can expand, contract, or change in accordance with the living and embodied form of canon, the guru. In this sense, even the most sacred scriptures should be viewed as derivative of the guru's genius to enliven and interpret them. How then do gurus acquire the prerogative to select their canon?

The Guru and the Canon: Mutual Confirmation and Skillful Means

The guru's authority is conferred by his or her own guru and either confirmed or called into question by the scriptures. In other words, the scriptures assert the guru's prerogative to select and interpret them. More significant is the scriptural claim that a guru possesses the extraordinary ability to obtain and interpret all forms of knowledge by virtue of Self-realization. The great Kashmiri Śaiva siddha Abhinavagupta, in his magnum opus the *Tantrāloka,* cites the *Svacchanda Tantra* to the effect that all thought, including the Vedic revelation, originates in Śiva who is none other than the perfect guru.[40] The same Tantra goes on to explain that all human experience is a form of Śiva's own thought.

> Wherever the mind goes in order to obtain knowledge, one should contemplate there alone; wandering so, where could it go? For what is the All but Śiva?[41]

Abhinavagupta's disciple Kṣemarāja quotes *The Garland of the Heart's Jewels* (*Śrīkularatnamāla*) to assert the extraordinary power of the guru to bring perfect insight to the disciple without resorting to any other means, such as scriptural study or ritual:

> When the best of Gurus explains entirely that [supreme reality] by which one is undoubtedly liberated at that very moment, [the disciple] remains but only as an instrument [of the divine]. And how much more the yogi who is of true understanding, fixed in singularity within the supreme absolute, liberated, and conferring liberation on disciples.[42]

Implicitly, knowledge is not possible without the guru's grace nor by self-study of the scriptures. While power seems to locate itself entirely in the guru's "limited" body as a person rather than in the extended body of the canon, this is because texts may not substitute for living gurus.

The transmission of the lineage's power and the authority to act as guru, however, requires a mutual confirmation in which gurus confirm canons and canons confirm gurus. There is no "third" party, no "council" of siddhas, nor any equivalent ecclesiastical board that can determine who is and who is not worthy of the title "siddha guru." A lineage, however, can set its own standards and any violation of those rules would constitute an abdication of the role. Even though texts assert that gurus and *not texts* are the source of power and authority, textual descriptions of gurus are a critical means by which to check unbridled power. The *Śiva Sūtra* makes it clear that "the guru is the means,"[43] and as Abhinavagupta says, ". . . He alone is a competent guru who has truly achieved the autonomy of Śiva's state and so is capable of conferring that initiation."[44] Such a guru "is an anointed one having been initiated by the Goddess of his own consciousness . . . and for him there arises spontaneously the knowledge of the meaning of all the scriptures, this according to the *Mālinīvijaya Tantra*."[45] Not only must the guru have the experience of Śiva, he or she must be able to confer grace on others so that they might achieve the same goal. This role as the grace-bestowing agent may be the single definitive feature of the siddha guru inasmuch as it distinguishes the siddha guru from any other sort of teacher. Muktananda writes, "Through a Siddha Guru's grace alone, many individuals are liberated. . . . The love that the entire world seeks in one thing or another I found within myself through the Guru's grace. . . . Sundardas says that whoever receives Gurudev's grace easily attains the knowledge of the Truth."[46]

Swami Muktananda asserts similarly the scriptural basis for the claim that all authority to define and interpret ultimate truth must originate first in the guru. He quotes the *Kulārṇava Tantra* to make his point:

> In the great scripture, the *Kularnavā Tantra*, it is said, *tataha shri Gururupayaha sakshat paraśivaya cha*—"Shri Guru is the means by which Parashiva Himself bestows knowledge." . . .
>
> Without the grace of such a Guru, there is no knowledge and no state of meditation.[47]

While a guru is a canon unto himself in the form of his words and deeds, and as such is the arbiter of scripture and tradition, the canon is not unto itself a guru. But neither can one be a guru without the authority of the tradition as it appears in the canon. Put differently, the scriptures depend on the guru even while one's claim to being a guru is inseparable from canonical authority. As Swami Muktananda states, "A true Guru is proficient at distinguishing between that which is correct and that which is incorrect according to scriptural doctrines."[48] This is because the guru is not a personality in the sense of one who creates idiosyncratic truths or interpretations. Rather, according to the Tantras, the guru is bereft of ego and personal desire and is nothing less than God, the supreme Śiva, the Self of all whose purpose is to enable the worthy to experience their intrinsic freedom. The *Kulārṇava Tantra* states, "As the manifest supreme Śiva himself bound in human skin, he wanders on earth in disguise for the sake of disposing grace to the true disciple."[49] Bhagavadutpala, in his *Lamp of Vibration* (*Spandapradīpikā*), establishes clearly the correct order of values regarding the guru, scripture, and the godhead. He states:

> He who desires to realize God should seek a Master because (the Lord) is known through scripture and scripture is known through the Master.
>
> By destroying ignorance, through an enlightened understanding (of the Master's teachings) knowledge is attained and He (the Lord) is realized. Therefore the Master is said to be even greater than both scripture and the Lord.[50]

In the *Pāñcarātra* also:

> One should behave toward the Master as one does toward the Lord Himself.[51]

Swami Muktananda describes such a *sadguru* in typical scriptural fashion:

> A true Guru is not trapped in anything, nor is he concealed. He has risen above both body and senses. With the coolness of imperishable peace and knowledge, he puts differences to flight. Through his perfection and his pure awareness of the all-pervasive and perfect Absolute, he roots out impure thoughts. Viewing everything as equal, he destroys the sense of duality and the other impediments to the perception of God's unity. In the fire of knowledge of unity, he consumes all the doubts that create duality and make one burn in agitation, jealousy, negligence, and desire.[52]

The mystical foundation of the guru's authority is crucial to understanding how the sources of a Śaiva lineage tradition are chosen and interpreted. Beginning with the assumption that the scriptures, like everything else, are nothing other than the divine, the guru alone experiences the universe as *wholly* divine. Therefore the guru is uniquely qualified to discriminate truth for those whose insight is yet limited. Commenting on the verse in the *Spandakārikā* in which it is said that ". . . there is no state in the thoughts of words or (their) meanings that is not Śiva," the medieval Kashmiri Śaiva philosopher Rājānaka Rāma states:

> This Self is indeed all things, for he is the source of everything and assumes as his body (all) that he experiences externally, because there is consciousness only of that which is experienced. . . . Thus, because one's own nature is all things in this way, there is no state in the thoughts of words or (of their) meanings that does not reveal Śiva's nature. . . . He whose state of awareness (*citta*) is . . . constantly attentive and perceiving everything as play, is for this reason, like the Lord, emancipated in this very life.[53]

Swami Muktananda describes how the guru's power of grace is actually the source of power that confers the ability to choose, interpret, and act upon tradition. The canon of teachings has come into existence and lives as an extension of the guru's grace, rather than as an autonomous being. He says:

> . . . [T]he Guru is not merely a human being but an eternal principle, the power of grace. A Shaivite text says, *guror gurutara shaktir guruvaktragata bhavet* [*Mantriśivobhairava*]—"The power of the Guru's grace inherent in his speech is greater than the Guru himself." Moreover, even though this power of grace is transmitted from one Guru to another, it is actually the power of God; in his commentary on the *Shiva Sutras*, Kshemaraja writes, *Gurur vā pārameshwarī anugrāhikā shaktihi* [*Śrī Malini Vijaya Tantra* 2.10]—"The Guru is the grace-bestowing power of God."[54]

This mystical claim, which makes the guru *the* foundational principle by which one pursues truth in scriptures, practices, and traditions, is viewed as a simple and rather pragmatic fact. Swami Muktananda makes the point clearly:

> In our life we learn everything from someone else. Whatever it is, we have to learn from someone else, or we learn from books. Our scriptures say that in order to have inner awakening, it is very necessary to have a Guru, and this is my own experience also.[55]

Learning only from books and without a qualified guru's guidance, he goes on to observe, is "lifeless." He writes:

> There is something you should remember: A person who becomes aware of his own ignorance is drawn to the Guru's feet, but the pride of knowledge gleaned from dry books leads one to look for scriptures rather than for a Guru. Although the scriptures emphasize surrender, vows, and discipline, they are lifeless, so one does not really have to surrender to them; one can interpret them in any way one likes. But one cannot interpret the Guru. You may change the scriptures, but the Guru will certainly change you.[56]

The *Gurugītā* elaborates this relationship between scriptural study with and without a guru:

> The Vedas, treatises (*śāstra*), ancient lore (*purāṇa*), epic accounts, and other sources; such works as those about the science of mantra and yantra; ritual and legal sources; and those entailing incantations; the scriptures (*āgama*) of the Śaivas and Śāktas as well as various other sources are cause for confusion in this world among those persons whose minds wander [because they are bereft of a guru].[57]

Here the warning is pointedly extended to the most sacred scriptures and does so, ironically, from within a scripture that affirms the primacy of the guru. Thus, scriptures affirming the *guruvāda* assert the guru's prerogatives over the scriptures but do not undermine scriptural preferences which are seen as having come through guru lineages. In fact, Śaiva gurus, such as Swami Muktananda, use all of the scriptural genres listed in the *Gurugītā* verse selectively to explicate their teachings and experiences.

It seems clear, also, that the guru-disciple relationship does not in itself restrict a lineage guru from using texts that were not used by an earlier lineage guru. While interpretations and scriptural choices may change to suit different circumstances, it is generally agreed that basic teachings do not.

The essential point is that gurus *rely* upon gurus and *resort* to scriptures and other resources to create, sustain, and cultivate their tradition's identity. A disciple's experiences will neither violate the guru's commands nor contradict the sources on which tradition is based and through which it is passed. Swami Muktananda, whose own guru, Bhagawan Nityananda, seems to have had little interest in scriptural learning per se, makes clear his own respect for scriptural learning while making sure not to equate it with Self-realization.[58]

> It is not my intention to criticize learning or the reading of books. What I want to convey is that when the same Shakti which made them write is awakened within us, all that is written is understood without effort. If the knowledge that you seek in these books can be obtained from within your Self, then you won't have to look for it outside.[59]

Similarly, Swami Chidvilasananda urges disciples to get beyond a mere intellectual understanding of the teachings:

> So many people understand the teachings intellectually. They know A comes from B and so on. They know the whole alphabet by heart. But their lifestyle does not match the teachings at all; and when you ask them the meaning of what they are saying, of what they are giving to others, they don't know.[60]

Siddha Yoga, like many other Indian spiritual traditions, is not preoccupied with texts but with teachings and practices. For example, in Swami Muktananda's case there are prominent aspects of the Vedic tradition and teaching that are *not* mentioned or necessarily endorsed, such as animal sacrifice or certain birthright prerogatives that restrict access on the basis of caste or gender. Disavowal of these teachings or traditions, however, is largely by omission rather than by an explicit rejection. While this process of scriptural selection and empowerment permits the endorsement of some ideas and suggests the condemnation of others *within the same text,* it reaffirms *the guru rather than the text as the canonical center.* One is confused about which teachings are canonical only when the living canon is missing, that is, in the absence of the living guru.

The Three Sources of Authority: Scriptures, the Guru, Direct Experience

A guru may use virtually any source selectively and thereby confer upon it some degree of authority, but this may or may not suggest the authority of any greater portion of it. Understanding the principles of choice as well as the selections made is crucial to establishing what is meant by a guru's own "tradition." The role and importance of a given teaching, practice, or text depends on three variables: first, the role that study has played for a guru in teaching disciples as well as his own use of scripture and tradition; second, the particular guru-disciple relationship; and third, the personal experiences of both gurus and disciples. From the guru's perspective, it seems the scriptural sources of tradition corroborate and describe rather than merely prescribe the experience of Self-realization. This triadic basis for establishing truth, as well as lineage traditions, places scriptural sources within the living canon of the teacher who then presents his own interpretation of teachings, symbols, and actions. Abhinavagupta in his *Tantrāloka* restates this triadic basis of authority by which one discriminates truth from falsehood, and (implicitly) one's own tradition from that of others:

> For knowledge to be fulfilled it must emanate from authoritative texts, from the investigation of a knowledgeable teacher, and directly from one's own Self-realization. Therefore it is said in the *Śrī Kiranāgama* and likewise in the *Niśatanāgama,* that this knowledge that emanates from the guru, from the scriptures, and from oneself has a threefold basis. That [basis] so reveals itself either as a whole, in some different order, or singly [as authoritative knowledge].[61]

All three sources of authority function simultaneously as expressions of the play (*līlā*) of the one Śiva with whom the true guru (*sadguru*) has merged. We are explicitly told that Śiva cannot be limited by any particular process of unfolding knowledge since the divine consciousness is utterly free by nature. Abhinavagupta says:

> As there is no succession (within consciousness), there is no simultaneity; as there is no simultaneity, there is no succession either. The perfectly pure conscious nature transcends all talk of succession and its absence.[62]

Rājānaka Rāma describes how such a guru perceives the world in his extensive *Spandakārikā* commentary:

> [The soul within whom] the manifestation of supreme Consciousness has dawned . . . knows the true nature of all existing things is nothing but the expanded power of his own essential nature (*svasvabhāva*). . . . He who perceives everything as play in this way is liberated while alive.[63]

Even though the authoritative basis of knowledge is triadic, its ultimate source remains singular: Śiva has taken the form of the guru *without sacrificing his freedom to take other forms, including the scriptures.* From the vantage point of a disciple, one's own guru is, as the *Jayākhya Saṃhitā* says, "God, the Lord of the Universe, fashioning (for himself) a mortal body, out of compassion, who lifts up with the hand of scripture those who have fallen. . . ."[64]

The Siddha Yoga gurus establish the basis of authoritative knowledge in essentially the same way. They use scriptures skillfully to establish the parameters of lineage tradition as well as to articulate their understanding of ultimate truth. Swami Muktananda begins by quoting a portion of the *Jñāneśvarī* on the 18th chapter of the *Bhagavadgītā*:

> "O Arjuna, because you have acquired countless merits, you have become worthy of receiving the teachings of the best of all scriptures. Now follow these the teachings completely and with unswerving faith. Otherwise, O Arjuna, if you do not pay sufficient attention to the divine knowledge which has come down through the lineage of the Guru . . . you will be in the same condition as those gods who churned the ocean. You may possess a fine, healthy, and beautiful cow, but you can drink its milk in the evening only if you know the art of milking it. Similarly, know that when the Guru becomes pleased the disciple attains knowledge, but that knowledge bears fruit only when the disciple properly follows the path shown by the Guru. Therefore, follow with great faith the divine teaching which has come down from the lineage of the Guru.[65]

Muktananda comments:

> Our time is different from the orthodox era when certain people were prohibited from studying the scriptures. Even in Vedic times, the yogini Gargi went to the place where King Janaka performed the fire sacrifices and entered into a great discussion with the sage Yajnavalkya. More recently, the sage Dayananda broke the bonds of the orthodox attitude toward women and

> people of lower caste. . . . It is obvious that the orthodox restrictions are not applied in Siddha Yoga Dham; everyone chants the *Rudram*, which is a portion of the *Rig Veda*. Everyone should read and understand the scriptures. By performing good actions, a person should make himself a pure temple of God and worship the Lord of the Self within.[66]

Swami Muktananda here follows the same pattern as Abhinavagupta. He offers a scriptural citation and exegesis followed by an imperative based on knowledge passed through the lineage of gurus. Swami Muktananda's reconfiguration of the parameters of orthodoxy with respect to the scriptures, including his rejection of caste and gender restrictions and his revolutionary egalitarianism, is derived from his interpretive prerogative as a guru but is placed *within* the contexts of scripture and his lineage tradition.[67] Thus, he employs the traditional triadic basis of authority as well as the instruments of valid knowledge (*pramāṇa*).

We see the same pattern of traditional exegesis and distinctive input in the work of Swami Chidvilasananda. Her entire discussion of virtue, for example, in *My Lord Loves a Pure Heart* can be considered a prolonged commentary on the 15th chapter of the *Bhagavadgītā*.

The Three Instruments of Valid Knowledge: Perception, Logic, and Scripture

As far as the means by which one acquires valid knowledge are concerned, the Siddha Yoga gurus assume a view familiar to Abhinavagupta's Trika school of Kashmiri Śaivism. Direct perception, inferential logic, and scripture or revelation provide three valid instruments of knowledge or *pramāṇas*.[68] Both Kashmiri Śaivism and Siddha Yoga base the *possibility* of knowledge on the guru, and the power of the lineage and the *use* of the instruments of knowledge on the guru-disciple relationship. The consequent use of these instruments of knowledge is ultimately validated as one's own experience (*svataḥ*).

In both cases, we see gurus deferring authority to gurus of their lineage as well as to ancient sources believed to contain timeless truths. One needs the guru to learn the canon and to verify the experiences the canon describes and prescribes. Thus, while the Trika Kashmiri Śaivism of both Abhinavagupta and the Siddha Yoga gurus affirms the incontrovertible authority of the Vedas as revelation (*śruti*) and as *the* fundamental expression of eternal truth, their choices and interpretations define for their disciples the scope and meaning of this mystical concept. At stake is not whether the Vedas or other resources and reflections (*smṛti*) within the Hindu spiritual traditions are expressions of timeless truth. That is largely assumed and only infrequently a topic for discussion. Rather, at stake is how to make the timeless truth of scripture and tradition timely and applicable.

The Guru as Synchronic and Diachronic Truth

The process of affirming an eternal reality not dependent upon historical developments or precedents of tradition might be termed *the guru's synchronic vision of truth.* A synchronic vision of truth opens a window that transcends the conditions of time, place, or location of any sort, including books or spoken words.[69] Being present at all times, the synchronic truth becomes, in effect, timeless. In this sense, the truth of scriptures, or of any teaching, is present in particular times but without concern for "mundane" matters that involve historical developments. The synchronic reality is ever-present even as it manifests within time and space, just as Śiva is immutable and ubiquitous though he assumes embodiment and becomes localized in particular places. On this synchronic basis of timeless truth revealed in time, the guru chooses texts and teachings selectively and invests in them importance, relevance, and applicability. This is the principle of *upāya,* "skillful means," by which a guru addresses the particular methods and concepts that effect the desired result according to the needs and abilities of the disciple.[70] Gurus therefore ignore their own uniqueness, deferring instead to their own guru, to tradition, and to the sacrality of scriptures.

Simultaneously, siddha gurus invest in the complement to synchronic truth which may be termed "diachronic truth." Diachronic truth makes clear the investment in history and particularly the continuity of relationships that exist within lineages and between gurus and traditional sources through time. Diachronic truth establishes the guru within time and space as part of the unfolding process of Śiva's power, or Śakti, particularly as it is understood to be the dynamic reality of consciousness (*citi-śakti*). *Truth is experienced as synchronic because it is not bound to time even though it exists within it. Truth is experienced as diachronic because it lasts through time as part of an unbroken but developing transmission.* Canonical teachings are synchronic when they require or demand no context; they are diachronic when they address specifically the context and circumstance in which they are true or authoritative. To put this another way, scriptures may be treated as applying at all times (because they are synchronically true) or they may be understood to apply in instances and so reveal the truth to be a matter of time (that is, diachronically as before/after or now/then).

Thus the guru, like the canon, is beyond the constraints of time and space and yet is established entirely within them and by means of them. The guru exists as a principle (synchronically) and simultaneously as a living person (diachronically). Similarly, the canon of the siddha scriptures is believed to embody eternal truth, regardless of time or space, and yet remain historical both in the texts themselves and the extended body of a living person. What is meant to remain, as it were, when the embodied gurus exit their bodies is the particular teachings of the historical lineage, preserved by the community of disciples and in chosen successors, *and* the timeless teachings upon which the gurus have so skillfully drawn. What makes this possible is that most fundamental assertion: All immanent and transcendent realities are nothing but Śiva. As the Śaiva philosopher Rājānaka Rāma asks rhetorically:

> Why is "there no state that is not Śiva"? [The reason for this is] because "the individual soul," that is, the Self, "is all things." . . . There is nothing, be it an action, perception, or their objects that does not derive its existence from the essential unity it attains with the [one] supreme reality. . . . The point is that the daily commerce of life [*vyavahāra*] that the individual soul [experiences] can only arise on the basis of an underlying unity between subject and object. . . . [And so,] by carefully attending to [the nature and basis] of the soul's daily life . . . one realizes this reality as it is.[71]

THE PRECONDITIONS AND PRINCIPLES OF CANONICAL CHOICE

The Role of Scriptural Study: Knowledge and Experience

Like many other Śaiva gurus, the Siddha Yoga gurus are deeply interested in the study and application of scriptural resources but also insist that the most essential reality is neither dependent upon nor obtainable by scriptural knowledge. Swami Muktananda once told a student:

> If you once experience the divine love shining in your sahasrar, you will understand everything. Mere book knowledge will be of no avail. You must have the direct experience. For one who keeps himself free from pride, free from anxiety, keeps directing his attention to his sahasrar, keeps praying inwardly, springs of love begin to flow inside. But that will be possible only by the grace of the One who dwells in the sahasrar.[72]

The Siddha Yoga gurus' view echoes the mainstream of Hindu spirituality: Self-taught scriptural study is insufficient to obtain the highest goals in life. In the *Bhagavadgītā*, for example, it is said:

> Not by Vedic sacrifice nor recitation, not by gifts, and not by ritual acts nor severe austerity, am I [the Lord] capable of being seen in the human world as such. . . . [73]

However, one should not take this to mean that scriptural knowledge or study is unworthy or unimportant to spiritual discipline. Instead the gurus, like the text, point out that the divine experience cannot be *reduced* to texts or teachings. The reason "everyone should read and understand the scriptures,"[74] as Muktananda writes, is that "by thinking about the scriptures over and over again, all that you have gained is the desire to attain God. . . . God is not words; He is an extraordinary inner experience. The scriptures belong to Him, but He cannot be confined to them."[75]

Choosing to study scriptures or to pay attention to anything has its consequences. Scriptural study is itself a choice with important consequences. In commenting on the way actions can lead one to Self-realization or delusion, Swami Chidvilasananda comments:

> Everything, even the news, affects you on a deep level. Haven't you often realized, hours after hearing a piece of news, that you are still saddened by it—or uplifted, as the case may be? . . . Whatever you feed your ears stays inside you.[76]

In Śaiva yoga, understanding the power and usefulness of scriptural knowledge depends not only on one's self-effort and discipline but on grace—an extraordinary gift of the guru, which the *Bhagavadgītā* represents as Kṛṣṇa's gift of the divine eye that permits Arjuna's extraordinary vision of the godhead. Just as basic, however, is the confusion of scholarship with insight into the immortal. As Jñāneśvar says in his verse commentary on the *Bhagavadgītā*:

> Though a person may be learned, if he scorns the knowledge by which Self-realization is attained he is also ignorant. He won't read the Upanishads, has no interest in yoga, and pays no attention to the knowledge of the supreme Self. . . . He is versed in the Smritis, knows the secrets of the juggler, and has at his command the whole glossary of Vedic roots. He is master of grammar and proficient in logic; nevertheless, he is blind to the understanding of the supreme Self. . . . Similarly, all sciences are invalid without the supreme science of the Self.[77]

The point that scriptural study is barren without knowledge of the Self does not diminish the role scripture should play in a spiritual discipline. In what seems to be a complete reversal of views, Jñāneśvar insists that knowledge is barren without scriptural studies:

> Therefore, O Arjuna, understand that a person who doesn't know the scriptures, who doesn't study this science with determination,
> Has a body in which the seed of ignorance is growing, and his learning is like the vines that spring from it.
> Everything he says is merely the flower of ignorance, and any meritorious actions he performs are its fruit.
> It goes without saying that a person who doesn't believe in this science can never realize the highest Truth.[78]

Nonetheless, one should not confuse direct experience (*anubhāva*) with intellectualism. Muktananda is emphatic in much the same way as Jñāneśvar. He writes in *The Perfect Relationship*:

> [T]he ultimate state of the perfect inner "I"-consciousness, the blissful thought-free state . . . does not need the scriptures and has nothing to do with them. Even if the scriptures were destroyed the Truth would be unaffected, because the Truth produced the scriptures; the scriptures did not produce the Truth. . . .
>
> One who tries to journey [to the thought-free state] by giving lectures will miss the path, for articulated speech is gross, and the gross can never grasp the subtle. Birth and death both take place in silence. Silence is the true life. . . . Once words go, language also goes, and one should understand that one has then learned everything.[79]

Yet this deference extended to the ultimacy of silence is, once again, not meant to diminish or subvert scriptural truths. Rather, scriptures themselves reinforce and confirm this claim as the testimony of seers, sages, and gods. Muktananda writes:

> Through the Guru, the knowledge of the scriptures, his own efforts, and the understanding that he is independent, all-pervasive, eternal, and perfect, he transcends all his ordinary experiences and feelings. . . . With the help of these things, a person's knowledge expands, and he experiences the bliss of Consciousness.[80]

Making Explicit the Implicit Scriptural Choices

Implicit in every guru's teachings are the ethical, religious, and philosophical values that shape his thought. These values create stipulations, boundaries, and important implications that help determine how and what a guru chooses to include within his canon. We might term these the "preconditions of canon formation" since they operate as the background against which scriptural choices and practical determinations are made. To use a metaphor familiar to Kashmiri Śaivite yogas, these preconditions are the screen onto which the canon of texts and practices is projected. In this way the preconditions create a format for understanding the scriptural choices themselves. Examining these preconditions we can then consider how they become principles that determine choices. Knowing the texts that the Siddha Yoga gurus have chosen allows us to consider which texts *could* be chosen on the basis of their deeper principles, values, and beliefs. Knowing the Siddha Yoga gurus' principles, values, and beliefs will enable us to understand the scriptural choices they have made.

The Preconditions of Scriptural Selection

We can identify three preconditions or principles that the Siddha Yoga gurus regularly employ in their choice of scriptures: (a) the principle of serving one guru (*ekagurūpāsti*); (b) the ethics of purity and the prefiguring of grace; and (c) the ultimate truth of unity and its manifestation in the siddha guru's nondual state. As we shall see, these ideas allow us to determine which scriptural sources within the larger, inclusive canon might appear in Siddha Yoga as the gurus continue to teach.

Ekagurūpāsti: Serving But One Master

One of the clear bases of Siddha Yoga belief is the notion that one's relationship with a single, ultimate guru is the most important means by which one obtains the grace necessary to achieve Self-realization. Achieving *ekabhakti,* or "singular love or devotion," as the *Bhagavadgītā* calls it, requires a relationship with the *ekaguru,* the one master. Swami Muktananda writes, "An ordinary teacher can give you a limited kind of knowledge and teach you different meditative techniques, but only a Guru can give you inner meditation."[81]

The relationship between guru and disciple becomes *the* critical basis for the choice and the interpretation of scriptures. In Swami Muktananda's case this guru was, of course, Bhagawan Nityananda, whose own brand of charismatic yoga seems both archetypal in form and mysterious in content. It is their relationship that sets the tone for scriptural interpretations, including the role texts play in Siddha Yoga practice and their potential in developing understanding of the guru-disciple relationship.

Nearly always wearing a simple loincloth and speaking only when it seemed to suit his divine whimsy, Nityananda was said to have been a siddha from birth (*janmasiddha, saṃsiddhika yogin*). This fact in itself is significant for understanding the canon of Siddha Yoga since the assumption is that his behavior, including whatever teachings and practices he may have set for himself, should not necessarily be imitated nor is it subject to further scrutiny. Like Śiva himself, Nityananda enacted outwardly the appearance of absolute freedom: sometimes speaking, sometimes silent; sometimes active, other times immobile; and always, it seemed, utterly unpredictable and beyond reproach. As Swami Muktananda says:

> Shree Gurudev's influence and presence were, in themselves, so powerful that he did not need to give lectures or teach explicitly. Even so, the devotees always hoped for a few words from him; they were eager to know how he would answer their questions. For their sake, Gurudev would occasionally speak a little.[82]

In this sense Nityananda was himself the "text" that his disciples studied and the embodied ideal of ultimacy behind the scriptures. To serve one guru (*ekagurūpāsti*) means, in a sense, to study but one text. For Muktananda this meant his Gurudev, Nityananda. Certainly it did not mean simply Nityananda's words or teachings. Just as one can become enlivened or brought to inner stillness by contemplating a scriptural passage, likewise a siddha guru can affect others by his mere presence. From Nityananda's example, we gain a critical insight: that the fundamental purpose of any endeavor, including scriptural study, is self-transformation. For Swami Muktananda the effect of the guru could be immediate or gradual, spontaneous or after long contemplation, and might occur within or beyond his physical presence. In any case, he says, the effect's cause is the grace-bestowing power that emanates from the goddess Citi Śakti and works through the guru. In his spiritual autobiography, *Play of Consciousness,* he writes:

> The Guru has the uncommon power to transform man completely. He bestows a new life in which there is no old age and no sorrow. He makes us attain perfection in this very world. Just as an owl cannot see by day nor a crow at night, without the grace of a Guru man does not see the world as heaven, but only as sorrow and suffering. . . .
>
> In Gurus, the Chiti Shakti of the Supreme is continually at play. Intoxicated in Shakti's dance, Gurus live enraptured, engulfed in the bliss of love. That beginningless energy, which comes from God and has been flowing until this moment, is still reveling. When She is set in motion in the disciple by the Guru, She burns all his impurities in the fire of yoga. She removes all his layers of ignorance and makes him completely pure. In the end, the disciple himself becomes a Guru.[83]

Texts or teachings become sacred and scriptural only if they fulfill or complement this transformative role. The more a text catalyzes Self-realization, the more important it becomes. Like the guru, a sacred text is a medium through which flows the divine Śakti. It is in this sense that we should emphasize that Swami Muktananda's first and ultimate "text" as well as his final canonical authority is his Gurudev Nityananda. "Reading" this most sacred of "texts" meant not only listening but seeing, that is, having the guru's darshan (Sanskrit, *darśana*) and recognizing the potential for awakening and insight beyond thought, words, or sights. As Muktananda writes, "Words can point the way to God, but He is far beyond them. He cannot be understood through the mind, . . . yet a true seeker attains Him within himself through the path and the wisdom of the Guru."[84]

Through the lens of Swami Muktananda we gain a glimpse of Nityananda's unfathomable powers to transform those around him. Even those without spiritual intentions were liable to his yogic influence. Muktananda writes:

> . . . [T]he surroundings of my supremely revered Guru Nityananda were still, silent, detached, and free of mental agitation. Anyone who came from Bombay would find his mind emptied of thought when he entered the ashram. This was because of the influence of the atmosphere around Gurudev Nityananda. Restless people from Bombay, people of all types, would lose their restlessness once they had bathed in the hot springs and come before Gurudev; they would become calm and still. The majesty of Bhagawan Nityananda's state permeated the surroundings. Under the influence of his perfect stillness, silence, and reticence, everyone sat peacefully observing discipline. Gurudev was the living ideal of detachment, stillness, freedom from thought, and silence. Sitting in his presence, everyone meditated spontaneously. As I meditated every day, both my enthusiasm and my experiences increased as if my divine spiritual journey were rapidly accelerating.[85]

Similar experiences are relayed by Muktananda's disciples as well as by those of Swami Chidvilasananda, all of whom report that it is the guru's own nature that effects the transformation of their entire being. And from Muktananda's descriptions of this transformative power as the grace of the shaktipat guru, we gain an insight into Nityananda's inner state. He writes:

> . . . [T]he whole world is a forn of God. And Shree Gurudev pervades all of it.
>
> "I am in everything," he used to say to people coming for darshan. Once a photographer asked permission to take his picture. "Take a picture of the world," replied Gurudev. "I am the world. Is there any place where I don't exist? In everything, there is a glimpse of me." The world is one with Nityananda, and Nityananda pervades the entire world.[86]

For Swami Muktananda the only true "textual" study is the experience of the guru. It is little wonder then that the study of sacred scriptures is a constant theme in the work of the Siddha Yoga gurus, all textual study being ultimately the study of their primary "text," the guru.

Swami Chidvilasananda relates her own experience with the guru-as-text in a selection from her poem, "Ashes at My Guru's Feet":

> Again Baba called me,
> He looked at me lovingly,
> And asked, "Have you heard the song,
> 'Become Ashes at the Guru's Feet?'
> Isn't it the sweetest song
> That you have ever heard?"
>
> Again I was consumed by a powerful agony.
> I wished I could disappear.
> I wished I weren't such a rock.

> All of a sudden, my Guru, my Baba,
> Placed his hand on my head.
> Streaks of fire exploded from his palm.
> The house of my individuality was set ablaze.
> Everything I had was burned away.[87]

Here we are led again into the deeply personal experience that characterizes the guru-disciple relationship. This experience remains at the center of Siddha Yoga practice and so at the basis of its understanding of scripture and study.

If texts become sacred or valuable to a disciple because they instruct and even manifest the guru's will (*saṅkalpa*) and power (*śakti*), it becomes increasingly important to distinguish those texts that possess the divine Śakti from those in which it is inert or inactive (*jaḍa*). One of the key elements from the standpoint of the Siddha Yoga gurus is whether a text or teaching is "pure," that is, whether it inspires actions, intentions, and values that are moral and just.

The Ethics of Purity

Bhagawan Nityananda's ethics further distinguished him from other siddhas. The Siddha Yoga gurus are unambiguous in their affirmation of ethically pure practice and in this way set themselves apart from so-called "*kaulikas*" or Tantrics of the "Left-Current" (*vāmācārin*), that is, siddhas who indulge in explicitly antinomian rituals that might include the use of intoxicants, nonvegetarian food, or illicit sexual pleasures. Swami Muktananda explicitly rejects these behaviors whether they are performed inside or outside the ritual context. Swami Chidvilasananda has made it a central part of her teaching to emphasize the cultivation of virtues and the need for a continuous cleansing of body, mind, and spirit.[88]

In this sense, Siddha Yoga should be considered a so-called "Right-Current" (*dakṣiṇācāra*) of mystical yoga in which strict rules of purity and moral conduct are seen as natural outward expressions of an inner spiritual state. This clear position quite interestingly sets the Siddha Yoga gurus apart from many of the historical philosopher-yogis of Kashmiri Śaivism who understand antisocial or morally ambivalent ritual as a *means* to transcendence. The difference between "right" and "left" is quite straightforward: For the yogis of the Left-Current, freedom is expressed as a boundary-defying act or intention; one transcends boundaries established by society or tradition through deliberate acts or indifference to social standards or reactions. The Right-Current practitioners, including the Siddha Yoga gurus, see no need for these deliberate acts of boundary-defiance and sustain a respectful view of social conventions. Their vision is one of boundless freedom for the siddha who simply chooses to act in ways that instruct, edify, and transform those who encounter them. Rather than view the Right-Current as *subject* to boundaries, we might rather see it as *accepting and choosing* boundaries for constructive purposes. The siddha concedes none of his absolute freedom even as he moves within frameworks that foster intelligibility. The relationship between ethical standards and spiritual practice offers an important instance in which we may distinguish those particular Left-Current teachings of Kashmiri Śaivism and Tantrism with the Right-Current thinking of the Siddha Yoga gurus. This structure also suggests how teachings or texts could be categorized as accepted and condoned and differentiated from those that would be rejected and condemned. Naturally, any selection of text that advocates or condones material or sensual indulgence without disciplined yoga as a guide is either rejected or dismissed by the Siddha Yoga gurus.

The command to ethical purity on the part of the guru indicates that the disciple should not discriminate against persons by caste, gender, race, or ethnicity; in addition, one must remain respectful of differing social and ethical conventions. An ethical standard is not a simple command to social conformity. Rather, the commitment to tolerance rejects ethical permissiveness while respecting those who follow a different but ascending spiritual path. This distinction is both practical and a matter of common sense. Ethical discipline is the key:

> The purity of a guru should always uplift his disciples. Some people become gurus, teach 108 different therapies, and lead a completely wanton life, without self-control or discipline. A seeker should evaluate such teachers. . . . An incomplete teacher who is pure and ethical and who puts his knowledge into practice is far better than an undisciplined person who poses as a perfect Guru.[89]

Swami Chidvilasananda succinctly makes the same point: "Purity of being, *sattva-samshuddhi*, evolves out of pure actions."[90]

Not intended necessarily as judgments or restrictions, these moral standards are considered the outward expression of an inner condition. Muktananda writes that "Siddha Yoga does not discriminate between men and women, for the One who has become man has also become woman."[91] Societal conventions are likewise posed in terms of this inner attitude of equality. He writes that "Siddha Yoga respects marriage and does not condemn disciplined pleasure. . . . One creates one's own pain and pleasure. Therefore, one should be vigilant about one's actions."[92]

Clearly the Siddha Yoga gurus understand the responsibility for a person's overall condition in terms of the relationship between the outward physical being and the inner subtle being. An ethical lapse, as it were, does not affect the intrinsic perfection of a person's deeper Self but rather reflects the nature of actions that have been deluded by the ego. A person's ultimate inner divinity is never in question. Swami Chidvilasananda makes this point explicitly:

> The vast Lord dwells in every heart. What stops a person from knowing this? The light of God burns brilliantly in every heart. As the poet-saint Kabir says, there is no such thing as a heart where there is no *sai,* no light. Then, what stops a person from seeing it? What weakens a person so much that he does not have the power to go within?
>
> The answer is, that person's own impurity—layers and layers of consequences, piles and piles of debris from the past. Not only is he staggering under the weight of his actions, he's attached to them.[93]

As far as the Siddha Yoga gurus are concerned, this fact makes people more rather than less responsible for their outward actions. To act immorally or to indulge in sensual pleasure for its own sake is to live counter to one's inborn divine nature. In this sense, ethical transgression is Self-violation or Self-forgetfulness. This position permits the yogi to see the divine Self as the permanent condition of every person even before the process of ethical purification is complete. It also functions as a command to disciples to treat all persons, and especially themselves, as forms of the divine. While there is room for constant improvement and correction on the spiritual path, there is no final judgment or condemnation. Human depravity results from a constellation of impurity, ignorance, and egoism. It is therefore an illness that can be cured, however chronic and persistent it appears to be.

Siddha Yoga, like many other forms of Indian spirituality, not only admits human perfection but believes it manifests as virtue. One notices how the Siddha Yoga gurus refrain from judging persons—whom they consider embodiments of the divine—and describe their actions in terms of the delusions of dualism. Dualism is that notion of the "other" as a separate, disconnected reality, apart and therefore an "object" different from one's own Self. Dualism is rooted in this delusion and its cause is the ego's desire for constant self-gratification, the ego's own selfishness. These delusions are not part of the true Self whose "natural state" is unattached to desire. Rather, the ego's delusions arise from the impurities known as the *mala*s and *kleśa*s. Yoga is the discipline by which these *mala*s and *kleśa*s are removed.

The notion of essential human perfectibility is reflected in the siddha's attitude toward the ethical lapses of others: Even the most fallen individual's deepest nature remains untainted by karma. Once purified, karma itself becomes one's ally. Swami Muktananda explains the position:

> One should perform actions considering them to be service to God. At the same time, one should renounce their fruits, knowing that to perform actions with a sense of detachment is the natural state of *prakriti,* or nature. Through

> the *ānava mala*, consciousness becomes contracted. Through the *māyīya mala*, one becomes aware of differences. Through the *kārma mala*, one performs good and bad actions. One who understands the mystery behind these things realizes that Shiva, through His play, is performing all the activities of the universe. With this understanding, a person pursues the miracle of seeing duality in unity and unity in duality. He finally attains the all-pervasive unity-awareness. . . . As long as a person lacks the understanding of the universe and his own true nature, as long as he fails to experience the multiplicity of the universe as the play of the *shakti chakra*, the group of powers, he is bound by *karma*. However, after the awakening of the knowledge of Truth, a person's *karmas* help to expand his knowledge.[94]

Swami Chidvilasananda offers further clarification:

> These impurities are the result of three constant, deep-seated feelings: "I am imperfect; I am different; I am the doer, the author, of my own actions." Nothing is more destructive than these feelings which Kashmir Shaivism calls the three *malas*. Because of them, a person goes round and round on the wheel of birth and death, trapped in his own limitations.[95]

Actions themselves, however, do not "produce" divine realization but create the conditions for it. Swami Muktananda writes:

> Many actions are performed by the physical body, the subtle senses, and the subtle body, which interconnects them. These actions can either bring about one's downfall or, when they cause the expansion of knowledge, improve one's welfare. However, actions are not the true cause of the expansion of knowledge. They can only make one worthy of it.[96]

Similarly Swami Chidvilasananda explains how the process of purification leads to the uncovering of the intrinsically pure Self:

> How can you purify your being? You begin with the simple things. First, purify your actions. When a thought arises, pause for a second before you act on it. If it is not a nourishing thought, let it dissolve back into Consciousness. Secondly, sever your false attachment to impure actions. . . . Finally, develop a healthy discipline. There is no other way to take control of your senses, your habits, your emotions, and your thoughts.[97]

The imperative to ethical action arises from a deeper human desire to experience one's own true Self. Muktananda says, "If greed lurks in the heart, that is vice enough for anyone. If one criticizes others, that is sin enough for anyone. But if the mind is pure, how can God be far away? If one possesses virtue, what other qualities does one need?"[98]

Swami Muktananda summarizes Siddha Yoga's ethics of purity without condemnation by first establishing the position within a scriptural framework:

A true Guru is proficient at distinguishing between that which is correct and that which is incorrect according to scriptural doctrines. . . .

He does not indulge in sense pleasures. He neither keeps bad company nor becomes ensnared in addictions. He is free of conflicts, desires, and thoughts. He is disciplined and possesses self-control, and he also makes his disciples observe discipline.[99]

These standards of basic conduct (*samaya*) are not to be confused with the siddha's perfect freedom, which may appear as a certain unpredictability or even an apparent eccentricity. One needs to distinguish between actions rooted in a consciousness that has attained perfection and actions based on the mistaken vision of the dualistic mind. From this standpoint, the siddha guru's actions are a divine play rather than a license to act according to whimsy or desire. In the siddha there is no longer the slightest disruption of mental equipoise brought about by desires or mental activities. The siddha has conquered the senses and mastered the wayward mind. Swami Chidvilasananda describes the difference between the siddha's state in which every motivation or action is a play of the divine Self and that of the aspirant bound to a false identification with the body and mind:

A person who is deluded in this way sees the entire world through a filter of his own distortions. From the standpoint of the knowers of Truth, this universe is a play of Consciousness. But for a person like this, the universe is a place of punishment.[100]

Muktananda states:

Everyone knows the actions performed by the body and experiences the feelings and thoughts of the mind. Enlightened beings fully experience the serene state, which is devoid of both bodily and mental activities, as their true nature. This serene Consciousness is the basis of all bodily and mental activities. This is called the knowledge of one's own Self.[101]

Moral purity is the result of this attainment of the "awareness of equality" and stands in contrast to the limitations of duality. Muktananda continues:

The awareness of equality is the highest attainment. Human beings are troubled by duality and a sense of differences. Disparity exists because of delusion, anger, attachment, and ignorance. When we keep the company of great beings, duality turns into unity and disparity into equality. When we have this understanding, we become worthy of receiving the grace of a Siddha.[102]

The urge to imitate the siddha's behavior, however, must arise in the disciple in the same way it arises in the siddha: without expectation for personal gain, without desire, and as a play of divine consciousness. Until the disciple has achieved this stage of personal realization—that is, a pure motivation without the constraints of an encumbered, dualistic mind—then he or she is cautioned to examine this desire to act as the siddha acts. Until one is a siddha, one should remain under a siddha's guiding discipline. Even then, the siddha guru is sustained by choosing the discipline of discipleship. Muktananda makes the difference between the siddha and the aspirant clear:

> One of the aspects of God's play is bliss. . . . All these actions are virtuous, all bring progress. By searching for faults in the behavior of such a Guru, the seeker hinders his own sadhana. One should never look for bad qualities in Gurus, saints, or Siddhas. . . .
>
> Such saints possess a divine radiance. Their way is such that they learn from the ignorant and teach the learned; they fight the brave and flee from the jackal. If they do not get anything, they demand it. If they get something, they give it away. Everybody wants something from these emperors of saints, who possess nothing but give everything to those who ask. The things that the world considers valuable are worthless to them. Siddhas are far, far away from ordinary life.[103]

Swami Muktananda's point is that one cannot merely mimic the siddha's outward actions and expect to achieve the inner state of nondualistic awareness. It can be misleading to dwell on his tales of siddhas whose outward actions seem either ethically questionable or bizarre. Before one "acts as the siddha acts" one must understand that the siddha's outward expressions of radical freedom are the result of an inner purity of heart that never lapses nor indulges in the abuse of others. Swami Chidvilasananda affirms that the fundamental responsibility remains in the individual's own choices:

> When you set your heart on something that is completely uplifting, you gradually become free from impurities. Wherever you place your heart, that is where you end up. It is very difficult for someone who is not able to stick to a steady and clean resolve to work his way out of delusion.[104]

Swami Muktananda has no aversion to making this point about inner purity with examples that might seem extreme if taken out of context. His description of the modern siddha Zipruanna offers one such case:

> Many are the ways of Siddhas. I knew a great Siddha, Zipruanna, who was always naked. He would lie on a heap of garbage. He ate whatever passersby gave him. Although he sat surrounded by filth, he was never affected by it. He saw only equality everywhere. He was always happy. Although he was in the body, he knew that he was totally different from it. He was an ecstatic Siddha.[105]

Muktananda insists, however, that the siddha's ecstasy is neither madness nor some sort of license to do simply as one pleases. Zipruanna, like other siddhas, had conquered the lure of the senses and the delusions of the mind. For the siddha, the pleasures of the world, like suffering, are no longer determining his experience, his motivation, or his actions. In *Play of Consciousness,* Muktananda describes what it takes to achieve this ascent to lasting freedom:

> As long as "possession and renunciation" control you, you will still be bound to the world. While they exist the world will exist for you, but a man who forgets about "possession and renunciation" goes beyond worldly existence. Neither renounce "possession/renunciation" nor accept it. Become absorbed in your inner reality. . . .
>
> The Siddha student who knows his true nature and remains absorbed in his Self, who lives in contact with his inner being and finds contentment there, who feels neither distaste for crowds nor any special taste for solitude, is a great and holy center of pilgrimage.[106]

He notes as well that Zipruanna's outward behaviors did not encourage others to imitate him. Rather, people of all types came to honor his inner awareness. "There were a large number of Hindus and Moslems in his village, and both groups respected him greatly."[107] This point is crucial to understanding the siddha's exemplary ethics, which go deeper than surfaces and outer examples. Those around Zipruanna never thought of imitating his behavior; they knew they could not. Swami Muktananda believes it is because they had not yet achieved the siddha's state of inner purity.

In his own case Swami Muktananda was careful to set an outward example that his disciples could comprehend and appreciate, one that advanced their own spiritual understanding and progress. Disciples grasped very clearly which sorts of behaviors they might imitate and where their own boundaries lay. Swami Chidvilasananda has fostered this tradition of exemplary action. What seems perfectly appropriate and even natural in the cultural and historical context of India, where ascetics like Zipruanna have been part of the social fabric for perhaps three thousand years, is more difficult for others, especially Westerners, to understand. The gurus of Siddha Yoga appear entirely aware of this fact. While Muktananda extolled the greatness of ascetical siddhas like Zipruanna, he did not himself behave that way or encourage others to use that example. In his own context, Muktananda understands Zipruanna to be anything but antisocial or morally suspect. Rather, his person in all aspects is a transformative spiritual force that leads to communal harmony and individual peace of mind. For Swami Muktananda, Zipruanna exemplifies the siddha's goal of effecting inner transformation; he quotes Zipruanna as saying, "It is your attitude that bears fruit according to your conviction."[108] There is no room for exploitation or abuse since the siddha guru seeks nothing for himself. Swami Chidvilasananda explains the siddha's unselfish love:

> One of the reasons the great ones can love everyone equally is that they have no selfish interest. They don't desire anyone's wealth or anyone's body or anyone's wife. There is nothing they want and they want for nothing. In this state it is possible to love everyone, because you have no regrets, you have no anger, and you have no fear. So you are able to experience love for all humankind. There is no transaction, no bargain. This is not a love of business, it is the love of God. And so, there is no duality and no separateness, but only and always the experience of oneness.[109]

In this relationship between guru and disciple there is no room for the manipulation of others. Muktananda says, "A true Guru will not try to control a disciple's life, yet he will make the disciple control himself."[110] Muktananda is constantly urging us to consider the inner life and the deeper, contemplative meaning of actions and intentions. This is a guiding principle for understanding the way the Siddha Yoga gurus make use of any text.

This distinction between ethical standards and the guru's divine play is a critical canonical principle of choice. There is no compromise when it comes to ethical ideals:

> Just as we expect a disciple to be high and ideal, we should expect a Guru to be high and ideal. The Guru should have the power to cause an inner awakening in his disciple. He should be well versed in all the scriptures, he should be able . . . to transmit knowledge directly. He should have extraordinary skill in instructing his disciples. This is what a true Guru is like.[111]

Scriptural passages that do not meet the Siddha Yoga gurus' standards of ethical conduct or are misleading are simply not taught. Passages within the same text, however, that do meet these ethical criteria may be held as authoritative. One important example of this is the *Kulārṇava Tantra,* which Swami Muktananda calls a "great scripture" and which he and Swami Chidvilasananda cite frequently *but selectively.*[112] The same *Kulārṇava Tantra* endorses practices that the Siddha Yoga gurus neither condone nor commend.[113] In short, ethical preconditions create criteria that inform the Siddha Yoga guru's scriptural choices. Put differently, it is not the text *as such* that they endorse but the teachings that reflect an understanding of the spiritual path and the inner state of the siddha.

Muktananda, renowned in his ashrams for the strict discipline of the daily schedule and insistence on ethical behavior and intention, offers admonitions to moral decency so frequently that this fundamental canonical principle is beyond any shadow of a doubt.[114] This tradition of sustaining standards of probity continues to highlight Siddha Yoga under Swami Chidvilasananda. The characteristic play that Muktananda asserts as the siddha's prerogative is presented as an example of the difference between those who are perfectly free (*svātantrya*) and those who have not yet reached this state of perfection.

Perfect freedom affirms the siddha's extraordinary self-control:

> He is never upset by suffering, nor does he desire happiness. He never leaves the path of virtue; he never follows the path of evil. His mind is always filled with the vibrations of Chiti. He is profound, steadfast, pure, and detached. He is compassionate, loving, and gracious. Such a Siddha student is liberated while living in the world.[115]

Swami Muktananda is careful to draw his own line between what a siddha *could* do because he or she is perfectly free, and what the siddhas of his lineage would never do. Similarly, he draws a distinction between those teachings that may have belonged to other lineages or that appear in the larger body of texts *for whatever reason* and those selections and interpretations of scriptures that match his own experience. This latter point is crucial: Siddha Yoga gurus cite scriptures because they reflect the siddha's own experiences and offer the best example for disciples, not because they appear in a given text or are part of the larger siddha traditions. The commands of siddhas outside one's own lineage may not be applicable to oneself.

The *sadguru*, according to swamis Muktananda and Chidvilasananda, will be recognized as much by the effects he produces in others as by the textual criteria that describe ethical boundaries and standards. Standing between appearance and reality, the guru acts primarily as the dynamic and transformative force of the divine rather than as a static, paradigmatic lawgiver. This unique role for the guru helps to explain how certain principles will predetermine textual selections and suggests to disciples which ideas are consistent with lineage teaching. Muktananda carefully explains the difference between divine surrender to the guru, which must be a constant state of awareness that creates a meaningful life in the world, and the static or passive attitude that reduces spiritual practice to a set of lifeless rules.

> I am a person who has surrendered to my Guru, yet I still have my individuality. . . . In surrender a person loses himself; however, he attains that person to whom he has surrendered. If you surrender to a great person, it is not that you lose your individuality—you too become a great person. . . . Submission does not mean that you give everything to God and then remain passive. What happens is that you submit your sense of self to Him and in return you absorb His vastness. Arjuna submitted himself to Lord Krishna, and after that he fought a violent war. All the *gopīs*—the milkmaids—had submitted themselves completely to Krishna, and yet they were living their family life, taking care of the children they had, and having more children.[116]

At the same time, the disciple remains reliant on the guru to make clear both what the scriptures prescribe and what the lineage teachings suggest is possible. Ultimately, the guru retains canon-making and interpretive prerogatives, and disciples are cautioned not to fall prey to the errors of intellectual pride. Clear ethical standards and the guru's exemplary behavior leave Siddha Yoga disciples with few doubts about expected norms of behavior.

There is a certain mutual responsibility that characterizes the guru-disciple relationship. Disciples are not required to abdicate their capacity for judgment any more than the guru may abuse the disciples' intrinsic right to freedom. Rather, the task of the disciple is to become the guru, not in the sense of gaining a position or a status, an ashram, or a following, but of attaining the guru's state of inner Self-perfection. The *position* of guru, with its specific powers and responsibilities, is always invested by the lineage-holder in a specific chosen successor, who is thus empowered to perform the function of guru. However, as Swami Muktananda explains, this does not mean that other disciples cannot attain the Self-realized state:

> A true Guru is not one who makes everybody his disciples and keeps them in that condition even after leaving his physical form. Only he is a true Guru who, having himself become a Guru, takes discipleship away from his disciples and turns them into beings like himself.[117]

The guru accepts the responsibility to lead disciples to their own divine Self-transformation. Both guru and disciple have roles in a process founded on mutual respect and ethical trust. Muktananda says:

> There is the teacher's grace and there is the student's grace. The teacher's grace is to teach the student with respect, and the student's grace is to study what the teacher has to say with respect and faith in the teacher.[118]

Certainly the Siddha Yoga gurus treat some issues as non-negotiable, whether they are ethical or conceptual. The crucial point is not simply the gurus' assumption of a moral high ground, but their insistence that the guru's spiritual power is a force for ultimate good. As Swami Muktananda states:

> . . . The Guru is simple, direct, and loving. He is the well-wisher of his disciples. He doesn't steal his disciples' money; instead, he takes their ignorance, or nescience. He doesn't seize their wealth and property, but he takes their sins and anxieties. . . . He shows the spiritual path in the midst of the world. . . . Such Gurus do not advise the wrongful renunciation of property and the wealth of this world but, instead, make us renounce our limited individuality. They are hostile to the limited self, jealous of individuality, and angry with differentiation. . . .

> Blessing him with divine favor, the Guru turns a person's ordinary life, with mother, father, and relatives, into a sacred existence. Then he follows his occupation in society and sees his life as a gift bestowed by God.[119]

Here we are signaled to another important canonical principle of choice: In the view of the Siddha Yoga gurus, the guru demands an inner discipline through which one controls desires, but he or she does not command that all should become formal renunciants.

The Siddha Yoga gurus connect the necessity of the guru's indispensable grace with the need for the aspirant's own self-effort. While this may seem common to yogic texts, this understanding sheds new light on the relationship between renunciation and the formal life of the renunciant *sannyāsi.* In sum, the Siddha Yoga gurus view renunciation as a universal requisite, an inner state of awareness and intention that liberates the Self from the delusions of the ego. In this sense everyone must achieve a state of inner renunciation in order to realize the Self. Formal renunciation, however, is appropriate only as an outward expression of this inner aspiration. Thus the Siddha Yoga gurus endorse the *sannyāsa* way of life but do not believe *sannyāsa* is necessary to attain enlightenment.

The siddha guru is one who has obtained this inner renunciation; the outward form is purely exemplary. The guru, Swami Muktananda says, "may be a householder or a renunciate, but he must be able to transmit Shakti. God's power of divine grace should dwell in him completely."[120] In order to become an effective shaktipat guru, however, one must conquer the senses entirely, especially any sensual urges or desires. Put in yogic terms this means one must "retain the sexual fluids" or become an *ūrdhvaretin.* Presumably even householder gurus must eventually abstain from sex if they are to transmit the divine power. Muktananda writes, "The source of power to give Shaktipat is this *ūrdhvaretas*, the rising of the sexual fluid." Once the *kuṇḍalinī-śakti,* the innate divine power, awakens, sexual desires eventually vanish and are transformed into pure love.[121]

While honoring *sannyāsa* as exemplary, the Siddha Yoga gurus chide those who view it as a lifestyle rather than as a skillful spiritual practice. Renouncing desires is an essential aspect of spiritual discipline that should become part of one's meditative reflections. He writes, "If your renunciation is purposeless or goes against the scriptures, you will get confusion instead of peace. . . . Whether you are a householder, an ascetic, a monk, or a mendicant, the world reflects your own state. . . . A man who has attained realization sees the Lord in the world—not emptiness or joylessness."[122] Here Swami Muktananda's point is that renunciation is not world-rejection any more than it is an external lifestyle. While formal renunciation requires the integrity of sustaining formal vows, the act itself will remain fruitless until one renounces the mistaken identification of the body, senses, and mind with the Self.

Muktananda's general view that a guru need not be a formal renunciant and that a disciple need not become a renunciant to obtain the highest realization is clearly a statement of principle about the siddha tradition in general. The Siddha Yoga canon upholds this value of inner renunciation as the key to liberation. However, Swami Muktananda is equally emphatic about the role renunciation, in both its inward and outward forms, must play in the leadership of his own siddha lineage. There is no question that Muktananda commanded that the Siddha Yoga gurus be lifelong celibates who take formal vows of *sannyāsa*.[123] The inner state of the renunciant guru should have its outward counterpart. Since the shaktipat guru is by nature one without sexual desires, the tradition of *sannyāsa* creates an example to sustain the spiritual discipline of aspirants. This is in keeping with Swami Muktananda's own standards of exemplary behavior: What is possible within the siddha tradition is not necessarily true for Siddha Yoga. Siddha Yoga students are taught to admire and contemplate the lives of siddhas, and particularly renunciants. Clearly, Muktananda sought to clarify any ambiguity concerning his ethical understanding of Siddha Yoga practice and its future leadership.[124]

This view of the role of renunciation and the guru's grace-bestowing power similarly affects Swami Muktananda's scriptural choices as he carves the middle ground between the generally anti-renunciant view of the yogic Tantras and Āgamas and the fiercely ascetical vision of Advaita Vedānta. Often drawing on examples of householders who achieved the state of the siddha, he likewise makes his view that true renunciation is particularly worthy of honor: "Siddha Yoga highly respects the sacred vows of all monks, *sannyāsins*, and other great souls who have renounced everything."[125] Drawing from both Tantra-Āgama and Vedānta scriptures, Muktananda places renunciation in the context of the exemplary *guru-vāda*.

Muktananda is careful to distance himself from texts or traditions that violate his understanding of renunciation's purpose, equate it with world rejection, or use tactics such as fear to impose moral standards. First he quotes the poet-saint Banārsi, whose effort he calls "an authoritative poem for Siddha students":

> Ram is not attained by renouncing wealth or life;
> Only he attains Narayana who renounces the pride of his body.
> God can never be attained by renouncing all worldly affairs,
> By renouncing wife, children, family, or household matters,
> By eating only roots, tubers, and fruit. . . .
> By renouncing all these things but not abandoning the constant pride of the body,
> Banarsi says, even after renouncing all life, still He is not attained.[126]

Next, he suggests that certain scriptures or teachings will lead to misunderstandings of renunciation.

> In some scriptures it is said that the world is unreal, and without joy, and that it is an obstacle. If a seeker, out of a spiritual impulse, devotes himself to the search for God, he is repeatedly told that the world is false, transient, and joyless. He starts believing it to be true. These concepts are very harmful, since the world becomes as you see it. . . . In the same way, the writers of some scriptures have for some reason described the world as unreal, harsh, empty, and futile, but it is in fact not so.[127]

The Siddha Yoga gurus teach that leading an ethical life and serving one master (*ekagurūpāsti*) is to become a renunciant. This is not the same as being a monk (*sannyāsī*). While everyone must become a renunciant, only a few should become monks. Moreover, realization of the Self is not equated with becoming a shaktipat guru. At the basis of this understanding of ethics and the renunciation of desires are two points: first, that the enlightened being and the spiritual seeker have the same intrinsically divine nature, and second, that true renunciation is an inner state that has as its outward manifestation an unmistakable integrity. One of its principle features is "steadfastness in yoga," as Swami Chidvilasananda explains:

> To be steadfast in yoga is to acknowledge your reverence for the goal of spiritual life. It means you know how important it is to hold on to the golden cup of yoga. It means you embrace the path with great care and gratitude; and the fact alone, the simple conscious recognition that you cherish yoga, is enough to fill you with the great yogic feelings: moderation, discipline, and regularity.[128]

Keeping in mind these yogic principles informing ethical values it is not particularly difficult to establish Siddha Yoga's canonical boundaries.

The Truth of Ultimate Unity, Practical Truth in a Diverse World, and the Siddha Guru's Realization

No textual selection or practice that runs counter to these ethical standards, denies the existence of God, or affirms a radical philosophical dualism will be part of the Siddha Yoga gurus' canon. This last point—the affirmation of the Oneness of all and the rejection of duality as the basis of ultimacy—is not the same as saying that other views are necessarily valueless, in error, or opposed to Siddha Yoga teaching. As Swami Muktananda says, "Siddha Yoga does not engage in arguments or debates about acceptance and rejection. When there is nothing different from Shiva, what can be accepted or rejected?"[129] Again, the point is: That which siddhas understand wholly, aspirants experience only partially. To put the matter differently, lesser truths are sublated by higher ones; lower knowledge has its place but is subordinate to higher knowledge. This vision creates different levels of understanding which occur before and after Self-realization and similarly provide a basis for understanding, scriptures, and scriptural choices. What was "true" for someone at one time or place may no longer be true at another, higher state of realization. Muktananda says:

> The ideas that arise during sadhana are discovered to be unauthentic in the state of realization. It is like the division in the scriptures between pre-revelation and post-revelation. Pre-revelation is weak, whereas post-revelation is strong. Pre-revelation states. . . "A man who has no son is not liberated after death." The question should then be asked, "Should a renunciant get married?" And how was it possible for celibates like Narada, Sanatkumara, and others to attain liberation? However, post-revelation states . . . "Immortality comes not from good deeds or a son or wealth; immortality can be attained only through renunciation."[130]

The difference between pre- and post-revelatory awareness, which underlies all of the Siddha Yoga gurus' scriptural choices and interpretations, is rooted in their understanding of the states of the siddha and the aspirant. Where the siddha sees perfect unity and therefore no contradiction, the aspirant is still fraught with the delusions of fragmented, dualistic consciousness.[131] Muktananda offers specific instruction when asked how one knows the difference between the guru's voice and the voice of the ego.

> If you have the knowledge of the Guru, certainly you'll know if it's the voice of the ego. Man should become free from ego. Ego is the worst enemy, the most wicked thing. . . .
>
> If you contemplate in this way, your ego melts. If the ego melts, what is left is God. Become free from ego just for a second. Then see what answer you get from within. It is due to ego that a person is far away from the Truth. It is due to ego that instead of experiencing peace, a person burns in the agitation of the mind. The success of every sadhana lies in getting rid of the ego. The enemy is within man—and that is the ego.[132]

Herein lies an important key to understanding the notion of pre- and post-revelatory awareness: Pre-revelatory awareness works within a realm still tainted by egoism. Pre-revelatory understandings of scriptures must be directed toward subverting the ego so that one can experience "what is left," God. Post-revelatory understanding, however, sheds a new light on those techniques and concepts that might have been useful for dismantling dualism.

Swami Muktananda's pre- and post-revelatory awareness restates the traditional Kashmiri Śaiva and Advaita Vedānta view of the simultaneity of ultimate (*paramārtha*) and ordinary (*vyavahāra*) levels of reality, *neither of which is true at the expense of the other.* Put simply, ultimate truth does not render conventional truths "false" but rather affirms the existence of multiple levels of conventional truth. Ordinary truth applies to an ordinary world, one which requires attention and care even after the realization of ultimate truth. The realization of ultimacy provides precisely the perspective that allows one to evaluate the ordinary world. Ultimacy is not a "level" of truth. Rather ultimacy includes all levels of conventional truth and something more than that, something that is *parā*, "beyond." Only the siddha has a full appreciation of ultimacy and so the capacity to apply conventional truth at its many levels simultaneously. This explains, in part, the reason why the Siddha Yoga gurus may at different moments cite textual sources that seem entirely at odds with one another. It also helps us to understand seemingly contradictory statements either in scriptures or in their works.

Understanding the distinction between pre- and post-revelatory awareness allows us to consider the whole of the guru's teaching rather than focus on any fragment. The guru's prerogative derives from his vision of the absolute which translates into his ability to choose which ordinary or "lower" truths will lead a particular aspirant to Self-realization. From the standpoint of Kashmiri Śaivism the ordinary or "lower" (*aparā*) world of multiplicity and convention does not exist apart from the supreme reality of oneness (*parā*). Both are real and both true simultaneously (*parāparā*). In other words, the oneness of reality includes those truths that apply to its multiple forms.

Understanding scriptures at different levels or drawing from them selectively under specific circumstances is not a relativizing ethic. Pre- and post-revelatory awareness does not permit arbitrary moral standards or a sliding scale of values. Simply because the ordinary world demands us to consider situations with an understanding of context does not compromise ethics or standards. Since the ordinary world consists of a plurality of things and of situations—all of which are manifestations of the one divine reality—it naturally requires multiple responses. For the Siddha Yoga gurus this is a practical matter of common sense as much as it is a metaphysical fact. Truth is not compromised because it has multiple forms any more than God is diminished or limited because he has assumed the expanding form of the universe. Similarly, the Hindu scriptures continually reiterate the importance of creating understanding instead of lifeless dogmatism.[133]

The Siddha Yoga gurus believe the relationship between the unified essence of God and God's multiple forms is reflected in the state of the siddha who is singular in essence but multiple as form and appearance. The guru, like the scriptures, empowers the remembrance or recognition (*pratyabhijñā*) of this highest truth while at the same time seeing fit to offer guidance through the world—neither task undermines the other. To put this into the language of Śaivite yoga, the guru makes all things *caitanya*, or filled with consciousness, and thereby distinguishes the false as *jaḍa*, or lifeless.

A more detailed examination of ordinary and ultimate truth in light of a model familiar in Kashmiri Śaivism will further our appreciation of the Siddha Yoga gurus' ability to see the world in light of the pre- and post-revelatory stages of awareness.

At the most mundane and worldly level of ordinary truth, called *aparā*, we see the Siddha Yoga gurus apply the greatest consistency *and* the greatest variation in teaching Siddha Yoga. For example, they will assert that sobriety and the restraint of desire are always better than drunkenness and sensual indulgence. While in this case there are clear and unambiguous means, tests, and results, there are also instances in which what is true for one person may not be true for another. For example, a medicine may be vital to sustaining the life of one person but be deadly to another. At the mundane level of truth things can be simultaneously true so that each operates in its own context or they can be ranked, such that one is superior to another.

There can be stages of truth or stages of understanding reality in which different forms of truth apply. To give an example of this, one might say that the scientific truths one might use to explain one level of reality (such as the laws of Newtonian physics) need not apply at all other levels of reality (such as those better explained by relativity or quantum mechanics). Both forms of truth retain their usefulness and veracity in their respective realms. A spiritual example of this is Swami Muktananda's description of the spiritual awakening of shaktipat which occurs "in any one of twenty-seven different strengths. . . . How a person receives it depends on his past actions, the actions that he is performing in this body, and his tendencies."[134] One can view these stages either sequentially and hierarchically, or cumulatively and simultaneously as they occur to different persons in different contexts. Thus, conventional truths that apply to the world will either overtake each other or serve to reveal higher levels of truth about different aspects of reality. Put simply, worldly truth always has *some* context and is governed by the constant and ultimate truth of oneness.

While this ascending ladder of ordinary truths may be complex, it is not confusing. The Siddha Yoga gurus establish certainty about the most fundamental levels of their teaching. Ethical boundaries, for example, are always clear: The guru should be a paradigm and an example of personal integrity who leads aspirants to their own birthright.[135] The guru's prerogative to assert multiple, ordinary truths depending on need, circumstance, and context is not fundamentally different than that of any teacher or parent who guides his charge to make appropriate choices. To the siddha different, ordinary truths are important because they lead the aspirant along the path to Self-realization and ultimate truth. Ordinary truth depends on the ultimate, and realizing the ultimate means one must deal with the practical ramifications of ordinary life. This is not the same as saying that ultimate truth is only understanding the ordinary world nor should one confuse one level of truth for the others. Swamis Muktananda and Chidvilasananda make clear that ultimate truth is in itself beyond all other forms of knowledge. Knowledge which is not ultimate is not incorrect or "wrong." Rather, it is limited. Muktananda makes this clear as well:

> What did Lord Shankaracharya, Lord Buddha, Nanakdev, Kabir, and Jnaneshwar not know? What did they not understand? They mapped out the entire world from top to bottom, in all its aspects. They fully understood time and its effects and extracted a single essence from everything they knew. But if we were to ask them questions about our mundane lives and activities, they would not be interested. If we were to try to draw them into long scientific discussions, they would consider us ignorant. . . . Truly, there would be no point in asking these great beings about worldly matters. Having come to understand that which contains all knowledge, they would find no reason to take interest in lesser forms of knowledge. . . . [136]

> Scientists are always disproving all theories and discovering new ones. People die. But the Truth is unfailing. It is old in the old and new in the new. It is the truth within the Supreme Truth; it is the you in you, the ultimate state of the perfect inner "I"-consciousness, the blissful thought-free state. . . . Even if the scriptures were destroyed the Truth would be unaffected, because the Truth produced the scriptures, the scriptures did not produce the Truth.[137]

As one ascends the ladder of spiritual understanding, one reaches next the distinction between ultimate and ordinary truth and so the point at which these levels of reality converge. Kashmiri Śaivism calls this level *parāparā* or ultimate-and-ordinary. Here *all* conventional truths are understood to be actually dependent upon the ultimate. Ultimate truth makes the pre-revelatory awareness a state preceding the higher understanding. What was once a matter of levels of truth is now perfect equality: The world is permeated with both ordinary truth and ultimate truth. God is both the forms of the world and a reality beyond all form. Post-revelatory awareness makes clear that there is nothing but God. Swami Muktananda writes:

> When a person's identification with the body is totally destroyed, he need do nothing else to become God because he has been completely saturated with God all along. His experience is "I am in God and God is in me." Moreover, he experiences the entire universe as being filled with God. This kind of understanding is *jñāna svarūpa*, the true nature of knowledge.[138]

Knowledge of the ultimate makes everything ordinary into something intelligible and it resolves any remaining questions or conflicts. Commenting on a verse from the *Chāndogya Upaniṣad* (6.1.3), Swami Muktananda writes:

> However, when one understands That, everything one was previously unable to understand becomes understandable. That has manifested in many aspects, all so different from one another that they do not appear to be connected. But when one knows That, the desire for all other kinds of knowledge is fulfilled. When That is known, whatever was not known becomes known.[139]

There is, however, yet another level at which the dichotomy of ultimate and ordinary completely vanishes. This is the *parā*, or "beyond," which encompasses all without distinction. Muktananda describes this as the persistent state of the siddha:

> Only one who has the supreme knowledge of unity and equality can know the state of an enlightened being. A Siddha understands that he himself is the force behind that power of knowledge. He also understands that he is the principle of the Self, beyond both unity and duality, beyond the beyond. There is no doubt about this.[140]

At this point the canon's highest truth is silence, embodied as the siddha himself. Swami Muktananda quotes an unattributed scripture to make his point. He writes:

> "The Guru lectures in silence, and the disciple's doubts are removed." The Guru's silent speech destroys all the disciples doubts. The glory of silence is limitless; nothing is so powerful. One who has observed the ancient truth of silence has nothing more to attain. In silence one realizes that one is the perfect Self, the embodiment of Truth and Consciousness.[141]

This triadic reality of ordinary (*aparā*), ordinary-and-ultimate (*parāparā*), and ultimate (*parā*) truth not only describes the metaphysical state of existence, it prescribes the principles of understanding that inform the siddha's scriptural choices and interpretations. Thus we will find scriptural choices that affirm radically different claims, or seemingly so, because multiple perspectives or levels of understanding exist simultaneously.

In the final phase, the highest scriptural truth is pure silence leaving only the siddha's incomparable divine consciousness or *anuttarabhairava-saṃvid.* At the point of complete Self-realization there is not only nothing left to say, there is nothing left to do. As Muktananda says:

> A seeker who is truly ripe does not need any *upāyas* to recognize that he is Shiva. Just as he can naturally recognize his parents, in the same way, he can recognize that he is Shiva through inference, scriptural truths, or a word from the Guru. He does not need to perform any spiritual practices. For him, the means to attainment (*upāya*) and the goal which is attained (*upeya*), the attain-

> ment (*prāpya*) and the one who attains (*prāpaka*), the enjoyer (*bhoktā*) and that which is enjoyed (*bhogya*) are all forms of Shiva.[142]

As an approach to the world and a means of choosing scriptural teachings, the underlying principle is that human beings are not forced to deny reality's diversity in order to affirm its oneness. Conversely, affirming oneness or affirming a particular truth does not necessarily mean rejecting other views. Instead the principle is rooted in the idea that we must have a direct experience of reality's oneness in order to live happily amidst its diversity.

The Siddha Yoga gurus state again and again that the world is nothing but the manifestation and movement of Citi or intelligence and consciousness, the Goddess Śakti herself, who is not constrained by any limitation whatsoever. She is not different from Śiva, the One who is eternal and unchanging, and yet there appears to be two and diversity is undeniable. Reality is the appearance of Śiva as Śakti. Muktananda states, "To one who has received the Guru's grace, whose inner Shakti is awakened, and who has seen the play of Chiti in his heart, the outside world is the blossoming of Chiti."[143]

We find precisely the same strategy for interpretation and understanding at work for traditional Kashmiri Śaivas, who root their canonical choices in this distinctive metaphysics that affirms oneness and diversity. The idea that truth or reality (*satya*) is one, many, and one-and-many is as much a principle informing canonical choices as it is a matter of canonical teaching. Thus, Abhinavagupta's well-known affirmation of the reality of the conventional world seems to stand in contrast to his dismissal of the world as an appearance consisting of only so much *māyā*. Compare these two statements:

> If daily life, which is useful to all persons at all times, places, and conditions, were not real, then we know of nothing else that may be represented as real.[144]

And,

> The world of transmigratory existence does not really exist, so how can there be any question of bondage for embodied beings? To one for whom there is no bondage, the act of liberation is, free as he is, false. [Both are] the products of delusion, the illusory appearance of goblins, ghosts, or the snake that is really a rope. Abandon nothing! Take up nothing! Rest; abide in yourself, just as you are![145]

It is the siddha's own experience and the record of the canon that stand behind both of these statements and deem them both to be true. While the canon of the siddhas offers a subtle and complex body of teachings, its most enduring and unambiguous form has always been the siddhas themselves. It is in their lives and their power to transform others that we observe their most powerful and convincing teaching. In these ways, the lineage of the Siddha Yoga gurus has offered examples that reflect the canon's most seminal teachings. At the same time, we can easily locate the Siddha Yoga gurus within that canon of Indian spirituality in which the ultimate unity of existence is affirmed, the meaningful examination of an ethical worldly life is central, and the critical role of the guru as example, guide, and goal is the primary subject.

Chapter Five

THE SELF

A Vedāntic Foundation for the Revelation of the Absolute

William K. Mahony

WHAT IS THE SELF?

Like an intricate tapestry formed of various interwoven threads, Siddha Yoga is a spiritual tradition in which a number of distinct indispensable elements are woven together to form a comprehensive whole. Some of the most important components of that tradition—some of the several strands in the tapestry, as it were—are discussed at length in other chapters in this book. In this chapter, we will examine the tapestry's foundation itself, the material from which all these various threads are spun. This is the experience and expression of what Swami Muktananda and Swami Chidvilasananda have called the "Self." We see reference to the Self in the remarkably succinct instruction that Muktananda repeated, with slight variations, over and over again and with which he crystallized the essential intentions of Siddha Yoga as a spiritual movement: "Meditate on your Self. Honor your Self. Understand your Self. God dwells within you as you."[1]

The discovery (or recovery) of the Self is the goal of Siddha Yoga and thus the intent of all its spiritual disciplines. Like those of her guru, Swami Chidvilasananda's words in this regard have been concise. She has said, for example, that the "experience of the light of the Self is the goal of our practice."[2] The experience of the Self stands as the very foundation and purpose of the guru-disciple relationship; without it, that relationship would be one of possibly harmful dependency and immature devotionalism. Knowledge of the Self is cultivated and refined through the practice of meditation; without it, such practice might well be nothing more than a technique to calm and focus the mind. Understanding of the Self is clarified and strengthened through diligent scriptural study; without it, such study might remain at a purely academic level. Siddha Yoga's basic ethic, including the fundamental teaching that genuine and deep respect for oneself and for others is the ground of human relationships, rests on the underlying and defining experience of the Self.

What is this "Self"? Why is the revelation and expression of the Self so important to Siddha Yoga as a spiritual movement? How does the experience of the Self connect to the Indian tradition at large? These questions will take some time to answer in any fullness. In this chapter we will discuss ways in which swamis Muktananda and Chidvilasananda have defined the Self, note some of the sources from which they draw their descriptions of the Self, and look briefly at how the experience of it informs the various spiritual disciplines and ethical stances of Siddha Yoga.

It should be noted at the outset that we could look at these issues through any number of conceptual frames. After some initial discussion of the nature of the Self as it is understood in Siddha Yoga, we will look at these various concerns from the particular perspective of Vedānta philosophy. (We will return to a definition of this philosophy in the next section of this chapter.) The reader is to understand that by choosing this particular frame we do *not* imply that Siddha Yoga is an exclusively Vedāntic religious tradition, at least if that tradition is defined in a narrow sense. To the contrary, Siddha Yoga also reflects deep affinities with Kashmir Śaivism and the Bhakti traditions of the Indian poet-saints, as well as with other traditions such as Sufism. However, when we look at the ways in which swamis Muktananda and Chidvilasananda express their understanding of the Self, we see that their vocabulary, metaphors, and references return repeatedly to Vedāntic texts—particularly the Upaniṣads and the *Bhagavadgītā*—as well as to the insights and lessons presented by such Vedāntic philosophers and theologians as Śaṅkarācārya.

But we must return to the initial question: What is the Self, as it is understood in Siddha Yoga? It is important to understand that, in this context, the Self is not the self as it normally might be understood and experienced in the West. The term *self* does not refer to a person's specific qualities, which distinguish him or her from others. It is not one's physical body, for example, although the body is considered sacred because it is the abode of the Self. Nor may the Self be identified as one's particular set of distinguishing qualities or psychological proclivities. Accordingly, in urging his students to honor and worship and meditate on the Self, Swami Muktananda is not asking them to practice a form of egoistical self-indulgence, and in stating that the goal of spiritual life is to experience the light of the Self, Swami Chidvilasananda is not advocating a narcissistic reverence for oneself at the expense or exclusion of others.

Muktananda and Chidvilasananda have described and taught of the Self in a number of ways. We will consider several of those various perspectives as we move through the following discussion. For our initial purposes, however, we will briefly look at five: the Self as the uncategorical subject, the "inner witness," by which any object is known; the Self as ultimate reality itself; the absolute Self as God; the Self as pure being, pure consciousness, and pure bliss; and the Self as universal love.

The Universal Subject and the "Inner Witness"

In a very general way, one could say that the idea of the Self distinguishes what might be called Hindu-based sensibilities from those associated with other major religious traditions of India. Viewed from the widest possible angle, the affirmation of the reality of the Self is what separates Hinduism from South Asian Buddhism, for example, for the latter is based in part on the idea that there is no real self. Such Buddhist terms as *anātman* (Pali, *anatta*: "nonself"), *nairātmya* (Pali, *niratta*: "void of selfhood"), and *niḥsvabhāva* ("without personal essence") mark the Buddhist teaching that since all things are constantly changing and thus impermanent (*anitya*, Pali *anicca*), there is no underlying reality or substratum to one's being that can be considered an eternal "soul" or "self." Islam, which is not of course Indian in origin, but is nevertheless another of India's major religious traditions, holds that there can be, and is, no creature whatsoever—no "self"—without the prior reality of a divine Creator, the latter being God (Allāh) himself. Islamic theology describes Allāh as "the Producer (from nothing)" (al-Bāri'), "the Creator" (al-Khāliq), "the Self-existent" (al-Qayyum), "the Maintainer" (al-Muqīṭ), "the Witness" (ash-Shahīd), and other terms that imply the belief that God fashions, sustains, and looks over all of creation, from which God stands eternally independent.[3]

Speaking very generally, what we might call Hinduism[4] is based on the idea that the *only* thing that is real in this universe is the Self. Similar in some ways to Platonic thought in classical Greek philosophy, Hinduism holds that what is fully or ultimately real is that which does not change. Plato identified that unchanging reality as the "True" and the "Good," which he held to be eternal in nature. Hinduism tends to identify that abiding reality not only as truth but also as Existence or Being. Hindu theologians generally hold that without the prior reality of Being, there can be none of the many and diverse beings who populate this world. It is this very "being-ness" of reality to which Hindu thinkers refer when they speak of the "Self." In one way or another, most forms of Hindu thought identify this universal "Self" as God. Accordingly, from the Hindu perspective, there is only one Self in the universe, and that is the Self of God. Without this, there is nothing. It is the divine *aham*, the universal "I," that creates and watches over and lives in the universe in the guise of the many things and beings who have their existence therein.

In recognizing the ultimacy of the divine *aham*, Hinduism holds that the world of distinct and separate beings is completely contingent on the reality of the absolute. Without the priority of the divine "I am", nothing exists. While Hinduism and Islam are quite different from each other in many ways, this is a theological position that would resonate favorably with orthodox Islamic thought. Furthermore, if Islam holds that Allāh—as al-Bāri' and as al-Khāliq and as al-Qayyum—has fashioned the human being, so too it teaches that God is in some ways vitally present within that glorious creation, for Allāh is said to be "closer to you than your own jugular vein."[5] Orthodox Islam will not affirm the autonomous divinity of the soul. But it will accept the idea that God reveals himself to the human heart. Indeed, the ninety-nine names of God in Islam include such epithets as al-Bāṭin: the "Inner."[6]

Similarly, in holding that there is only one Self, and that this truth is the source and foundation and ultimate resting place of all things, Hinduism—at least the forms of Hinduism that are consistent with the Siddha Yoga gurus' experience and expression of the Self[7]—is not in the end so different from some forms of Indian Buddhism, especially those Mahāyāna schools of thought that hold that ultimate reality is none other than the plethoral, universal "emptiness" (*śūnya, śūnyatā*) from which all forms emerge. According to the Śūnyavāda (the "Emptiness-School" of Buddhism), it is precisely on this emptiness that all forms are grounded, and this universal truth is therefore identical to its manifest expressions. As the opening of the *Prajñāpāramitāhṛdaya* (the "Heart of the Perfection of Wisdom," more commonly known as the "Heart Sūtra") asserts, "Form is emptiness, and emptiness is form; emptiness does not differ from form, and form does not differ from emptiness. Whatever is form, that is emptiness, and whatever is emptiness, that is form." Some Mahāyāna schools associated with the Śūnyavāda compare this emptiness with the *tathāgatagarbha*, that is, with the formless "womb of suchness" which nourishes and gives birth, as it were, to the world of manifest being. According to some Mahāyāna schools, this very emptiness is none other than the infinite Buddha-Mind itself. Although the specific language does not appear in Buddhist texts, one might say from such a perspective that there is only one formless Self in the universe of form and that this is the Self of the Buddha-Mind.

The experience of a universal Self appears in some Buddhist traditions beyond southern Asia, as well. We see it, for instance, in the influential Sōtō Zen tradition of Japan. While still maintaining the final unreality of any particular "conscious self" (Japanese, *ishikiteki jiko*), as well as of a conditioned "self" or "self-conscious self" (Japanese, *rikoteki jiko*) which experiences itself as "me" as distinct from "others" and which seeks to gratify that me-ness, Sōtō Zen teaches of the experience of an "all-encompassing self" (*jinissai jiko*) which is beyond any egoistic or conditioned consciousness. Sōtō Zen holds that one comes to understand and experience the *jinissai jiko*—the all-encompassing Self—through meditation and the cultivation of mindfulness.[8] That it is an important element of Zen Buddhist teaching is suggested by the fact that Zen texts and commentaries have used a number of terms as synonyms for *jinissai jiko*.[9] These texts also describe such a reality not only as the "highest truth" (Japanese, *daiichi gitai*; Sanskrit, *paramārtha*) but also as "nondual" (Japanese, *funi*), the latter of which is the equivalent of the Sanskrit term *advaita*.

This is all to say that Indian spirituality in general (as well as various theological, philosophical, and experiential traditions outside of India) holds that, even if the physical body and particular personality that one might normally regard as the "self" is not of itself ultimately real, there is still some notion of an uncategorial truth, some foundational state of being—some universal Self—that gives rise to and supports all beings.

It is in this larger context that we may begin to look at the way the Siddha Yoga gurus define the true Self. Swami Chidvilasananda has said:

> Right in the beginning one should understand this Self is not the body, this Self is not the ego. Meditation on the Self is meditation on the depth of the soul, on the great Self that is pure, that is love, that is filled with bliss.[10]

Her words are similar to these by Swami Muktananda:

> We think of ourselves as the body. We think that we are a certain physical structure, with hands, feet, legs, and eyes. We think of ourselves as a man or a woman, as belonging to a particular class or country. We identify ourselves with our thoughts, our talents, our good or bad actions. But none of these things is what we are.[11]

Muktananda distinguished the physical, mental, and social identity from an inward presence that in some way watches over the various workings of one's body and mind. Quoting the *Bhagavadgītā*—"this body is called a field, and the one who knows it is called the knower of the field"[12]—he wrote:

> Within us is a being who knows all the actions of the body and the mind and remains untouched by them. . . .
>
> [The] one who knows the field must be different from the field. For example, one who says "my book" must be different from the book; one who says "my table" must be different from the table. In the same way, one who says "my body" must be different from the body; one who says "my mind" must be different from the mind. Who is that being who observes the activities of our waking hours? At night, when we go to sleep, that being does not sleep, but stays awake and in the morning reports to us on our dreams.[13]

Who is this one who "knows the field?" Who is this inward presence who "knows all the actions of the body and the mind and remains untouched by them"? In the following passage Muktananda identified that untouched knower as the Self, which he characterized as "pure consciousness" and of the "form of bliss":

> The one who lives in the body but who is apart from the body as the knower of it is our real Self. That Self is beyond the body, beyond the mind, beyond distinctions of name, color, and sex. It is the pure "I," the original "I"-consciousness which has been with us since we came into the world. We have superimposed different notions onto that "I"-awareness, notions like, "I am black," "I am white," "I am a man," "I am a woman," "I am American," "I am Indian." Yet, when we wipe away those superimpositions, that "I" is nothing but pure Consciousness, and it is of the form of bliss.[14]

According to Swami Muktananda, the Self is not to be identified with whatever one might otherwise regard as one's own personal characteristics. It is neither the body nor the mind, and it resides beyond all of one's otherwise idiosyncratic qualities. Muktananda held, in fact, that to identify the Self with any personal characteristics is actually to superimpose those qualities onto it. As he said elsewhere, the Self is *neti neti*: "Not this, not this."[15] The Self cannot therefore be known as an object among other objects in the world. Free of all such superimpositions, the Self is that which, although having no characteristics itself, is nevertheless aware of any and all characteristics. The Self is the "knower" rather than the known. This "knower"—this "witness" (Sanskrit, *sākṣin*; nominative, *sākṣī*)—never leaves us and has been with us since our birth; it is the abiding "I" that has resided within our being "since we came into the world."

"The Self is the witness," Muktananda said.[16] The Self is that silent inner presence who watches compassionately over the body and mind. "What is your idea of yourself?" he asked. "You think that you are just a constantly flowing stream of thoughts. Don't identify with your thoughts but with their root, their source, the Self, who is beyond all these thoughts which arise around the Self, who is beyond the mind. Your reality is that you are the witness of all these thoughts, the constant witness, so identify with the Self."[17] In a collection of poems on spiritual life, Swami Muktananda wrote:

> He remains with you, and protects you.
> He is the source of all your actions.
> The Witness, the knower of all,
> He transcends the mind.
> Always love Him, your true friend.[18]

"The Self is our dearest friend," he wrote elsewhere. "It exists inside us in its fullness, right within the heart. Though the Self is always with us, it is so subtle that most people cannot see or hear it. The Self is the formless substratum of everything, the foundation of our lives." Continuing on the theme that it is the inward presence that abides beyond all categories, Muktananda said of the Self: "We cannot see it through the eyes, nor can we attain it through speech. The tongue can speak about it, but the true description of its nature is silence." He added that one, therefore, comes to know the Self through meditation: "The Self cannot be attained through the mind or through the senses. Yet when the inner psychic instruments are purified through meditation, it reveals itself on its own. . . . Just by meditating peacefully, we can make the Self manifest to us."[19]

Swami Chidvilasananda similarly distinguishes the essential Self from all of the various categories by which one might normally identify oneself. In speaking of the Self, she has quoted this passage from the *Yogavāsiṣṭha*:

> When the truth is known, all descriptions cease,
> And silence alone remains.
> Not until one renounces everything
> is knowledge of the Self attained.
> When all viewpoints are abandoned,
> What remains is the Self.[20]

According to Chidvilasananda, the recovery of the uncategorical Self liberates one from attachment to the vagaries of life that one might otherwise experience. "Once we have become established in the Self," she explains,

> . . . we become free from all worries and all anxieties. Baba [Muktananda] used to say, this doesn't mean that there won't be worries or anxieties or difficulties. All it means is that we are free from them. When you're a witness, when you're an observer, you're able to take something in more easily than when you are involved in it. So become a witness. . . . Then you'll realize the Truth.[21]

Swami Chidvilasananda notes that to see oneself and one's life from the perspective of the inner witness is also to be free from the entrapping effect of harmful patterns of thought. Using the term *saṃskāra* to refer to such latent psychological templates, and the phrase "great Seer" to indicate the inner witness who is not bound by the constraints of those patterned ways of thinking, she states:

> When you experience oneness with the great Seer, the flame merges with the flame, the water merges with the water, you merge with your own Self. When this state of the Witness is attained, all the *samskaras,* all the past impressions, are nothing more than burned seeds. Then you live freely, truly independent.[22]

For Swami Chidvilasananda, it is only the Self that remains stable in one's otherwise changing physical and psychological being. Its firm and abiding nature marks the Self's unwavering integrity; and the Self's integrity is inseparable from its inherent unity, which is itself wisdom. "Because of its stability," she writes, "we are able to return to the experience of oneness, where we understand everything. If it weren't for the Self, our whole life would fall apart. The Self, the witness, brings everything together and keeps it in check. So become the witness. As you do this, you merge into the Self."[23]

The realization of the Self is said to bring a conviction of the inherent dignity of one's being as well as that of others. The Siddha Yoga gurus teach that to experience the Self as the witness is to see one's life from such a perspective. "As you become established in the state of the Witness," Chidvilasananda says, "you experience yourself as becoming purer. You develop a sense of worthiness. Pettiness falls away. You see yourself as an instrument of God rather than a burden on this earth."[24]

The Supreme, Divine Reality

In the passage just quoted, Swami Chidvilasananda makes use of explicitly theological language. Her words suggest the idea that there is an effective bond between the dignity of the human soul and the power of divinity. Siddha Yoga gurus hold that an individual's inherent, God-given integrity of being is an expression of the integrity of God. Like God, being is indivisible; for, while there may be many beings, being is One. Therefore, it is not to particular beings but to being itself that the siddha gurus refer when they speak of the Self.

From the perspective of Siddha Yoga, the very "being-ness" that is inherent within one's own being is, thus, the indivisible Self, and one who knows that Self within himself or herself also sees the same Self in all beings. To be firmly established in the experience of the Self is the goal of Siddha Yoga sadhana. The siddha is described as one who has reached this goal and thereby remains constant in the awareness of the indivisible universal Self playing within all of the many and diverse manifest selves. Swami Muktananda reminded his followers that his own guru, Bhagawan Nityananda,

> . . . treated all people alike, regardless of their color, their importance in the world, their education. Rich and poor, educated and illiterate—all of them were the same in Gurudev's eyes. For him, this entire universe was a reflection of the same divine Self. He used to say that the world is a play of Consciousness.[25]

For Nityananda the Self is the single divine consciousness, which he saw to be residing in and masked by the multiplicity of beings in the world. Nityananda seems to have loved all people, not for their individual personalities but precisely because they each embodied this single reality. The world of apparent diversity was, for Nityananda, the blissful play of a single, abiding, and universal Self. Muktananda himself said, "We should look directly at the Self, which is the same in everyone. Riches, poverty, literacy, illiteracy, these are all external things and do not affect the internal reality of man which transcends these distinctions."[26] Similarly, Swami Chidvilasananda says, "It is quite important to recognize that everybody around you is a form of the Self. It does not matter how gorgeous or how ugly they may be on the outside; the supreme Self is beyond all that. It is in everyone."[27]

For these siddha gurus the Self is thus the comprehensive unity of being. It is the singular integrity of the absolute. As that which gives rise to and supports the universe in its entirety, the Self gives rise to and supports each and every being in that universe. Swami Chidvilasananda has quoted the sage Aṣṭāvakra in urging her followers to "know that the Self is one and enter into the state of the Absolute. In this way, you regard the universe as being one with your own Self."[28] She commented, "To recognize that very Self, we have to have the absolute experience that the universe and we are one and the same."[29]

The Manifestation of God

Referring to the Self as "That" and as "Brahman" (a word to which we will turn our attention at some length later), Swami Muktananda declared to his devotees:

> You are That, more wondrous than all.
> You are Brahman, one with everything.
> You alone exist everywhere.
> Neither birth nor death exists in you.
> You are without cause, unborn.
> You are the death of mortality.
> You are free of faults and cares.
> Immense freedom is yours.[30]

Both Swami Muktananda and Swami Chidvilasananda make use of explicitly theological language in identifying the Self not only as the divine absolute reality but also as the supreme being, that is to say, as God. Muktananda said, for example, that the Self "is an unchanging form of the manifestation of God."[31] Again quoting the *Bhagavadgītā,* which he did quite frequently, he reminded his followers that God himself—here in the form of Kṛṣṇa—says in that sacred text, "I am the knower of all these fields."[32] Muktananda also quoted Indian religious texts dating to roughly the eighth to fifth centuries B.C.E. in teaching that the divine Self "lives in the mind, but the mind cannot know it, because the mind is its body," and "that is God who makes the mind think but who can never be apprehended by the mind."[33] According to this line of thought, the "I" that resides within all beings and within all forms of awareness is therefore the divine *aham* ("I") of God. Referring to an influential Indian philosopher and theologian from the eighth and ninth centuries, Muktananda said, "It was with the awareness of that 'I' that the great Shankaracharya proclaimed, *Aham Brahmasmi*, 'I am the Absolute.' That 'I' is God."[34]

Using the Sanskrit word *ātman* (a term usually translated as "Self" or "soul"), Swami Chidvilasananda has taught, "When we become one with the Self, the Atman, we experience God in everything and everyone. Then we know that we belong to God, and this entire world is His family. If we have this firm conviction about God and about the world, we experience His presence all the time."[35] According to Muktananda and Chidvilasananda, the term *Self* therefore refers to none other than God. Said to be the inward Self of the universe as a whole, the "unchanging form" of the absolute is said to abide within all beings, and all beings are said to stand as "the manifestation of God."[36] The Self is the divinity of being itself.

One implication of this idea is that if one honors and worships and meditates on the Self, then one honors and worships and meditates on God. To know the Self is, in Swami Chidvilasananda's words, to "experience God in everything and everyone." In a set of poems on spiritual life entitled *Reflections of the Self*, Swami Muktananda wrote:

> The all-pervasive Lord
> manifests throughout the universe.
> The elixir of love pulsates through all things,
> radiates through every tree and branch.
> Welcome that bliss;
> get rid of fear and grief.
>
> O dear one, keep chanting God's name
> while sitting, or standing,
> or involved in the world.
> Never forget Him.
> Unite your mind with the Self.[37]

Muktananda taught that the Self is not constrained by the limits of time and space. Accordingly, for Muktananda, the Self is infinite, pervasive, and eternal in nature. "[T]he Self exists in the east, in the west, in the north, and in the south," he said. "It exists in all countries. It is here today, it was here yesterday, and it will be here tomorrow. The Self is not bound by any place, thing, or time."[38] God's very eternality means that the Self is present in all time, and therefore within each and every moment. And God's very pervasiveness means that the Self is present in all places. Therefore, God—

the Self—lives within all things. As Muktananda once said, "God, the Self, exists everywhere in His fullness. Being present in everything, He is also present within us."[39] Swami Chidvilasananda makes a similar point in a short statement in which she encourages spiritual seekers to "bathe in the nectarean knowledge that the Self and the world are one."[40]

Being, Consciousness, and Bliss

We have already seen reference to the Self as absolute being, understood here to be God. Both Swamis Muktananda and Chidvilasananda have also said repeatedly that the divine Self is of the nature of both consciousness and bliss. For example, in a verse in which he urged his students to seek an experiential understanding of the Self, Swami Muktananda wrote:

> With your own eyes,
> see the treasure of delight and peace.
> Contemplate the supreme Essence.
> Merge into all,
> meditate on your inner Self.
> It is Existence, Consciousness,
> and supreme Bliss.
> It is the one Consciousness in its totality.[41]

The underlying idea here is that the whole universe and everything in it—the "all" into which one merges—is a reflection of a single truth ("the supreme Essence"), which Muktananda characterizes as of the nature of "Existence, Consciousness, and supreme Bliss." As we will see, the bliss of which Muktananda speaks is not to be mistaken for the transient happiness one feels when one's desires have in some way been gratified. The latter kind of contentment is conditioned by external circumstances, which are subject to change and decay. Such happiness cannot last and therefore cannot be considered to constitute an abiding joy. When Muktananda and Chidvilasananda use the word *bliss*, they are not speaking of a quality that is in any way dependent on outer conditions. On this point, Swami Chidvilasananda says:

> The joy that we are talking about is an inner state. It is the *antarāvasthā*, the state of one's own elevated mind and purified heart. It is not just a certain feeling or a giddy emotion; it is the way you conduct yourself in the privacy of your own being. Joy is the natural state of the Self. It is constant and it can be experienced. Then, just as the space inside a pot and the space outside it are one and the same, similarly, joy is within and joy is without.[42]

Using vocabulary drawn from traditional Indian spirituality, Swami Muktananda said not only that God is the Self but that "God, the Self, is of the form of sat, chit, and ananda"[43] Doing so, he drew on a well-known Vedāntic formula, that characterizes ultimate reality as *sat-cit-ānanda*, which may be rendered as "absolute being, absolute consciousness, and absolute bliss."

Commenting on this description of the Self as *sat-cit-ānanda*, Muktananda said, "*Sat* means Truth," by which he meant a universal, pervasive, and unchanging truth:

> Sat means Truth, that which exists in all places, in all things, and at all times. If Truth were not omnipresent, it would not be the Truth; it would not have absolute existence. For example, if you are in New York, you are real in New York; but since you are not in Los Angeles, you are not real there. But God, being sat, is not bound by place or time, nor is He restricted to one particular object.[44]

Muktananda similarly noted the qualities of the Self as consciousness. "Chit means Consciousness, or that which illuminates everything. Chit is the light of the Self, which destroys ignorance. Chit makes us aware of outer objects, and it also makes us aware that God exists inside."[45] The very fact that a person can think that God is *not* real proves, for Muktananda, the reality of consciousness; for the very fact that one thinks anything at all means that consciousness is real. "[I]f we think that God does not exist because we cannot see Him," Muktananda said, "it is chit which illuminates that understanding. Chit is the discloser of the knowledge that something exists or does not exist. Chit is that which illuminates all places and all things at all times; therefore chit also illuminates our inner being."[46]

For Swami Muktananda, the Self was also of the nature of bliss. He held that—like truth and consciousness—bliss exists in all places and at all times and remains unconditioned and free of any limitations. He described how the pleasure one gains from looking at a beautiful shape disappears once that form disappears, or how the pleasure that comes from hearing a melodious sound disappears when that sound fades, or how one no longer feels pleasure from a soft touch when that touch is removed. "But," he said, "ananda does not depend on any external factor. It arises, unconditioned, from within. When the mind and intellect come close to the Self, they are able to experience bliss."[47]

The Self is pure and unconditioned because it is neither delimited by the structures of time and space nor distorted by any of the superimpositions otherwise placed onto it. The Self is, therefore, possessed of its own inherent nature, unstained by extraneous forces and unbound by external constraints. That inherent nature is *sat-cit-ānanda*: pure being, pure consciousness, and pure bliss. Muktananda states:

> The Self is the most subtle of all subtle things. It is highly secret and mysterious, and it has no name, no color, and no form. Even though it is without

> attributes, the sages have described its nature as *sat chid ānanda*—existence, consciousness, and bliss absolute.[48]

Referring to the Self, Muktananda could therefore say, "Inside us lies divine happiness."[49] Swami Chidvilasananda has similarly affirmed the idea, "Joy is great and it is great to experience joy. But you must also know that *you* are great. Never forget that. It is where true joy lives—in the secret of your greatness, in the Self that makes you great."[50]

Universal Love

It is of primary importance to Siddha Yoga as a spiritual tradition that the Self of which its gurus teach is also of the nature of pure and universal love. This has significance not only for the practice of inward meditation and prayerful contemplation but also for the essential Siddha Yoga ethic, which revolves around respect for others. According to Siddha Yoga theology, when one seeks God one thereby seeks not only the very source, foundation, and sustaining power of the universe, but the source of one's own life within that wondrous creation as well. Swami Chidvilasananda writes:

> . . . [W]hen the scriptures and the sages tell us: "Dissolve your identification with the body and the mind," they don't mean give them up. How can we give up our bodies and our minds? After all, God gave these things to us. It's just that we have to expand our awareness a little bit beyond what we are seeing and thinking. That is what gives the experience of the Self, that is what gives the experience of love, that is what takes us deeper and deeper inside. When you really see beyond all the senses, all the bodies, all the objects, what you discover is that one thing that is within all of this. And this energy, it is love. And to feel that love wherever we are, we contemplate and we meditate.[51]

Speaking of her guru, Chidvilasananda has said, "Baba Muktananda lived with great reverence for everything in God's creation. Respect was one of his principal teachings—respect for the Self that dwells within all things, sentient and insentient." Quoting Muktananda's own words, she explains:

> Every day during my lectures I say, respect everybody. To do this, first of all, you must respect yourself. Only then can you also respect others. You are not what you appear to be on the outside. You are something else on the inside, so discover that. Within a person there is the effulgence of God; each of you should see that radiance. Along with this light of God, there is so much joy. The purpose of human life is to attain that joy.[52]

For Swami Muktananda, a key to the attainment of this joy, which is the "purpose of human life," is to offer one's devotion and love to others, and thus to God. Muktananda accordingly gave his followers a principal teaching that has broad, ethical implications and deep, contemplative significance for the practice of Siddha Yoga: "See God in one another."[53] He believed that to cultivate and express such love—he used the Hindi word *prem*—is a vital element of spiritual discipline. In his autobiography he wrote, "The *sādhanā* ['spiritual discipline'] of love is a very high sadhana. Love is also called *bhakti,* or devotion. Love is a dynamic and inspiring throbbing of the heart."[54]

The centrality of love, therefore, stands as a foundation of the theology of Siddha Yoga, for the divine power and presence residing within one's own heart as well as within the hearts of all others is identified not only as being, consciousness, and bliss, but also as love. According to the Siddha Yoga gurus, God *is* love. Swami Muktananda wrote, "Love is of the very nature of God, whom the scriptural authors have called supreme Bliss, and *Sat chid ānanda.*"[55] Following Indian tradition in general and quoting a medieval text composed by the devotional philosopher Nārada, Muktananda said that the experience of the "sweet and beautiful love" of God cannot be described in words: "Love is God. That is why Narada says in the *Bhakti Sūtras, anirvacanīyaṃ premasvarūpam,* 'Love is indescribable in its very nature.'"[56] For Muktananda, love is the ground of being itself, without which nothing would exist. He taught spiritual seekers that in order to experience that ineffable divine love in its most immediate form they were to seek the presence of God within their own hearts. For Muktananda, and for Siddha Yoga in general, love is associated specifically with the *ānanda,* or "bliss", component of the Self as *sat-cit-ānanda.* "A human being cannot live without inner love," he taught. "The Self is called *satchidananda*—absolute existence, consciousness, and bliss. It is the Supreme Truth. To attain love, we have to turn within. By doing this, we discover the vastness of love."[57]

VEDĀNTIC TEXTUAL SOURCES

In speaking of the Self as the inner witness; the universal and divine Creator and foundation of all that is; and ultimate reality, which they experience as *sat-cit-ānanda,* swamis Muktananda and Chidvilasananda signal to their devotees that the reality to which they refer has also been revealed in the lessons and texts associated with the Indian religious and philosophical tradition known as the Vedānta. We see a reference to the Vedāntic tradition in a verse Swami Muktananda wrote concerning the universal Self, which he here calls Brahman:

> With eyes brimming with love, sing His name.
> All inner mysteries will be disclosed.
> Every bird and plant
> will reveal itself to you as Brahman.
> The knowledge of Vedanta will manifest everywhere.[58]

Swami Chidvilasananda refers to key Vedāntic teachings and texts when she notes:

> The *Ṛig Veda* declares: *prajñānam brahma,* "Consciousness is Brahman, the Absolute."
>
> The *Atharva Veda* declares: *ayam ātmā brahma,* "The Self is Brahman, the Absolute, the supreme transcendent Reality."
>
> The *Sāma Veda* declares: *tat tvam asi,* "Thou art That."
>
> The *Yajur Veda* declares: *aham brahmāsmi,* "I am Brahman. I am the Absolute."[59]

As we mentioned at the opening of this chapter, swamis Muktananda and Chidvilasananda have encountered discussions of the Self in other religious traditions besides the Vedānta. They have seen such revelations in the Śaiva theologies of Kashmir, for example. They have also seen the Self discussed in the classical yoga of Patañjali, in the interior and charismatic traditions of the Nātha yogis, in the devotional warmth and ecstasies of the *bhakti*-oriented sensibilities of the medieval Indian poet-saints, and in other spiritual traditions from India and beyond.[60] However, our attention here will be directed specifically to the Vedāntic understanding of the Self, because in many ways Vedānta stands as the primary source of the Siddha Yoga teachings regarding the nature and experience of that Self. Viewed historically, the Vedānta precedes all of the other religious and spiritual traditions just mentioned. Viewed thematically, the great insights and practices that drive these latter traditions lie implicitly if not explicitly in Vedāntic theology, metaphysics, spiritual disciplines, and ethics. Abhinavagupta and other theologians of Kashmir Śaivism were well-versed in Vedāntic thought. The Śaiva mantra *Śivo 'ham,* "I am Śiva," expresses an experience of nondualism that is fully consonant with the Vedāntic experience. Four of the great poet-saints of Maharashtra—Jñāneśvar, Nāmdev, Eknāth, and Tukārām—were deeply familiar with the Vedāntic ideas of the unity of all being and the illusion of the separation between God and soul; they sang of this notion in their *abhaṅga*s (Marathi devotional songs) that were to become popular with the often illiterate people of the Maharashtrian countryside. Jñāneśvar and Eknāth themselves wrote commentaries on major Vedāntic texts.

It is not insignificant that most of Swami Muktananda's books have substantial sections and sometimes entire chapters dedicated to the Vedānta and Vedāntic teachings, even in the context of discussions explicitly addressing what might otherwise be regarded as non-Vedāntic teachings and perspectives.[61] One could argue that Muktananda's description of the Self is essentially Vedāntic in nature, although the understanding is presented by means of various ideas, metaphors, practices, and values drawn from Kashmir Śaivism, classical yoga, Hindu devotionalism, and other forms of Indian spirituality. Kashmir Śaivism, in particular, places vital importance on the Self, which it identifies with supreme consciousness.[62] But even here the general notion of the Self, if not the vocabulary (*ātman*), is based on Vedāntic ideas. And the Siddha Yoga lifestyle and general worldview—which revolve around the idea that true enjoyment (*bhukti*) and true renunciation (*mukti*) are related to each other or even the same thing since one can truly take delight in the world when one does not allow oneself to be trapped by it—are much closer to the perspective and values presented by Kashmir Śaivism than, say, the classical yoga taught by Patañjali and his followers or some of the more austere forms of the Vedānta. Nevertheless, we can still say that such *bhukti* and *mukti* are possible only because of the underlying reality of the Self; for it is the Self that truly delights in the world while at the same time remaining fully free from all forms of bondage. Like Kashmir Śaivism, Siddha Yoga places emphasis on seeing God through the delightful play of the senses rather than retreating completely from the sensual world. Like Kashmir Śaivism, Siddha Yoga stresses the value of family life and the need to engage responsibly in the marketplace. Here, too, Siddha Yoga varies from some of the more stridently ascetic forms of the Vedānta. Yet, it could be argued that even such values derive ultimately from a deep sense of the integrity of the divine Self dwelling within all beings and that one is to offer one's life to the expansive celebration and reverence of that divine truth. As we will see, this is a thoroughly Vedāntic idea.

And what is the Vedānta? Said briefly, it is a highly regarded and influential set of principles and practices centered on the insights presented by a set of sacred texts known as the Upaniṣads and on a number of philosophical and commentarial texts based on those works. The Sanskrit term *vedānta* literally means "the end [*anta*] of the Veda," the Veda ("sacred knowledge") referring here to a large body of sacred songs, verses, ritual instructions, and theological teachings dating from roughly 1500 to 300 B.C.E. which are said to reveal eternal truths. The Vedānta is honored as the "end of the Veda," in the sense of the "fulfillment" or "completion" or "intended meaning"—in a word, the "culmination"—of all forms of sacred knowledge.

The Upaniṣads are collections of teachings in prose and verse form given to spiritual seekers by mostly anonymous sages, the earliest of which date to roughly the eighth century B.C.E. With a few exceptions, those to which we will refer in this chapter were first taught between that time and about the fourth century B.C.E.

It is somewhat difficult to arrive at an exact number of Upaniṣads, since several works refer to themselves as Upaniṣads but may not be regarded as such by the larger Vedāntic tradition as a whole. Perhaps some of the latter call themselves "Upaniṣads" as a way to align themselves with a respected literary genre or religious tradition. Of the nearly 250 texts which claim to be Upaniṣads, slightly more than 120 can be regarded as genuine, that is, as emerging from or expressing the Vedāntic tradition itself. This is not to say the others are not worthwhile; it is simply that they are not particularly Vedāntic in their perspective. The *Muktikā Upaniṣad* (ca. fifteenth century C.E.) and other late south Indian works mention 108 separate Upaniṣads in an enumeration that has become somewhat of a stock list.

The Upaniṣads present complicated and quite densely packed teachings. This is not the occasion to review the larger contours and subtle implications of those lessons. But we will in this chapter consider a few of the central points and the way in which they express similar insights regarding the nature and experience of the Self as taught by swamis Muktananda and Chidvilasananda. The core teaching of the Upaniṣads as a whole articulates the realization that behind or within all of the apparent spatial swirl and temporal flux of the world of multiplicity, as it is experienced by the senses, is a singular, sublime, pervasive, eternal, and unchanging ultimate reality that gives rise to, envelops, and sustains all things. This reality is Being itself. Without it, there can be no separate beings, just as without an ocean there can be no waves. It is the Godhead, without which there is nothing. The Upaniṣads hold that this imperishable world soul resides within each and every form, hidden, as it were, "like oil in sesame seeds" or "like butter in cream."[63]

The Upaniṣads call this Self of the universe Brahman or Ātman. As we will see, the former applies more typically to the Godhead dwelling within the macrocosm, and the latter signifies the divine Self residing at the deepest levels of one's person. Theistic Upaniṣads teach that this Brahman or Ātman is a single deity known generically as Īśvara or Īśa or Īśāna (all of which may be rendered as "Lord"), living deep within one's being and identified as Śiva, Viṣṇu, or the Goddess by particular sectarian communities. Muktananda and Chidvilasananda have referred to the universal Godhead in a number of ways: not only as Brahman and Ātman but also, most frequently, as Śiva, the "Benevolent One." But use of one name of God to the exclusion of another seems not to be of interest to these siddha gurus. What *is* important, it seems, is that both regard God as the divine, universal Self who enlivens and gives meaning to all beings.

That the Upaniṣads are considered *vedānta* marks the traditional Hindu understanding not only that the lessons they give regarding the nature of Brahman and Ātman constitute the completion of the Veda but also that one who truly understands those teachings finds an inward fulfillment and completion. The realization of one's inner integrity frees one from the doubt and fear engendered by what the Upaniṣads hold to be the false identification with one's physical body and particular personality, both of which are buffeted by the vicissitudes of life, and both of which ultimately stand helpless before the inevitability of decease. Upaniṣadic sages taught that knowing and experiencing the undying universal Self within one's own being, one is "liberated from the jaws of death."[64]

In addition to the Upaniṣads, the canon of the Vedānta also includes the *Bhagavadgītā* (ca. 300-100 B.C.E) a didactic poem appearing in the Indian epic the *Mahābhārata*, and perhaps the best known and therefore most influential of all Hindu sacred texts. The *Bhagavadgītā* puts to voice what are considered eternal truths in the form of a conversation between God in the form of Kṛṣṇa and his disciple, the devout yet ethically troubled Arjuna.

The Vedāntic canon also traditionally includes what are regarded as revealed truths presented by the *Brahma Sūtra* ("Aphorisms on Brahman," ca. third to second centuries B.C.E, attributed to the sage Bādarāyaṇa), which consists of terse and somewhat abstruse teachings regarding the nature of the absolute. The *Brahma Sūtra* is also known as the *Vedānta Sūtra* and as the *Śārīraka Sūtra*, the latter because the text pertains to Brahman as *śārīraka*, that is, the absolute "embodied" in the universe.

These three sets of religious teachings—the Upaniṣads, the *Bhagavadgītā*, and the *Brahma Sūtra*—serve as the "triple foundation" (*prasthānatrayī*) of the Vedānta as a spiritual tradition. Those who have listened to their talks and those who have read their published writings will agree that swamis Muktananda and Chidvilasananda have made extensive reference to the Upaniṣads and the *Bhagavadgītā*. Neither has referred with much frequency to the *Brahma Sūtra*.

Both siddha gurus have also directed their followers' attention to a set of works by Indian commentators on these honored texts. Of particular interest to them are works attributed to the great philosopher-sage, Śaṅkarācārya, who lived in the eighth and ninth centuries. A skilled and honored teacher (*ācārya*) named after the god Śiva (one of whose many epithets is Śaṅkara, "Auspicious One"), Śaṅkarācārya is considered by many to be preeminent among the Vedāntic sages who taught the unity of the Godhead and thus the essential identity of Brahman and Ātman. The particular form of Vedānta he taught is known therefore as Advaita Vedānta (*a-dvaita*: "nondual").

Śaṅkarācārya's particular form of Advaita Vedānta is sometimes known as Kevala Advaita or "absolute nondualism." Here, ultimate reality is said to be eternally unchanging. Any seeming change is the result of a superimposition (*adhyāsa*) or the appearance (*vivarta*) of such on what is in fact an abiding and stable reality; the change comes only because of one's ignorance (*avidyā*) of that steadfast truth. Śaṅkarācārya's absolute nondualism is similar in many ways to the Śuddha Advaita or "pure nondualism" later presented by the fifteenth- and sixteenth-century theologian Vallabhācārya, who held that the one God, who pervades the whole world, is untouched by any such ignorance. According to Vallabha, the single universal divinity becomes all worldly objects as well as human souls through a process of transformation. Throughout this process, however, God remains unchanged, just as gold remains gold no matter what the shape of ornament into which it may be formed.

There are other forms of Vedānta besides Advaita, as well. There is, for example, the Viśiṣṭādvaita Vedānta or "qualified nondualism" of the influential eleventh- to twelfth-century theologian Rāmānuja, who held that while God is absolute reality, physical matter and individual souls have distinct qualities (*viśeṣanas*) that are also real; the difference is that the reality of the latter is dependent on the prior reality of God. The Viśiṣṭādvaita concludes that there is one God, qualified by matter and souls. According to Viśiṣṭādvaita, the unity of being (*advaita*) is therefore a complex (*viśiṣṭa*), consisting of God, matter, and individual souls. So, too, there is the Acintyabhedābheda ("different-yet-not-different") Vedānta based on the teachings of the fifteenth- to sixteenth-century Bengali Gauḍīya Vaiṣṇava theologian Caitanya, whose philosopher-followers held the position that God and the soul exist and are distinct from one another but within a larger context of divine unity, as perhaps the sparks of a fire are at once different and also not different from the fire itself. And there is also the Dvaita Vedānta represented by Madhva in the twelfth and thirteenth centuries, who took a dualistic (*dvaita*) and salvation-oriented theological stance, maintaining that God and individual souls are, in kind, essentially different and eternally distinct from one another and that the only reconciliation possible between the two is through God's grace. There is also the Śabda Advaita associated with the seventh-century philosopher-poet Bhartṛhari, who held that ultimate reality is essentially of the nature of the sacred Word (*vāc*) and that all things emerge from the primordial "sound" (*śabda*) made manifest in the Vedic mantras.

One hears little reference to these latter schools of Vedāntic thought in the words of swamis Muktananda and Chidvilasananda. Some of this may be due to the generally Śaiva- and Śākta-oriented theologies around which Siddha Yoga teachings largely revolve.[65] The closest Vedāntic vision to Siddha Yoga's besides Śaṅkarācārya's Kevala Advaita Vedānta would be Vallabhācārya's Śuddha Advaita. Muktananda and Chidvilasananda share Vallabha's fondness for the playful sport of God as Lord Kṛṣṇa within the complicated drama of the world, though the Siddha Yoga gurus are more likely to identify the playful Lord with the god Śiva or the goddess Kuṇḍalinī. Vallabha held that it is through the spiritual nourishment (*puṣṭi*) one gains by sharing in God's bliss (*ānanda*) that one comes to live a sublimely textured life. The religious tradition based on Vallabha's Śuddha Advaita is, therefore, sometimes known as the Puṣṭimārga, the "way of spiritual nourishment." Siddha Yoga does not share the "left-current" Tantric associations that characterize some of the Puṣṭimārga. The dualism of Madhva's Dvaita Vedānta is not consistent with Siddha Yoga's foundational nondualistic theologies and philosophies. The legacy of Rāmānuja's thought finds its home more in Śrī Vaiṣṇavism, the followers of which worship God as Viṣṇu, especially in association with Viṣṇu's feminine counterpart, Lakṣmī or Śrī. To be sure, Swami Muktananda and Swami Chidvilasananda have spoken with great reverence of Viṣṇu and Lakṣmī. But they do so from a nondualistic perspective. Similarly, the devotional tenor of Caitanya's Gauḍīya Vaiṣṇavism and other Bhakti traditions finds an echo reverberating through Siddha Yoga's affectionate and reverential praise of the Lord's joyful, liberating play in the world. But here, too, God's divinity is not, according to the perspective of Siddha Yoga, to be separated from the divinity of the Self. We may conclude from this that, for these siddha gurus, the Advaita Vedānta revelation of the Self more closely resembles that of Siddha Yoga than do such revelations presented by other forms of Vedānta.

Śaṅkarācārya, as was mentioned earlier, is generally acknowledged to be the most influential of Advaita theologians. His place in the larger history of Indian religious thought is approached perhaps only by that of Siddhārtha Gautama (whose teachings form the basis of Buddhism), Mahāvīra Vārdhamāna (the founder of Jainism), and Rāmānuja (whose ideas stand as the basis for Śrī Vaiṣṇavism). Śaṅkarācārya founded four monasteries (*maṭha*), which have stood as the model of Indian monasticism throughout the centuries. He also established ten orders of renunciant monks (*sannyāsin*), including the Sārasvatī Order, the monastic lineage into which swamis Muktananda and Chidvilasananda and all Siddha Yoga swamis have been initiated. Śaṅkarācārya's thorough nondualism finds a sympathetic voice in that of the magnificent Abhinavagupta, whose work stands as one of the pillars of Kashmir Śaivism. Śaṅkarācārya was a prolific writer who wrote astute and systematic commentaries (*bhāṣya*) on several of the Upaniṣads as well as on the *Bhagavadgītā* and the *Brahma Sūtra*. Advaita Vedānta as a religious tradition holds that he wrote a total of 117 works, consisting not only of these commentaries but also of a number of independent philosophical works (*prakaraṇa*) and devotional songs (*stotra*). The influence of Śaṅkarācārya's thought in the history of Indian religion has been extensive. Following an honored Indian tradition, a number of otherwise anonymous Indian philosophers and poets who were deeply affected by his teachings may have composed a number of those works in his name, including a number of *prakaraṇa*s and *stotra*s that are both philosophically astute and aesthetically pleasing. In their own teachings Swami Muktananda and Swami Chidvilasananda have referred with some frequency to a few of these latter works, particularly but not limited to the *Vivekacūḍāmaṇi*, the "Crest-Jewel of Discrimination," which outlines the difference between the real and the unreal; the *Aparokṣānubhūti*, "Direct Realization," which teaches the importance and means of knowing the Self as a "means of liberation";[66] and the *Ātmabodha,* "Self-Knowledge," a poem consisting of sixty-eight verses telling of the nature of the Self and of the way to come to know it. Śaṅkarācārya is also said to have composed the *Dakṣiṇāmūrti Stotra,* a devotional hymn to God as guru, from which are drawn some of the verses Siddha Yoga devotees sing twice each day as they chant the "Āratī."

Swamis Muktananda and Chidvilasananda encourage their students to look at the world from a nondualistic perspective. It is in the spirit of Advaita that Muktananda taught:

> With nondual vision, see only totality.
> In the many, see the One
> in whom all are contained.
> There is no division, no change.[67]

The nondual perspective similarly appears in Muktananda's encouragement to those who yearn to understand the absolute:

> O seeker, hear the immortal voice of the Self,
> and wake up!
> Balanced and serene in the world, pursue yoga.
> When you attain the true Principle
> through lengthy practice,
> your experience will teach you thus:
> . . . "What is fundamentally one cannot become many.
> If Brahman alone exists,
> how can there possibly be duality?
> Nothing that you hear or see is separate from Him.
> He is undifferentiated.
> I am Brahman, I am the Self."[68]

The importance of the Vedāntic perspective in Swami Muktananda's experience is indicated historically, in that his early spiritual training was primarily Vedāntic. He has said that he studied Vedānta from a teacher named Kabīrdās while practicing his initial sadhana (Sanskrit, *sādhana*) at Siddharuddha Swami's ashram near Hubli.[69] This would have been roughly from 1923 through 1928, although we cannot be absolutely certain of the dates. He studied Vedānta and Sanskrit for a number of years in the ashram of one of Siddharuddha's chief disciples, Muppinarya Swami. As Muktananda subsequently traveled throughout India, studying with teachers aligned with various spiritual traditions, his understanding of the scope of Vedānta seems to have expanded to include the essential teachings of a number of otherwise non-Vedāntic traditions. Wherever he saw nondual theological ideas and values, he embraced them, regardless of their outward presentation. He was attracted to the mysticism of the Sufi saints, for example, and came to cherish the thoroughly devotional religious sensibilities of the Marathi- and Hindi-speaking poet-saints of the eleventh through seventeenth centuries—the youthful Jñāneśvar, the tailor Nāmdev, the householder Eknāth, the shopkeeper Tukārām, the weaver Kabīr, the princess Mīrābāī, the scholar Tulsīdās, the outcaste leatherworker Ravidās, and the blind visionary Sūrdās. He found deep agreement with the nondual Śaivism of Kashmir as presented by such profound theologians, philosophers, and aesthetes as Kallaṭabhaṭṭa, Abhinavagupta, Bhāskara, Kṣemarāja, and Utpaladeva.

THE NOTION OF BRAHMAN

In order to understand more fully the Vedāntic perspective on the Self and its importance in Siddha Yoga tradition we need to look briefly at the history and use of the term *brahman*, beginning in Vedic literature before the time of the Upaniṣads. The Vedic tradition of which the Upaniṣads are said to be the fulfillment (*anta*) consists of a wide range of religious sensibilities, ideas, and practices. The Vedic worldview includes the following related ideas: that the forces of nature, the many deities who are said to have formed and to give life to the world, the structure and patterns of society, and the nature and destiny of the individual person are somehow all connected to one another through a universal order and harmony of being; that the integrating forces of vitality and truth, which express this power of being, are threatened by forces of disintegration and decay and thus need to be revitalized and supported; that because of the interconnectedness of all things, actions performed in any realm or place affect the condition of all others; and, finally, that by recognizing the presence and influence of that timeless and unchanging power of Being deep within one's own being, one thereby frees one's spirit from the vicissitudes of life and the constraints of death.

Within all of these Vedic ideas lies a common assumption or experience: It is possible to see and thereby to know this otherwise invisible power or principle that links all things. This presupposition stands behind the meaning of the Sanskrit word *veda*, which is based on a verbal root meaning to "know" (*vid-*) and which serves as both a verb and a noun. *Ya evaṃ veda*, ancient teachers asserted, that is: "One who thus knows" sees hidden foundational truths within the otherwise incomprehensible forces in the world of existence.

A Brahman *as Prayer*

The mysterious, hidden, unifying power that supports the wondrously intricate and complicated universe and keeps it from falling apart was known in Vedic India as the *brahman*. Based on the verbal root *bṛh-*, to "swell" or to "increase," the word literally means "possessing the power of pervasive expansiveness." In its earliest use, *brahman* referred to a powerfully transformative verse or phrase—a prayer, if you will—spoken by a priest. Singing forth a *brahman*, such a priest thereby sent vitality and strength to whomever or whatever the words of the *brahman* were directed. If spoken correctly, the object of this transformation was then pervaded and enlivened with expansive power. As a transformative word or phrase, a *brahman* was therefore similar in a way to a mantra, for both a *brahman* and a mantra possessed an inherent effective force which infused its object with sacred power. Priests directed their *brahmans* primarily to the many deities with whom the human community was understood to share the world as a home. A verse from the *Ṛgveda* (ca. 1200 B.C.E) illustrates this idea that, like an in-flowing stream swells the size of a lake, the power of a *brahman* "fills" the god Indra and causes his strength to increase: "O Indra, just as waves fill a [body] of water, so too *brahmans* fill you and cause you to expand."[70] Likewise, the gods Agni and Soma are said to be strengthened by the power of a *brahman*.[71] The opening verse in the fond and appreciative "Hymn to the Earth" (ca. 1000 B.C.E) has a poet-priest sing: "O purifying Earth, I invoke you! Bearer of nourishment and strength . . . O patient earth, which grows strong by means of the *brahman*. O Earth, we honor you with proper adoration."[72]

The Brahman *as Sacred Power*

A *brahman* as a sacred phrase or prayer thus effectively linked the human spirit with the larger divine and natural worlds. All *brahmans*, therefore, possessed a common power, namely, to unify an otherwise fractured world. Accordingly, the word *brahman* came to refer not only to a prayerful phrase but also to that cosmic power that made these sacred words effective. It is in this sense that we may therefore speak not only of *a brahman* but also of *the brahman*. The opening verse of the "Hymn to the Earth" lists *brahman* with other forces that maintain the world itself: "Expansive truth, unwavering universal order, consecration, contemplative fervor, sacrifice, and the *brahman* support the Earth."[73]

Vedic visionary sages came to see that the vital and revitalizing force of the *brahman*—understood now not only as a sacred mantra but also as the transformative cosmic power embodied by the mantra—extended invisibly throughout all of existence, joining all things together in an intricate tapestry of being. Experienced in this way, the *brahman* is the universal thread of which that tapestry is woven, warp and woof. As a Vedic song proclaims:

> One who knows the finely drawn thread on which
> the creatures are woven;

> one who knows the thread of that very thread:
> that person also knows the great *brahman.*[74]

From the Vedic perspective, the *brahman* is, thus, the hidden cosmic force and structure that supports and sustains all things in the universe. Without this *brahman,* the universe would disintegrate into a lifeless chaos, much as the pattern of a beautiful tapestry couldn't exist without the underlying threads. Even the passage of time itself depends on the hidden structure of being that connects otherwise discrete events. From the Vedic perspective, the fact that there is any effect whatsoever resulting from any cause whatsoever reveals *brahman,* for it is the underlying, eternal presence of the *brahman* that links the moments of time and all the events within it. Because the *brahman* is the source of time, it cannot be said to have been created in time; it is *svayambhū,* "self-existent." Uncreated as well as unaffected by the fluctuations of time, the *brahman* may be regarded as *nitya,* "unchanging" and thus "eternal."

Brahman as the Ground of Being

It was not long before Vedic philosopher-teachers came to regard the self-existent, eternal, and unchanging *brahman* on which all things are grounded and by which they are linked as the supreme Godhead itself. Accordingly, we may now speak not only of *the brahman* but also of Brahman, a word usually capitalized in English translations to mark the sanctity and divine power of its referent. Brahman is now ultimate reality; it is the ground of being, the absolute. The eternal power and presence that makes the universe possible, Brahman is the source of all beings. It is, in the words of the *Ṛgveda,* that "by which the earth is established, the heavenly realm is set firmly above, and the expansive atmosphere spread high and wide."[75]

We quoted a moment ago from a Vedic song that describes this ground of being as the "finely drawn thread on which the creatures are woven." These lines were first sung in India no later than 1000 B.C.E. It is a beautiful hymn worth translating at some length. Other verses of this song reflect the Vedic idea that, as the foundation and source of all beings, Brahman alone sustains the many different creatures of the world. They describe Brahman not only as the universal thread but also as a single, universal pillar on which all things in all times find their hidden support. From this hymn we hear the following reverential proclamation:

> Homage to that supreme Brahman who presides over all things—
> that which already exists and
> that which is yet to be—
> and to whom alone belongs heaven. . . .
> In him dwell all things that live and breathe,

all that open and close the eye. . . .
Though manifest, it is hidden and secret.
Its name is "Ancient." It is the Great Way of Being.
On that pillar is formed this whole universe:
on it is established all that moves and breathes.

The infinite stretches in all directions.
The infinite and the finite share a common boundary.
The protector of the heavens alone can separate the two;
he who knows what is, and what is to become. . . .
A hundred, a thousand, tens of thousands, a hundred million:
countless are the forms of his own entered into him.
They die; he looks on.
Thus shines this God. Thus is he.[76]

The poet-sages who sang this hymn noted that just as it is not bound by the constraints of time ("They die; he looks on."), the absolute—described in the following verse as feminine—is not bound by the constraints and definitions of space.

The One is smaller than a child;
the One is nearly invisible.
And yet this deity—she who is so dear to me—
is vaster than the whole expansive universe.[77]

The "One" of which the poet sings is said to live *within* all things and thus appears *as* all things. Addressing that divine presence, the poet proclaims:

You are woman. You are man.
You are boy, and young girl, too.
When old, you lean on a staff as you totter.
When born, you reveal your face in all directions.
He is their father, and also their son.
He is the largest and smallest of them.
He is the one God, who has entered into the mind:
the firstborn, yet even now within the womb.[78]

According to this hymn, all things in the world possess their own particular essence—and thus their own particular being—due to the underlying reality of the One. The following verses further explain, for example, that "It is because of her form that these trees are green, and green the garland of flowers." We also will see that the enveloping unity of the One is not diminished by the fact that it abides within each and every thing:

From fullness he spreads forth the full;
the full is poured with the full. . . .[79]

The deity, whose name is "Helpful," sits
enveloped by universal Order.
It is because of her form that these trees are green,
and green the garland of flowers.
See! The marvelous wisdom of God!
Near though he is, one cannot leave him!
Near though he is, one cannot see him!
He neither dies nor grows old![80]

Vedic sages came to realize that even the many gods and goddesses of the Vedic pantheon were actually manifold reflections or expressions of the singular Brahman. Referring to "the One" addressed variously by the names of several Vedic deities, the visionary sage Dīrghatamas, for example, proclaimed, "They call him Indra, Mitra, Varuṇa, Agni, and he is the heavenly Garutmān. The wise speak of what is One in many ways; they call it Agni, Yama, Mātariśvan."[81]

This idea that the many reflect or embody the One came to be a key element of Vedāntic thought. Teachers whose lessons form the early Upaniṣads tended not to assign a personal name to the absolute. Rather, they referred to it as "that One" (*tad ekam*), or simply as "That" (*tat*). The *Bṛhadāraṇyaka Upaniṣad* (ca. eighth century B.C.E) includes a conversation reported to have taken place between a sage and a seeker of the truth, here in edited form:

Then Vidagdha Śākalya asked him: "How many gods are there, Yājñavalkya?"
"Three hundred and thirty-three," [Yājñavalkya replied].
"Yes, but how many gods are there really?"
"Thirty-three."
"Yes, but how many gods are there really?"
"Six."
"Yes, but how many gods are there really?"
"Three."
"Yes, but how many gods are there really?"
"Two."
"Yes, but how many gods are there really?"
"One and a half."
"Yes, but how many gods are there really, Yājñavalkya?"
"One."
"Which is that one god?"
"He is the breath of life," [Yājñavalkya said]. "He is Brahman. He is what they call 'That.'"[82]

By leading him in this way, Yājñavalkya helps the seeker to understand that all of the many gods otherwise worshiped in the divine pantheon are, in fact, various powers or personifications of one ultimate reality, namely, Brahman.

Manifestations of Brahman

As the "breath of life" (*prāṇa*), Brahman gives beingness to all that lives. Remaining One, it is manifest in the many. And Upaniṣadic teachers described Brahman in other ways besides "breath." Brahman is also "wind" (*vāyu*), perhaps because the single wind refreshes the whole world as it blows throughout all places. As universal breath, the wind of being, the absolute is at times described as "life" or the "life-principle" or "life-energy" (all three of which translate the Sanskrit *āyu*), and also as "intelligence" (*prajñā*) and "immortality" (*amṛta*). In the *Kauṣītaki Brāhmaṇa Upaniṣad*, for example, God says: "I am the universal breath. Worship me as the intelligent self, as life, as immortality. Life is breath and breath is life. As long as breath remains in the body, so long is there life."[83] The instruction continues, "The breath of life is One," and thus:

> When we speak, the breaths of life speak.
> When we see, the breaths of life see.
> When we hear, the breaths of life hear.
> When we think, the breaths of life think.
> When we breathe, the breaths of life breathe.[84]

Some Upaniṣadic sages describe Brahman as "space" (*ākāśa*), for all things exist within the encompassing expanse of space. According to the *Muṇḍaka Upaniṣad* (ca. sixth to fifth centuries B.C.E), Brahman is the primordial light that illumines all things and by which all things are brought into existence: "There the sun does not shine, nor the moon, nor the stars. Neither there do the bolts of lightning shine, far less earthly flames. But all [these] shine because of him, the Shining One. From his light is illumined this whole world!"[85] Accordingly, Bādarāyaṇa said in his *Brahma Sūtra*, "Brahman is the primordial light."[86]

Elsewhere, teachers whose lessons form the *Kaṭha Upaniṣad* (ca. fifth century B.C.E) speak of Brahman as the hidden yet powerful energy of heat and fire which, having entered the universe, becomes all forms.[87] The *Chāndogya Upaniṣad* (ca. eighth century B.C.E) states that fire is the first element to emerge from the primordial reality that is Being itself—*sat*—and that from fire came water and from water emerged earth; accordingly, at the time of dissolution, earth returns to water, water returns to fire, and fire returns to the reality of pure Being, the substratum or foundation (*mūla*) of the universe, which the Upaniṣad calls the "highest divinity."[88] The sages of the *Chāndogya Upaniṣad* equate Brahman not only with breath and space, but also equate these two with bliss (*ānanda*). "Brahman is breath. Brahman is bliss. Brahman is expansive space."[89]

The *Taittirīya Upaniṣad* (ca. seventh century B.C.E) declares: "The knower of Brahman attains the Supreme"; for "one who knows Brahman as the real, as knowledge, and as the infinite [*satya, jñāna, ananta*], established in the secret place of the heart and in the highest realm, realizes . . . Brahman, the intelligent."[90] A story told in the same Upaniṣad recounts a conversation between a student and his father, whom the young man had asked to explain the nature of Brahman. The father tells him that Brahman is not only "physical matter, life-force, sight, hearing, mind, speech," but furthermore Brahman is "truly, that from which these beings are born; that by which, once born, they live; that into which, when departing, they enter." The teacher, Varuṇa, tells Bhṛgu, his son, *tad vijijñāsava tad brahmeti*: "That, seek to know; for That is Brahman."[91] Bhṛgu contemplates this teaching and eventually realizes that Brahman may be known in increasingly subtle and sublime ways. First he comprehends, "Physical matter is Brahman, for truly, beings are born from physical matter when they are born; they live on physical matter, and into physical matter they enter when departing." Further contemplating this, he understands that the life-force itself is Brahman, for "Truly, beings are born of the life-force when they are born; they live by means of the life-force; and they return to the life-force when they depart." Bhṛgu's continuing reflection leads him to discover increasingly subtle forms of Brahman. More subtle than the life-force is mind. More subtle than mind is intelligence. Bhṛgu comes finally to realize that Brahman is more subtle even than intelligence itself. Brahman is *ānanda*. "He knew that Brahman is bliss. For truly beings are born of bliss when they are born, they live by bliss, and they enter into bliss when they depart." The Upaniṣad then says that "one who knows this, the wisdom of Varuṇa and Bhṛgu, becomes established in the highest heaven. . . . One becomes great . . . in the splendor of sacred wisdom [*brahmavarcasa*]."[92]

A similar story appears in the *Chāndogya Upaniṣad*. Here an accomplished yet humble scholar-seeker, Nārada, asks the sage Sanatkumāra to teach him of the nature of Brahman. Sanatkumāra asks Nārada what he already knows and then promises to teach him "what is beyond that." The scholar replies that he knows all of the Vedas and all of the ancient sacred literature. He knows philosophy and mathematics and astronomy. He knows logic, ethics, and politics. He knows the fine arts. "But," he admits, "I am like one who simply knows words," and he adds, "I do not know the Self." To this, Sanatkumāra replies: "Truly, whatever you have learned here is only a name. . . . Meditate on name itself. One who meditates on name as Brahman becomes free as far as name goes."[93] In other words, Sanatkumāra teaches Nārada a threefold lesson: Words cannot fully reveal Brahman; nevertheless, to one who is attentive to it, Brahman *is* revealed in words (as it is in all things); and that, knowing this, one is liberated from the constraints of language. Sanatkumāra brings Nārada's attention to increasingly subtle and sublime forms of the absolute. Brahman as speech is more subtle than Brahman as name. Mind is more sublime than speech. Will or intention is more subtle than mind; thought is more subtle than will. Contemplation is more sublime than thought, while understanding is more sublime than contemplation. The progression moves onward to include other increasingly subtle forms of Brahman, including, among others, memory, hope, and the basic life principle. Sanatkumāra teaches Nārada that infinite abundance (*bhūman*) is more sublime and encompassing than the life principle, and that such abundance is of the nature of joy (*sukha*). He then teaches Nārada that such infinite joy pervades the whole universe: "Truly, it is below. It is above. It is behind. It is in front. It is to the south, it is to the north. Truly, it is this all [*sa evedaṃ sarvam iti*]."[94]

Drawing on all of these different ways of speaking about Brahman and condensing them into perhaps their most sublime form, Vedāntic teachers in general came to teach that Brahman is *sat-cit-ānanda*: being, consciousness, and bliss.

Despite the different ways they described it, Vedāntic teachers held that the absolute resides within all things as the beingness of being, and that this eternal reality is not bound by the constraints of death. Upaniṣadic sages were at times to state this lesson quite poetically, as in the following passage from the *Brahmabindu Upaniṣad*:

> There is only a single Being-Self.
> It lives in each and every being.
> Uniform, yet multiform, it appears like the [reflections of the single] moon
> on [the many ripples of] a pond.
>
> [Think of] the empty space enclosed by a jar.
> When the jar is broken into pieces,
> the jar alone breaks, not the space.
> Life is like the jar.
>
> All [manifest] forms are like the jar.
> They constantly break into pieces.
> When gone, they are unaware.
> Yet, he is aware, eternally.[95]

Brahman Behind the Veil of Ignorance

The nondual Vedānta holds that Brahman is the sole Self of the universe. According to Advaita, not only is Brahman the universal Self, it is also the real, as opposed to the unreal. From this perspective, the real is therefore unchanging. One implication of this line of thought is that whatever changes must in some way be unreal. If this is the case, then what is one to think of life in a world that is constantly changing? Is the world therefore unreal?

Advaita thinkers resolved this problem by teaching that the world as we normally experience it—a world of manifold multiplicity and change and, therefore, of decay, misery, and bondage to death—is actually a result of the human mind's tendency to "project" or "superimpose" its habitual ways of understanding things onto the essentially changeless Brahman. Such a projection or superimposition is a result of one's ignorance (*avidyā*) of the actual unchanging reality of Brahman. In order to know Brahman, in order to know the undying Self, one must therefore remove the veil of ignorance and discern the difference between the real and the unreal, the eternal and the momentary, the infinite and the finite. Advaita Vedānta describes such a superimposition (*vivarta, adhyāsa*) and the suffering it brings as being similar to the way one is frightened by a snake that, upon closer inspection, is seen to be in fact a coiled rope. Śaṅkarācārya alludes to this phenomenon of the snake and the rope when he says:

> The veil of ignorance vanishes only when one has a vision of the real. As long as there is false perception, that mistake causes distraction and misery. Misery ends when false perception is corrected. These three [ignorance, false perception, and misery] appear, for example, in the case of a rope [which is mistaken for a snake. As soon as one realizes that the rope is a rope, the snake vanishes, and one is no longer tormented by the fear it caused.] Therefore, the wise person who wishes to be liberated from bondage must know the Real.[96]

Advaita Vedānta holds that the mind superimposes an apparent world of multiplicity and change onto the singular and stable Brahman, just as it superimposes a snake onto what is in fact a rope. We might think of the visual illusion often presented in the study of psychology in which a picture depicting the silhouette of a vase may, from another perspective, look like the profile of two faces. What is real? Is it the vase? Or is it the two faces? In a sense, neither is real. Both are projections, superimpositions, onto the paper of the mind's habitual ways of organizing the world. What is "real" in this example is the ink on the page. The vase and faces are therefore imaginary forms that "disappear" when the actual reality is known. This is true for the recognition of the eternal Brahman within the changing contours of our lives, as well. Advaita holds the position that what we experience as the world of different personalities and forms is actually a complicated image of what we *want* to see or have *become accustomed* to seeing. Swami Muktananda expresses a similar perspective when he says, "That Self is . . . beyond distinctions of name, color, and sex. . . . We have superimposed different notions onto that [Self], notions like, 'I am black,' 'I am white,' 'I am a man,' 'I am a woman,' 'I am American,' 'I am Indian.'"[97]

Understood from this perspective, we live in a world that we have created ourselves through our own ignorance of Brahman. This is a world in which apparently distinct beings live in isolation from each other. It is a world of change, marked by birth and death and rebirth and, once again, death. It is an inexorable cycle of momentary happiness followed inevitably by loss and disappointment. Vedānta calls this cycle *saṃsāra,* the turning "wheel of life," the "disease of worldliness." According to Advaita Vedānta, the world of *saṃsāra* is a result of what it calls *māyā,* a word often translated in this context as "illusion." The power of *māyā* is therefore inextricably connected with the force of ignorance (*avidyā*). Vedāntic thinkers in general hold that one cannot find true contentment and joy until one no longer lives in the fruitless redundancy brought on through the forces of illusion and ignorance. One is urged, therefore, to seek freedom or liberation (*mukti, mokṣa*) from this cycle. It is for this reason that the Vedānta teaches that one is to know Brahman. Said differently, one is to know the Self.

THE SELF AS ĀTMAN

From the Vedāntic perspective, Brahman is the absolute, the ground of being that supports the very beingness of all things. But the Vedānta also uses the term *ātman* to refer to the abiding, essential "Self" of the universe. The derivation of the word *ātman* remains uncertain. The classical Indian etymologist Yāska held that the term comes from two verbal roots, one meaning to "move constantly" and the other to "pervade."[98] The great Sanskrit grammarian Pāṇini (sixth or fifth century B.C.E) also derived the word from a verbal root meaning to "move constantly."[99] Śaṅkarācārya traced the word to a verbal root meaning to "obtain" or to "enjoy" and thus by extension, similarly, to "pervade" all.[100] More recently, various scholars have traced what they felt to be the origin of *ātman* to verbal roots meaning to "go," to "blow," and to "breathe."[101] Just what its actual derivation may be is not of particular interest to us in our present concern. But it is notable that, in each possibility, we see the suggestion of an expansive and animating power. In fact, the earliest use in the *Ṛgveda* of the word *ātman* likely implied "wind," with which is quite understandably associated the sense of "breath."[102] Breath is then connected with the sense of "life force" and thus of "spirit" as distinct from physical body.

In the earliest literatures of the Vedic canon, the word *ātman* is associated with the vital "spirit" of a deity whose body is the physical universe. The *Ṛgveda* (ca. 1200 B.C.E) mentions a divine and universal "Self" identified as Puruṣa or Bṛhaspati or Viśvakarman. We hear, too, of Hiraṇyagarbha, the "Golden Embryo," whose Self takes birth as the world. Beginning with the *Atharvaveda* (ca. 1000 B.C.E), we see the term used in reference to the sublime, hidden, and essential nature of not only a universal deity but other beings as well.[103] It is in this way that the word *ātman* entered late Vedic and early Vedāntic texts to refer to the inward "essence" or "self" of anything.[104]

The Enlivening Inward Presence of the Divine

In their wider connotations, the meaning of the words *ātman* and *brahman* were, therefore, quite similar. But whereas the essence of Brahman is impersonal, Ātman is more personal in nature. If *brahman* referred to the ground of being—what Radhakrishnan called the "eternal quiet underneath the drive and activity of the universe"[105]—*ātman* came to stand for "the foundational reality underlying the conscious powers of the individual, the inward ground of the human soul."[106] We might say that if Brahman is the divine Self abiding in the macrocosm as a whole, Ātman is the Self dwelling within the microcosm. This is an enlivening, vital presence. According to the *Aitareya Upaniṣad*, even after its various physical organs have been fashioned, a person's material body cannot function without the indwelling presence of the power of life. Perceiving this, the universal Creator, the very power of being itself, entered into the various physical and mental organs—"This is a dwelling place," he declared—where it watches over the body as a whole.[107]

The Self as Ātman was, therefore, to be distinguished from the self as manifest body and personality, the latter being infused with the reality and power of the Ātman. The *Taittirīya Upaniṣad* speaks repeatedly of the various dimensions of the spiritual, mental, and physical body as being "full of" or "filled by" the sublime Self.[108] According to the Upaniṣadic sages, a true seeker is therefore to discern and honor and revere that vital, abiding Self rather than the transitory physical or psychological self.

We see an example of this teaching in a conversation between the sage Yājñavalkya and his wife, Maitreyī, as reported in the *Bṛhadāraṇyaka Upaniṣad*. Yājñavalkya has informed his wife that he plans to depart for the forest, where he will practice contemplation in solitude, and that he has arranged his affairs so that Maitreyī will be well cared for in his absence. She responds by saying that she is not interested in material wealth and comfort but would rather he give her his wisdom instead: "What can I do with things that do not bring immortality?" she asks. "Your understanding, sir: this, please tell me!" Yājñavalkya treats her request with respect—"You speak dear words"—and agrees to share his knowledge with her.[109] He then proceeds to teach her:

Truly, it is not for the love of a husband that a husband is dear;
rather, it is for the love of the Self [Ātman] that a husband is dear.
It is not for the love of a wife that a wife is dear;
rather, it is for the love of the Self that a wife is dear.
It is not for the love of children that children are dear,
rather it is for the love of the Self that children are dear.

. . .

Truly, O Maitreyī, it is the Self that
is to be seen, heard, reflected on, and meditated upon.[110]

The lesson here seems to be, in part, that one cannot truly love another until one uncategorically and unconditionally loves the Self—the Soul—residing within the other. Yājñavalkya's body is transient and subject to change, but the Self residing within that body is not. True love recognizes and honors the eternal within the temporal. All other forms of love are simply superimpositions of one's own conditions and expectations and desires onto the divine Self.

The Uncategorical, Sublime, and Essential Being

As the underlying universal reality on which all otherwise individual realities are superimposed, Ātman must necessarily be without form. To think of it as having physical qualities is to misunderstand or misperceive the true nature of the Self. As Yājñavalkya repeatedly taught his disciples, the Self is *neti neti*: "not this, not this!"[111]

That Self, which stands as the fundamental principle of one's very being, is without any qualities. As Prajāpati tells Indra in the *Chāndogya Upaniṣad*, the Self is like the empty sky into which clouds of various shapes momentarily form, through which they briefly move, and from which they disappear. Physical bodies are like the clouds: they come and go while the Self remains.[112]

The Self is said to be the foundational awareness that never sleeps, even though the body and mind slumber. An early Vedāntic example of this teaching appears in the *Māṇḍūkya Upaniṣad*, which holds that there are four increasingly subtle levels of consciousness.[113] In waking consciousness, one is aware of the world in its objective multiplicity. In dream consciousness, one lives in a world of similar multiplicity, but does so within one's own mind. In dreamless sleep, even those many mentally formed objects disappear into the steady, quiet, and abiding Self that sustains the sleeper while he or she rests. In this third level of consciousness, however, there is no awareness per se, and thus no experience of being. But the Upaniṣad goes on to describe a deeper and more encompassing level of consciousness it calls *caturtha* (the "fourth") in which the Self knows itself as the supreme subject, the source of all objects. This deepest and most subtle state of consciousness is "unseen, indescribable, ungraspable, without distinguishing characteristics, beyond thought, without name, the essence of the knowledge of the one Self, that into which the world is resolved, peaceful, benevolent, nondual."[114] The *Māṇḍūkya* identifies the fourth level of consciousness with the sacred syllable *auṃ*.[115] Other Upaniṣads refer to this level of consciousness as *turya* and as *turīya*, both of which also mean "the fourth."[116] Later Vedāntic works invariably refer to the state as *turīya*. In any case, the Upaniṣads identify this sublime level of awareness as the Self: "This is the Ātman. It is to be known. . . . One who knows this thus enters into the Self with one's self."[117]

The Ātman is therefore the invisible yet vital source and essence of one's being. This lesson finds articulate expression in a set of teachings given in the form of analogies by the wise Uddālaka to his son Śvetaketu, as recorded in the *Chāndogya Upaniṣad*. The conversation between the two is a long one. The following exchange is representative.

> "Bring me a fruit from that sacred fig tree there," [Uddālaka tells Śvetaketu].
> "Here it is, sir," [Śvetaketu replies].
> "Break it open."
> "It is broken open, sir."
> "What do you see there?"
> "These extremely small seeds, sir."
> "Of these, please break one open."
> "It is broken open, sir."
> "What do you see there?"
> "Nothing at all, sir."

Uddālaka then ceases his questions and points out to Śvetaketu:

> "That subtle essence which you do not perceive, my dear: truly, it is from that subtle essence that this immense fig tree arises! Believe me, my dear!"

The teacher then shifts his disciple's attention to the nature of the sublime universal essence that similarly resides within all being, including his own being:

> "That which is the subtle essence: this whole world has as its Self! That is Reality. That is Ātman. O Śvetaketu, you are That!" [*tat tvam asi*][118]

The Layering of the Self from Manifest to Sublime

That which brings life to and sustains life in the material body, Ātman is itself not of a material nature. Like Brahman, Ātman is a sublime presence and power, without which physical matter remains inert and lifeless. Accordingly, the more sublime aspects of one's being are closer to the soul than are the manifest parts. Vedāntic thinkers therefore saw a certain "layering" of the Ātman, as it were. A good example appears in a set of teachings presented by the *Taittirīya Upaniṣad,* which speaks of different levels of the Self. The external world beyond the confines of the physical body it calls the realm of "food" (*anna*), for all creatures must necessarily gain nutrition and vitality from food, and it is therefore "from food [that] all creatures whatsoever dwell on earth." The Upaniṣad calls the physical body itself *ātmā prāṇamayaḥ,* the "self that consists of the life force." Within the material body, however, is a series of increasingly more subtle bodies arranged in a concentric order, if you will. More subtle than the physical self is the "self consisting of mind" (*ātmā manomayaḥ*). More subtle than the mind is the "self consisting of understanding" (*ātmā vijñānamayaḥ*). The Upaniṣad thus far identifies four layers of the self: the outer world, the physical body, the mental self, and the wisdom-self. It also notes that there is a fifth layer: *ātmā ānandamayaḥ,* the "Self consisting of bliss."[119]

According to the sages whose teachings form the *Taittirīya Upaniṣad,* the most sublime and true quality of one's being is that of bliss. From this perspective, *ānanda* is the Self's original and deepest nature. The Self, therefore, reveals its true form in bliss.

Ātman and the Individual "Self" (Jīva, Bhūtātman)

Upaniṣadic teachers spoke of the individual "self"—one's particular being rather than the Self of the universe—as *jīva,* a word we may translate as "the living one." It is the *jīva* that thinks of itself as an individual person with a particular body and distinct personality. It is the *jīva* that identifies itself as "male" or "female" or "tall" or "short." Later Upaniṣadic thought, influenced by a complicated philosophical system known as the Sāṃkhya, came to associate the *jīva* with various aspects of *prakṛti,* "physical existence" or, more literally, "that which has emerged" into manifest form. Most particularly, *jīva* resembles the function of what Sāṃkhya calls *ahaṃkāra,* the "ego," which suggests an awareness of oneself as separate or different from others. The *jīva* is therefore the "self" (lower case) as it is normally experienced. Upaniṣadic and Vedāntic thought in general hold that one's *jīva* mistakenly regards itself as the agent and benefactor of one's actions. It is the *jīva,* then, that benefits and suffers from the forces of karma and thus undergoes the cycles of *saṃsāra.*

The *jīva* is to the Ātman as a particular individual wave is to the abiding and deep ocean across which it moves. The wave exists in and is precisely the same as the ocean, yet it cannot be said to *be* the ocean in its entirety. Similarly, the *jīva* is both the Ātman and not the Ātman at one and the same time. To help clear up possible confusion, perhaps, Vedāntic teachers sometimes called the lower-case "self" *bhūtātman,* that is to say, the "elemental self" or "self consisting of the physical elements." We read in the *Maitrī Upaniṣad* (ca. fifth century B.C.E), for example, of the distinction between Ātman and *bhūtātman.* It begins with a description of Ātman:

> Truly, wise seers declare that this Ātman wanders here on earth in all bodies, unaffected as it were by the light or dark effects of karma. Because of this, its unmanifest and subtle nature, imperceptibility, ungraspability, and freedom from a sense of separate self [*nirmamatva*], it appears that [the Ātman] does things and undergoes change. But, truly, it is pure, steadfast, unswerving, unstained, unagitated, and free from craving. It remains fixed, like a witness, and abiding in its own Self.[120]

The passage then turns to an outline of the nature of *bhūtātman:*

> There is another [self] called the "elemental self." He is different. He is overcome by the light and dark effects of karma and thus enters a good or an evil womb, so that his course [from birth to birth] is downward or upward and he wanders about, overcome by the nature of opposites. . . . Now, because he is overcome, he goes on to become confused, and because of this confusion he does not see the Lord [*prabhu*], the [true] source of action, who stands within himself. Carried along and defiled by the stream of [physical] qualities, unsteady, wavering, befuddled, filled by craving, distracted, he falls into the state of self-infatuation [*abhimānatva*]. By thinking, "This is me" and "That is mine," he binds himself with his self, like a bird [caught] in a snare.[121]

Vedāntic thought, therefore, holds that the various forms of fear and doubt and dismay—and the experience of life that such debilitating and alienating forces engender—result from the *jīva*'s or *bhūtātman*'s mistaken conclusion that it is all that the "self" is. The *jīva* thinks of itself as *ātman,* the true self. According to Advaita Vedānta, this is not entirely wrong, for the *jīva* is an embodiment, albeit a contracted and ignorant embodiment, of the true Ātman. But it is not all that the Ātman is. Whereas the *jīva* mistakenly *thinks* it is a self, the Ātman *is,* always was, and always will be the Self. As the *Bṛhadāraṇyaka Upaniṣad* says, "The priest, the soldier, and these various worlds, these Vedas and all of these beings: All this is the Self!" (*idaṃ sarvam yad ayam ātmā*).[122]

This of course leads us to one of the basic and most fundamental of Indian religious ideas, namely, that it is one's mistaken identification with one's body and mind that leads a person to confusion, addiction, conceit, and the recurring cycles of birth and death. From the general Hindu perspective, the way out of such *saṃsāra* is therefore to be free of one's mistaken identity and to recognize the true Self. Attached to the false idea that one can gratify the *bhūtātman,* which is constantly changing, the foolish person seeks meaning and a sense of identity from outside sources. The Upaniṣads are firm in pointing out both the futility of doing this and the value of looking within to find the true Self. According to the *Kaṭha Upaniṣad*, for example:

> Seeking life eternal, a wise person
> beholds the Ātman with his gaze turned inward.
> The [spiritually] immature seek outward pleasures;
> they walk into the widespread snare of death.
> But wise people, knowing life eternal,
> seek not the changeless among those things that change.[123]

BRAHMAN IS ĀTMAN

Coming inwardly to know the Ātman, Upaniṣadic seekers thereby came to know the universal Self that resides within all beings. And knowing that Self, they came to know the very ground of being. Accordingly, in a revelation that has reverberated in Indian spirituality through the many centuries since it was first declared, Upaniṣadic teachers proclaimed that the essence of Ātman and the essence of Brahman are one and the same. Nowhere in the early Vedānta is the identity of Ātman and Brahman more succinctly stated than in the *Māṇḍūkya Upaniṣad* (ca. fifth century B.C.E), which states, *sarvaṃ hy etad brahma ayam ātmā brahma,* "Truly, all this is verily Brahman! This Atman is Brahman."[124]

Said differently, the soul within one's heart is the same as the universal, divine Self. As the *Muṇḍaka Upaniṣad* says:

> Enthroned behind an excellent, golden veil
> sits Brahman, untainted and undivided.
> Brilliant, it is the light of lights.
> One who knows Ātman, knows it.
> It shines forth: vast, transcendent, of unthinkable form,
> and yet more minute than the minute.
> For those who behold it, it is farther than the far
> yet here, near at hand, abiding in the cave of the heart.[125]

Vedāntic thought thus came to regard the revelation of the Svayambhū Ātman—the self-existent and thus uncreated, eternal Soul residing within one's own being[126]—as equivalent to the revelation of the Svayambhū Brahman,[127] the self-existent absolute. There is only one Self.

The Vedāntic understanding that the absolute alone is real means that this reality abides also within (or as) the human soul; the ignorance found in the human mind cannot stain or lessen its glory. This idea finds expression in the following lines attributed to Śaṅkarācārya from the *Vivekacūḍāmaṇi*:

> Brahman is existence, knowledge, infinity.
> It is sure, supreme, self-existent, eternal.
> It is unbroken bliss, not separate from the individual soul,
> and having neither exterior nor interior,
> it is eternally triumphant.
>
> This supreme Unity alone is real,
> since there is nothing else but the Self.
> Truly, there remains no other independent entity
> in the experience of the highest truth.[128]

The realization that there is only one Self in the universe led to the quintessentially Vedāntic teaching: To experience one's fundamental identity with the eternal Brahman brings freedom from the recurring cycles of birth and death and an unbounded magnificent joy. As Śaṅkarācārya is reported to have taught:

> The realization of one's undivided union with Brahman brings liberation from the [repeated return to] birth;
> [such revelation] is the means by which the awakened attain Brahman,
> the One without a second, bliss itself.[129]

The *Aitareya Upaniṣad* (ca. eighth century B.C.E), which mentions the body is the "dwelling place" of the Self,[130] offers us another perspective on the nature of this great inner being. According to this text, the Creator is said to have entered the body and mind, whence he "looked at" those creations, ("He perceived this very person," the Upaniṣad notes) and said, "I have perceived this." The Creator is therefore known as Idandra, a name the Upaniṣad glosses as *idaṃ-dra*, "the perceiver of this."[131] According to this line of thought, therefore, the inner Soul is the divine "Witness" who looks out onto the physical and mental self. Vedāntic thought in general has described this inner Witness as *sākṣin*, "the one who observes."

The Witness is the universal subject by which any and all objects are known. As the vital principle of life and being, the Self is that from which all objects emerge and in which all objects find their existence. But, being *svayambhū*, "self-existent" and therefore uncreated, the Self is not itself an object. Accordingly, it cannot be known in objective ways. How is one therefore to know it? The *Kena Upaniṣad* (ca. fifth century B.C.E) reports a similar set of queries from a seeker:

By whose will and direction does the mind descend [onto its object
of thought]?
By whose command does the first breath of life stir?
By whose will do people speak forth language?
Please, what god is it that prompts the eye [to see] and the ear [to
hear]?[132]

The teachers whose lessons form that Upaniṣad state that they cannot describe this universal Subject by which all objects are known:

There the eye goes not,
speech goes not, nor the mind.
We do not know, we do not understand,
how one can teach this![133]

Acknowledging the ineffable nature of the Self, those teachers say the reason one cannot know the Self through the senses and mind is that the Self is not an object; it is the very foundation and power that gives rise to and supports not only worldly objects but also the senses and the mind. The Self is therefore that "by whom" (*kena*) the world exists and comes to be known (hence the title of the *Kena Upaniṣad*). The Self is that power and underlying truth by which the ear hears, the mind thinks, the eye sees.

It is That which is the hearing of the ear, the thought of the mind,
the speech, truly, of speech, the breathing of the breath,
and the sight of the eye. Freeing themselves [from attachment to
these]
the wise become immortal upon leaving behind this [conditioned]
world. . . .
That which is not expressed by speech
but by which speech is expressed: know That as Brahman.
That which is not thought by the mind
but by which, they say, the mind thinks: truly, know That as Brahman.
That which is not seen by the eye
but which the eyes see: truly, know That as Brahman.[134]

Knowledge of Brahman thus demands a paradoxical shift in the direction of one's awareness. Brahman is not an object to be known—it is "That which is not thought by the mind"—and yet one is to "know That as Brahman." The shift takes one away from concentrating on the Self as an object and reveals it as the supreme Subject—the effective power of being that allows one to know anything. It is that "by which the mind thinks."

Yājñavalkya presents a similar teaching to an inquiring seeker who has asked, "Explain to me just who is Brahman here and now and not beyond our comprehension, he who is the Self in all things." Yājñavalkya replies, "He is your Self, which is in all things." Still confused, the seeker asks, "Which one, O Yājñavalkya, is in all things?" The teacher answers by pointing out:

> He who breathes in with your breathing is the Self of yours, which is in all things. He who breathes out with your breathing is the Self of yours, which is in all things. . . . You cannot see the Seer of seeing. You cannot hear the Hearer of hearing. You cannot think the Thinker of thinking. You cannot understand the Understander of understanding. He is your Self, which is in all things.[135]

If this is true—that "you cannot think the Thinker of thinking"—then how does one come to know the Self? As we will see shortly, the Upaniṣads give seekers the ways by which they are to know the intellectually unknowable Self, namely, through meditation and through being open to the grace of God.

Although the Upaniṣads warn the spiritual seeker not to identify the Self with the physical body, many passages throughout Vedāntic texts speak with particular emphasis of the "secret place of the heart" or the "lotus of the heart" as the abode of this divine presence.[136] The Upaniṣads sometimes call the body the "city of Brahman," much as other religious traditions speak of the body as the "temple of God." The *Chāndogya Upaniṣad* says:

> Within this city of Brahman is a small house or lotus flower, and within this lotus flower is a small space. That which is within this space, that should be sought, for truly that is what one should yearn to understand.[137]

The realm of the heart is said to encompass all things:

> Truly, as far as the space of this [universe] extends, that far extends the space within the heart. Within it are held both heaven and earth, both fire and air, both sun and moon, lightning and the stars. Whatever there is of him [in the outer world] and whatever there is not: all of that is held within [the heart].[138]

Just as it is infinite in scope, the lotus of the heart as the abode of the Self is eternal in nature. It is therefore not buffeted by change. It seeks that which is abiding rather than transient:

> The Self does not age and does not die at the death [of the body]. . . . The Self is free from taint, free from old age, free from death, free from sorrow, free from hunger and thirst. Its yearnings are for the Real. Its thoughts are for the Real.[139]

Entering into the heart, the abode of the Self, one thereby enters the divinity of Being. One returns to Brahman:

> Truly, the Self abides in the heart. Knowing this, the [wise person] enters daily into the heavenly world. The Self is the immortal, the fearless. That is Brahman. The name of that Brahman is Truth.[140]

ĀTMAN AS UNIVERSAL LORD

The related Vedāntic insights that the Self alone is real and that this Self—the absolute reality on which the whole universe is grounded—resides within the human heart lead us to another realization that is of unparalleled significance, not only to Vedānta but also to many other religious traditions of India and certainly to Siddha Yoga: Ātman is none other than the universal "Lord". The sage Yājñavalkya, for example, is said to have used royal or monarchic imagery to describe the universal Self:

> Truly, this Ātman is the Overlord [*adhipati*] of all beings. He is the king [*rājan*] of all beings. Just as all of the spokes are held together in the hub and felly of a wheel, so in this Self all beings, all gods, all worlds, all breathing creatures, all these selves are held together.[141]

Other Upaniṣadic teachers describe the one Self residing within all beings using similarly majestic terms. The sages of the *Śvetāśvatara Upaniṣad* (ca. fifth century B.C.E.), for example, believed:

> Higher than this [world] is Brahman, the supreme, the great,
> hidden in all things according to their [particular] bodies.
> The One who embraces the universe:
> by knowing him, the Lord [*īśa*], people become immortal.[142]

According to the *Śvetāśvatara Upaniṣad,* the Self as universal Lord or King reveals itself in and through the forms of the many gods. Here, the Self is not only Brahman and Ātman, but the One who creates the universe, the One into which that universe dissolves, and the One who gives the sage the wisdom to know this.

> The One—who himself has no color—
> by the manifest exercise of his transformative power [*śakti*]
> distributes the many colors in his hidden purpose
> and into whom the universe is gathered in the beginning and end:
> may he endow us with clear understanding!
> Truly, that is Agni. Truly, that is Āditya,
> that is Vāyu, and that is the moon.

Truly, that is the pure. That is Brahmā.
That is the waters. That is Prajāpati.[143]

The *Śvetāśvatara Upaniṣad* refers to different aspects of that universal One. For example, it speaks of the One as the Lord, the bestower of blessings, the adorable, the creator of all things, the embracer of all things; it also speaks of the One as God and describes that divinity as *śiva,* a word which in this instance serves not as a proper noun but rather as an adjective meaning "kind" or "benevolent" or "auspicious." The Upaniṣad teaches that one attains unending peace if one knows God as *śiva*:

The One who rules each and every source,
in whom this whole universe comes together and dissolves,
the Lord, the bestower of blessings, God, the adorable:
by discerning him, one goes forever to this peace. . . .
More minute than the minute, in the midst of confusion
the creator of all, of many forms,
the one embracer of all things:
by knowing him as kind [*śiva*] one attains peace forever.
. . .
By knowing him as benevolent [*śiva*], he who is hidden in all things,
like the exceedingly fine cream that rises from clarified butter:
By knowing God, one is liberated from all fetters.[144]

The word *śiva* also stands, of course, as a sectarian epithet for God as Śiva, whose name accordingly means the "Auspicious One" or the "Benevolent One." Later sectarian Upaniṣads continue in this identification of the absolute with a supreme deity. Some Śaiva teachers follow the *Śvetāśvatara Upaniṣad* in urging their students to know Lord Śiva or sometimes Rudra, the latter being a Vedic precursor to the former.[145] Vaiṣṇava teachers referred to the supreme deity as Viṣṇu, usually in one or another of his incarnations.[146] For still others—notably those aligned with the Śākta Tantric tradition, which worships God as feminine power[147]—the absolute is not the universal Lord but rather the universal Lady, as it were. The *Tripurā Upaniṣad,* for example, praises the Goddess as "the abode of all, deathless, ancient, great [and] the principal cause of the greatness of the gods." She is "the Joyous, the Proud, the Auspicious, and the Prosperous. And she is the Beautiful and the Pure One; the Modest, the Intelligent, the Satisfied, the Desired, the Thriving, the Wealthy, Lalitā [the Lovely]." She is the "Mother of the Universe."[148] Referring to four of the teachings of the Vedānta represented by various *mahāvākyas* ("great statements"), the *Bahvṛcā Upaniṣad* says this of her:

> She alone is Ātman. . . . She is Brahman. . . . The holy, revealed texts have said that "You are That" and "This Ātman is Brahman" and "I am Brahman" and "Brahman alone am I." But she who is contemplated as "That which I Am" . . . is the Beautiful Great Goddess of the Three Cities, the Virgin, the Mother, the Lady of the Universe.[149]

Whether God is honored as Śiva, Viṣṇu, the Goddess, or any other name for the supreme deity, the theistic Vedāntic view holds that these deities are nothing but forms of the absolute truth, Brahman, and therefore they are also Ātman. From this perspective, God is the Self, and the Self is God.

THE EMPHASIS ON MEDITATION

We have already noted the Vedāntic understanding that to know the eternal and unchanging Self, and to know of its essential unity with the divinity of being, delivers one from the constraining and fractious cycle of constant becoming. As the *Śvetāśvatara Upaniṣad* puts it:

> Like a mirror clouded by dust
> shines brilliantly when it has been cleaned,
> the embodied one—upon seeing the nature of Ātman—
> becomes integrated, of fulfilled purpose, and liberated from sorrow.
> When one who is integrated beholds, as if by [the light of] a lamp,
> the essence of Brahman by seeing the essence of the soul as
> unborn, abiding, free of all [limiting] characteristics:
> By knowing God, one is released from all fetters.[150]

To answer the crucial question: How can this glorious Self be known?, the Upaniṣads give one overriding prescription: Meditate on the universal divinity residing within the heart. The *Taittirīya Upaniṣad*, for example, proclaims:

> One who knows Brahman reaches the supreme [state of being]. As to this, the following has been declared: One who knows Brahman as the real, as knowledge, and as infinity,[151] abiding in the cave of the heart and in the highest heaven, he realizes all desires, along with Brahman, the intelligent one.[152]

A later Upaniṣad, the *Varāha Upaniṣad*, makes a similar point but from a theistic perspective. In this passage the teacher is God himself, here in the form of Viṣṇu:

> Concentrating on consciousness as unwavering, meditate on my abode in your heart. . . . All that is conscious in the universe is actually [a reflection] of

> absolute Consciousness. This universe is absolute Consciousness only. You are Consciousness. I am Consciousness. Meditate on the world as Consciousness.[154]

The great lesson the Upaniṣadic sages taught their students was that the same consciousness that upholds the universe also resides within the human spirit, and that by knowing one's own inner world one comes thereby to know the divine foundation of being itself.

From this we can see that Vedāntic teachers taught their students to practice inward contemplation as a way of attaining the acuity and subtlety necessary to recognize abiding truths. Such contemplation facilitates the control and focus of one's otherwise active and unfocused mind. The *Śvetāśvatara Upaniṣad* presents a set of instructions to such a seeker:

> Holding one's body steady with the three upper parts in a line [that is, with the back straight], and bringing the senses and the mind into the heart, a wise person should cross over all of the rivers of anxiety with the boat of the holy power [*brahman*]. Having controlled one's breathing here [in the body], let one restrain the mind without distraction, the way a chariot is yoked to wild horses. One should practice meditation in a hidden retreat that is protected from the wind; in a clean and level place that is free from pebbles, fire, and gravel; that is near the sound of water and other features; that is conducive to thought; and that is pleasing to the eye.[154]

According to the *Kṣurikā Upaniṣad,* a later work, the workings of the mind are to be enfolded into the deeper and more sublime heart. The contemplative does this, in part, by closing his or her eyes and mouth ("shutting the doors") and slowly calming the breath by inwardly pronouncing the sacred syllable *auṃ*:[155]

> Like a tortoise drawing in its limbs,
> [the seeker] encloses the mind within the heart.
> Slowly pronouncing the twelve sounds[156]
> within the syllable *auṃ*
> he fills his whole body with one breath
> and shuts all of its doors.[157]

Such advice appears, too, in the *Yogaśikhā Upaniṣad*:

> Choosing a posture such as the lotus position,
> or whatever else may please him, . . .
> controlling the mind at all times,
> the wise should meditate
> continuously on the syllable *auṃ*,
> enthroning the highest God in their hearts.[158]

What we have here, of course, is a description of a yogi in meditation. Sitting in a posture suitable for long periods of concentration and calming the fluctuations of the mind, the contemplative enfolds his awareness into the heart and slowly pronounces the sacred syllable *aum* (or *om*), which, as we have seen earlier, is the sound of the universal Self.

Meditation is said to bring the calmness and steadiness of mind that is necessary for one to see beyond the mind. One might compare meditation to letting a jar of muddy water lie still for a period of time in order to allow the silt to settle; as the water clears one is better able to see through it. Similarly, by cultivating a tranquil and clarified mind, one is better able to transcend the mind. The *Kaṭha Upaniṣad* notes that it is "through the tranquility of the mind [*dhātu-prasādāt*]" that one sees the "greatness of the Self."[159]

The Upaniṣads note that there is another means besides meditation through which one may come to know the Self. This is the way of grace (*prasāda, kṛpā,* and other terms). Here, the universal Self chooses of its own nature to reveal itself. Using similar language to the passage from the *Kaṭha Upaniṣad* just quoted, (substituting the phrase *dhātuḥ prasādāt* for the compound *dhātu-prasādāt*), the *Śvetāśvatara Upaniṣad* teaches:

> Subtler than the subtle, greater than the great
> is the Self abiding in the cave of the heart of the creature.
> One sees him as actionless and one becomes free from sorrow when,
> through the grace of the creator [*dhātuḥ prasādāt*],
> one sees the Lord and his magnificence.[160]

Both personal discipline (in the form of meditation) and the help of God (in the form of divine grace) are necessary for genuine spiritual growth, realization, and fulfillment. Meditation and grace are distinct from each other, and yet they are closely connected to one another. Meditation allows one to refine the attention and sharpen one's focus so that it is possible to recognize the grace of God that is constantly showering into everyday life and infusing one's very being with love.

MORAL RESPONSIBILITY, EQUALITY-CONSCIOUSNESS, AND EGOLESS DHARMA

Now the question is: How can a seeker put the Vedāntic revelation of the Self into action in his or her relationship to the outer world? The common, even stereotypical, but not entirely inaccurate, understanding of the classical Vedānta is that it is directed toward the renunciant who relinquishes all ties to the world. However, there is another side to the Vedānta which stresses the importance of remaining open to the world, as it were, and of living one's life in a socially and morally responsible way based on the understanding that all beings are equally valuable embodiments of the universal Self.

As we have seen, Vedāntic spirituality in general holds that the Self one comes to know in meditation is the very same Self that fashions and maintains the universe as a whole and that this Self may be known in all things. Such an idea is presented by the *Yogatattva Upaniṣad*, which teaches:

> Whatever one sees with one's eyes, let one regard as the Self [Ātman].
> Whatever one hears with one's ears, let one regard as the Self.
> Whatever one smells with one's nose, let one regard as the Self.
> Whatever one tastes with one's tongue, let one regard as the Self.
> Whatever one touches with one's skin, let one regard as the Self.[161]

Despite the widespread perception that it is based on a world-renouncing practice of inward meditation, the fuller truth is that the Vedānta as a contemplative tradition generally maintains an ethic which holds that one is not to neglect one's responsibilities to the world. The philosophical basis of this perspective stands in the assertion that just as the Self resides within one's own heart, so too it abides within the hearts of all others. One very effective form of meditation, in fact, is suggested by such lines as those from the *Yogatattva Upaniṣad* just quoted—"Whatever one sees with one's eyes, let one regard as the Self." Understood from this point of view, to turn away from others is, in a very real sense, to turn away from the Self. Put into theological terms, to turn away from others is to turn away from God.

The most influential of Vedāntic texts presenting this ethic of responsibility is undoubtedly the *Bhagavadgītā*, a text which we will recall forms fully one-third of the "triple foundation" of Vedāntic thought and values. Here, the supreme Self is identified as God, known in this poetic song as Kṛṣṇa. Based on the Vedāntic idea that there is only one true Self in the universe, the song reminds its listener, "The Lord abides in the heart of all beings and through his mysterious power makes all creatures revolve."[162] This "eternal Lord" is the "Highest Self [*paramātman*], who enters into and supports the three worlds."[163]

The *Bhagavadgītā* presents its teachings in the form of a conversation between Lord Kṛṣṇa and Arjuna, the latter of whom seeks to understand the nature of his moral responsibility in the world. Kṛṣṇa reminds Arjuna, "I reside in the heart of all";[164] "There is nothing higher than I am; on me all this is strung, like pearls on a thread";[165] and "I am the seed of all beings. There is no creature, moving or motionless, that is without Me."[166]

Drawing on this idea, one who truly loves God necessarily honors and respects not only his or her own self but others, as well; for, just as a person lives within the inherent integrity of his own soul, so too God lives within others and stands as the foundation of their inner dignity. Alternatively, one who shows disrespect for others shows disrespect not only for himself but also for God. As Kṛṣṇa instructs Arjuna, "You shall see all beings in yourself and in me."[167]

True spiritual discipline—a phrase that translates what the text calls *yoga*—centers on the vision of the presence of God in others: "He whose soul is disciplined in yoga, who regards all things equally, sees himself in all beings and all beings in himself."[168] Seeing the Self in everyone, the truly disciplined yogi would not purposely harm anyone, for to do so would be to harm the Self residing within his or her own being. Therefore, "Seeing the Lord dwelling equally in all beings, he does not injure the Self and thus he takes the highest path."[169] Knowing this and treating others as one's Self, one returns to God. Kṛṣṇa declares to Arjuna:

> He who sees me in everything
> and everything in me,
> for him I am not lost
> and he is not lost for me.[170]

One ethical implication of such a stance is that a person who knows God sees the same Self in all beings no matter how "high" or "low" they might otherwise be; that Self resides as much within an outcaste as it does within a scholarly and cultivated brahmin or, for that matter, within a cow or an elephant.[171] One who would seek to know God therefore must necessarily regard all creatures with respect.[172] According to Kṛṣṇa:

> He who is grounded in oneness,
> who reveres me as dwelling in all beings,
> whatever his life's work or otherwise:
> That yogi abides in me.
> He who by comparison with his own self
> sees the same everywhere, O Arjuna,
> whether pleasurable or painful:
> He is considered a supreme yogi.[173]

The *Bhagavadgītā* holds that the perfected seeker is not, therefore, one who turns away from the world but rather one who "delights in the welfare of all beings."[174] Accordingly, this foundational Vedāntic text teaches that one is to engage oneself actively in the welfare of others, for to do so is to honor the Self within them. One is to do this, moreover, from a genuinely unselfish perspective, that is to say, without hope of reward or fear of punishment. Such service to others contributes to the well-being of the world. Such selfless action constitutes one's *dharma*, a word that essentially refers to action that supports the integrity and dignity of the universe as a whole. One person's mode of *dharma* may be different from another, for we all have different sets of responsibilities to each other, to society, and to the world. The *Bhagavadgītā* holds, however, that it is essential that each person undertake his or her own responsibilities as fully as is possible, even though he or she might not feel willing or especially adept at doing so. Twice the text notes, "It is better to perform one's own responsibilities, however imperfectly, than to perform another's perfectly."[175]

A religious tradition based to any degree on the teachings of the *Bhagavadgītā* would thus hold that one honors and worships God, in part, by selflessly meeting one's responsibilities to others and by fulfilling one's moral obligations to the larger world. At the same time, one undertakes such activity without any ulterior motives. The *Bhagavadgītā* teaches that a person is to perform his or her *dharma* simply and precisely because it is the right thing to do, for such right action serves the universal Self.

In this way, to honor and respect others is to love God. Through such devotion (*bhakti*) to God, the spiritual seeker finds himself or herself enveloped in the loving grace of that supreme Self. "Through devotion he recognizes me, how great I am and who I truly am," the *Bhagavadgītā* has Kṛṣṇa teach Arjuna; "then, having known me as I truly am, he enters immediately into me."[176] God's protecting grace is said to help the seeker through all forms of difficulty and trouble: "If your mind is on me, through my grace you will cross all obstacles."[177]

The universal, divine Self that is worshiped through love returns to the worshiper that very same, divine love. In the *Bhagavadgītā* Kṛṣṇa tells Arjuna, "Those devotees of mine who are of faith, who are intent on me, who accept this nectar of truth as I have spoken it: they are dear to me beyond measure."[178]

CONTOURS IN THE SIDDHA YOGA EXPERIENCE OF THE SELF

With the perspective outlined in the previous pages, we may return now to Swami Muktananda's and Swami Chidvilasananda's teachings regarding the nature and experience of the Self. As we do so we will now be able to recognize both implicit and explicit signs of the Vedānta in those teachings. Reading their words with a Vedāntic eye, we recognize how much of their teaching is anchored in the language and imagery of the Upaniṣads and the *Bhagavadgītā*.

For example, like Śaṅkarācārya, Swami Muktananda believed that the origins of suffering—all "pain, disappointment, weakness, mental disturbance, jealousy, enmity, envy, and so on,"[179]—are a result of ignorance. Quoting Śaṅkara's *Aparokṣānubhūti,* Muktananda defined ignorance as *svasvarūpa vismaraṇa,* the "forgetfulness of one's own Self."[180] And who is one's own Self? Borrowing a line from the *Bhagavadgītā,* Muktananda described one's own Self as the "One [who] pervades all beings, inside and outside, movable and immovable."[181] This One is, of course, the universal Self, Ātman as Brahman, the "indestructible One [who] permeates everything in a subtle form. . . . [T]he One without a second."[182]

"A human being's predicament," Muktananda wrote, "is that he has forgotten himself. He thinks about others and dwells on their faults, wasting the priceless years of his life by uselessly envying and criticizing others. What greater ignorance can there be? Ignorance is the city of utter darkness."[183] Because of ignorance, he said, we superimpose false distinctions on the absolute, thus unnecessarily alienating ourselves from the eternal and ubiquitous presence of the divine. Using the classic Vedāntic metaphor, Muktananda likened such ignorance to the misapprehension of a snake in what is in truth a coiled rope. "Suppose a rope is lying on the ground and we see it as a snake and become afraid," he wrote. "There was never a snake in the rope. The snake appeared because of an optical illusion, a delusion on the part of the observer. In this way, we fear our own imaginary snake and become the cause of our own pain or pleasure."[184]

Seen from this thoroughly Vedāntic point of view, the way to end disappointment and fear and alienation is to remove the ignorance of the Self. Voicing a perspective that is in this instance closer to Vallabhācārya's Śuddha Advaita than to Śaṅkarācārya's Kevala Advaita, Muktananda pointed out, however, that "the real teaching of Vedānta is that the ignorance which is destroyed never really existed,"[185] just like the snake did not exist in the rope. "To destroy ignorance and attain bliss is to destroy what never was and to attain what we have always had," for the "Self of all, which is extremely subtle, is forever attained."[186] Following Advaita Vedāntic thought in general—whether Kevala Advaita or Śuddha Advaita—Muktananda held that although the Self may appear to be many, it is One, and the essence of that One suffuses all things. As he put it, "The moon may be reflected in thousands of pots, yet it is only one. Although there are countless grains of salt, they all share the same quality of saltiness."[187] Quoting again from the *Bhagavadgītā,* Muktananda said that the "same Parabrahman [that is, the supreme Brahman] exists eternally in the hearts of all. One who sees no differences among all existing creatures attains the bliss of Parabrahman in this very body."[188]

According to Muktananda, that Self is the supreme principle of the universe, and the "creation of forms, their expansion, preservation, and destruction all proceed from That. That supports the earth through its own power. . . . We should come to know that Supreme Principle. It has not the slightest trace of duality. By perceiving it, the seer, the process of seeing, and the seen merge together."[189]

Like the teachers of the Vedānta, Swami Muktananda held that, knowing the Self, one is released from the recurrent cycles of suffering. "The true nature of the Self is supreme bliss, not sorrow," he taught. "The Self always remains as it is. Just as day and night come and go in the heavens, similarly, countless bodies come and go in the Self."[190] One who thus knows the Self "does not get caught on the wheel of birth and death. With this wisdom of equality and oneness, he sleeps comfortably in a bed of bliss and fearlessness."[191] Referring once more to the *Bhagavadgītā*, he taught that such a person "sees God equally everywhere."[192]

Using similarly explicit theological language, Swami Chidvilasananda has suggested that it is in fact precisely this vision of the divine in all things that God himself wishes for the human soul, for this vision allows the soul to break free from the cycles of *saṃsāra* and to return to its divine source. "All that God wants," she has written,

> . . . is that we go back to Him, we understand Him, we recognize Him. For that, we turn within and have that experience. If we don't have the experience of the Truth, then it doesn't matter how much we talk about God or the Self. If we haven't had the experience of the Self, if we haven't become established in the Self, then we are born again and again and again.[193]

Like earlier Vedāntic teachers, these siddha gurus proclaim that the experience of the Self is a truly liberating and transforming one. As Swami Chidvilasananda has said, "Once you see the face of the Truth, even for a second, you can never forget it. In that brief moment, the Self fills your heart with its own essence, which is ambrosia. It fills your mind with its essence, which is knowledge, and your understanding of life is permanently altered. Even one glimpse of that Reality is enough."[194]

Swami Chidvilasananda's words in the lines just quoted reverberate with a sense of the infusive and yet also expansive power of the divine as it enters into and transforms the human spirit, giving one a taste of the sublime—ambrosial—undying truth. The Self "fills your heart with its own essence, which is ambrosia . . . and your understanding of life is permanently altered." This very experience lies at the core of the Vedāntic experience of Brahman. We remember that, in the earliest Vedic texts, *brahman* was a forceful, flowing, divine power that brought life and vigor to its recipient. We remember, too, that the very word *brahman* literally means "that which is possessed of the nature of expansive power." As we have seen, the Vedānta recognizes this universal power of being as the universal power and substratum of being—Brahman—which grounds and pervades (*bṛh-*) all things. We have also seen that Vedāntic sages maintained that the sublime essence of this pervasive and universal Brahman is identical to that of the abiding Self—Ātman—whose very breath of being infuses all that exists. Similarly, some Vedāntic teachers regard this divine Self dwelling in the hearts of all beings as God himself. Such teachers hold that to experience the presence of the Self is therefore to experience the presence of God.

Chidvilasananda teaches that even hearing of the possibility of such an experience can itself be a transformative moment. Quoting her guru's central message, which she describes as "very simple"—"Honor your own Self. Meditate on your own Self. Worship your own Self. Kneel down to your own Self. Understand your own Self. Your God dwells within you as you"—she says, "Even if you haven't had the experience of this great Self, just by hearing that it exists within, you can actually feel the layers of ignorance falling away; you can feel the wisdom sprouting within. It's always amazing how a Master can do this: he tells you something very simple, and the heavens open wide."[195]

Shaktipat

Here we arrive at a crucial point: Swami Chidvilasananda has described Siddha Yoga's characteristic means for Self-revelation, namely, the grace of the guru. It is through this compassionate gift of grace, a transmission of power from the guru to the seeker known as shaktipat (Sanskrit, *śaktipāta:* "descent of power"), that one experiences a powerfully transformative, pervasive, expansive divine reality.[196] To locate the experience of shaktipat textually, swamis Muktananda and Chidvilasananda have turned to the scriptures of Kashmir Śaivism, yet they maintain that the experience of shaktipat is described, at least implicitly, in several notable stories told by Vedāntic texts. Perhaps the best known of such narratives tells of Kṛṣṇa's overpowering revelation of his universal form (*viśvarūpa*) to Arjuna in chapter 11 of the *Bhagavadgītā.* Swami Muktananda also liked to tell a story recounting the moment when Śaṅkarācārya told his disciple Hastāmalaka, "You are That," and Hastāmalaka instantly realized the divine within himself. Muktananda used to say that this realization could have only come through shaktipat.[197]

Siddha Yoga holds that this experience of the divinity of being takes place through the compassionate grace of the guru. And who is the guru? There are several ways to answer this question,[198] one of which is that the guru is none other than the Self. The *Gurugītā* describes the guru as the "eternal witness" (*nityasākṣin*),[199] who "pervades this entire world, consisting of the movable and immovable and also the animate and inanimate," the "Lord of the universe" and "Self of all beings" who is "Brahman, eternal and pure" and of the nature of "eternal knowledge, consciousness, and bliss." From the Vedāntic perspective, the guru as the universal Self is therefore none other than God. According to Siddha Yoga, *gururātmā īśvareti*: "The Guru is the Self as well as God,"[200] and *īśvaro gururātmeti*: "the Lord is the Guru and the Self."[201] To receive the grace of the guru is therefore to receive the grace of God; and to receive the grace of God is to receive the grace of the Self.

Vedāntic thought holds that since the mind cannot comprehend its own divine source, one can only come to know the Self through the grace of the Self.[202] According to this line of thought, as one returns to the Self by means of the guru's grace, one thereby returns to the experience of the divine unity of being. Swami Muktananda seems to have felt the same way, for he said:

> Only those who have received the grace of the Guru and are adept at discriminating between the Self and the non-Self can grasp the Supreme Principle. One who has merged into the Guru, the embodiment of wisdom, who has become him, who has merged into the all-pervasive Consciousness, who has become both immanent and transcendent, who has lost his sense of duality, and who has become ecstatic in supreme bliss and complete in his perfection dwells in all and all dwell in him.[203]

Drawing on Tantric ideas as she associates the experience of grace with the awakening of spiritual energy, *kuṇḍalinī*,[204] Swami Chidvilasananda explains:

> So when you receive shaktipat, that's when it happens. When the Kundalini awakens, that's when it happens. It is said in the Upanishads that the Atma, the Self, is not attained by listening to lectures nor by great learning. When the Self is contented with us, that is the time when we attain the Self. In the same way, when the Kundalini Shakti is contented, then the Kundalini arises. That's when we reach the Guru.[205]

Allowing the Self's graceful presence to direct one's life, one becomes, the Siddha Yoga gurus say, less rigid and more flexible, less contracted and more expansive, less insecure and more confident. According to Swami Chidvilasananda:

> We must learn how to accept grace when it comes. Grace is nothing but the Self; it is that divine energy. The work it can do is far greater than we can accomplish just through the mind or the intellect. When grace manifests itself in our bodies . . . we feel very expanded. We feel we can envelop the universe. . . . In that state of entire grace there is a greater ability to do things, and it happens naturally. It's not like when you have to push yourself to do things. It's almost the feeling that there is a hand supporting our life, a hand protecting us completely. That is grace.[206]

Sadhana and Meditation

For Siddha Yoga students, the experience of the expansive Self takes place as a result of some form of shaktipat. But this is only the beginning; shaktipat begins the process of Self-discovery. Siddha Yoga gurus place great emphasis on the importance of the seeker's own cultivation of the strength of inner character and the practice of spiritual disciplines—meditation, selfless service, repetition of mantras, worship, study, self-inquiry, and so on—that will strengthen and clarify the essential realization of the Self. Swami Chidvilasananda has pointed out that the "saints and great beings keep telling us the same Truth over and over again. . . . Become one with the Self." But, she adds, "Somehow when we hear these teachings, we do not connect them to our life; we do not try to apply them in a practical way."[207] The Siddha Yoga gurus hold that, in order for God's unconditional grace to take hold in one's life, one must undertake sadhana, that is, the practice of spiritual discipline. As Chidvilasananda has said:

> You know, there's a saying which has become a cliche, yet it is the absolute truth: that grace and effort are the two wings of a bird, the two wings of our sadhana. . . . When we keep both grace as well as effort completely tuned up, and if we remain in tune with them, then certainly this is a great way to become one with the Self.[208]

She warns her followers against merely talking about the Self, and urges them to undertake spiritual discipline in order to know the Self:

> If you are only clever at theorizing about God, the Truth, or the Self, you do not attain any of them. You need the practical aspect of *sādhanā*, the direct realization of God. Without this direct realization, there is no attainment. We read and read, we listen and listen, yet we do not feel anything because we have neglected the practical aspect. Without direct realization, theory cannot really do much to help us.[209]

Quoting a Vedāntic teaching—"The Ātman can always be won by truth, self-discipline, knowledge, and by a life of purity"[210]—she notes:

> These qualities portray the nature of *sadhana.* They summon the drive to follow spiritual practices.
>
> *Sadhana,* spiritual practice, has a way of creating a boundaryless boundary to hold the experience of the Infinite.
>
> When you have discipline, you can experience ecstasy without allowing it to dissipate.[211]

For Siddha Yoga students, the core element of that spiritual discipline is the practice of meditation. Swami Muktananda noted, "There are many techniques which are supposed to lead us to God, but of all these, meditation is the one recognized by all the saints and sages, because only in meditation can we see the inner Self directly."[212] He saw a congruity between meditation and intense concentration of any sort. Thus he said, "Meditation is not something difficult or strange. . . . All our arts and skills, from driving a car to cooking a meal to painting a picture to solving a mathematical problem, are perfected through the power of concentration, which is nothing but meditation." The difference between these disciplines and true meditation, however, is that the former are external forms of concentration while meditation directs that concentration inward. "When we turn our attention within," he said, "and focus on our inner being, just as we focus on external objects, we are meditating on the Self."[213]

Swami Chidvilasananda teaches that it is precisely this inward contemplation that allows a person to know the Self, and thus to remember the guiding presence of God in his or her life:

> As we contemplate and contemplate the imperishable Self, this contemplation takes us very deep inside. When we do not contemplate at all, our energies run everywhere and go to waste. As we contemplate the Self more and more, all our energies return to their source, and there is a greater strength, greater devotion and love. . . .
>
> This is just a simple analogy, but it is the same thing that happens with us and the Self, with us and God. Everything else interests us more than the One who has created us, the One who has given us life, the One who has infused our being with energy. To maintain our interest in God, we need constant contemplation. The human mind is such that if we do not contemplate, we can forget.[214]

The practice of meditation on the Self draws one's attention inward and, thus away from the outer physical body. Despite their emphasis on identifying with the Self rather than with the physical body—a perspective that is consistent with Vedāntic thought in general—Siddha Yoga gurus have been careful to warn their students against mistreating their bodies. Taking a perspective that shares much with Kashmir Śaivism, Swami Muktananda has taught his followers:

> O Siddha students! Your live body is the temple of Goddess Chiti. Treat it with respect by being pure and chaste, by eating good, wholesome food, and by wearing beautiful, simple, clean clothes.
>
> O Siddha students! If others call this body low, let them. You should not forget that salvation is attained through this very body. If you want to attain your beloved God and Guru and unfold the inner source of love, you must first love yourself. Only love will take you to God. You desire inner peace, but hate your body and senses. You long for inner joy, but are hostile to the body, which is a means to that joy, as if it were your worst enemy. . . . Once you know

your inner being, you will realize that the body is not illusory but a beautiful temple filled with knowledge; by loving it you will make your own spring of love flow.[215]

According to Muktananda, this liberating inner love that is tapped through meditation is then to be shared with others:

> Understand that the ever-new joy that reveals itself in meditation dwells in the heart as a free, inspiring force. Develop this love, and let it flow from you to others.[216]

Swami Chidvilasananda similarly teaches that "the human body is the temple of God," and, accordingly:

> One must take care of it. When you are on the spiritual path, it is easy to feel, "What is the body? I want to know God. I want to know the Self. This body is just an obstacle." When you have this attitude you begin to think that if you starve the body until it becomes invisible you will be able to know God. You start torturing the body and putting it through many ordeals. You forget that it must be protected and taken care of, that God dwells within it.[217]

The same holds true for the care of the mind:

> If you do not keep your mind very beautiful, if you do not polish it again and again with the mantra, with meditation, with respect, with understanding, with worship, then the mind does not shine; it does not reflect the Self at all. Because it has not been bathed in the light of God, it reflects only ugliness and darkness. You do not allow the light of God to shine through it. . . .
>
> When you keep the state of your mind very beautiful, you enjoy an ecstasy greater than anything this entire world can offer. The sages have said there is great ecstasy in your own being. Experience the ecstasy of the Self; there is nothing higher than this.[218]

The disciple's diligent practice of inward spiritual disciplines thus strengthens, clarifies, and makes firm the experience of the Self known first as a result of the guru's infusive gift of grace in the form of shaktipat. The Siddha Yoga gurus hold that such discipline leads to a third level or stage of the experience of pure Being: Here a disciple expresses the divine Self through the love of others and dedication to the welfare of the world as a whole.

Compassion and Responsibility

The social vision of the Siddha Yoga gurus is based entirely on their fundamental realization of the Self as love. This love is known inwardly and expressed outwardly. Accordingly, the cultivation of love constitutes an important part of one's spiritual discipline. Love, in fact, stands as the foundation of all such discipline. "Dear seekers!" Swami Muktananda wrote, "Learning without love is useless. Yoga without love is meaningless. Sadhana without love, whatever sadhana is, cannot take you to the joy of the Self."[219] He characterized the Self as of the nature of love. "Love is man's very Self, his true beauty, and the glory of his human existence," he wrote; he believed therefore that "Man should love his Self, which is all-embracing."[220] Swami Chidvilasananda teaches that the Self is by nature compassionate. For her, compassion is an "innate capacity" of the human spirit, an inherent virtue "which is so simple and yet so far-reaching in its effects."[221] In her view, compassion both characterizes and reveals the Self. Drawing on the Vedāntic teaching that the Self resides in the heart, she reminds her followers that "you carry the tenderness of the heart, the loving heart," and that

> [t]his supreme compassion exists in everyone. Therefore, all the great beings say, come into the realm of your heart. Bathe in the light of your own heart. Drink the nectar of compassion from the wellspring of your own heart. Don't look for compassion anywhere else, from anyone else. It is inside you. You are the owner of this great virtue.[222]

Chidvilasananda does not equate compassion with a condescending attitude or patronizing pity toward others. Compassion, in her view, arises out of deep and genuine respect both for oneself and for others. "To be compassionate," she says, "you must learn to think well of yourself and others. Therefore a bleeding heart, which sees other people as helpless, is not a sign of compassion."[223] Compassion arises not out of a degrading self-righteousness, but rather out of the righteousness of the true Self, which is "so stirring that it is said to make even rocks weep with love."[224] True compassion has no trace of ego in it. From the perspective of Siddha Yoga, to cultivate and practice compassion is therefore an important element of one's sadhana. As Swami Chidvilasananda has said, "The practice of compassion is so potent that one tiny service has the power to purify your thoughts and burn your selfishness to a crisp."[225] True compassion breaks down the barriers between people, thus making manifest the true unity of being grounded on the integrity of the Self. Compassion therefore allows one to discover and recover one's true Self. Chidvilasananda teaches:

> As you make the effort to let compassion be your guide, instead of your self-centered judgment of a situation or a person, then you find yourself being rocked in the cradle of your own divine heart. Your heart will never have walls again. Compassion is such a great virtue that it melts the walls around the heart.[226]

Siddha Yoga gurus recognize a kind of reciprocal loop between action based on compassion and the inward revelation of the Self. In other words, compassion is both an outward expression of one's inward awareness of the Self and an avenue that leads to that very recognition. Swami Muktananda maintained that egoless service can and does require inner strength and steadfastness. Restating the revelation of the Self as it appears in the Vedāntic tradition, Muktananda urged his followers to pursue a sadhana based on meditation on the Self and supported by responsible moral action. Such practice of meditation and commitment to ethical living are consistent with the *yamas* and *niyamas*—modes of self-discipline and moral conduct—of classical Yoga which, like Vedānta, stresses the importance of virtuous action on the path to inner revelation of the Self.

In the following passage, Muktananda refers to the Self as "That" and identifies "That" as the Lord, known here as Śiva:

> Cherish good conduct.
> Become established on the path of morality.
> Earn virtue; shun defects.
> One who is anchored in the Self
> attains bravery and courage.
> If you meditate on That,
> you will never depart from it.
>
> Perform righteous deeds,
> and you will develop courage. . . .
>
> Perform all actions for the sake of Shiva;
> do nothing for yourself.
> By serving the world, you serve the Lord.
> Take no delight in duality;
> consider all to be the Lord.
> Recognize only Him in all,
> sentient and insentient.[227]

In this set of teachings, which is quintessentially Siddha Yoga, Swami Muktananda says much that is consonant with Vedāntic values and ideas. The theistic Advaita Vedānta perspective finds expression in his urging devotees to "take no delight in duality; consider all to be the Lord. Recognize only Him in all, sentient and insentient." Muktananda strikes a general Vedāntic note when he teaches, for instance, that when one takes refuge in that Self one gains inner strength and steadfastness—"One who is anchored in the Self attains bravery and courage"—and also when he asserts that constant awareness of the Self links one with that Self: "If you meditate on That, you will never depart from it." Although he here identifies the Lord as Śiva rather than as Kṛṣṇa, he is consistent with the ethical teachings of the *Bhagavadgītā* when he encourages devotees to "cherish good conduct. Become established on the path of morality. Earn virtue; shun defects. . . ." He is in perfect harmony with that text's perspective regarding the spiritual discipline of *karma-phala-tyāga* ("renunciation of the fruits of action") when he instructs the devotee to "perform all actions for the sake of Shiva; do nothing for yourself." The *Bhagavagītā*'s vision of the sacramental nature of ethical human conduct is reflected in Muktananda's assertion that "by serving the world, you serve the Lord." Vedāntic views and values thus infuse this short but quite representative passage.

Swami Muktananda taught that one way to act morally in the world is to imagine what a siddha would do in any given circumstance and then to act *as if* one were oneself such a siddha. "Siddha students, watch carefully," he said:

> Take good care of the Siddha Shakti spreading throughout your body, the Shakti that has been set in motion by a Siddha. Never look on one another with anger or resentment, or with an eye to see sin or differences. . . . Control your bad habits and don't behave in a way that is contrary to the behavior of Siddhas. Live as a Siddha would live.[228]

Performing all of one's responsibilities in the world as an expression of the universal Self, which is love, one returns the heart's gift of joy to an otherwise dry and parched world. Swami Chidvilasananda remembers her guru repeatedly urging people to "know your own Self. Follow the dharma, the duties, of your own life and find God there."[229] Muktananda encouraged his followers to "work as selflessly as the clouds / that shower rain,"[230] and thereby reflect or make manifest the work of the universal Lord, for—

> Just as rain is the life of all—
> the moving and the unmoving—
> the universal Lord is the life of all.
> He showers compassion equally on all.
> To Him, the ignorant and wise are the same.
> He removes the suffering of all,
> and gives knowledge to all.[231]

Following the voice of her own guru, Swami Chidvilasananda has been careful to caution her followers against turning away from their responsibilities to the world as they seek the Self. Indeed, for her, there is no place, no time, no person in which God does not dwell. She teaches, therefore, that it is important to honor God by respecting others:

> There is nothing that is not God. There is nowhere where you do not exist. Therefore, when you give your blessings to one another, you are recognizing the Self within yourself and in others.[232]

CONCLUSIONS

As we hope by now is clear, an essential element of the Vedānta centers around the revelation and experience of the eternal and abiding absolute, which the Vedānta describes in terms denoting a universal "Self." The fact that the Siddha Yoga gurus describe the divine in similar terms indicates that they recognize that the Vedānta teachings regarding ultimate reality are consistent with their own experience. We may recall that swamis Muktananda and Chidvilasananda also have seen reflections of the Self in other religious traditions of India besides Vedānta, notably in Kashmir Śaivism and the devotional sensibilities of the poet-saints. But since the Vedānta as a spiritual tradition precedes and informs Kashmir Śaivism and the great Bhakti movements of classical India, we can say that the revelation of the Self, as it has been defined by Siddha Yoga gurus, finds its foundational sources in the Vedāntic tradition.

In consonance with the larger Vedāntic tradition, Siddha Yoga gurus hold that the path to the Self takes one across increasingly expansive terrain. If the Upaniṣadic sages taught their students not only that *aham brahmāsmi* ("I am Brahman") and *ayam ātmā brahma* ("This Self is Brahman") but also that *sarvaṃ khalvidam brahma* ("Truly, this whole world is Brahman") and *tat tvam asi* ("You are That"), so too the shaktipat initiation given through the grace of a siddha guru ultimately gives one the vision of the powerful reality of the eternal Self abiding not only within the inherent dignity and integrity of one's own heart but also within the heart of all others. The disciplined practice of meditation and other forms of sadhana allow one to cultivate a deeper understanding of the nature of that universal Self and to refine one's experience of it as pure being, consciousness, and bliss. The clarity of one's vision of the Self allows one to regard others with equality-consciousness and to treat all beings with honor and respect. As Swami Muktananda said, "First love yourself, then your neighbors, and then the whole world."[233]

The Siddha Yoga teachings hold that by honoring the Self within all beings, one comes to undertake all of one's actions as external worship of the divine love that supports the world as a whole. According to Swami Muktananda, "Love is God; love is the universe."[234] One's egoless and loving service to others thus stands as the full outward expression of the inner realization of the absolute. The whole of one's spiritual life returns finally to the experience and expression of the love that *is* the universal Self. "Love is your very nature," he wrote. "It is your sadhana and your highest attainment. Love is God; love is the universe."[235]

Chapter Six

SHAKTIPAT
The Initiatory Descent of Power

Paul E. Muller-Ortega

yasmād anugraham labdhvā
mahadajñānamutsṛjet
tasmai śrīdeśikendrāya
namaścābhīṣṭasiddhaye

Receiving his grace
One gives up great ignorance
Salutations to the highest Guru
For the attainment of the object of desire.

Gurugītā 56

INTRODUCTION: THE EXPERIENCE OF SHAKTIPAT

In the context of the Indian yogic and spiritual traditions, shaktipat (Sanskrit, *śaktipāta* or sometimes *śaktinipāta*) is understood to be the highest form of spiritual initiation, an initiation that bestows immediate and spontaneous entry into spiritual life. The term *śaktipāta* literally means "the descent of the *śakti*," and this has traditionally been understood as the descent of the power of ultimate consciousness itself. The concept of shaktipat has been documented in textual sources since about the sixth or seventh century onward.[1] It appears to have accrued widespread fame very rapidly as perhaps the rarest form of esoteric or secret initiation practiced in these traditions. The earliest references to shaktipat indicate that its authentic experience was always considered to be very difficult to locate and to secure.

The transmission and reception of shaktipat are thought to constitute the essence of the process of initiation (*dīkṣā*).[2] In the traditional, interpretive etymologies of Sanskrit pandits or textual commentators, the meaning of the term *dīkṣā* is often expounded by being broken down into two verbal roots: *dā-*, "to give"; and *kṣi-*, "to destroy."[3] In this way, initiation is understood to give liberation or ultimate freedom (*mokṣa*) by removing or destroying the impediment of the root ignorance or impurity (*ajñāna* or *mala*).

The agent who performs and bestows shaktipat is the *sadguru*, the "true teacher," or the siddha guru (Sanskrit, *siddha guru*: the "perfected teacher" or the "teacher belonging to the lineage of the siddhas"). Therefore, shaktipat confers the highest form of what is more widely known as *gurukṛpā*, the "grace of the awakened and consecrated teacher."[4] Traditionally, it had always been considered that teachers capable of granting authentic shaktipat were extremely rare. Even when a prospective aspirant for shaktipat could locate a teacher who was appropriately empowered to bestow it, it was never an easy matter to receive shaktipat. Most often, the teacher would impose various tests, austerities, and preliminary disciplines as prerequisites. Moreover, these were always prescribed with no guarantee that the desired initiation would *ever* be forthcoming.

In the tradition of Siddha Yoga, the bestowal of shaktipat is thought to be one of the primary and most important functions of the siddha guru. Indeed, the siddha guru is often known as a shaktipat guru. Swami Muktananda explains it as follows:

> The grace of the Guru is itself a process of initiation known as *shaktipāt dīkshā*. This is the same process of grace whereby Shri Ramakrishna Paramahamsa gave a direct experience of divinity to Swami Vivekananda the moment he touched him. Indeed, the process of *shaktipāt dīkshā* is highly mysterious, secret and amazing. It is a very ancient tradition practiced in India.[5]

What actually occurs during shaktipat—or rather, the elaboration of the conceptual universe within which shaktipat is embedded—is the subject of sustained inquiry in the philosophical and ritual texts of several of the spiritual traditions of India. It will be our purpose in what follows to inquire into that universe of meaning, as it has been historically elaborated as well as in its more modern and contemporary expressions. One of the results obtained from such an inquiry is evidence of a profound continuity between what we know about shaktipat from historical texts, such as those of the Śaivism of Kashmir, and the practice of shaktipat initiation as it is currently exemplified in the siddha lineage of Siddha Yoga.

It is important to note that in the early traditions the technical details surrounding shaktipat are first narrated in terms of external ritual performances (*kriyā*). Nevertheless, within several centuries, the definitive occurrences resulting from shaktipat are theoretically located as occurring wholly inwardly in the deepest consciousness of the initiate and, therefore, in some sense are seen as independent of outer ritual actions. This should not be construed to mean that external rituals of various sorts do not continue to be present, as they certainly do. But the shift of focus from external rituals to deep, inner events is highly significant (echoing as it does early shifts in Indian religious praxis), and seems to have taken place certainly by the tenth century as evidenced by the writings of the Kashmiri teachers on shaktipat.

In any case, whether by means of obvious ritual procedures (*kriyā*) or not, shaktipat is thought to constitute a transmission of spiritual power from the *sadguru* to the initiate. When the essential, enlightened consciousness of the *sadguru* enters the disciple, shaktipat occurs, and it is thought to destroy the root or foundational impurity of spiritual ignorance. In this way, shaktipat ignites the fire that will culminate in the achievement of liberation and enlightenment. Swami Chidvilasananda describes it this way:

> The Guru purges the seeker of worldly ignorance and bestows upon him the direct experience of the light of the Supreme Reality. Through Shaktipat, the Guru transmits his own fully awakened energy into the seeker, and the seeker's own inner energy, the kundalini, is awakened in turn. Thus, the process of Siddha Yoga begins to unfold.[6]

For the disciple, the occasion of shaktipat sets in motion an unprecedented journey of spiritual discovery. Though often received in the absence of formal, external rituals of initiation, shaktipat is essentially initiatory in character. It provokes a profound, experiential awakening. Having received shaktipat, the disciple finds that yogic sadhana (Sanskrit, *sādhana*: "practice") then begins to unfold naturally as he cultivates through his own efforts the liberating impulse of grace that is given in shaktipat.

It is traditionally said that there are four ways to grant shaktipat: by means of the guru's look, touch, word, or will.[7] This last is probably the most important. It is called *siddha-saṃkalpa*, the "intention of the perfected master." We will see that the early philosophies of shaktipat identify this purified and potent will of the guru with the divine will of Lord Śiva. Here Śiva is understood by the tradition both as the absolute consciousness as well as the primordial guru who is the fountainhead of shaktipat. It is important to emphasize that the guru is understood to embody Śiva and thus to be capable of wielding this divine will that functions as the essential mechanism of the initiatory process.

It is therefore quite significant that one of the primary ways in which Swami Muktananda characterized the purpose of his work, the mission of Siddha Yoga, was in terms of bringing the knowledge and power of shaktipat to the world. Early in his first world tour, Muktananda responded to an Australian woman's request for shaktipat in the following way:

> Certainly, *Shaktipat* is meant for everybody. What else do I have to give you? Babaji belongs to everyone, and so do his followers. I don't follow a religion.

> All people are my people. My only reason for travelling is that people receive *Shaktipat*, nothing else.[8]

Because of shaktipat's historical rarity and relative unavailability, the notion that Swami Muktananda should have made shaktipat attainable on a wide scale around the world is quite noteworthy. After many centuries of barely being available even in India, its sudden and relatively easy accessibility marks an unprecedented and significant historical shift. It is only when we fathom the rarity of what Swami Muktananda professed to be offering to the world that we can begin to appreciate the boldness and genius of his decision to bring shaktipat out of its millennial obscurity. He began quietly giving shaktipat to the seekers who found their way to his ashram in the early 1960s. With the decision in 1970 to launch his first world tour, Muktananda appears to have decided to make shaktipat the centerpiece of a worldwide movement of spiritual awakening, which later he was to call, quite forthrightly, the "meditation revolution." In this he was inspired, he always said, by the inner command of his own guru, Bhagawan Nityananda.

In the following account Gurumayi Chidvilasananda gives us a brief portrait of this meditation revolution in action. Though the account depicts but one of the countless occasions during which Swami Muktananda gave shaktipat, it gives us insight into the immediate experiential and transforming impact that shaktipat has. She says:

> When Baba was in Germany in 1976, he was giving evening program after evening program. Of course, Baba spoke in Hindi, then he gave me the grace to translate his words into English, and then that was translated into German, all one after the other. Of course, there were some Indians, and they got to understand Baba right away. Then there were some English-speaking people, one or two, so they got my translation right away. And then all the Germans had to wait until the other translator spoke, but by this time they had gone into deep meditation; they were not really there to listen to the talk. So even though Baba was giving this high wisdom night after night, everybody looked the same. There was no change.
>
> So four days later, Baba got fed up. But he did not get fed up in the way we do, where we give up. No, he would not give up. He said, "Tonight, no talk. Turn the lights off." He had everybody close their eyes, and he went around giving Shaktipat.
>
> The Germans had not heard about Shaktipat before. Now, they were already inside the hall, and they were very polite, they were not going to run away. So they closed their eyes and Baba went around with his peacock feathers awakening the inner energy.
>
> Lo and behold, within five minutes the room, and every person in it, began to change. The manager of the hotel where Baba was holding the program came running up. He thought something had really gone wrong. So he tried

to come in, wondering, what is going on? What has happened to all my people? Baba went out and told the manager, "There is nothing to worry about. Everything is going very well." The manager was happy to know that, and he went away.

An hour later, when everybody came out of meditation, they were able to understand what Baba was saying, because initiation had taken place. After that, we had to have a security system, because everybody began to follow Baba. And in their own language, they began to say, "Give more initiation. More."

The next night Baba said, "As long as your inner energy was not awakened, you took this life so seriously; now you know what this life is all about." And truly for the first time—after the initiation—they were able to understand what Baba said. Now they did not need any translation. In fact, Baba was just speaking in Hindi at times and everybody understood what he was saying, because his words were vehicles for the same energy, the same truth, the same love that they had experienced.[9]

What is it that occurred in that room that so radically changed the understanding of Swami Muktananda's audience? We are told that the manager of the hotel came running up to see what was going on. He did so because as Muktananda bestowed shaktipat the room erupted into an ocean of sound. Almost everyone in the room began to have *kriyās*, the spontaneous manifestations of initiation: shouting in joy, erupting in mantric sounds, engaging in spontaneous loud breathing or *prāṇāyāma* of a particularly noisy sort, spontaneously assuming difficult *haṭhayoga* poses, and much more. This noisy surface transformation of his audience registered the immediate, experiential impact of the initiation that Swami Muktananda was bestowing.[10] It should be noted that often those who are engaged in such noisy *kriyās* externally describe their inward state as one of absorption in a peace and recollection of the spirit that is of an entirely different nature from the visible, outward agitation. *Kriyās* of this sort tend to be part of the early stages of spiritual practice.

The term *kriyā* that is used to name these reactions to initiation literally means "action." In this sense, *kriyās* are generally understood to be secondary reactions to the process of initiation. They are not shaktipat itself but rather one of its by-products. As the awakened energy of *kuṇḍalinī* seeks to move and free itself within the person, it encounters obstacles and blockages. The *kriyās* are understood to be the result of an ongoing process of purification by means of which these obstacles and blockages are automatically removed.

As well, this vivid passage provides an early glimpse of Swami Muktananda's process of bringing shaktipat out of India. It alludes to some of the obstacles that he was to encounter continuously in such a process:

language and cultural barriers but, more importantly, the state of unawareness of his audience, their almost total lack of understanding of the significance and uniqueness of what he was offering to them. Much of Muktananda's work, as will be discussed later, was to give his students a conceptual understanding of shaktipat. The passage also depicts the immediate experiential impact of shaktipat, which seems to be what allowed Swami Muktananda to transcend and override many of the barriers that might otherwise have stood implacably in the way of students understanding and taking in what he was teaching. This depiction also gives us insight into another innovation of what might be termed "mass" shaktipat, the granting of shaktipat to many people at once. All of these elements constitute important aspects for an understanding of Muktananda's work as he instituted his "meditation revolution."

In the early days of the foundation of his ashram in Ganeshpuri, India, shaktipat was given individually and often in an unstructured way. In later years, Swami Muktananda gradually evolved the format of the Siddha Yoga Intensive as a vehicle for granting shaktipat to many hundreds of people at once. But at the beginning of his time as the guru, no such program existed. Like his teacher before him, when Muktananda first began giving shaktipat, it was almost always received by what could be called a process of divine contagion. Arriving at his ashram in Ganeshpuri in the early years, people would be welcomed by Muktananda and invited by him to enter into the quiet, daily routine of ashram life. Caught up in the mysterious and highly attractive presence of this guru, early seekers describe their experience of the spiritual fullness and sacredness that saturated the atmosphere of the ashram. With a minimum of outer guidance or direction, they were slowly enticed into the discovery of inwardness. Without formally performing any outward rituals of initiation and, most often, without even alluding to the process that was taking place, Swami Muktananda would grant shaktipat, and people would experience themselves going into spontaneous states of deep meditation. One early witness to these days describes his own experience:

> Bestowing grace was child's play for Baba. He gave off grace as naturally as the sun gives light. Sometimes you were not aware of it at first. It would happen while he was casually chatting with you, joking with you, playing with one of the ashram dogs, or talking to someone else. Grace flowed out of everything he did. At the same time, he always acted with meticulous care, and no detail escaped his attention.
>
> I first met Baba in 1960. I had gone to see Nityananda Swami at the insistence of a friend, who knew that I meditated regularly but was dissatisfied with my progress. I went for Nityananda's darshan twice, but he never even glanced at me. My anger grew as hot as the scorching sun outside. Seeing how upset I

> was, my friend told me that there was another swami down the road who would answer my questions. I was in no mood for another swami, but my curiosity got the better of me, and soon I found myself in the hall of Baba's ashram. The hall was almost full of devotees, and Baba was answering their questions. "Well," I thought, "at least this swami talks." My friend approached Baba, but I preferred to keep my distance. I folded my hands out of mere courtesy and sat on the marble floor. Baba was chatting with an elderly couple who had just been to England for the first time, and was inquiring about the details of their trip. I was barely paying attention.
>
> As I sat on the floor, I started to feel more and more comfortable and relaxed. All my anger and tension vanished. Soon I was totally relaxed. The atmosphere around me felt thick and soothing. All of a sudden a feeling of bliss began to well up from deep within me. This state was deepened and deepened, until I felt as though I were floating on waves of joy. I had known joy before, but nothing remotely like what I was now experiencing. When I became conscious, I thought, "He must be a Siddha. Let me know that you are responsible for what just happened to me." Just at that moment he looked me right in the eye. He laughed out loud with his rich, hearty laugh and pointed his finger right toward me.
>
> Though my feet were numb from having sat so long on the marble floor, somehow I managed to approach Baba. I bowed and touched his feet. I felt just like a child. He looked at me with the tenderest, most loving eyes, just like a mother looking at her son. Then he asked me, "Are you returning to Bombay?" I said, "Yes, Baba. I have to go." Baba said, "Okay, Okay. But do come again, huh? Return soon." He was like a mother telling a son not to stay out after sundown. Come home, my son, come home before sundown. That is how we parted.[11]

This passage typifies the experience of so many early seekers who seem to have stumbled into Swami Muktananda's ashram as if by accident or coincidence. Some came from nearby Bombay; others were intrepid world travelers who had somehow found their way to the isolated ashram where Muktananda lived. There they encountered his almost informal and nonritualistic style of giving shaktipat. In this, he was emulating the style of his own teacher, Bhagawan Nityananda. As Swami Muktananda says:

> [T]he power of a Siddha Guru is so great that one can receive his Shakti without any deliberate initiation. The Shakti that saturates his being also pervades the atmosphere around him, including the things he has used or worn. Therefore, if a person is receptive, it is enough for him simply to come near the Guru to receive that energy. It was like this with my own Guru. He would rarely give formal initiation. But so much Shakti flowed from him that people received Shaktipat even from his abusive words. Sometimes he would ask someone to leave, and the person would linger. Then my Guru would raise his arm

and throw a towel or some other object at him shouting, "Go now!" At that instant, the person would receive Shaktipat.[12]

With a kind of easeful spontaneity and seeming effortlessness, the siddha guru grants initiation. Nevertheless, as growing numbers of spiritual seekers arrived at the ashram, Swami Muktananda began to formalize and thus demarcate the process of shaktipat in a more overt manner. Beginning in 1970, he began signaling the granting of shaktipat by the giving of the "touch," either indirectly by the vigorous and repeated brushing of devotees with a wand of perfumed peacock feathers, or more directly by himself touching the head, forehead, or back of seekers with his hand in order to transmit into them the divine energy of his fully awakened consciousness.[13]

This manner of granting shaktipat finally evolved in 1974, at the beginning of Swami Muktananda's second world tour, into the format of the structured Intensive as the formal vehicle for shaktipat. The Intensive is a one- or two-day program that teaches all of the major elements of Siddha Yoga sadhana, and in the context of which people now more formally receive shaktipat. The following is a participant's account of an early Intensive given by Swami Muktananda in India in 1978:

> I received Shaktipat in the spring of 1978 in Ganeshpuri, India, when I first met Baba. It was very exciting being in India and meeting Baba for the first time there. In fact, there were old-timers in 1978. But things like Intensives were still very new and very exciting. I remember sitting in the Intensive as Baba had just finished an exquisite talk about the breath and the balancing of the energies. He was going around and beginning to give the touch. I was sitting there with my spine completely straight feeling a cool, shimmery, silvery light passing all the way from the top of my head to the base of my spine. The breath seemed to unite with this energy in a completely effortless way. It seemed as though my breath was just as much on the outside of my body as it was on the inside of my body. It almost felt as if my body itself was a permeable membrane that this breath and energy were both moving into and out of.
>
> As Baba was going around and giving the touch, I was in that state as I was sitting for meditation. When he came to me, he placed his hand on my forehead. It just lingered there for a moment. It was the softest touch. I felt this incredible "ah" inside myself as his hand was on my head.
>
> As his hand came off of my head, suddenly, there was an explosion of light inside. It was as if the whole field of vision, my whole field of awareness, burst into a brilliant red light. And then it burst into a brilliant golden light, and just as quickly, it burst into a brilliant blue light. There were no more thoughts, and I felt that I was not breathing. I was lost in a field of blue light where there were no thoughts and there was nothing but the sensation of pure awareness. There was simply the experience of "I am."

> At the end of the meditation, I was in a state of complete awe that I had met such a Guru for the first time, and that I had had this experience—so beyond my imagination or anything I could create. It is amazing.[14]

Powerful as this experience is, it is quite typical of the experiences of many thousands of people who received shaktipat from Swami Muktananda. As we have seen, upon receiving shaktipat, people say that dramatic and powerful experiences of very deep meditation often begin to manifest spontaneously. More importantly, the power of shaktipat is not limited to these immediate, dramatic experiences. Rather, shaktipat is felt as an opening to an ongoing, intense, and highly positive journey into spirituality and the evolving transformation of life.

The structure of the Siddha Yoga Intensive has continued to evolve and progress under the direction of Swami Chidvilasananda, who has instituted a number of thoughtful and insightful innovations. These are intended to clarify and further assist those who are receiving shaktipat and to instruct them about the nature of the experience and process. It is important to note that the fundamental experience of shaktipat remains a wholly inner event, which is apprehended privately and differently by each individual. In one of Chidvilasananda's Intensives in the mid-1990s, a woman wrote of her experience in the following way:

> On the last day of the Intensive during meditation, I experienced a piercing of the lower *cakra* [a center of energy], and it was like a laser beam, just a tiny point—very, very pointed like a laser beam. It was white and it went "shhhh" into that *cakra*. Well, . . . it was like an earthquake, and I started literally rumbling, like "bruuuu" at the base of the spine. Then I saw a shaft, it was like a *śivaliṅga*, but white—pure white—light at the base of my spine, beginning to push up my spine. The light was really exactly like the shape of a *śivaliṅga*. It was a very powerful, very solid light. It started pushing up my spine. At the second *cakra*, it found tremendous resistance to go through. I really started shaking up and down, very strongly. Then it finally got through and went very easily up until the heart *cakra*. There I felt resistance again, and pushed again very, very forcibly. Then it moved up to the throat *cakra*. There again resistance and pushing, pushing, pushing. Then it got to the crown *cakra*, to the head *cakra*, and there it became tiny, little blue lights that were falling like a fountain out of the crown *cakra*. It was just pure bliss, just complete bliss.[15]

This very classic experience of the ascent of the *kuṇḍalinī* energy, the piercing of the *cakras* (spiritual centers), and the entry into the highest space of consciousness, reveals an intriguing continuity with the most ancient sources of yoga in India. It will be one of our purposes here to explore this continuity with what we know from the traditional texts of India and to examine the nature of shaktipat, which has emerged from the obscurity and almost total unavailability that was the case less than fifty years ago.

SOURCES AND INITIAL CONCEPTS

In order to approach an understanding of the concept of shaktipat, the worldview and theoretical matrix within which this deeply esoteric subject is embedded must be explored. As well, it is important to keep in mind that there are several possible direct and indirect sources for such a practice in the broader sweep of the Indian tradition. Perhaps because shaktipat traditionally has been considered to be secret and rare, there occur relatively few direct references to it in the Indian scriptures. Nevertheless, we do find it treated in such geographically distant and chronologically disparate texts as the *Tirumantiram*, the *Yogavāsiṣṭha*, the *Kulārṇava Tantra*, the *Tantrāloka*, and Jñāneśwar's commentary on the *Bhagavadgītā*, to name just a few of the more salient examples. Moreover, in examining the meaning of shaktipat, it is useful to remember that there are several analogous initiatory and revelatory practices in the early phases of the Indian tradition.[16]

The clearest scriptural explication of the nature of shaktipat, however, is inherited primarily from the Śaiva Tantric traditions. It is in these traditions, in the writings of the tenth-century Kashmiri sage Abhinavagupta, that we find the most extended, early exposition of shaktipat. To explore what these and other Indian traditions have to say about the nature and necessity of shaktipat is to approach simultaneously one of the theoretical structures lying at the core of the worldview of Siddha Yoga.

In the Indian tradition, the freedom that resides in the power of grace and expresses itself as shaktipat contains a mystery that is as profound as that which is expressed by the bondage engendered by karma. The philosophical and religious traditions of India have puzzled over these mysteries and asked: How can the ultimate freedom and fullness of the primordial and absolute consciousness give rise to bondage and emptiness? How can ultimate consciousness be bound by the power of karma, or "action"? And once consciousness has been bound, how then does the state of liberation occur; how does the experience of freedom rise once again?

In attempting to address these queries, the Śaiva traditions create an elaborate soteriology, a conceptual structure in which both freedom and bondage are thought to arise from the will of Śiva, the supreme consciousness. Shaktipat resides very close to the center of these deliberations because it is thought to hold the experiential key that unlocks the knowledge of both bondage and liberation.

It might be noted that in certain of the earlier traditions of Indian religious practice, the notion of *dīkṣā*, or initiation, initially seems to have named an essentially ritual practice that was not necessarily attended by any experiential results. For example, it appears that the Kashmiri traditions of Śaiva Siddhānta understood it in this way.[17] *Dīkṣā* in this earlier sense was conceived as the formal, ritual entry into a life of ritual performances and of sectarian allegiance to a religious group, and it was thought to lead to a state of liberation only in the afterlife.[18]

It is only later that it begins to be conceived much more broadly than simply as a symbolic or performative ritual act marking the entry into a particular form of religious praxis. Since the time of Abhinavagupta and possibly even earlier, shaktipat has been understood to involve a fundamental spiritual transmission that carries a powerful and, in many cases, immediate experiential impact. As we have already mentioned, insofar as this transmissive or even transactional element comes to the fore, the performative aspects of the ritual of initiation tend to recede to a background position. This is evident already in the texts of the tradition that speak of the possibilities of initiation as something that can occur from seemingly casual contact with a master, or from dreams, or in other nonritualized ways. The focus thus shifts from the performance of an external ritual to the inner transmission of the awakening power, a transmission that may, but need not, occur in a formally ritualized way. In this way, there is a shift from the outer formalities of ritual to the inner domain of experiential awareness.

When shaktipat takes place, something moves from the guru to the disciple, and that is understood to be the *mantravīrya*, the "potency of the enlightened consciousness" of the guru, encapsulated in the sonic form of the initiatory mantra. The reception of the *mantravīrya* as the initiation mantra awakens the initiate to a journey of transformation that eventually results in the awakening characterized as *jīvanmukti*, liberation in this very life. In the *Tantrāloka*, Abhinavagupta describes in just such terms the transmission of the empowered mantra. He says:

> The subtle breath, which rises from the heart of the Master and which is like the moon or a crystal or a very fine thread, is composed of sound that serenely travels along the series of centers until it comes to rest at last in the *dvādaśānta*. The *dvādaśānta* is the terminal point where the *suṣumṇā* comes to an end. The *suṣumṇā* is the central pathway of the three paths. At this point, after having caused his heart to overflow, the teacher must recite the mantra, which then blazes brightly like an undersea fire and bursts forth from his eye sockets and the pores of his skin, until filling the tranquil topknot, in which are melted the streams of clarified butter, which has been propitiated and satisfied by the streams of clarified butter. The mantra then reaches the disciple's heart. In this way *mantras* give liberation when they are awakened and completely purified.[19]

This passage describes the inner processes performed by the guru in highly technical terms. For our purposes, it should be noted that the transmission of the guru's enlightenment is mediated to the disciple by the charged mantra that has been infused with the potency that dwells in the guru's heart. When this mantra is received, it functions like a sprouting seed from which there will unfold the new life of spirituality as the growth and development of the sequences of yogic sadhana. We will see that this passage from tenth-century Kashmir bears a striking resemblance to Swami Muktananda's description of his own shaktipat. For example, in his book *Secret of the Siddhas,* Muktananda says:

> That Siddha gave me one word [the mantra] which completely transformed me, but I had to spend such a long time with him to receive it. That word which I received after so many years spread through my body from head to toe like wildfire carried by the wind. It produced in me both inner heat and the coolness of joy.
>
> After the awakening of the Shakti, this process of yogic movements began to take place within my entire body. What power that word had! I almost hesitate to write all of this. It revealed whatever was within me—in my heart and in my head. I saw my own double many times. In the *sahasrāra* at the crown of the head, I perceived the brilliance of a thousand suns.[20]

Thus, shaktipat is essentially initiatory in character: It creates a new beginning that sets in motion a process of yogic sadhana. For this reason, the theoretical construction of shaktipat as elaborated in the Śaiva traditions gives us entry as well into the practice and phenomenology of yogic meditation. For if shaktipat is understood as a discrete initiatory event, it is an event with continuously operative and persistent consequences. It is through shaktipat that the ongoing process of experiential transformation and adaptation to the awakened energies of consciousness is set in motion. As Swami Chidvilasananda has described it:

> Shaktipat diksha is the master key that allows entry into the temple of truth.
>
> Shaktipat initiation, the awakening of the Kundalini Shakti, is the supreme act of the Master's grace. It is the lightning bolt that reveals the greatest treasure within. It is the ultimate gesture of compassion, the breath of the Absolute that breaks the chains of endless death and rebirth and sets you free once and for all. When Kundalini Shakti is awakened by the Master's grace, the knot of the heart is released. All karmas, all sins, are washed away and the pure Being is revealed within. This Being is the embodiment of wisdom, light, and truth.[21]

Let us explore and illustrate these initial theoretical considerations by turning to the specific example of Swami Muktananda's understanding of shaktipat.

SWAMI MUKTANANDA AND SHAKTIPAT

In his spiritual autobiography, *Play of Consciousness*, Swami Muktananda describes the initiation that he received from his guru, Bhagawan Nityananda.[22] After many decades of performing his own spiritual practices and after visiting most of the major teachers in India at that time, Muktananda spent a number of years paying prolonged visits to his guru. It was only then that he received the shaktipat that he later described as a "divine fortune." On the morning of August 15, 1947, after having spent the night in meditation in his guru's ashram, Muktananda received this initiation not in a formalized and ritualistic manner but rather by means of a series of seemingly impromptu yet overwhelmingly powerful actions by his guru.[23]

On that morning, Bhagawan Nityananda offered Swami Muktananda the pair of wooden sandals that he was uncharacteristically wearing that day, saying, "You'll wear my sandals?" Muktananda describes his amazement at this unprecedented and inexplicable gesture, and says he answered by saying:

> Gurudev, these sandals are not to be worn by my feet. Babaji, they are for me to worship all my life. I'll spread my shawl, and then please be so gracious as to put your feet on it and leave your sandals there.[24]

Swami Muktananda continues, describing what then took place:

> Gurudev agreed. Making the same humming sounds, he lifted his left foot, and its sandal, and placed it on the edge of my outspread shawl. Then he put his foot down, raised his right foot, and placed the other sandal on the shawl. He stood directly in front of me. He looked into my eyes once more. I watched him very attentively. A ray of light was coming from his pupils, and going right inside me. Its touch was searing, red hot, and its brilliance dazzled my eyes like a high-powered bulb. As this ray flowed from Bhagawan Nityananda's eyes into my own, the very hair on my body rose in wonder, awe, ecstasy, and fear. I went on repeating his mantra *Guru Om*, watching the colors of this ray. It was an unbroken stream of divine radiance. Sometimes it was the color of molten gold, sometimes saffron, sometimes a deep blue, more lustrous than a shining star. I stood there, stunned, watching the brilliant rays passing into me. My body was completely motionless. Then Gurudev moved a little and again made his "hunh, hunh." I became conscious again. I bowed my head upon the sandals, wrapped them in the shawl, prostrated myself on the ground. Then I got up, full of joy.[25]

Swami Muktananda's beautiful and charged description of his initiation continues with several other highly significant events—most importantly the reception of the *Oṃ Namaḥ Śivāya* mantra from his guru.

This remarkable account contains several important elements for the understanding of shaktipat. First, it might be noted that what is described is not a formal ritual in the usual sense in which Indian religious rituals are understood. The focus is entirely on the "transmission" of the divine energy, here meant in concrete, experiential terms. Swami Muktananda's rich description of the event reveals the intensity of this process, as he describes the searing, red-hot ray of light that enters him from his guru's eyes. This description parallels certain textual descriptions of initiation found in other places in the Indian tradition. The most remarkable parallel is found in the writings of Abhinavagupta when he describes the ritual of initiation that makes a new teacher.

However much the event of shaktipat was a cause of rejoicing for Swami Muktananda, those who continue reading his autobiography find out that it is really the beginning of a remarkable journey. It was followed by nine years of intense meditation practice and other forms of yogic sadhana. During those years, the gift of grace that Muktananda had received from his guru unfolded a series of extraordinary and even overwhelming spiritual experiences, visions, and states of advanced meditation. Finally, through his perseverance and practice, Muktananda received the ultimate gift that was contained in the moment of shaktipat: the achievement of the permanent state of liberation and fulfillment.

In later years, he became a world-famous teacher and himself a bestower of shaktipat to many tens of thousands of seekers. In order to explain the value and significance of what he was offering, Swami Muktananda would lavish effort on explaining and clarifying the process of shaktipat. In his mind, shaktipat constituted the most essential secret of spirituality—and not just Indian spirituality. Rather, he postulated the universality of shaktipat, pointing to its hidden or forgotten presence in all of the religious and spiritual traditions of the world. He would say, for example:

> All the great beings who expounded their own religions had this inner energy awakened. Some of them spoke about it, while others did not. If Jesus moved his hand over someone, that person would be completely transformed. What else was this but Shaktipat?[26]

Nevertheless, he recognized that its essential practice was either largely misunderstood or had been essentially lost. This was not only the case in the many religious traditions around the world, where, of course, the term *shaktipat* itself would not have been used, but also in India.

It is fair to say that Swami Muktananda's vigorous reestablishment of the practice of shaktipat initiation, as well as his detailed explanations of this extremely esoteric practice, revived and once again brought to light a secret of yoga that had been long hidden and, indeed, was largely lost even in India.

It is not just that Swami Muktananda brought shaktipat to the West. He could also be said to have brought shaktipat to contemporary India, by rekindling an understanding of the practice as well as by imparting, on a wide basis, this secret key to the highest form of yoga. In many ways, it might be said that the primary and most important contribution that Swami Muktananda made was to reestablish the practice of shaktipat. He says:

> For countless ages, *shaktipāt* has been used as a secret means of initiation by the great sages. To transmit one's own glory and luster of divine enlightenment into a disciple and give him an instantaneous, direct experience of Brahman, the Eternal Spirit, is the secret meaning of *shaktipāt.*[27]

In order to explain this "secret means of initiation," Muktananda connects shaktipat with the *kuṇḍalinī,* saying:

> In every human being there dwells a divine energy, the *kundalinī shakti.* This energy has two aspects: one manifests *samsāra,* the ephemeral worldly existence; the other leads to the highest Truth. When the Guru transmits his soul power to a disciple, the latter aspect of the Kundalini Shakti is automatically activated in the disciple and set into operation. This is known as *shaktipāt dīkshā* [initiation] or *gurukripā* [the grace of the guru].[28]

As we have already seen, the term *shaktipat* means the "descent of the *śakti,*" the spiritual energy or cosmic power. As Swami Muktananda tells us, shaktipat is directly related to the awakening or activation of what is termed the *kuṇḍalinī-śakti,* which is the coiled energy or power that lies dormant in the subtle body. With the awakening or activation of this dormant power, the process of yoga is set in motion. The awakened inner power sets the foundation for the life of spirituality.

It seems evident that the conceptual and intellectual understanding of shaktipat that Muktananda later would bestow on his own students was not a knowledge that necessarily came easily or immediately to him. Part of his struggle during the nine years that he spent immersed in meditation following his initiation involved precisely his attempt to understand what it was that he had received. It also involved his attempt to locate and identify the historical presence of shaktipat in the philosophical and religious writings of the Indian tradition. Thus, there is a useful distinction between the experiential knowledge of the inner Self awakened by shaktipat as given to Swami Muktananda by Bhagawan Nityananda, and the gathering up of the conceptual knowledge about shaktipat from a variety of sources. Obviously, these written sources did not give Muktananda shaktipat and would have been—for his purposes—useless to him without shaktipat itself. Nevertheless, the textual and scriptural sources that he gradually discovered were invaluable in helping him to understand his experiences. This relationship between the primacy of a direct, experiential knowledge of the Self given by shaktipat and the assistance received from a conceptual understanding and intellectual knowledge *about* shaktipat itself is very important. It is in examining this relationship that the place and function of study and insight in assisting the work of shaktipat are brought to light. Although he never defined himself as such, Swami Muktananda was himself something of a scholar, but only insofar as scholarship and scriptural study were able to illuminate the direct experiential knowledge that unfolds from yoga. Muktananda always criticized a "dry" (i.e., unilluminated) scholarly knowledge.

It is in this particular combination of someone who had received the very powerful impact of shaktipat from his guru—as Swami Muktananda had—and an existing body of traditional knowledge about such an initiation that the revival of the knowledge of shaktipat was able to occur. Muktananda candidly recounts the series of events in the years following his initiation by means of which he gradually discovered and identified what it was that he had so dramatically received from his guru.

It is interesting to look into the precise textual *sources* by means of which this conceptual understanding of shaktipat was mediated to him. There is a difference between the reception of shaktipat and the mediation to Swami Muktananda of the *concept* of shaktipat and its various theoretical components. It is important to understand that the experience itself initiated an intellectual search for understanding, contextualization, connection to the larger tradition, and a progressive understanding of the universality of the phenomenon that had been granted to him by his guru. Especially in portions of *Play of Consciousness*, we witness Swami Muktananda's perplexity (which threatens to undermine all that he has received) and his search for a means of understanding what is happening to him. He says:

> At this time, I understood nothing about the various experiences, such as the vision of dissolution and the radiant light, that had come to me on the first day. Only afterward did I learn that they were all part of a process pertaining to Shaktipat. Shaktipat is simply another name for the full grace of the supreme Guru, the blessing of a Siddha, or *shāmbhava* initiation. People who have experienced it call it the awakening of the Kundalini.[29]

It is very interesting to see the candidness with which Muktananda confesses that he "understood nothing about the various experiences" he was having. He experienced himself as being in the grip of an overwhelming power that was revealing the mysteries of the inner worlds to him, but he had not yet received a conceptual category within which he could categorize and understand the phenomenon of shaktipat. He continues, saying:

> At this time I did not know that I had received the sacred Shaktipat. For two consecutive days I saw a number of different lights along with the red light. I

was fully conscious of everything that was happening in meditation, and I was also happy. As I watched the lights, I would see naked men and children, cows and herds of splendid war-horses. Sometimes I would see the images of deities in the temples in neighboring villages. I meditated without fail every morning and every evening for two hours or sometimes longer, and I meditated with great love. Sometimes a very pure intoxication would come over me—what ecstasy that was!—but I did not have the strength to bear it; as I became absorbed in that intoxication, I would fall asleep.[30]

In this revealing passage, Muktananda describes some of the varied phenomena of meditation that were erupting in his consciousness as a result of shaktipat and because of his own assiduous cultivation of its power through meditation. It is important to note here that the intense fervor and dedication with which he cultivated his spiritual practices is itself something that in later years he would recognize as a gift of the process of shaktipat. But, as he so clearly stipulates here, though shaktipat was working its intense process within him, he still says, "At this time I did not know that I had received the sacred Shaktipat." He then gives us a few details of the process by means of which he finally comes to identify and recognize that he has received shaktipat from his guru. He says:

There was a cupboard in that hut. As I was sitting there, I heard a voice within me asking me to open the cupboard and read the book lying inside. First I did not pay much attention to it but I heard the same words two or three times. It became impossible for me to ignore them so I opened the cupboard and picked up the book. The very same page I opened described the yogic experiences I was passing through. It also explained how a person who had received Shaktipat by the grace of a *siddha* Guru and whose Kundalini was thereby awakened, got different kinds of wonderful experiences. Reading a few pages of the book, I was relieved of all mental disturbance and became peaceful. No doubt I had passed several days in a state of great anxiety and dejection; but when I read that book I was fully convinced that I was experiencing the reward of virtuous actions, not the bitter fruit of sinful deeds.[31]

It is important to note that it is this intellectual knowledge about shaktipat, derived from his readings of various scriptures, that sets his mind greatly at ease. He goes from anxiety and dejection to a state of peace and a reinforced commitment to his spiritual practices. Now he is able to pursue his meditation vigorously once again, and simultaneously, it is clear, he continues to search the scriptures for descriptions and clarifications of the highly mysterious nature of shaktipat. His description continues:

Nagad was a solitary and beautiful place. My meditation progressed automatically. I studied books such as *Mahāyoga Vijñāna*, containing descriptions of some experiences which are helpful for the yoga of meditation. I sent for

> other, similar books, such as *Yogavāni* and *Shaktipāt*. Mahā Yoga has a very important place in Shaivite philosophy. In the *Shiva Sūtras, Pratyabhijñā-hridyayam, Tantrāloka, Shiva Drishti*, and other works, one can read what the saints say, in the light of their own experiences, about Shaktipat, the grace of a Siddha, and the dynamic play of mother Kundalini.[32]

The fervor of meditation and its varied and fascinating experiential fruits now clearly impel Swami Muktananda to identify and understand intellectually what is happening to him. In this passage, he describes how he begins to reach out to connect with the textual traditions of Indian spirituality. He is seeking to recognize himself and his experiences in the authoritative spiritual texts, in the scriptures of India. Having done so, Muktananda renews his practice and sets it on a firm foundation. He says:

> Now my practice of yoga started to progress very quickly. Three things had combined to bring this about: divine Shaktipat, the grace of a great Siddha, and a burning desire to attain God. Before I had lacked one thing: knowledge about the experiences and the yogic *kriyās* that happen after Shaktipat. Now that I had read the books that explained it all to me, what was there to hold me back? My *sādhanā* advanced with the speed of a river in flood. I had new kriyas every day.[33]

This statement is very important. Having received intellectual clarification of the mysterious nature of shaktipat and of the many powerful, even overwhelming spiritual phenomena that had been unleashed within him by his guru's initiation, Swami Muktananda now feels fully capable of pursuing his sadhana with great force and dedication.

These descriptions by Swami Muktananda of his gradual identification and discovery of the knowledge about shaktipat are very important, for they exemplify and certify the relationship of initiation to intellectual knowledge. Moreover, they describe the very process by which Muktananda was ultimately able to revive the understanding of shaktipat. We now proceed to further explore the nature of what the scriptural traditions of India have to say about shaktipat.

SHAKTIPAT PIVOTS THE DIVINE PLAY OF ŚIVA AND ŚAKTI

In order to understand further the notion of shaktipat, it is crucial to look more deeply into the understanding of Śiva and Śakti. As has already been said, shaktipat—both as a notion and as an esoteric secret of a salvational path—is embedded in a conceptual structure. This structure attempts to make sense of and bring an overarching dimension of coherent meaning to the existential situations and predicaments of life. The conceptual structure—it might be called Śaivite theology or philosophy—narrates the play of cosmic forces and the intrinsic and fundamental reality behind the panorama of life.

In the usual parlance of Hinduism, the term *śiva* names a primordial and awesome deity, anthropomorphically portrayed in many forms and guises. He appears as a great and dynamic dancer, the four-armed Naṭarāja; or as a blue-throated ascetic, the transcendentally calm and trident-armed supreme yogi; or as a terrifying and remote being named Bhairava, who is at once the cosmic guru or supreme teacher as well as the overseer of the process of cosmic destruction at the end of time.

However, the great theologians and philosophers of the traditions of Śaivism expand and broaden the meaning of *śiva*. Without contradicting or subverting the images of this personified deity, the term *śiva* is additionally used to name the absolute consciousness, a reality of superb unboundedness and of incomparable freedom. Śiva, in this deeper, less personalized sense, refers to the ultimate reality. It is the foundation of being and of all becoming, the intrinsic and eternal truth behind the façade of the ever-changing display of life.

Most importantly, Śaivite philosophy asserts that Śiva, in this absolute sense, constitutes the true and most profound identity of all human beings.[34] Indeed, it is finally Śiva who is the living and percipient consciousness concealed *in* and *as* all living beings. The purpose of all Śaivite philosophy (and of its attendant yogas and sadhanas) is precisely the experiential realization of this truth. Such a realization—gained perhaps over many lifetimes of effort and achieved with profound existential consequences—uncovers the complete, permanent, and ecstatic awareness that "I am Śiva," (*Śivo 'ham*). The achievement of this realization—which reveals a truth that is always and already the case—constitutes the highest purpose of Śaivism known as *mukti* or *mokṣa*, "freedom" or "liberation." The achievement of *mokṣa*—as conceived by these schools and lineages and, indeed, by all Hindu schools—is the highest purpose or aim of human existence. Shaktipat plays a crucial and pivotal role in the achievement of this goal.

Śaivite philosophy tells us that, impelled by the will of Śiva, the intricate and complex dance of existence continuously arises. By setting in motion this cosmogonic impulse, Śiva apparently fragments his intrinsic fullness and seems to lose himself in a forgetfulness that then appears as the life experience of the myriad beings that inhabit countless universes. Nonetheless, impelled by a countervailing impulse of his own supreme will, Śiva, as these myriad beings, must find a way back to himself—back to the totality and wholeness of the absolute consciousness. It is here that shaktipat plays a crucial role. By impelling the journey of yogic sadhana, shaktipat initiates the journey of remembrance and recognition (*pratyabhijñā*). In this cosmic sense, shaktipat sets in motion the journey of Śiva's return to himself. In this cosmic play, the guru—who is considered to be none other than the embodiment of Śiva or the absolute consciousness—gives shaktipat to the disciple, who thereby recognizes and remembers his true identity as Śiva. In this way, the Śaivite traditions of India understand that it is by means of what is called *anugraha-śakti*, the "power of grace," that the supreme Lord as the guru bestows shaktipat on himself as the disciple.

As we have seen, the term *śakti* names the intrinsic power of this absolute consciousness. Just as Śiva is conceived both anthropomorphically as well as in terms of an ineffable and formless absolute consciousness, so too is the *śakti*. There are many forms of the Goddess, or *devī*, in the Indian tradition: Kālī, Durgā, Lakṣmī, Sarasvatī, Lalitā, and many other images of the primordial Śakti, who is the supreme mother of creation and who is intimately and intricately involved in its functioning. But simultaneously, in the nondual Śaiva and in the later Śākta traditions, the power, or *śakti*, of the absolute consciousness is thought of as an intrinsic and inseparable power that is nondifferent from Śiva himself. The power-holder and the power are likened to the flower and its fragrance or the fire and its heat.

Moreover, in the Indian tradition this cosmic and ultimate power of consciousness known as the *śakti* is always conceived as having two sides or aspects. One aspect of this cosmic energy is always involved in the continuously creative process of manifesting the relative and ever-changing world of our daily experience. The *śakti* creates and sustains the myriad forms of life. It creates and sustains the very fabric of existence within which both animate beings and inanimate objects can exist. By creating the transitory worlds of relative experience, however, this aspect of the *śakti* is also responsible for obscuring from view the eternal and absolute consciousness that is known as Śiva.

The second aspect of the *śakti* is continuously involved in revealing once again the absolute consciousness that it has initially concealed. This happens by means of the operation of shaktipat. Once activated and released by the operation of the guru, the *śakti* begins to reveal a deeper and more fundamental reality, the reality of the absolute consciousness that underlies and informs our daily experience. In the most advanced practitioner, the activated *kuṇḍalinī* awakened by shaktipat will reveal the vision of this absolute and irreducible reality and, indeed, finally stabilize the practitioner in a state of its permanent and omnipresent awareness.

This energy, which is called *śakti*, gives its name to the form of initiation that we have been considering. Shaktipat as the "descent of *śakti*" is described by Swami Muktananda in classic terms that hearken back to the great Tantras and Āgamas of medieval India. He says:

> That energy which has the supreme capacity to create the universe independently, is called the *chiti shakti*. This pure Consciousness, which is full of absolute bliss, dwells in the Guru in its fullness.[35]

He continues tracing the cosmic nature of the *śakti* saying:

> When the attributeless, formless, changeless Reality which underlies the entire universe, and which is pure, ultimate Consciousness, is stirred up, this divine energy begins to operate in it. She is the power of becoming, released out of the Eternal Being and expressing herself through all names, all forms, and all changes that we call the world. Indeed, She is the most magnificent power—Shri Kundalini Shakti—of the Supreme Reality.[35]

This description locates the most fundamental, cosmic creative energy of consciousness as that which is being awakened in some new way by shaktipat. The very energy that has created the visible cosmos and all the beings that dwell in it is the energy of the primordial and absolute consciousness. Indeed, it is not so much that the energy has created the world as that the world is the concretization of Śakti, who reveals herself tangibly in the spectacular and endless display of visible reality. It is for this reason that Muktananda considers this universal energy to be present in every religious and spiritual tradition. Again, Swami Muktananda synthesizes all of the traditions with which he is familiar and points out the intrinsic unity of their discourse about the ultimate, saying:

> This active energy has many names—Chiti, Mahamaya, Shiva's Gauri, Narayana's Lakshmi, Rama's Sita, Krishna's Radha, the yogi's Kundalini, the poet's inspiration, and the blissful stream of joy of the *ātman*—and an infinite number of aspects. This divine energy is not in any way different from or independent of the highest reality.[37]

So the meaning of shaktipat revolves around this great power of consciousness. Just as this power has been set free to display herself as the visible cosmos and all the beings that dwell therein, she has however in that process obscured the primordial attributeless and ultimate consciousness. So, in the dialectic of these traditions, the creative or manifestational impulse of Śakti is seen also as the operation of the power of concealment (*tirodhāna*). The ultimate becomes hidden, lost from sight, unavailable to experience. The theoretical crux of shaktipat revolves, then, around the need for some new impulse that will begin the phase of revelation of the ultimate consciousness.

Shaktipat is understood as this new and highly secret phase of the operation of the divine energy. It begins a new process of creativity and intelligence, one that will ultimately result in the tangible revelation of the ultimate consciousness. The "great and perfect yoga," the "yoga of the perfected ones," Siddha Yoga is the name that Swami Muktananda gave to this process. In it the very same energy that has operated to conceal the ultimate consciousness behind the visible cosmos now begins to operate intelligently and spontaneously, as well as tenderly and ferociously, implacably and—ultimately—unstoppably to reveal the experience of the ultimate consciousness. This is what is called shaktipat: the "great descent of the *śakti.*" Because the great energy of consciousness is said to be fully present in the guru, to receive such an initiation is to receive what is conceived of as the highest and the most potent and effective initiation into spirituality. Historically, then, such an initiation was rare even in India, and was considered one of the most closely guarded secrets of the millennial teachings of yoga. As Swami Chidvilasananda has said:

> With the initiation called *shaktipat,* the Guru transmits his own fully awakened, conscious energy into the disciple. Through this action, the Guru ignites the same Kundalini energy that lies dormant in the disciple, waiting to catch fire. Putting this divine act into words makes it sound so simple and easy, but what actually happens within, hidden from the senses, is something marvelous. It can only be deciphered by the deepest part of you, yet your whole being is rejuvenated by its light.[38]

After receiving such an initiation, what before was attempted with great effort now begins to happen of its own accord. An account of just such a shift from difficult practice to effortless success is given by an early recipient of shaktipat from Swami Muktananda:

> When I received shaktipat I had been practicing a very complicated technique of visualization. One feature of it was that I had to visualize little fiery balls of energy moving from my navel center to the heart and then to the *ājñā cakra.* I could never get it. It was torturous trying to visualize something that I could never see! The day after I got shaktipat I sat to meditate and to my amazement the little red balls were there and not only were they there, they were full of heat and glowing with a luminescent radiance, and moving by themselves up to the heart and *ājñā cakra* and back again. It was extraordinary to me to see that the inner world was actually real and not just a subject for books.[39]

The reception of shaktipat opens a new vista on spiritual practice, which becomes a process of allowing the great energy to do its work, of cooperating, even of getting out of the way so that the *śakti* can carry out its purification and upliftment. Swami Muktananda says:

> After a disciple is initiated by such a Guru, various types of internal activities occur. Some disciples experience great joy, while others become either apparently dull and stupefied, or restless. With certain disciples a variety of strange bodily reactions, such as yogic postures, gestures, tremors, or dancing

> poses, begin to take place involuntarily in every part of the body. This may cause wonder.[40]

These initial symptoms can be of the most varied kinds. As we have seen, they are already talked about and classified in the esoteric texts of the medieval Śaivism of Kashmir. Swami Muktananda continues:

> Some disciples get frightened. For a short period of time, one may feel pain in almost every part of the body. Various stirrings may occur in the heart, head, and abdomen; and throbbing of the muscles and fascinating, thrilling sensations may be experienced. One may feel drowsy and may even enter a state of deep meditation without making any effort.[41]

What should be emphasized is that shaktipat is the releasing into operation of an autonomous and intelligent energy that will accomplish its purposes independently of the will of the practitioner. This is why the Siddha Yoga gurus speak of the "spontaneous yoga," the "yoga of grace." As it moves into operation, this energy reveals the deeper structures of consciousness, the mechanisms of liberation that are secretly present in the makeup of a human being. This is not to say that nothing need be done by the practitioner. On the contrary, he or she must learn how to cooperate intelligently with the operation of this energy before it may succeed in accomplishing its revelatory and liberating purpose. Swami Chidvilasananda comments on this saying:

> It is your destiny that brings you to the Guru to receive *shaktipat*, but then you must make the right self-effort to cultivate the golden virtues. With this partnership, you conserve the energy that has been awakened within you so that it can transmute all your inferior qualities into sublime ones.[42]

Once activated by the power of the siddha guru, however, the *śakti* will continue irresistibly to operate until it leads the practitioner to the highest state of spirituality. Swami Muktananda describes this process saying:

> When a disciple begins to see lights of different colors—red, white, black and azure—in meditation, his joy increases day by day, and he follows his spiritual discipline with greater enthusiasm. Sometimes during meditation one may see temples, mountains, caves, and even other worlds. Thereafter, a divine light of indescribable luster is always visible during meditation.[43]

This is the context for an understanding of the process of shaktipat: an ancient, secret, and esoteric form of initiation into the highest, most authentic, and spontaneously liberating spiritual discipline or yoga. As Swami Muktananda emphasizes:

> The Shakti, the active aspect of the Supreme Lord, which brings about the creation, continued existence, and absorption of the universe, is the Supreme

> Shakti Uma, also described in the *Shiva Sūtra Vimarshini* as follows: *paraiva pārameshvarī svātantryarūpā*, "She is absolute and of independent will." She creates an infinite number of worlds out of nothing. She is the same Shakti which is awakened in a disciple by the Guru's grace. Can any spiritual practices be difficult for those whose Kundalini is awakened by the Guru's grace? Even salvation is within their easy reach. Such favored ones practice the easiest of the easy means of discipline. The power of *gurukripā* always saves them from degradation.[44]

To appreciate the genius of Swami Muktananda's synthesis and exposition of the concept of shaktipat, as well as to understand further its theoretical backdrop, we may now turn to the older Śaiva traditions of Kashmir to explore what they have to say about this subject.

SHAKTIPAT IN THE ŚAIVISM OF KASHMIR

The earliest, sophisticated theoretical exploration of shaktipat in the Indian scriptural tradition occurs in the writings of the tenth-century Kashmiri philosopher and teacher Abhinavagupta. In his massive work entitled, "Light on the Tantras" (*Tantrāloka*), Abhinavagupta discusses in some detail both the theory within which the process of shaktipat becomes meaningful as well as some of the technical points that explain the great variety of experiences that its reception can precipitate. It is important to note that Abhinavagupta attributes his own intellectual and spiritual attainments to the receiving of shaktipat. In *Tantrāloka*, Abhinavagupta explains:

> The highest Reality, the nature of which is a free Consciousness, the supreme Light, out of its own enjoyment of the sport of concealing his own true nature, becomes the atomic, finite self, of which there are very many. He himself, as a result of his own freedom, binds himself here by means of karma, actions, the nature of which are composed of imaginary differentiations. Such is the power of the Lord's freedom that, even though he has become the finite self, he once more truly attains his own true form in all its purity.[45]

This passage sets up the fundamental notion that it is Śiva himself who has concealed himself as all living beings. This is the nature of his divine sport or play (*krīḍā*), which arises purely as an expression of his own supremely unimpeded freedom. As part of his play, Śiva proceeds to bind himself—that is apparently to lose the supremely free and unbounded consciousness that is his true nature—and thus he appears as the limited and bound consciousness that, in different measures, characterizes the awareness of all transmigrating beings. Abhinavagupta continues:

> The cause of grace is therefore Śiva himself, pure, whose essence is the free and autonomous light. The fact that there exist several grades of such an illumination is also due to his freedom alone.[46]

In this passage, Abhinavagupta asserts that though it is by his own will that Śiva has bound himself in sport, it is also by his own supreme will that he now bestows his grace on any particular limited and transmigrating being. It is by means of this bestowal of grace that the unbounded consciousness, concealed and hidden behind the play of limitations of form, will once again reveal itself as the true reality.

This passage also alludes to the notion that there are several different grades of illuminative experience that arise as an immediate result of shaktipat. This too is asserted by Abhinavagupta to be an expression of the freedom of the Śiva. In an organizational schema of some subtlety, Abhinavagupta discusses three "levels" of intensity of shaktipat. These are labeled "mild," "medium," and "intense." Each of these is further subdivided into three sub-levels and three sub-sub-levels for a total of twenty-seven.[47] The details of this schema are not as interesting as the essential implication of what is conveyed by this graduated spectrum of possible levels of what is actually experienced by the person who receives shaktipat initiation. Those who experience the most intense varieties of shaktipat reception are very strongly moved to spiritual life in an irrevocable and totally focused manner. Indeed, it is thought that the most intense form of shaktipat precipitates enlightenment itself as an immediate consequence. In a slightly less intense form, the reception of shaktipat inspires the desire to pursue spiritual practices with great zeal.

In the median and less intense fashion, the reception of shaktipat plants a seed of spirituality that will bear fruit in the person in corresponding degrees of effortful turning toward spirituality. It is important to realize that these distinctions of experiential result do not subvert the notion that from the highest perspective there is really only one shaktipat, as the descent of divine grace and as the shattering of the *āṇavamala* (which is discussed in some detail in what follows). These grades of shaktipat classify the perceived "experience" of shaktipat on the side of the receiver, so to speak. It is also important to note that in terms of this schema, it appears to be the case that when Swami Muktananda refers to shaktipat, he seems to be referring primarily to the most intense varieties.

Stating the matter in a slightly different way in his *Parātrīśikālaghuvṛtti*, Abhinavagupta says:

> He who obtains this seed-mantra, in the very moment he obtains it, is no longer a bound creature. Because when this seed-mantra is obtained for him, this Heart is produced. This Heart is the very condition of Bhairava. For that reason, as long as he is not born from the union of the pair—from the union

> of Rudra and the yoginī—that is to say, as long as he has not opened his vision to the very Self or, in other words, if "descent of energy" (*śaktipāta*) has not fallen on him, how then could this Heart appear to him?[48]

In this passage Abhinavagupta reasserts the unique centrality and importance of the initiation mantra to the process of shaktipat. It is clear as well from this passage that it is not just a random sequence of sounds that constitutes the liberating and transmissive power of the mantra. It is the fact that the mantra is somehow charged with the expressly revealing, liberating, and graceful power of the enlightenment of the guru that allows it to function as an instrument of grace.

An important element in this consideration has to do with what are called the *pañcavidha-kṛtya*, the "fivefold cosmic actions" of Lord Śiva. These are generally enumerated as: (1) creation or manifestation (*sṛṣṭi*), (2) maintenance (*sthiti*), (3) destruction or dissolution (*saṃhāra*), (4) concealment (*vilaya, tirodhāna*), and (5) the revealing power that grants grace (*anugraha*). Each of these functions or actions is understood as a *śakti*, a power of the Lord. The Śaivite traditions emphasize that he is perennially and simultaneously involved in the process of performing these five great cosmic actions. In the "Doctrine of Recognition" (*Pratyabhijñāhṛdayam*), Kṣemarāja, the primary disciple of Abhinavagupta, says:

> Here, the distinction between the *Īśvarādvaya* [i.e. Śaivite] philosophy from (that of) the Brahmavādins [i.e. the Vedāntins] lies in this—that the divine whose essence is consciousness always retains his authorship of the fivefold act which is in accordance with what has been stated by the grand *Svacchanda* and other disciplines (of Śaiva Philosophy), viz., (Vide. *Svacchanda Tantra* 1st Paṭala, 3rd verse) "(I bow to the) Divine who brings about (1) emanation (*sṛṣṭi*), (2) re-absorption (*saṃhāra*), (3) concealment (*vilaya*), (4) maintenance (of the world) (*sthiti*), who dispenses, (5) grace (*anugraha*), and who destroys the affliction of those who have bowed down (to Him)."[49]

Of these five functions there is much to say, including the interesting analysis Śaivism makes of their inherent presence in every moment of individual perception. But for our present purposes, it is the fifth function, the *anugraha-śakti*, that is of greatest relevance. There are several pertinent questions that are posed and answered in the texts of Śaivism. The first inquires: How does the Lord bestow this power of grace? A second important question further queries, Why is it necessary to receive this grace?

The response as proposed by Śaivism to the first question has already been considered in some detail. Shaktipat initiation (and the resultant journey of yoga) implements the specific operation of the *anugraha-śakti*, the supreme Lord's revealing power of grace. It is specifically through the *sadguru* that the *anugraha-śakti* functions most explicitly and palpably. In his comment on the *Śiva Sūtra*, Kṣemarāja makes the famous statement, which is often quoted by both Swami Muktananda and Swami Chidvilasananda:

> The Guru is the grace-bestowing power of the Lord [*gurur vā pārameśvarī anugrāhikā śaktiḥ*].[50]

The *Kulārṇava Tantra* mentions the process of shaktipat in a chapter devoted to the nature of initiation, saying quite explicitly:

> The disciple receives the Guru according to the impact of the *śakti* (*śaktipāta*); where there is no impact of the *śakti*, there is no fulfillment.[51]

Once again, this passage emphasizes the unique importance of the *sadguru* for the process of initiation. It also reiterates the notion that it is shaktipat alone that sets the stage for the achievement of spiritual fulfillment. Why this is the case from a technical perspective is the consideration taken up in the next section.

WHY IS SHAKTIPAT NECESSARY? THE NATURE OF THE THREE *MALA*S

The traditional argument for the necessity of shaktipat to be found in some expositions of Śaivite philosophy revolves around the notion of the three *mala*s, the three "impurities."[52] Śaivite philosophy (particularly of the nondual variety) asserts that it is only shaktipat that can overcome what is called the *āṇavamala*, the impurity of limitation or smallness. In order to understand what this is, we must return to analyze the fourth cosmic power of Śiva. This is called the *tirodhāna-śakti*: the power that conceals, the power that obscures or binds. Within the transmigrating individual, the *tirodhāna-śakti* functions by means of three powerful shackles that imprison Śiva himself within the *jīva*, the "transmigrating soul." These shackles are the three *mala*s, three encircling forms of limitation that Śiva creates to imprison himself in bondage—the *āṇavamala*, the "limitation of smallness"; the *māyīyamala*, the "limitation of illusion"; and the *kārmamala*, the "limitation of action and the illusion of doership."[53]

Śaivite philosophy asserts that these shackles are so powerful that once Śiva freely imprisons himself in them, he becomes the small self, the *jīva*. It is as if Śiva, the great and unbounded consciousness, impelled by his desire to sport or play (*krīḍā*), locks himself in a prison and then hides the key. The *jīva* then cannot release itself, even though in its deepest essence it is still the infinite light of consciousness. Only someone who is no longer bound by the three *mala*s can open the door that liberates the *jīva*.

The basic and deepest shackle is called the *āṇavamala*, the self-limitation that the infinite Śiva imposes on himself to become small. The supreme consciousness contracts into what is called a *cidaṇu*, an "atom of consciousness." Śaivite philosophy asserts that each human being is a *cidaṇu*, a "small self." *Aṇu* means "atom"; *āṇava* is an adjectival form meaning "atomic"; so the *āṇavamala* is the "limitation of smallness." As a result, Śiva's essential nature is veiled. His omnipotence, omniscience, fullness, eternity, and freedom become concealed.

The *cidaṇu*, or small self, begins to experience itself as an emptiness that desires very powerfully to be filled. At this point there arises the limitation known as the *māyīyamala*, the "limitation of *māyā*, or cosmic illusion." It is described as a darkening or a veiling. It darkens the *cidaṇu* which then lies submerged in a state of total ignorance of its true nature, almost like a piece of inert matter. The *māyīyamala*, the second limitation, compounds the difficulties of the small self because it begins to encompass it with the great universe and the experiences of difference and diversity, polarities and dualities. Where there was only oneness, twoness begins to spring up: light and dark, pleasure and pain, male and female, good and evil, heat and cold. Also, it is within *māyā*, or illusion, that the seeds of *karma*, of "action," lie latent. *Māyā* arouses the impulse toward action and the vast possibilities inherent within Śiva begin to emerge. The small self draws to itself the material elements suitable for the creation of a body.

This is actually accomplished by the third limitation, the *kārmamala*, the "limitation of action," which impels the creation of the limited mind and physical body that will permit the performance of actions. The *kārmamala* results in even further concealment of the true nature of the Self as the activities of body, senses, and mind are superimposed on it. The result is a transmigrating being associated with a body.

The technical term for such a being is a *sakala*, that is, one who is associated only with what is fragmented, limited, partial, and incomplete. Because such a being is completely oblivious of the true Self, there occurs complete identification with the temporary coverings of the body, the transitory experiences of the senses, and the ever-shifting display of the personality and limited ego. This is called ignorance or delusion: the compact mass of delusion that covers over the Self and involves the *cidaṇu* in karma, or pleasurable and painful actions. These actions produce reactions, which the limited self is bound to experience, and so the *jīva* falls deeper and deeper into the net of karma. This is Indra's cosmic net. The more one struggles to escape, the tighter its ropes cut and bind one. The result is the immensely long journey of transmigration, as the small self restlessly moves from one plane of existence to another impelled by its karma and the results of its karma.

"Shaktipat" is the name of the process that comes to rescue the small self from its dilemma. "Shaktipat" is the name that is given to the operation of the fifth of the five powers of Śiva, the *anugraha-śakti*, the "power of revealing" and the "power of grace." It is so important to understand the nature of the *tirodhāna-śakti*, the "power of concealing," precisely in order to understand the functioning of this power of grace. When he hides himself in the small self through the power of concealing, Śiva becomes the supreme secret of reality, the hidden and precious secret of life. In the game of cosmic hide-and-seek that is Śiva's eternal sport, Śiva has hidden himself so well that finally the small self will only find its way back to Śiva if Śiva wants it to. Just as Śiva wills his self-concealing in the small self, so too it is only Śiva who can wield the *anugraha-śakti*, the power that reveals himself to himself within the limited being. Only Śiva removes the blindfold, loosens the knot of the heart, and gives the imprisoned small self the vision of the reality outside its prison cell. This is shaktipat. Through it, Śiva in the form of the *sadguru* ignites the fire of knowledge, the fire of wisdom. Through it, the small self will regain its primordial and noble greatness, and a human being will come to overwhelming recognition of God within. Shaktipat initiates this second and supremely sweet act in Śiva's play, the unfolding of supreme consciousness through the process of sadhana.

This is the philosophy of shaktipat as it is narrated in the texts of Śaivism. Śaivism asserts again and again that shaktipat is an act of divine freedom. It is the impulse of liberation that is released by the *sadguru* from within the supreme consciousness, which is the guru's most intimate reality. That impulse of freedom enters from within, from the deepest, highest, subtlest regions of the inner being.

BY WHOM AND HOW IS SHAKTIPAT GIVEN? INITIATION, *SADGURU*, MANTRA

A medieval work of the Hindu Tantras (ca. tenth to fourteenth century C.E.) known as the *Kulārṇava Tantra* makes a powerful point about the nature of the *sadguru* in the following passage:

> Śiva has no binding form, Śiva is not perceivable by the human eye; therefore he protects the disciple conforming to dharma in the form of the Guru. The Guru is none other than the supreme Śiva enclosed in human skin; he walks the earth concealed, for bestowing grace on the good disciples. Though formless, Śiva, the store of compassion, takes form for the protection of the good devotees and acts in the world as though he were a householder. He conceals his eye on the forehead, his crescent moon and two of his hands and functions in the form of the Guru on the earth.
>
> The Guru is none other than Śiva without his three eyes, Viṣṇu without his four arms, Brahmā without his four faces. To him who is loaded with sinful karma, the Guru appears to be human; but to him whose karma is auspicious, meritful, the Guru appears as Śiva. The less fortunate do not recognize the

> Guru [as the] embodiment of the supreme Truth even when face-to-face with him, like the blind before the risen sun.
>
> Verily, the Guru is none else than Sadāśiva; that is the truth; there is no doubt about it. Śiva himself is the Guru; otherwise, who is it that gives fulfillment and liberation? There is no difference between God [Sadāśiva] and the Guru; it is sinful to make a distinction. He is the Guru because taking the form of the Preceptor, he cuts asunder all bonds of the *paśu* and leads to the supreme status. The store of compassion, Īśvara, being the fount of all grace, takes the form of the Guru, and releases the "animal" by his initiation.[54]

This passage articulates the perspective of the Indian tradition on the reality of the *sadguru.* The *sadguru* as envisioned here is the embodiment of the divine consciousness. Far from being considered limited by his human form, the *sadguru* uses his embodiment in a human body for the sake of granting grace to his disciples. God conceals himself as human without forgetting that he is God. Such is the idea of the *sadguru* and the one who is fit to give shaktipat initiation.

Passages such as the one above offer a different vantage point from which to contemplate the seriousness of shaktipat. In Śaivite philosophy it is understood as a unique and precious treasure that can be received only from one who has walked the ascending path of Śiva to its final heights. Even then, such a one must receive a special consecration that enables the liberated one to become a *sadguru.* Of teachers there are many in life. The tradition often points out that everyone can be considered to be a teacher in one way or another. The universe sees to it that people learn certain lessons and puts those people in our path who can teach what is needed to be learned.

But in the context of ancient India, the *sadguru* was considered to be extremely rare and only a *sadguru* can bestow shaktipat. Once shaktipat is bestowed, the path of yoga unfolds spontaneously and ineluctably within. Shaktipat does not simply teach a method or a technique. Rather, it is thought to inject into the deepest being the very seed of the tree of the *sadguru*'s liberation. That seed will inevitably grow, eventually to blossom and bear its precious fruit. Shaktipat fills the initiate with such power of yoga that then any yogic technique that is practiced will prove effective and powerful.

The *sadguru,* the siddha guru, is described in the *Yogavāsiṣṭha* as one at whose touch a person experiences supreme bliss and finds life transformed. Indeed, the siddha guru is one in whose mere presence yoga begins to happen spontaneously within. Swami Muktananda says:

> Indescribable bliss is the very goal of meditation, of Shaktipat. When you are experiencing this bliss, let your mind merge into it completely. There is a

place inside where supreme bliss constantly vibrates; when your mind reaches that place, it experiences this indescribable bliss. When it returns from there, it leaves the bliss behind. As your mind returns, hold on to the Guru and repeat *Guru Om, Guru Om, Guru Om,* and then that bliss will come back. It is that state of bliss which people like me live in. We are continually drunk on that bliss.[55]

When the prospective initiate approaches such a being with deep reverence and simplicity, the *sadguru* bestows *dīkṣā,* the liberating initiation. We can recall the traditional analysis of the term *dīkṣā,* which is often broken down into the two verbal roots *dā-* and *kṣi-*. *Dā-* means "to give," and *kṣi-* means "to destroy." In order to understand what is given and what is destroyed, the idea of the three *mala*s, the three limitations within which Śiva binds himself, must be recalled: the limitation of smallness (*āṇavamala*), the limitation of illusion (*māyīyamala*), and the limitation of action or doership (*kārmamala*). It must be remembered that for Śaivite philosophy these three limitations are self-imposed. Śiva imposes the *mala*s on himself in an instantaneous process that, in fact, occurs outside of time. Technically, therefore, the *mala*s are the beginningless bonds that structure the limitation of the small, transmigrating self. By diligent spiritual practices of various sorts, even *before* receiving shaktipat, the yogi will certainly begin to reduce the impact of the limitation of action and the limitation of illusion. These two bonds can be worn down or thinned out by diligent and sustained yogic effort. But the crucial point, Śaivite philosophy asserts, is that without shaktipat the first and fundamental limitation, the *āṇavamala,* will never yield before even the most heroic of yogic assaults. On its own, the small self will *never* be able to escape from its imprisonment. The *āṇavamala* is the impulse of Śiva's will to dance in the waves of karma. Nothing that is not Śiva's will itself can reverse the power that holds the small self bound by the *āṇavamala.* Swami Muktananda explains:

When one receives the Guru's grace, when one's karmas are burned in the fire of knowledge, then one does not take birth again. When the causal body is in bondage, it is called *āṇavamala.* When the inner *śakti* unfolds, the fire of love for God arises and this fire burns this *āṇavamala.* This fire is also called the fire of knowledge, and the fire of knowledge burns all the karmas. After all his karmas are burned to ashes, man becomes free from sins, faults, and he becomes free from rebirth and redeath.[56]

"Shaktipat" is the name that is given to that impulse of Śiva's will that makes possible the destruction of the *āṇavamala.* This is why it is such a precious and unique process. Only the *sadguru,* who *is* Śiva, can bestow that impulse of freedom that will break the bondage of the *āṇavamala.* In the absence of shaktipat, the yogi will never reach the summit of liberation no matter what furious and repeated assaults he launches.

For the Śaivite schools, then, it is the gift of shaktipat and shaktipat alone that leads to the destruction of the *āṇavamala.* In one moment, instantaneously, its binding power is done away with. Of course, this does *not* mean (in most cases!) that liberation is immediately achieved. It is through sadhana that the destruction of the other two *malas* is thought to occur. That is why it is always taught that there must be a balance between grace and yogic effort. *Both* are absolutely essential. But in truth, it is the *anugraha-śakti,* the power of revealing, the power of grace, that is truly indispensable. Without it, at best only preliminary practices are possible. With it, the destruction of the other two *malas* is assured and will eventually occur. Indeed for the Śaivite teachers, if liberation is *impossible* before shaktipat, it is *inevitable* after it. Nothing can stop or impede the power of Śiva. Once Śiva begins the journey that returns him home, the person *will* eventually reach the destination.

Shaktipat gives what is technically known as the *pratibhājñāna,* the "illuminating knowledge" in whose light *everything* becomes clear. This is the knowledge of the fullness of the Self, of the ecstatic unboundedness of Śiva that is the Self. As this knowledge unfolds more and more within, Śaivite philosophy asserts that it leads the yogi eventually to the culmination of sadhana which is called *mokṣa:* "liberation," the complete and total recovery of Śiva from the power of forgetfulness, from limitation, from delusion, from the indignity of ignorance, from the bondage of karma. This recovery from the cosmic amnesia, from the lulling fog of forgetfulness, occurs in the heart of a human being. One day the illuminating light of freedom reaches such a level of intensity that a human being exclaims in astonished and exulting recognition: *Śivo'ham,* "I am Śiva." The pilgrimage of Śiva is then completed.

We have considered above the schema by which Abhinavagupta categorizes the different experiential consequences of shaktipat. It is useful to revisit this schema both in the context of the Śaivite philosophy of Abhinavagupta as well as in terms of Swami Muktananda's understanding of shaktipat. It seems that different people have different experiences of shaktipat. How can we understand these differences? It is true that from the level of the individual's subjective experience there *are* great variations in the intensity of shaktipat. Some people have truly overwhelming sensations and visions, and seem to have a very intense experience of shaktipat. For others, the experience is milder and while still strong, not so intense. For yet others, there may be very little immediate experience. It is important to understand that the tradition holds that in all cases what has been accomplished is exactly the same: the beginning of the destruction of the *āṇavamala.* The differences in the subjective experience of shaktipat are based essentially on how much or how little the *kārma* and *māyīyamalas* have been reduced by previous spiritual practices. If they have been greatly reduced by yogic efforts, either in this life or in a previous life, then the veil of delusion has been thinned sufficiently that one can experience the destruction of the *āṇavamala*. In this case, shaktipat is experienced as being immediately very intense in its effects. If the *kārma* and *māyīyamalas* have been reduced only slightly, then the experience of the shaktipat is correspondingly less intense. If they have hardly been reduced at all, then it is like the dawning sun that shines above very thick clouds. Below all appears to still be in darkness. But it is no longer the deep darkness of the night.

One of the effects of shaktipat is that it may provoke a series of psychophysiological responses as the awakened energies released by the destruction of the *āṇavamala* begin to operate. These are sometimes called *kriyās*, "actions," in the yogic literature. When asked about *kriyās*, the physical movements that sometimes occur as a result of shaktipat, and whether one should try to stop them, Swami Muktananda said:

> You don't have to stop them. Let them happen for a while and then after a while they will stop on their own. Shaivism says, "In each person there are three types of malas, impurities. . . . So in this way, this body is covered or enveloped by three different types of impurities: *kārmamala*, *māyīyamala*, and *āṇavamala*. These three *malas* exist in three bodies. Don't think that you only have one physical body; that's wrong understanding. There are four bodies within the outer body. Therefore, the four bodies, the physical body, the subtle body, the causal body and the super causal body. These three *malas* exist in the three different bodies. For this reason, the moment the Kundalini is awakened it begins to work in all the three bodies and it starts purifying all the three bodies. These kriyas take place for the inner purification. For this reason, don't stop them and let them happen.[57]

This statement by Swami Muktananda reflects and summarizes much of what we have been discussing at some length above. It is clear that Muktananda envisioned the operation of the revealing *śakti* as a complex and all-encompassing process that was more to be cooperated with rather than directed by the yogi. The passage also typifies the understanding that the *kriyās* are part of a complex process of purification and readaptation of the entire being of the yogi. It is this process that will allow the *śakti* progressively to reveal and establish new levels of vision, understanding, and perception as it operates further and further. It is important, however, to understand that crucial as this process of purification is, the *kriyās* are a by-product or epiphenomenon of the operation of the *śakti* and are therefore not ends in themselves. We now turn to a consideration of notions surrounding the understanding of when and why a person receives shaktipat.

WHEN AND WHY DOES A PERSON RECEIVE SHAKTIPAT?

One of the questions that arises in the Śaivite tradition centers on the circumstances that determine the causes and conditions surrounding the reception of shaktipat. If, as has been said, shaktipat opens the doorway to liberation, why is it that some people receive it and others do not? This is a somewhat vexed and complex issue about which there are a variety of opinions and positions in the traditions of Śaivism. One might say that it can be understood from two different perspectives—the individual's perspective and the perspective of the absolute reality. From the individual's perspective, it is thought to be due to the performance of many meritorious actions, which accumulate to such a point that the supreme Lord sees fit to single out this person for the divine gift of shaktipat. There is no harm in thinking this way, as it induces a person always to perform pure and uplifting actions that will improve his or her karma.

However, from the perspective of the highest reality, the reception of shaktipat cannot be explained solely on the basis of the performance of good actions. There is a mystery to the will of Śiva. Shaktipat is understood to be an act of the infinite and supreme freedom of the Lord. It is the beneficent movement of the autonomous will of Lord Śiva. As such, the Kashmiri tradition, represented by Abhinavagupta, holds that the will of Śiva cannot be limited or constrained in any way, more especially by the finite and bounded field of karma.

> The cause of *karma* and of the *mala* [impurity] is the very desire for self- obscuring of the Lord. Their existence thus has no beginning within time. The self-obscuring of a reality that is full consists in its becoming not-full. This not-fullness is a longing to fill itself up by means of the differentiated reality. That is the reason why the *mala* is a tremulous agitation [*lolikā*].[58] Without Śiva, [who is] pure and whose essence is the light of freedom, nothing can logically exist. The cause of the *mala* and the rest is therefore Maheśvara [Śiva].[59]

> In the emission, maintenance, and reabsorption, he remains or abides so firmly that the will of Śiva takes recourse for its action to the power of illusion [*māyā*], and to action [*karma*], and the limiting impurity [*mala*]. When instead Śiva enlightens himself in all of his fullness, then he does not depend on such actions born of the limiting impurity arising from karma, which only concern the finite self. How can the limiting impurity, which is the cause of the condition of the finite self, be the cause of the abandonment of this very state? This same reasoning allows us to affirm that the Lord is in such actions independent of *māyā*.[60]

The reasonings that are compressed into the above statements deserve some unpacking. Śaivite scholars argue this point in the following way:

If the reception of shaktipat is explained on the basis of good karma, then it might be asked what *those* good karmas, in turn, are based on. The answer is that they are based on previous good actions, performed by the person in the past. And again, one might ask, what are *those* karmas based on, and again, the same answer is received. In this way, nothing has been explained because there has simply been set up a logical chain of infinite regression. In other words, it comes down to the following question: Why didn't the original good karmas suffice to merit the person's shaktipat? If shaktipat is based on good karmas, and good karmas are based on good karmas, and so on, in that case the person would have received shaktipat long ago on the basis of those original good actions. Therefore, why does shaktipat come at a certain point and not earlier or later? This is the nub of the mystery, and the only answer that can be given is that it is the free will of Lord Śiva that it be so.

This argument, however, is immediately liable to misunderstanding and misinterpretation. Such a scholastic or theological argument should not be taken as an inducement to stop performing good actions. That would be a wrong understanding of the intent of the argument, whose purpose is not to undermine the performance of pure and uplifting actions but rather to make clear the total autonomy and freedom of the will of Śiva. Grace arises from grace and nothing else. It is the pure and unblemished impulse of freedom.

Nevertheless, the recipients of shaktipat say that there always does seem to be a perfect appropriateness to the Lord's grace when it descends. It seems to come at exactly the right moment, just when the person is truly capable of receiving it. From the perspective of the supreme Lord, however, if he wishes to bestow his grace on the world's biggest scoundrel, then that is exactly what he will do. Besides, who knows what is accumulated in their own karmic records! A person might feel pure and upstanding at the present moment and yet have a large and heavy karmic debt hidden away and still pending. Therefore, it is some consolation that the reception of shaktipat does not directly depend on an individual's karma. It *is* grace. It is not earned. It cannot be compelled. The Śaivite tradition refuses to contemplate entering into a bargain or compact with God. Shaktipat is simply received with gratitude as the supreme gift. The tradition always emphasizes the mysterious will of Śiva.

On the other hand, because some of the Śaivite traditions *don't* want to say that the reception of shaktipat is an entirely random or chance event, they propose the theory of the maturation or "cooking" of the *malas*. These traditions (primarily the forms of both Kashmiri and Southern Śaiva Siddhānta) teach that the *malas*, the limitations that hold a person in bondage, are, like all other things, subject to the wearying pressure of time. Like a powerful tide pulling all things toward it, the supreme reality exerts, through the influence of time, a ripening effect on the *malas*. These schools teach that when the transmigrating soul has traversed a sufficient number of lifetimes, the *malas* begin to weaken. It is not that the *malas* would ever drop off on their own, but such a soul *will* begin to feel very powerfully a disenchantment with its present condition. It may even undergo a deep disillusionment and despair as it casts about blindly for some way to move beyond the constraining boundaries of illusion, the iron law of karma, and the repetitive experiences of suffering, death, and transmigration. Such a soul is said to be ripe for the return and ascending journey to Śiva.

The Śaiva Siddhānta traditions teach that Śiva out of his beneficent compassion arranges matters so that that soul finds its way to a *sadguru* and receives the liberating impulse of shaktipat. We can here recall the passage already quoted which asserts that the *sadguru* is Lord Śiva himself encased in human skin for the purpose of bestowing grace. These considerations, then, outline the difficulties involved in talking about the moment of the reception of shaktipat. If, in the Śaivite traditions, the reception of shaktipat is an event of transcendent importance in the long career of the transmigrating being, its reception nevertheless remains a profound mystery. To limit or constrain the will of Śiva in any way, is, as we have seen, finally unacceptable to the precise philosophers of Kashmiri Śaivism. On the other hand, to have declared that the reception of shaktipat is a random event would have been to invite a fatalistic and even possibly nihilistic attitude, and so the more conservative philosophers of the Śaiva Siddhānta clearly found this an unacceptable option. In either case, the contemplation of these matters raises interesting questions.

It is clear that Swami Muktananda was aware of the difficulties inherent in both of these positions. Nevertheless, he seems always to have emphasized that the reception of shaktipat was based on the accumulated merits of many lifetimes.

CONCLUSIONS

There is no doubt that the ancient roots of shaktipat in the initiatory traditions of India are very important. From an intellectual point of view, it is clear that the process of shaktipat stands as a pivotal and essential component of the Śaivite theological formulations. Without some notion that the expansive and liberating power of consciousness can be awakened in this way, the Śaivite conception of its own path of spirituality cannot succeed. But finally, these theological and intellectual concerns must give way to a more tangible argument, the argument of experience.

For many who have received shaktipat in the last decades, it has inspired a profound change in their lives.[61] Their work, their family life, their experience of themselves, their perspective on life and its purposes—any or all of these may be altered as the seemingly magical alchemy of shaktipat gradually does its work. In addition to transformation in the practical dimensions of their lives, modern recipients of shaktipat say they have found themselves launched on a definitive voyage of spirituality, embracing with fervor spiritual practices that might have seemed quite difficult or unappealing to them previously. The reception of shaktipat may open an expanded horizon of understanding of the world's many religious and spiritual traditions, a sense that what is most profound and important in all of them can now more clearly be heard. For many people, shaktipat as well opens the heart and illuminates the mind, engendering an instinctive knowledge of the unfolding presence of a living and sacred force, of the divinity that dwells within everything, and of the sheer magnificence of life.

In the end, it might be said that the culmination of all of these transformations wrought by shaktipat leads to the awakening of the deep heart of love. Swami Chidvilasananda encapsulates the nature of shaktipat in terms of love as follows:

> Shaktipat is the descent of love from the Guru and the ascent of love from the disciple.[62]

This statement alludes to the very core of shaktipat, a notion that may have gotten somewhat lost in the midst of such a prolonged consideration of the philosophical details surrounding this form of spiritual initiation. What is at stake is the awakening of the deepest love that abides within a human being. Many times, when people receive shaktipat they anticipate that new and marvelous experiences will awaken with them. And, indeed, they often do. But by focusing on the exotic or visionary experiences they desire to have, people may lose sight of a more fundamental dimension, the very heart of love that is awakened.[63] Upon receiving shaktipat, many people experience an upsurge of streams of love within themselves without realizing that this is, in fact, the most potent, valid, and important indication that they have indeed received shaktipat. It is precisely the spontaneous awakening of love or devotion, *bhakti*, that is finally the deepest result of shaktipat.

Shaktipat initiates the process by which a human being recognizes the intrinsic unboundedness of love that already dwells within his or her very own heart. It can set into motion a path of contemplation, service, sacrifice, and surrender. It is in following this path that a person can come to realize that there is nothing anywhere that is not lovable, that the very fabric of reality is secretly steeped in love, that the purpose of human life is not the arrogance of power but the humility of love. This higher love awakened by shaktipat is not mild or casual but enflamed and ecstatic. It is not a mutable love that fluctuates and alternates with jealousy, pride, or other negative emotions. Rather, the love that is awakened by shaktipat is profound, steadfast, and pure. It is liberating and consoling. It is this love awakened by shaktipat that will ultimately reveal the secrets of existence. What is most remarkable about this love is that it is awakened spontaneously by shaktipat. It is true that once awakened it must be cultivated. Nevertheless, its intrinsic nature is that it arrives unbidden: The upsurge of such powerful love in the heart is the graceful gift of shaktipat. When the hard shell of limitation that encases the human heart is cracked open, there results an outpouring of intoxicating love, unimaginable in its nature. In some ultimate sense, borne out by the experiences of so many people, shaktipat is a new birth. It initiates the path to liberation. It is the intervention in a human life of the force of ultimacy, of that deepest, holiest, and most sacred reality. Speaking about this, Swami Chidvilasananda has said:

> Shaktipat is like a volcano erupting. The brilliant red-orange molten lava that pours out of the crater is like the love that is suddenly released from the core of your being. This great love streams into the ocean of your life, seeps all the way to the bottom, where it continues to burn. Water cannot put this fire out. The current of events that beats against it like waves cannot stop it from burning nor quench the heat of this love.[64]

Chapter Seven

KUṆḌALINĪ
Awakening the Divinity Within

Douglas Renfrew Brooks and Constantina Rhodes Bailly

This is the highest principle, without beginning and beyond measure, the beauty of the state beyond the mind, and the dawning of the experience of the soul's oneness with God.

Jñāneśvarī 6.320

Selecting from the vast array of traditional resources that describe the phenomenon of Kuṇḍalinī, divine power, Swami Muktananda and Swami Chidvilasananda have cultivated an understanding that is remarkable both for its simplicity and its subtlety. They have distinguished their teaching without discounting or abandoning the wealth of the Indian classical and esoteric traditions and the myriad interpretations that inform this enormously complex subject.

Central to their presentation of Siddha Yoga, Kuṇḍalinī will be discussed in two distinctive yet related ways. First, Kuṇḍalinī informs the gurus' explanations of the creation and order of the universe. She is the Goddess Citi Śakti, the living divinity who as power and consciousness manifests the universe in both form and substance. Her relationship with Śiva and her role as the Self's own creative awareness are central to Siddha Yoga's world view. More specifically, Kuṇḍalinī is the "coiled one," the serpentine divinity who sleeps within every human being's subtle body until awakened. Second, the Siddha Yoga gurus discuss Kuṇḍalinī in the very practical terms of awakening divinity within through yoga and meditation. Closely aligned with the visionaries of Kashmiri Śaivism, and especially Abhinavagupta and Kṣemarāja, the Siddha Yoga gurus emphasize the crucial place of shaktipat in the process of Kuṇḍalinī's awakening and the guru's role as the protective and guiding force throughout this process.

Rather than offer yet another survey of the subject, this article focuses on the presentation of Kuṇḍalinī in the works of swamis Muktananda and Chidvilasananda. While we have included reiterations of the most fundamental elements of the Kuṇḍalinī phenomenon, our conversation focuses on describing the relationship between the traditional Indian sources from which the Siddha Yoga gurus draw and the ways in which Kuṇḍalinī appears within Siddha Yoga.

WHO IS KUṆḌALINĪ?

Kuṇḍalinī Śakti as the Deity of Siddha Yoga: Concepts and Sources

In his book *Secret of the Siddhas,* Swami Muktananda wrote of the Kuṇḍalinī energy as the primal and fully conscious power of divinity itself. He said:

> The principal deity of Siddha Yoga is the great Kuṇḍalinī Shakti, who is also known as Chiti or Supreme Consciousness. She has assumed the form of the entire universe.

He goes on in *Kuṇḍalini: The Secret of Life* to describe the infinite forms that are taken on by this divine energy, who is the universal creatrix:

> People who follow the tradition of bliss call her *Ānanda. Yogis* make Her the goal of their yoga. Devotees sing Her name with love, and She becomes the object of their love. Enlightened people of knowledge perceive Her in all the forms and objects in the universe, and seeing everything as one in That, they merge in That. There is nothing higher, nothing greater, nothing more sublime and beautiful than Shakti.[1]

The Siddha Yoga gurus' descriptions of Kuṇḍalinī's multifarious divine activity, as well as the fundamentals of the yoga of her awakening, are closely patterned after the teachings of Kashmiri Śaivism. Kashmiri Śaivism, especially in the hands of Abhinavagupta and his disciple Kṣemarāja, assumes virtually every text and teaching of the classical yoga tradition, and must be seen as well in light of the highly sophisticated and elaborate teachings of the Tantras and Āgamas. While we would be mistaken to identify Siddha Yoga with every feature of the Kuṇḍalinī phenomenon presented by the Kashmiri Śaivite sages or the Tantric yogis, the Siddha Yoga gurus similarly assume the wealth of these traditions, creating from them a vision true to their siddha lineage.[2]

Swami Muktananda writes:

> O Goddess Chitshakti! O Mother! O Father! You are Shakti. You are Shiva. You are the soul vibrating in the heart. . . . As long as they lack full knowledge

> of You, ignorant people project onto You various dualistic ideas such as Shiva-Shakti, world-illusion, bondage-liberation, indulgence-renunciation, spiritual-worldly.[3]

Elsewhere, in his collection of aphorisms known as *Mukteshwari*, Swami Muktananda further indicates the crossing of boundaries between male/god and female/goddess, for ultimately both forms are subsumed within the transcendent form of the primordial mantra *Oṃ*:

> Kundalini has the form of *Om*. She is the river of perfect bliss. She is both male and female. She is the all-knowing Yogini. She is the Goddess of yoga.[4]

Thus Kuṇḍalinī is perceived in a variety of forms, for it is she who is said to embody the whole universe. She is variously referred to as consciousness, a "serpent power," a goddess, a mantra. None of these is mutually exclusive, but rather each one amplifies the myriad variegations possible in all forms of life in the universe. Reiterating the intensity and majesty of the Goddess's all-encompassing presence and influence, Swami Chidvilasananda states:

> The ancient sages glorified the goddess Kundalini as the Divine Mother. She is the source, the womb of the world, the origin of everything that is, and everything that is not. Kundalini is both compassionate and terrifying at the same time. She is the greatest giver and the most ferocious slayer, simultaneously. What does she give? The freedom of the Self. What does she slay? Everything that holds us down.[5]

Siddha Yoga as the Awakened Knowledge of Kuṇḍalinī

At the very heart of Siddha Yoga are core concepts that contain within them the vast store of its teachings. First, the guru as a Self-realized being is said to awaken by the grace-bestowing initiation called shaktipat a latent spiritual yearning and inner conscious force in the disciple that lead to the liberating knowledge: God dwells in you as your own Self.[6] The guru's distinguishing feature is not simply that he or she is able to confer this blessing, but rather that the guru, in the deepest and most mysterious sense, *is identical with this divine and liberating śakti.*[7] This process of liberation unfolds "the great knowledge of the Kundalini," the One "filled with supreme energy," and so it "is called Siddha *vidyā*, the science of perfection."[8] In this way, Siddha Yoga can be defined as the awakening and unfolding of the all-encompassing divinity known as Kuṇḍalinī Śakti who lives—awake or asleep—within each of us.

Historically speaking, the discussion of the mystical process of awakening *kuṇḍalinī* energy within the subtle body begins sometime around the fifth or sixth centuries C.E. It is in this period that traditions that are likely far more ancient begin to appear in texts written in Sanskrit and other Indian languages.[9] What is important to note is that the assumptions, theories, and practices involving *kuṇḍalinīyoga* follow certain basic models shared across India's mystical traditions. There are few sectarian disputes or important theological differences that center on the Kuṇḍalinī phenomenon. Certainly no later than the early eighth century we engage the familiar systematic geography of the subtle body with its three main vertical channels (*nāḍī*) of *iḍā* (left), *suṣumṇā* (center, parallel to the spine), and *piṅgalā* (right), seventy-two thousand (or more) lesser channels crisscrossing the entire body, and six main centers (*cakra*).[10] This basic model persists even as it develops and evolves through the esoteric Tantras and Āgamas, particularly those of the Śiva-centered and Goddess-centered (i.e., Śākta) traditions. For example, later Śākta traditions describe a system of nine main centers, adding three to the well-known six, and then nine more from the forehead center to the top of the skull.[11] The Siddha Yoga gurus follow the more standard pattern of six cakras and three channels in their presentations, preferring to emphasize Kuṇḍalinī as a form of the living Goddess who is the living conscious power within the subtle body. The details of subtle body physiology are certainly well-known and even occasionally taught or mentioned by the Siddha Yoga gurus. However, there is little interest expressed in the elaborate symbolisms or mechanisms that seem to preoccupy the discussions of other teachers of mystical yoga. These features of *kuṇḍalinīyoga* are instead simply assumed and left to a rather secondary level of importance.

Kuṇḍalinī is neither an abstraction nor some sort of force or power that one learns to manipulate or control. Rather, in Siddha Yoga, as in other traditions of esoteric yoga, Kuṇḍalinī is a name given to the Power of God; she is the living deity whose special place is within one's body and, more specifically, within the subtle body. The subtle body exists within the physical; the relationship between the two bodies is usually described in terms of five coverings or sheaths (*pañcakañcuka*) which both protect and obscure the subtle body from our ordinary experience. While one can gain a certain access to the subtle body through the avenue of the physical, the *siddhavidyā* or *kuṇḍalinīyoga* begins with the assumption that it is the subtle body that directs the physical, not vice-versa.[12]

In Siddha Yoga one is not required first to do *haṭhayoga* or some other physically oriented practice before beginning *kuṇḍalinīyoga*. Rather, one begins with the awakening of Kuṇḍalinī through the guru's grace-bestowing power; other yogas and practices are developed and cultivated as a natural and sometimes spontaneous consequence of this initiation. Mastery of the physical body, from the standpoint of many Kuṇḍalinī yogis, is important and, according to some, a necessary prerequisite to the higher practices. However, from the standpoint of Siddha Yoga and other comparable *siddhavidyās*, awakening the intelligent Kuṇḍalinī through the guru's grace brings the yogi to the self-conscious awareness of the subtle body's primacy. One does not so much "master" Kuṇḍalinī as become her perfect disciple and eventually become one with her. Attuned to her subtle workings as the very substance and motive of our deepest being, the yogi creates an increasingly cooperative relationship rooted in devotion. Devotion is the key to fostering ultimate identification.

In Kuṇḍalinī traditions, awakening the goddess Kuṇḍalinī is following the spiritual path itself. For Swami Muktananda this awakening requires precisely what it confers: knowledge, action, and devotion. By becoming one with her, the yogi experiences the perfect harmony of these characteristics and goals. The final goal is, in this sense, a perfectly loving relationship that is utterly intimate, ecstatic, and fulfilling. Muktananda writes:

> The speed of one's progress on the spiritual path is in direct proportion to one's faith, love, and devotion for Kundalini. She is the form of God, the universal Mother. She is Shakti, the dynamic aspect of the Absolute. She is awakened through the grace of the Guru, who is himself Kundalini.[13]

Envisioned as like a coiled (*kuṇḍalin*) serpent, Kuṇḍalinī is said to sleep within the subtle body at the "root base" (*mūlādhāra*), near the base of the spine. As she unwraps herself to rise, her passage is in the subtle body's central channel or *suṣumṇā nāḍī*. In some descriptions, she is both that which moves and the medium through which she moves, thus completing the image that the entire subtle body is an extension of her own form. Continuing however with the symbolism of the rising serpent, as she progresses vertically up the *suṣumṇā nāḍī*, she not only penetrates three critical "knots" (*grantha*) but takes up residence in five vital centers—each of which represents a level of increasing awareness in the yogi as the divine manifests more explicitly and subtly as the content of one's experience. Through each level of yogic awareness, represented by a *cakra* ("wheel") pictured primarily in the form of lotus petals, there are detailed descriptions of the number of petals of each, the accompanying shapes within them, along with colors, smells, tastes, elements, and the divinities who make up the subtle experience which Kuṇḍalinī makes increasingly vivid and palpable. In an important sense, this rather well-known symbology of *cakras* and Kuṇḍalinī passage suggests how the experience of the subtle body becomes increasingly manifest as an experience available and connected to the outer world of the body and mind.

As Kuṇḍalinī moves toward her reunion with Śiva in the thousand-petaled lotus (*sahasrāra*) at the cap of the skull, she sojourns until the conditions prevail in which she might continue unimpeded by the karmic limitations of her host. It is not so much that Kuṇḍalinī is directed or impelled by the yogi, as if she were some sort of entity or mechanism that is made to "work"; rather it is that she chooses the course of her own awakening and movement as it suits her will and benefits the yogi. The very core of *kuṇḍalinīyoga* is rooted in the notion that she is intelligent, free, and beneficent. The imagery of vertical movement, awakening from sleep, residence in the *cakras*, penetration of obstacles, and serpentine form all suggest the notion of a gradual, systematic, and progressive ascent to divine consciousness and a deepening human awareness on the part of the yogi.

While it is traditional to discuss her ascent as successive, beginning at the "root base" (*mūlādhāra*) and moving through the central spinal column—through the subtle body centers located at the sacrum, navel, heart, throat, and brow, (*svādhiṣṭhāna, maṇipūra, anāhata, viśuddha,* and *ājñā*), texts and traditionalists also speak of her awakening in other ways. She may begin at any number of different points, just as her journey may reach its ultimate conclusion in the *sahasrāra,* in the heart, or between the eyebrows.[14] The key to Kuṇḍalinī's movements—at any stage of the spiritual path—is simply to remember that the Goddess, as the *Pratyabhijñāhṛdayam* states, "brings about the universe of her own free will."[15] This means that she appears everywhere *and* anywhere as she pleases; and that she is intelligent, discriminating, loving, and compassionate by nature, though sometimes this compassion manifests in "fierce" ways. Above all, Goddess Kuṇḍalinī is perfectly free (*svātantrya*) and so decides the course of her own progress. *Kuṇḍalinīyoga* is, from this standpoint, not so much a technique or method but rather a process of cooperation, surrender, and union with an innate divine reality.

Kuṇḍalinī and the Inner and Outer Guru

To obtain this "great knowledge" is both to experience Kuṇḍalinī directly as one's Self and to learn the "science of perfection" that brings about this realization. Both the experience and the practical teaching are aspects of the guru's grace. The guru exemplifies the person whose Kuṇḍalinī *is* awake and fully "unfolded" or accessible; thus the siddha guru is capable of instructing the seeker whose Kuṇḍalinī he or she awakens and then guides. The crucial feature of the Siddha Yoga gurus' understanding is that the highest and most subtle form of the guru is identical with Kuṇḍalinī who is none other than in-dwelling divinity. Just as there is a physical and a subtle body, there is an outer and inner guru. The goal of spiritual discipline is to experience the guru as one's own inner being, not simply as a person or as apart from one's divine Self. Swami Muktananda makes this point by clarifying the goal of the guru-disciple relationship as a transformation by which this inner state becomes one's constant experience *within the ordinary world.* This is crucial to understanding Siddha Yoga's teachings about Kuṇḍalinī. About the guru and disciple he says:

> A true Guru is not one who makes everybody his disciples and keeps them in that condition even after leaving his physical form. Only he is a true Guru who, having himself become a Guru, takes discipleship away from his disciples and turns them into beings like himself.[16]

For the guru to turn others "into beings like himself" requires not only his awakening the disciple's Kuṇḍalinī, but also the disciple's own identification of the inner guru as the Kuṇḍalinī. To put this another way, the disciple must achieve the recognition that the guru *is* that Śakti of his or her own Self-awakening, both as the awakening itself and the one who does the waking. The guru as Śakti is thus one's own realized Self and the indispensable agent or initiator of that realization. It is this Śakti, the guru within, Kuṇḍalinī, who is the divine vital energy permeating all things and whose manifestation develops within us as a growing awareness of her pervasive form. Kuṇḍalinī growing or awakening in us is the increasing recognition of God's ubiquity.

Though eternal by nature and revealing of herself as all things, Kuṇḍalinī as Śakti is divine energy simultaneously changing and concealing herself. By definition, Śakti is that which reveals, conceals, and transforms the world out of her own being (*svabhāva*) and her very own form (*svasvarūpa*),[17] even as she remains the constant beyond and within all of these processes. This is her play, her *līlā*. Kuṇḍalinī assumes this playful posture, appearing to "sleep" and then to "awake" within one's consciousness and in one's experiences of body, mind, and speech. She does so not because she has anything to "gain" or "accomplish"—because she is literally *siddha*; she has already "accomplished" or "perfected" everything. Rather, she "plays" merely for the sake of her and our own enjoyment, that is, so that we as human beings can experience the divine as the divine experiences itself—freely moving, creating, and interacting under its own terms and self-imposed commands. Whereas Kuṇḍalinī willfully directs the pulsation of consciousness that creates diversity from unity, we as unrealized beings do not have that experience of witnessing, controlling, and directing our experience, that is, until we experience the Self as identical with the inner guru who is God within us.

This identification of the disciple with the inner guru and Kuṇḍalinī is called *sāmarasya*, literally the "experience of sharing sameness."[18] It is an experience that is direct, not bound to words or concepts, and manifestly real to the experiencer. A simple analogy is to the "taste" or *rasa* of a delicious fruit which one experiences directly and cannot reduce to mere descriptions or sensations, such as sweet or juicy. *Describing* the taste of a fruit is not the same as experiencing that taste. Therefore we know that the *taste* of the fruit is not the same thing as its sweetness or any of its other qualities and yet the taste is unmistakable as an experience of that fruit. Kuṇḍalinī is not only the experience of the sweetness of the fruit but is the *one who experiences* that sweetness. She is the inner "experiencer" in the disciple. It is this notion that there is an experiencer to experiences, a knower to the things we know, and an essential reality *within* the realm-of-things-that-change that defines Kuṇḍalinī as the playful divinity whom we experience as the Self.

In Siddha Yoga, the purpose of any of the infinite forms through which the divine is experienced is to bring the *sādhaka* to an awareness of the highest Self, to attain the recognition (*pratyabhijñā*) that God dwells within each individual.

One Siddha Yoga devotee reports an experience in which the goddess appeared not merely for the sake of darshan (Sanskrit, *darśana*: "auspicious viewing") but in order to make the *sādhaka* aware that the splendor and power of the goddess, the guru, and the Self are one:

> While in India I had a very beautiful dream vision of the Goddess. In the dream I saw a stunningly beautiful female form made entirely of light. I looked at her and thought, This is the woman I have always wanted to meet, the woman of my dreams. I approached her, and then finally I had to cover my eyes. I said, "Who are you?" She replied, "I am your own Self." Then the dream ended. Afterward, I felt that I had approached her a bit too casually, had not treated her with the reverence befitting a goddess. About a week later she appeared again. I thought, This time I'm going to do it right. I did a full *pranam*, stretching myself out before her. She walked over to me and picked me up again. I threw myself down again. I kept going up and down like a yo-yo. Finally she grabbed me really hard, lifted me up, and said, "Why don't you see who you really are?" I looked down and saw my own form on the ground, only it had become her form, and it too was radiating a dazzling light. She embraced me, I embraced her, and we dissolved into one another, whereupon there was an explosion of golden light. Then the dream ended. But this experience made the Goddess very real for me. I became extremely conscious of the Kuṇḍalinī, the divine Mother, the spiritual energy within, and knew that I should take every opportunity to honor her through the practices and through my relationship to the Guru.[19]

The guru is Kuṇḍalinī Śakti assuming the role of one who effects divine revelation and brings it to outward manifestation. The guru is also that inner form of the Self which, in some sense, willfully remains concealed even when awakened within the subtle body. This is why, in some sense, the guru continues to appear before the disciple as the physical guru of one's worldly experience. But this continuing appearance is not the entirety of the guru's reality, even as it cannot and should not be denied. The idea is that one must penetrate to the deepest reality of one's own Self and that this journey inward reveals the guru as one's own innate divinity. Thus, Kuṇḍalinī is the form of the guru-within just as she is one's Self; in this sense, she is not a "serpentine" Goddess, or a particular aspect or method of yoga, nor is she a reality apart from one's own ordinary levels of experience. Rather, Kuṇḍalinī is that which reveals the experience that guru, Self, and God are, in the deepest and most direct sense, ultimately one. Kuṇḍalinī is, at this level of yogic awareness, both the *revealer* of that ultimate truth and the *revelation* or the ultimate truth itself. The inner guru is that aspect of Kuṇḍalinī who penetrates ordinary dualistic appearances, those that *merely appear* to define the Self, guru, or God as truly "other."

Kuṇḍalinī is spiritual experience itself. When she is "asleep," one's experience is of limited body, consciousness, and self-awareness. As she awakens, these limitations and experiences, which are conditioned by the misconstrual and misidentification of the Self and are the result of myriad karmic impressions, give way to an increasing recognition of the divine as the source, substance, and form of everything. Swami Muktananda's distinctive interpretation of Kuṇḍalinī and the yoga of her awakening is an extension of his subtle understanding of shaktipat as the divine force of Kuṇḍalinī's increasing self-awareness, and also the role of the siddha as shaktipat guru who effects this awareness in disciples.[20]

The Outer and Inner Kuṇḍalinī: The Language and Symbolism of Inversion

To appreciate the subtlety of the Kuṇḍalinī Śakti is to begin with this basic understanding: that she is both the Goddess who becomes the entire universe and the innate spiritual presence of that Goddess within every person. Swami Muktananda distinguishes these two features by calling Kuṇḍalinī-as-the-universe the "outer Kuṇḍalinī" and Kuṇḍalinī-as-yoga the "inner Kuṇḍalinī." He writes:

> The truth is that everyone's Kundalini is already awake. Just as she has created the external universe and dwells within it, she has created this human body and pervades it. . . .
>
> Kundalinī is the support of our lives; it is she who makes everything work in our bodies. When her flow is external, Kundalini functions through the mind and the senses.[21]

Thus, the outer Kuṇḍalinī, or external form of Kuṇḍalinī, is that which defines us as living, growing, thinking, organic beings; she is the form and shape of our sentience, of our being as *living* beings. This is important because it affirms Kuṇḍalinī's role as the manifesting divinity that becomes the "outer" or external universe. She is not, however, only this level of physical reality or of our human experience. Swami Muktananda continues:

> It is the inner aspect of Kundalini which has to be awakened. Kundalini in Her outer aspect is all-pervasive, and that is why even though She is functioning

> inside us, we don't perceive Her. Only through subtle understanding can we come to know Her; without understanding, we cannot find Her. This understanding arises when the inner Kundalini becomes active.[22]

Muktananda's point about our *not* perceiving Kuṇḍalinī in our usual awareness of ordinary experience is subtle: We do not notice that which is everywhere and everything. The "obvious," even if it be God, is precisely that which we do not see or pay attention to. Ignorance of Kuṇḍalinī as the form and shape of all things is, in part, the process of taking for granted that which is right before our eyes. That is, ignorance of the divine is our inability to see and to appreciate fully the reality that *permeates* appearances. For example, one does not notice that there is an experiencer who witnesses experience unless and until one contemplates more deeply the "obvious" experience that there *must be an experiencer within the very experiences.* To trace Kuṇḍalinī's outer and inner activity, her various passages and movements, as well as the effects of her awakening, is to detail the spiritual journey itself. It begins when we start with our experience of the "obvious," and move from simply taking for granted that the world is not divine to that deeper level of awareness in which one experiences nothing other than the divine. In this sense, Kuṇḍalinī is the very core of human experience itself, whether it is superficial and "obvious" or that deeper, inner reality of experience which makes the external reality appear before our senses and mind. This might be called Kuṇḍalinī in her microcosm, Kuṇḍalinī as the content and form of human experience.

Kuṇḍalinī's activity also describes the macrocosmic process by which the universe is created. Viewed from this macrocosmic perspective, as Kuṇḍalinī descends into sleep and then arises to rejoin her beloved Śiva, so the universe comes into being, sustains itself, and is eventually dissolved back into its primordial being. Thus her descent, that is, her "going to sleep," symbolizes creation, which is nothing other than the divine's desire to assume the guise of self-imposed limitation. The simultaneity of the symbolism is important: even as there is an expansion and transformation that creates the universe, so there is, at the same time, a process which is described as "divine slumber" or increasing *māyā*. As the *Śiva Sūtra* puts it laconically, "The Self is the actor. The stage is the inner Self. The spectators are the senses."[23] This divine act of assumed limitation is the power of *māyā* or illusion, which is not confusion but rather the gift of the creator becoming creation. Were the divine awareness not "falling asleep," as it were, there would be no world as such to experience and no ecstasy of "reunion" after the process of awakening has been completed.

We should notice here how the entire discussion of macrocosmic creation, persistence, and dissolution, and the individual's microcosmic process of physical and subtle awareness, is represented through the important symbolic strategy of inversion or reversal. This strategy is the primary mode of symbolic discourse throughout the yoga traditions and is crucial to understanding the language that surrounds *kuṇḍalinīyoga.* Thus, for example, the activity of creation, of "coming into being," depends on the divine "going to sleep." When Kuṇḍalinī sleeps, we as individuals are created, that is, we "wake up" into existence. Yet this existence with which we identify on the physical level is not the fully awakened state of the subtle body—it is not real or "true" awakening—but merely the conditions of waking, dreaming, and sleeping consciousness that belong to the physical body; it is *māyā.* Kṛṣṇa in the *Bhagavadgītā* restates this symbolism of inversion by distinguishing the yogi's higher state from that of an "unawakened" ordinary consciousness. Though he does not explicitly use the imagery of Kuṇḍalinī, he makes the point that the yogi's experience is the direct inversion of appearances. The *Bhagavadgītā* states, "The controlled one wakes in what is night for all creatures, as it is night for the visionary seer when other creatures are awake."[24]

To restate this in terms of Kuṇḍalinī, as the yogi becomes more deeply immersed and identified with Kuṇḍalinī and so more perfectly aware, he experiences various states of yogic trance that appear physically to be more like "sleep" than waking consciousness. In other words, ultimate reality is the direct opposite of appearances, which *seem* to be real. This is Kuṇḍalinī's *māyā,* her illusion, played out in the language and appearance of inverted realities. In his *Play of Consciousness* Swami Muktananda describes many of these yogic states of trance that are more fully aware than what is ordinarily called "waking consciousness." Muktananda's exacting descriptions of these states are one of his distinctive contributions to understanding the yogic processes that are described elsewhere in traditional sources but in veiled language. He is especially vivid in his description of what he calls the *tandra* state and the higher states associated with one-pointedness, that is, *samādhi.* Important to note here as well is the commonality with which this experiential state appears in Siddha Yoga devotees. It is often associated with the shaktipat experience and the sensation of identity with the guru's inner state. To give one example:

> Baba touched me. For a couple of seconds, nothing happened. Then I was catapulted into a perfectly still state. No self-consciousness, no awareness of anybody else—just me. For the first time in my life I was just there, existing, totally content and desireless. It was fabulous; I could have stayed there forever. Then I felt an inner explosion, and my heart seemed to burst open. It was very pleasurable. It stretched out to my sides and filled my whole body, and I became a big, open heart. Into this heart came three-dimensional pictures of all kinds of people. They were very lifelike: family, friends, people I worked with, people I had seen for maybe a second at a supermarket counter years ago. I felt total love for them filling me, and then, every seven or eight pictures, there would be a picture of me, and I would be just loving myself.[25]

To complete the imagery of inversion we discover that to experience the inner Kuṇḍalinī as fully activated is to enter *samādhi,* a unified state of inner absorption. (The word literally means to have one's "consciousness ever the same.") The more one is aware of change as the constant of ordinary experience, the more stable and unaltering one's experience becomes, at every level of consciousness. Thus the yogi is fully aware and active, while appearing to do nothing at all. Like Kṛṣṇa in the *Bhagavadgītā,* the yogi experiences the reality that, "I have no task at all to accomplish in these three worlds. . . . I have nothing to obtain that I do not have already. Yet I move in action . . . [because] the wise should take kindly to all acts, but himself do them in a disciplined fashion."[26] Thus, the yogi does everything by "not doing" and yet continues to act! At every level of yogic imagery we find such inversions of ordinary associations and expectations. But why? Why does the divine turn on itself and appear to do "contradictory" things? Why does Kuṇḍalinī "go to sleep" to create? What happens when she does?

According to the Kashmiri Śaivite view, shared by the Siddha Yoga gurus, God assumes the guise of the universe for the sake of enjoyment, both divine and human. Kuṇḍalinī's sleeping dreams reveal the universe creating and sustaining itself. Her sleep is the Śakti's dreamlike activity and so expresses itself to ordinary consciousness as the universe's state of constant change, appearing as her ever-increasing and unfolding self-manifestation. Kuṇḍalinī's activity is Viṣṇu's sleep which, as the Purāṇas explain, is what keeps the universe "going."[27] Kuṇḍalinī's awakening in the human being, on the other hand, is her penetration (*samāveśa*) of the subtle body's centers and the pervasion (*vyāpti*) of her divine energy throughout the subtle body's channels, or *nāḍīs*. Her eventual reunion with Śiva within the individual yogi dissolves the guise of limitation and differentiation that creates the facade of reality. It does not, however, dissolve ordinary reality itself, which continues unabated. Thus the yogi is no longer subject to the misconceptions of dualism even as he continues to live within a world predicated on dualism. This is the guru's *māyā,* that is the guru maintains the outer façade of an ordinary life while basking in the unified realm of inner divinity.

The goal of *kuṇḍalinīyoga,* then, is dissolution of duality and ignorance, which is why it is often equated with the term *layayoga* (literally, the "yoga of dissolution"). To awaken Kuṇḍalinī is to dissolve any trace of egoism, liberating the divine Self by creating the recognition (*pratyabhijñā*) of the eternal witness who is simultaneously assuming form and embodiment. Kuṇḍalinī's process of dissolution is not death or annihilation but rather the blissful destruction of dualistic consciousness. With such dissolution becomes the yogi's awakened experience of the universe not merely as a changing and effervescent reality but as a perfect eternality. The blissful dissolution of plurality into oneness is symbolized by the reunion of Śakti with Śiva, following the ascent in the body of the serpentine Kuṇḍalinī to the pinnacle of the thousand-petalled lotus at the crown of the head. Here, it is said, Śiva awaits her, immersed in his own perfect meditation atop "Mount Kailasa."

This symbolic language of dissolution also suggests the origin of much of the traditional erotic imagery associated with Kuṇḍalinī. Kuṇḍalinī's reunion with Śiva is nothing less, however, than their ecstatic and loving embrace which dissolves the appearance of their separation within the subtle body and brings the yogi to the blissful "fourth state" (*turya, turīya*) beyond all levels of ordinary consciousness. The notion of their erotic union is likewise an inversion of roles and an exchange of identities. Kuṇḍalinī becomes Śiva as her serpentine form elongates to become the *śivaliṅga* while Śiva becomes the *yoni,* or womb, of the *sahasrāra* into which Kuṇḍalinī enters. Kuṇḍalinī in this sense takes on Śiva's form, exchanges identities with Him, and finally merges their divine complement into their original state of undifferentiated unity. There the two enjoy each other as one; put into yogic terms, the interpenetration of the Lord and his power (*samāveśa,* literally, "moving into sameness") gives way to their perfect experience of "enjoying sameness" (*sāmarasya*).

It is little wonder that many traditional Kuṇḍalinī sources analogize this union of Śakti with Śiva in almost exclusively erotic terms and images, and also how rarely the sublime and subtle point is lost on traditional writers. Modern descriptions of this imagery have not always been as interested or as aware of its deeper meanings, thus the crude identification of *kuṇḍalinīyoga* with sex or Tantra. Some scholars, taking a "higher road," have chosen to reduce the erotic imagery to purely Freudian terms.[28] Unfortunately, this approach, like other more superficial descriptions, fails to take into account the esoteric meanings these texts most often assume must accompany their interpretation. Few aspects of Indian spirituality have been more gravely misunderstood.[29]

The Siddha Yoga gurus, we should note, express little interest in elaborating the tradition's erotic symbolism nor do they use any of the explicitly sexual connotations of the art and literature associated with Kuṇḍalinī. This position is not uncommon nor does it mean that such symbols are entirely abandoned. Rather, it is a matter of meaning, interpretation, and the practical messages conveyed about yogic practice.[30] Even further beyond their interest are any of the erotic or sexual aspects of ritual or yoga that have come to be associated with the Tantra of the Left-Current (*vāmācāra*). Rather the Siddha Yoga gurus internalize these symbols, just as they internalize the guru-disciple relationship, rejecting any metaphors or behaviors that would compromise their ethics or prove misleading or fruitless for devotees. Their rejection of these images or practices is not some modern or contemporary effort to massage, puritanize, or compensate for the excesses of others or their misunderstandings. Instead it is a trait of the Yoga and Tantric traditions of the Right (*dakṣiṇācāra*).[31]

Kuṇḍalinī is portrayed sometimes as the beloved and ever-loving wife of Śiva—here is called the loving Mother of the universe who nurtures and guides all aspects of one's existence from within the subtle body. Similarly, the guru—like Kuṇḍalinī—first gives life to the disciple through shaktipat and then guides that child with love, direction, and discipline to an inner, divine mystery. Kuṇḍalinī's awakening within the seeker dissolves all vestiges of the ego, leaving only the original, pure nature of the eternal Self as one's constant experience. It is this great potential for Self-awakening that Swami Muktananda asserts is possible in everyone who seeks Kuṇḍalinī with devoted discipline.

> O Mother of the world, when You manifest within, even an ordinary person becomes like Shiva. . . . Not only do You fulfill all the desires of the one who meditates on You with love, but You also grant him Your own form, making seekers merge into You.[32]

Swami Chidvilasananda similarly affirms this potential for Self-realization and identifies it as Kuṇḍalinī's awakening:

> So when you receive Shaktipat diksha, Shaktipat initiation, from the Guru, the central channel starts unfolding from the base of the spine to the crown of the head, and it is startled into wakefulness. And I like to use the phrase, "you are startled into wakefulness"—whether it's subtle or very, very dynamic—because that's how I experienced Shaktipat. I was totally startled into a new dimension in my own being. And that's when joy begins to reveal itself in a seeker. . . . This ecstasy is not relative to anything that you feel. It is complete within itself.[33]

In addition to the extraordinary descriptions of the yogic states associated with Kuṇḍalinī, it is this claim that Kuṇḍalinī can and should be awakened in all persons that sets apart the Siddha Yoga gurus. Theirs is not a "break" from tradition in the sense of a rejection, but rather an innovation in which the experience of shaktipat and Kuṇḍalinī's awakening are understood as universal to the spiritual path. Swami Chidvilasananda made this point clearly in a rather spontaneous remark, saying, "Last night someone gave me a little Mexican statue, and on its head was a snake. In every country, on every path, the image of Kundalini, the serpent power, is found."[34] Though the path of *kuṇḍalinīyoga* has been traditionally secretive and exclusive, this notion of Kuṇḍalinī's egalitarian love offered in shaktipat all around the world is distinctive to the teaching of Siddha Yoga.

THE COSMOGONIC KUṆḌALINĪ AS CITI ŚAKTI

Not a mere symbol or allegory, Kuṇḍalinī is a living presence awaiting our attention; she longs to express her own true nature and so confer the experience of liberation while the yogi is yet embodied; this is *jīvanmukti.* Thus, even as she sleeps within the unrealized individual she simultaneously enacts the outer universe as the play of her own consciousness by constantly pulsating, emitting, and withdrawing herself as reality's form and even as our own limited consciousness. When fully awakened within the realized being, her play continues, but now it is experienced with the perfect awareness that "the whole visible world is complete in God."[35]

The Siddha Yoga gurus go to great lengths to describe this divine power of consciousness, or Citi Śakti, who presents herself as the very form (*svarūpa*) and essence (*svabhāva*) of the universe and within the subtle body. But it is not for the mere sake of discussing metaphysics that Citi Śakti receives this attention. Rather it is to foster the science (*vidyā*) or discipline (*yoga*) of the latent Kuṇḍalinī who "is awakened by the Guru's grace, performs new tasks every day . . . purifies the body . . . enters the sushumna within the spinal column and, piercing the chakras through Her own force, changes the whole condition of the body and makes it fit for the spiritual path."[36] This process of Kuṇḍalinī's awakening is accompanied by mental and bodily purification, which Swami Muktananda describes as part of Kuṇḍalinī's subtle movement:

> Eventually, as the Kundalini works within, She gives rise to more and more profound experiences. As She purifies the *nadis,* She purifies one of latent diseases as well as of such feelings as aversion, hatred, and greed. When the *nadis* are purified, the mind becomes still, and one begins to enter the state of *samadhi.* Rising through the *sushumna nadi,* the central channel within the spinal column, the Shakti pierces and purifies the six *chakras.* . . . The Shakti gives the yogi control over his senses, so that he remains free of the pull of outer sense objects.[37]

Swami Chidvilasananda describes the process similarly, translating the technical vocabulary into terms and categories more intelligible to an audience not steeped in the original, ancient texts. She writes:

> When the Kundalini Shakti is awakened through the Guru's grace, she begins her upward journey through the sushumna nadi, the central channel of the subtle body, to meet the supreme Lord at the crown of the head. Along the way, she stations herself in the spiritual centers called chakras. While purifying them, she cuts through different blocks and knots that keep a person from experiencing her real nature. As she does her work in different centers of the body, you do experience different kinds of feelings, emotions, and sensations.

> Sometimes you feel you never even knew such a thing existed within yourself; you thought you were so pure. And all kinds of impurities come up, too; all kinds of thoughts and feelings come up. The best thing to do is just watch. Be a witness. It is a purification. It is going to be expelled from your system. Before that, the dust flies in the air and you feel suffocated, but the Shakti clears all this.[38]

By perfecting the practice of *kuṇḍalinīyoga*, one obtains the insight that "the world is permeated by Chiti, belongs to Chiti, *is* Chiti."[39] All other aspects of sadhana, from meditation and chanting the divine names to disciplined ethics and selfless service to the guru (*gurusevā*), are performed in order to serve and to awaken Kuṇḍalinī, and to nurture her unfolding until one can experience the world and oneself as divine.

The seeker's goal is to make life a continuous expression of the divine Kuṇḍalinī's will (*icchā*), activity (*kriyā*), and knowledge (*jñāna*) and so to experience the pulsating awareness "I am That," which as Swami Chidvilasananda states is "accompanied by great bliss and light."[40] When "through meditation [disciples] have awakened their inner Shakti . . . and through their dedicated practice of the great yoga, Kundalini yoga, they have become God," then "they are holy people. Mahashakti Chiti plays within them . . . [and] they are completely absorbed in the supreme Lord."[41] To become "holy" is to make the body a sacred vessel of Kuṇḍalinī by the practice of *kuṇḍalinīyoga* and so experience the world as nothing but her.

Part of the process of understanding the goddess Kuṇḍalinī—who unfolds the universe as her playful consciousness *and* as the discipline of yoga—is to consider her divine manifestations. Swami Muktananda lists these various manifestations to make clear that her inherent perfection remains unaffected by her assuming different forms and appearances. He writes:

> By nature, the power of the Self has absolute freedom of knowledge and activity. *Svaatantryam etanmukhyam* [*Ishwara Pratyabhijñā*, 7, 4, 13]—"Above all, it is absolutely free." It is also called the *svatantra shakti*, the independent power, *chetana shakti*, the conscious power, *spanda shakti*, the vibrating power, *vimarsha sara*, the pure essence of "I"-consciousness, *hridaya*, the heart, *samvit*, Universal Consciousness, *para shakti*, the supreme power, and *jaganmata*, the Mother of the world.[42]

Elsewhere Swami Muktananda writes:

> Chitshakti is completely free. She performs all actions and gives the fruit of all disciplines. She bestows both worldly fulfillment and liberation; she grants an easy means to happiness. Self-luminous, transcending time, space, and form, she is the creative aspect of Parashiva, the basis of all forms of energy.

> . . . The glory of this supreme Shakti is marvelous. She is the knowledge of the enlightened and the fruit of action of the active. She is the ecstatic state of *bhaktas* and the dynamic Kundalini of yogis. In fact, she is the beauty of the whole world. . . . The entire functioning of this universe, from worldly to spiritual, is carried on by Chiti.

As if transported by recollection of that ecstatic state of experiencing Citi Śakti, he now addresses the Goddess herself as he continues the description:

> O Mother Chiti, beloved wife of Parashiva and His dynamic expression, You are His throbbing vibrations. You are the essence of the five elements that compose the universe. You are the sun, the moon, the stars, the planets. O Goddess Kundalini, You are heaven, Vaikuntha, and the nether worlds; You are the three worlds and the four directions. . . .
>
> O Mother Kundalini, You are the blissful Shakti that came from Nityananda. . . . O Mother Kundalini, the embodiment of Chiti, You are the pure-souled Guru of all great Gurus. . . . O Guru, O abode of love, dynamic energy, You are the grace that came from Nityananda. You are the two-syllabled *So 'ham,* his gift to me. Because of You, I am. Mother, You were the consummation of my initiation. With the Blue Pearl as Your vehicle, You appear to my devotees in my form and, through these visions, give them faith.[43]

Though *kuṇḍalinīyoga* as the process of Self-realization is a discipline, a teaching, and a body of practices, the Siddha Yoga gurus explain Kuṇḍalinī's awakening as part of the divine destiny of those who seek God within themselves. In other words, God's deepest intention is to become every sentient being's own experience of him or herself. The divine has no wish to remain veiled behind the clouds of desire or self-deception. Like the sun, it shines no matter what appears to obscure it. In this sense, the seeker's increasing awareness of Kuṇḍalinī as the divine reality within him, as the principle of life, and as consciousness itself, is an unfolding vision of God as the Self and the absolute. This energy is both omnipresent and omniscient by nature and yet she appears within the world and *as the world.* We are aware of her divine splendor and attuned to her subtle manifestation to the degree to which she is awakened and has unfolded her splendor within us.

Kuṇḍalinīyoga is not so much a discipline of mastering the inherent form of Śakti but rather of creating an appropriate vessel through which she may operate and thereby enter, with the disciple, into a life-giving and loving relationship of cooperation and continuous worship. To awaken Kuṇḍalinī through the process of yoga is to worship her, to become her trusted and loving disciple, and to do her divine bidding. Meditation is understood to be the key to this deepening of awareness. In this sense, meditation on one's own Self is the process by which Kuṇḍalinī is recognized as the divine awakening through one's own body and in one's own awareness.

More must be said about the role of meditation in this process, especially in light of its importance to Siddha Yoga. First, however, we must consider its relationship to the love of the Self, the guru, and God—for meditation begins and ends as an expression of devotion and respect for all of these aspects of reality. Without the disciple's devotion and self-respect, Kuṇḍalinī's grace remains hidden behind the veil of ego.

Swami Muktananda revels in this exaltation of Kuṇḍalinī and experiences it as part of the guru's command to praise her and obtain her grace:

> Yogis pray to Her in the following way: "O goal of yogis! O supremely beautiful and effulgent one! O Mother! You are the beloved consort of the supreme primordial Guru Parashiva and are one with Him. I serve You with total absorption and humility, taking full refuge in You. . . . Through Your grace, even an ordinary person becomes blessed and is able to realize the Supreme Principle within himself. Then, being immersed in supreme bliss, he can lead a godly life.[44]

The task of Siddha Yoga, quite simply, is the awakening of Kuṇḍalinī and has as its aim the unfolding and fulfilling experience of Kuṇḍalinī as one's own Self, one's own deepest nature, and the nature of the universe. Awakening Kuṇḍalinī and guiding her to her final destination is the most important role of the guru. Gaining the insight that one's own Kuṇḍalinī Śakti is identical with the guru and the Self is the liberating knowledge about which Swami Muktananda speaks and writes so eloquently.

Swami Muktananda writes:

> [I]n order to experience Kundalinī Shakti one must use the instrument of the human body. One also needs the grace of the Guru and the compassion of Kundalinī. . . .
>
> It is very important for a human being to awaken his Kundalinī. It is a power, a vibration, an extraordinary energy. It is the soul of an individual and his vital force. It is the conscious power behind his senses. It is that which inspires the intellect and makes the mind contemplate. Siddha Yoga teaches that this entire universe is pervaded by the great Shakti.[45]

Swami Muktananda sets forth in these few lines both the essentials of Siddha Yoga's understanding of God and creation, and the highest goal of human beings to experience divinity within. At the core of Muktananda's vision is the relationship between the great macrocosmic deity Citi Śakti, literally the conscious power who surges forth as the entirety of the universe, and her microcosmic presence within the subtle body of each human being as the serpentine Kuṇḍalinī. He writes in *Secret of the Siddhas*:

> It is a philosophical premise that the microcosm is identical to the macrocosm. The great Shakti, the mother of the world, lives in the body as the microcosm. The entire universe exists in the seed of the heart, the inner Self.[46]

To awaken Kuṇḍalinī within oneself is, in effect, to reenact the very process of creation and so to mirror the playful relationship of the eternal and unchanging Śiva with his creative and volatile energy, his complementary Śakti. To experience Kuṇḍalinī within oneself is to experience the universe as the divine experiences itself.[47]

Despite their great affinity to Kashmiri Śaivite understanding, the Siddha Yoga gurus make no effort to identify themselves doctrinally with particular yogic schools or interpretations, such as the Trika, Krama, or Pratyabhijñā.[48] They also evince no interest in identifying with any particular Tantras or Tantric schools—major resources for the elaboration of Kuṇḍalinī theory and practice—and refrain from any language that suggests a dogmatic or textual identity. Rather, in the tradition of the *guruvāda*, which centers on the guru's interpretation of scriptural sources, they draw upon the most deeply rooted vision these schools and texts offer. As Baba Muktananda explains:

> . . . Chiti, the cosmic energy, becomes this manifold universe. She doesn't create this universe the way a human being builds a house, using different kinds of materials. She creates the universe out of Her own being, and it is She Herself who becomes this universe. She becomes all the elements of the universe and enters into all the different forms that we see around us.[49]

To put the matter in a slightly different light, Swami Chidvilasananda explains that the external world and the inner world are mirrored realities, each an aspect of the divine Śakti. The key to understanding this is the awakening of Kuṇḍalinī:

> The supreme truth is that we are not separate from nature. What is inside is outside. What is outside is inside. We meditate to maintain this experience at all times. We receive *shaktipāt* to awaken Kundalini Shakti, and once She is awakened, She remains bright, illuminating our minds, our intellects, our hearts, and our entire being.[50]

These insights of the Siddha Yoga gurus, historically first elaborated in the Tantras and then refined by Kashmiri Śaivism, are not sectarian as such. We find a similar vision in the works of the poet-saint Jñāneśvar, whose particular point of divine reference is the god Kṛṣṇa and especially the cult of Viṭṭhala in Pandharpur, Maharashtra.[51] (One need not take a particular sectarian position to incorporate Kuṇḍalinī into a body of teachings—Jñāneśvar is a particularly fine example of this phenomenon.) Like other traditional gurus, the Siddha Yoga gurus are interested only in making their teachings clear; their ultimate source, along with the particular sectarian interests of historical commentators, is secondary.

While it is possible to draw important ideological and practical distinctions between the classical systems of yoga that begin formally with the sage

Patañjali and especially those of *haṭha* and *kuṇḍalinīyoga*, the Indian tradition rarely shares the scholar's interest in these differences and historical developments.[52] The Siddha Yoga gurus frequently invoke the austere and comprehensive teaching on yogic discipline associated with Patañjali's *Yoga Sūtra*, though they do so from within a context that includes Kuṇḍalinī. This is not a context familiar to Patañjali. From the standpoint of those for whom Kuṇḍalinī is an important teaching, including the Siddha Yoga gurus, the classical sources of yoga serve as foundations, prerequisites, and indispensable aids to their understanding and practice. As if to further complicate the matter, traditional efforts to categorize various yogas and so draw distinctions among so-called *rāja, mantra, laya, haṭha, and kuṇḍalinī yoga*s are largely idiosyncratic. In other words, such schemes may set apart *aspects of a larger tradition of yoga but do not necessarily represent autonomous or independent teachings or movements.* Siddha Yoga draws liberally from all facets of the yoga traditions but retains its distinctive vision by centering on particular facets of siddha lore, many of which are described in the elegant language of the Kashmiri Śaivites. With Swami Muktananda's introduction of the term *mahāyoga* or the "great yoga," as we shall see in the following chapter, he places all of these various yoga teachings into the specific context of Siddha Yoga.

The feature common to all of the traditional sources in which Kuṇḍalinī is mentioned is that she is simultaneously the cosmogonic source of the universe and that same creative power within every human being. The macrocosmic process by which reality itself unfolds is mirrored within the human being in the relationship between the multiple aspects of the embodied self (*jīva*) and the witness-consciousness of the eternal soul, or Ātman. To bring out this particular point, Swami Muktananda makes frequent reference to the sources of nondualist or Advaita Vedānta tradition, which describe at length how the Self is the unchanging witness (*sākṣin*) of all activity. According to Śaṅkara, Advaita Vedānta's chief proponent, there is nothing other than the Self. Any perception or appearance that is not seen with the unifying vision of the absolute is mere illusion or error. According to Swami Muktananda, Kuṇḍalinī is ultimately nothing other than one's own Self. Muktananda's use of Vedānta sources is noteworthy since they are themselves decidedly disinterested in the subject of Kuṇḍalinī.[53] Yet one of the basic Vedānta teachings is easily incorporated here to explain how Kuṇḍalinī's own nature remains unaffected even as she descends into sleep or ascends to awaken.

The Siddha Yoga gurus, deftly moving from one scriptural tradition to another, should be understood within a larger historical context in which describing the *experience* is paramount rather than adhering to any dogmatic or sectarian consistency. When Vedānta can explain a subtle point of *kuṇḍalinīyoga*, it is drawn into the larger picture of the spiritual path. To sum up the Siddha Yoga gurus' view: Understanding *kuṇḍalinīyoga* enables one to know how the Self (*ātman*) becomes all the facets of oneself and yet remains untainted; *experiencing* Kuṇḍalinī is recognizing (*pratyabhijñā*) what has always been ultimately true, that within one's own eternal Self exists the plentitude of selves and, indeed, of all things.

Kuṇḍalinī and Other Yogic Traditions in Siddha Yoga

In addition, the Siddha Yoga gurus draw from sources that range far beyond those that explain Kuṇḍalinī's metaphysics. Both Swami Muktananda and Gurumayi Chidvilasananda have expressed serious interests in the physical practices of *haṭhayoga* as an aid to *kuṇḍalinīyoga. Haṭhayoga* is, in fact, as much a result of Kuṇḍalinī as it is a means to her awakening. Muktananda states:

> As the great Shakti begins to unfold, one may experience movements of the body such as shaking or rotation of the head, or one may perform spontaneous Hatha Yoga postures.[54]

However, according to the Siddha Yoga gurus, Kuṇḍalinī is not the handmaiden of *haṭhayogic* practices. Thus while one can rather unwittingly stir Kuṇḍalinī through *haṭhayoga*—or by other spiritual disciplines such as undirected meditation or asceticism (*tapasya*)—one cannot affect her progress in any significant fashion without the guru's grace of inspiration and guidance. Muktananda explains:

> There are some people who by means of Hatha Yogic processes, particularly mudras and the three bandhas (locks), try to arouse the Kundalini. Even if the Kundalini were awakened, it would be very difficult for one to lead it upwards, because that is not so easy. If the Kundalini were not to rise in a proper manner then it may prove to be harmful. Besides, in such a case a seeker, right from the moment his Kundalini is awakened, up to the moment when it finally merges in the sahasrar, has to depend on exercises all the time. . . . But when Kundalini awakening takes place through grace, it is most natural and spontaneous. Moreover, She works of Her own accord in those centres where her work is necessary. And She stops Her activity at the right time. . . . Therefore it is always better to have the Kundalini aroused by one who has already achieved perfection.[55]

Haṭhayoga, therefore, is no means unto itself to awaken Kuṇḍalinī though its practice affects a physical harmony that encourages and nurtures subtle body awareness. In contrast, one can spontaneously enact yogic postures as the latent impressions (*saṃskāras*, *vāsanās*) erupt with Kuṇḍalinī awakening through the guru's grace-bestowing power (*anugraha-śakti*). Swami Chidvilasananda explains:

> Through grace, the experience comes easily. Without grace, you have to do many complicated things. This is why Siddha Yoga is called spontaneous yoga. Through the awakened Kundalini, by the grace and will of the Master, all the yogic postures that are needed to mold and transform the body into gold happen spontaneously.[56]

This is reiterated in the *Gurugītā*, which is chanted daily in Siddha Yoga ashrams:

> (What is the use of) practicing for so long all those hundreds of windy *prāṇāyāmas*, which are difficult and bring diseases, and the many exercises, which are painful and difficult to master. Constantly serve only one Guru to attain that spontaneous and natural state. When it arises, the powerful *prāṇa* immediately stills of its own accord.[57]

In addition to *haṭhayoga* teachings, the powerfully charismatic images and concepts associated with the so-called Nātha yogis seem part of the deep background of Siddha Yoga tradition. These traditions center on their founding figures, the famous medieval siddhas Matsyendranātha and Gorakṣanātha who are associated with the origin and development of Indian alchemy and medicine. The Nātha tradition is, in these ways, helpful for understanding the Siddha Yoga gurus' traditional affirmation that *kuṇḍalinīyoga* transforms and transmutes both mind and body.[58] The Nāthas' influence on yoga traditions cannot be understated: they are, and continue to be, a primary conversant in the discussion of esoteric practices and teachings.[59]

The Nātha siddhas' interests in bodily and spiritual alchemy that effect a complete change in the experience of the realized yogi are indirectly echoed by Swami Muktananda. The Siddha Yoga gurus are not, however, interested in the Nāthas' scriptural sources nor their keen concern to transmute of the body through the use of mercury and other substances. Further, they do not speak of the Nāthas' link between physical alchemy and bodily immortality. Nātha tradition is virtually preoccupied with bodily transmutation as the primary expression of spiritual achievement. While the Siddha Yoga gurus accept the claim that the subtle body's development has physical consequences, they express no confidence in any of the Nātha claims of physical immortality nor do they share their interest in any form of bodily immortality.[60] Rather, it is the Nāthas' insistence that the state of the siddha is reflected in *every* aspect of existence, and more particularly that the transformation of the subtle body affects the material and physical body, that interests the Siddha Yoga gurus. Awakening Kuṇḍalinī, we are told, may bring all sorts of bodily symptoms and reactions, each as distinctive as the individual in which they appear. This is because, as Swami Chidvilasananda explains, it is Kuṇḍalinī's process of purifying us each according to our own natures:

> We are all motivated or animated by our nature. People have different natures, different temperaments, qualities, moods. When the Shakti is awakened and the Kundalini is at work, people have different *kriyas*. . . .
>
> When Kundalini Shakti is awakened by the Master's grace, the knot of the heart is released. All karmas, all sins, are washed away and the purest being is revealed within. This being is the embodiment of wisdom, light, and truth.[61]

Furthermore, Siddha Yoga practitioners often report experiences that corroborate transformation within the subtle body, with very particularized references to the symbols of *kuṇḍalinīyoga*. Some have experienced the "serpent power" literally in the subtle form of a snake, in meditative, dream, and even waking states. Such encounters are considered to be particularly auspicious.[62]

One practitioner expresses his experience of Kuṇḍalinī as a serpent power:

> Throughout the Mahashakti Kuṇḍalinī six-day Intensive, John Friend was teaching us to do the Mountain Pose [tāḍāsana], and as far as I could tell I wasn't really getting it. There were hundreds of intricate details, about where each muscle should be, which seemed impossible to follow.
>
> On the fourth day we did the Mountain Pose again. Shortly after, Gurumayi had us standing while she talked softly, preparing us for meditation. I was standing, the lights were dim, and I had my eyes open and I was watching Gurumayi. At that point I felt a huge "snake" as thick as my wrist—powerful, dark green, and shiny—enter my body at the bottom of my spine, and move right up my spine. When it reached the top of my head, its head curved over so that it was looking out through my forehead. It opened its hood so that the top of the hood was flush up against the inside of my skull.
>
> At that point my body went into perfect *tāḍāsana*, down to every detail that John had been giving for the last four days, including things he hadn't even mentioned. I could feel all of the muscles and bones align themselves from the feet up. I felt fascinated and thought, This is not just a vision; it is a tangible reality—my eyes are open and the effect manifests physically in my body.
>
> This "snake" is still there five days later, as I sit in my office. Again, it does not appear as a vision, it is a tangible reality—it is looking through my eyes. As I talk about it I can feel it from the bottom of my spine to the top of my head.[63]

For the Siddha Yoga gurus, Kuṇḍalinī's alchemy is one of inner transformation. It is not surprising then that they show no interest in the other facet of Indian alchemy made famous (or infamous) by the Nāthas, that is, in the use of the physical substances or alchemical experiments to produce inner, subtle changes or desired physical effects. Swami Muktananda is explicit in his rejection of the use of any foreign substances to bring about the inner awakening, whether these involve the traditional chemistries such as those discussed in Nātha *rasāyana* (alchemy) or drugs of any sort.

As he invokes Kuṇḍalinī in his commentary on the *Kuṇḍalinī Stavaḥ*, which is very likely a text with connections to the Nātha tradition, Swami Muktananda beseeches the Goddess to perform this inner alchemy by her own accord:

> May Your grace transform my ephemeral body into one which is blissful and eternal.[64]

Thus, we see in the writings of swamis Muktananda and Chidvilasananda a broad range of sources and concepts about Kuṇḍalinī, ranging from references to the achievements of ancient Vedic yogis, seers, and gods to the mature speculative insights of medieval India.

The Vision of Kashmiri Śaivism on Kuṇḍalinī and the Siddha Yoga Interpretation

To explain Kuṇḍalinī's mysterious work Swami Muktananda often evokes the cosmogonic vision of Kashmiri Śaivism. According to one of its primary sources, the *Stanzas on Vibration* (*Spandakārikā*), the universe is the pulsation, the *spanda*, of divine consciousness or Citi; it is nothing other than the eternal Śiva becoming Śakti. The one primordial reality called Śiva by the very act of becoming two—Śiva and Śakti—creates a process of emission and withdrawal, of expansion and contraction, which assumes the character of being (*sat*), consciousness (*cit*), and bliss (*ānanda*). While there is no ultimate difference between Śiva and Śakti, their play (*līlā*) begins when Śiva, who conceals Śakti within himself as the undifferentiated (*abheda*), offers this conscious power of his own being as his sacrificial oblation. Reality as such is set into motion as a gift of God in the form of a sacrifice, a *yajña*. Śiva, who is the sacrificial fire, is inseparable from the fire's heat, which is Śakti.[65] The offering of this sacrifice—its substances (*dravya*), sacred sound (*mantra*), and liberating intention (*tyāga*)—is Kuṇḍalinī.[66] In other words, Śiva offers himself by assuming the form of Kuṇḍalinī. Put in terms of the sacrifice, Kuṇḍalinī becomes the manifest world at all levels of being; her subtle expression is the sonic forms or mantras; and her intention is the perfectly free offering of grace-giving power of the sacrificer. It is by her compassion that we experience the various movements of body, speech, and mind and awaken to their divine origin. Thus, Kuṇḍalinī is both the offering and the sacrificer; she thus becomes God's own experience of himself as pure delight (*sukha*). To awaken Kuṇḍalinī is to share in the divine's very own nature (*svasvabhāva*) as an experience of encompassing aesthetic rapture (*camatkāra*) bereft of motive or of need. So, as the *Bhagavadgītā* states, "The Absolute is the offering, the Absolute is the oblation that is poured into the Absolute fire by the Absolute. One who contemplates the act as nothing but the Absolute reaches the Absolute."[67]

The great Kashmiri Śaiva writer Kṣemarāja, often cited by swamis Muktananda and Chidvilasananda, explains that describing the relationship between Śiva and Śakti is a means of orienting ourselves in terms of the divine.

> The Supreme Lord is both the Great Light [of universal consciousness] and the perfect medium of reflection [*vimarśa*]. His one power is motion and so is proclaimed in the scriptures by means of countless names including, "vibration" [*spanda*], "radiance" [*sphurattā*], "wave" [*ūrmi*], "strength" [*bala*], "exertion" [*udyoga*], "the Heart" [*hṛdaya*], "the essence" [*sāra*], "*Malini*" and "the supreme Power" [*para*]. Although this [power] is one, it is at once both expansion and contraction.[68]

The language of Kuṇḍalinī is yet another powerful tool of orientation. Kuṇḍalinī is the name and the form of the goddess Citi envisioned as the vital, organic, and divine power (*śakti*) or force (*bala*) that willfully and deliberately orchestrates these expanding (*unmeṣa*) and contracting (*nimeṣa*) movements of the universe. She is likewise the subtle form of consciousness who manifests within the human being. Put differently, both the material and subtle forms of the universe, like those of human beings, are nothing but the divine consciousness assuming postures and engaging in movements toward revelation and concealment. This vision of the universe as an unfolding divinity is mirrored in the experience of the seekers in whom Kuṇḍalinī has been awakened. Swami Muktananda describes this as a process of subtle body purification:

> . . . Kundalini inspires various hatha yogic movements or kriyas, which take place in the physical body. In the form of prana, She penetrates all 720 million nadis, consumes all the old decaying fluids, then releases vital energy into them all. As the nadis become filled with prana, the body becomes rejuvenated from within. It becomes strong and firm, with all the suppleness of a child.[69]

In Citi's pure stateless union with Śiva as the absolute "I" (or Aham) nothing moves or changes, and yet there is projected from this source by her powers of will (*icchā*), activity (*kriyā*), and knowledge (*jñāna*) the experience of the delimited "I" (or *aham*). Creation as such is a process in which we experience our own evolving "creature consciousness," but it is, in fact, Kuṇḍalinī's own devolving of her original higher and purer form as absolute consciousness.

In this language of Kashmiri Śaivism, so prevalent in the works of the Siddha Yoga gurus, we find further descriptions of Kuṇḍalinī's activity and explanations as to why she "goes to sleep" inside us only to signal us that we should awaken her. Her process is described as twofold. First, her "constantly awakened" and "asleep until awakened" natures reside ultimately in one nature, in Śiva; second, her power of *māyā,* or her manifestation as the great māyā (*mahāmāyā*), is the cause of all appearances. That Kuṇḍalinī is the "sleeping," not-yet-awakened experience of the Self *and* the constant pulsation (*spanda*) that is the universe's very form (*svarūpa*) is to affirm that nothing manifests that is not Śiva.[70] There is then but one reality who deliberately assumes the form of plurality. This is not, however, to say that this one reality becomes dualistic. Dualism is misunderstanding the divine's true nature which is both one and many.

Further, Kuṇḍalinī's sleep can be identified as *māyā. Māyā* is neither inexplicable (*anirvacanīya*) nor is it a cruel and deliberate effort on the part of God to delude or mislead.[71] *Māyā* is that aspect of the power of manifestation in which embodied beings fall prey to the triad of impurities, or *mala*s, that create ignorance (*avidyā*).[72] Ignorance, like a smudge obscuring a mirror, exists only until that time when it is removed; just as the smudge itself is not the mirror, so ignorance sullies the pure soul into thinking that there is a reality apart and distinct from itself. Kuṇḍalinī's awakening removes these impurities, and as Swami Muktananda describes, the three impurities (*mala*) are within Kuṇḍalinī's reach as she rises through the body:

> This veil of ignorance, which has taken the form of the world, hides one's own true nature, converts the state of Shiva into the state of individuality, and makes one undergo great suffering. This veil consists of the three impurities and is also known as the knot of the heart. . . .
>
> When Maha Shakti Kundalini unfolds within, the knot of the heart is automatically pierced, all thoughts and doubts are destroyed, and all *karmas* are weakened. Kundalini gives a seeker true understanding of all the worldly pleasures which appear so wonderful, and, knowing them to be the cause of the seeker's bondage, She roots them out for his own good. When Parakundalini Shakti, who is subtler than the subtlest, pierces all the knots which sustain the sense of limitation, the knowledge of the Absolute arises.[73]

Swami Chidvilasananda describes this process experientially:

> Sometimes you have the experience that somebody is holding a sparkler and literally lighting one of the chakras—and from that, another chakra, from that, another. It is Kundalini awakening. You become totally absorbed in these experiences. . . . There are so many colors, so many facets. So it's very important to rise higher and higher, and not get stuck in any of the chakras, either.[74]

At the basis of our adventitious self-delusion is a misunderstanding of Śakti's innately dynamic nature. She is constantly unfolding and withdrawing as both the objective manifestations of the world and as our own processes of subjective perception. This power of obscuring occurs because Kuṇḍalinī creates appearances which are themselves real though the differences between them are not. Thus while appearances change, change is itself only an appearance or, to put it differently, it is an illusion or a dream. Gurumayi explains Kuṇḍalinī as the great māyā who sleeps within and creates the world simultaneously:

> Shakti is called Kundalini by seekers and by those who realize Her within. When She is dormant, coiled at the base of the spine, she is also called Mahamaya, the great illusion. Due to Her great spellbinding power, sometimes Mahamaya makes us blind, sometimes deaf. Then we are not able to see Her true greatness or hear of it. But it is also Shakti who allows us to see; it is Shakti who allows us to hear. For this reason, one prays, "O Goddess, bestow grace upon me. Allow me to see Your true form. Allow me to hear about Your true form."[75]

Kuṇḍalinī's "true form," as the great Abhinavagupta further reminds us, is the absolute which is never actually obscured. Kuṇḍalinī's sleep is itself another play of God, another momentary dream in divine consciousness.

> Even that which, acting as an obscuring element, is considered to be an obstruction (to absolute consciousness) is nothing but the Supreme Lord, Whose nature is (pure) knowledge and action, and Who manifests by virtue of His freedom to assume the form of that very obscuration and the rest.[76]

In this sense, Kuṇḍalinī is never actually asleep nor is there an awakening. This perception of Kuṇḍalinī as sleeping or awake is also *māyā*—a matter of real appearances that produce their own effect on our limited understanding. There is a way to turn this power of self-deception into a lucid awareness. It begins with a certain insight that, as Swami Muktananda explains, becomes one's direct experience:

> This divine power is the power of our own Self. Though we talk about awakening the Kundalini, the truth is that everyone's Kundalini is already awake. Just as She has created the external universe and dwells within it, She has created this human body and pervades it from head to toe. Dwelling at the center of the universe, She holds it together and maintains it. In the same way, dwelling at the center of the body, in the *mūlādhāra* chakra at the base of the spine, She controls and maintains our whole physiological system, through its network of 720 million *nādīs.*[77]

To experience Kuṇḍalinī is to bring the mysterious power of *māyā* into the forefront of the physical and psychic reality of one's own individuated consciousness. Since Kuṇḍalinī is constantly manifesting as the universe, the task of the yogi is this inner awakening. Swami Muktananda states:

> The awakening of the inner Kundalini is the true beginning of the spiritual journey. Just as when She is directed outward, Kundalini enables us to explore the outer world, when Her inner aspect is activated, we are able to experience the inner, spiritual world. . . . In our present state, we identify ourselves with this body which has a certain size and shape. We are not aware that we are all-pervasive. It is only when the Kundalini is awakened that we become aware of our true nature, of our greatness, of the fact that not only do we belong to God, but we *are* God.[78]

In his commentary on the *Spandakārikā*, Kṣemarāja explains that as Kuṇḍalinī gradually crystallizes in the yogi's consciousness in her own form (*svarūpa*) as consciousness (*cinmaya*), individuation dissolves entirely. Residing in the great void (*mahāśūnya*), no longer shrouded by the mysterious veil of *māyā*, the yogi enjoys (*bhoga*) the inherent freedom (*svatantra*) of being liberated while yet living (*jīvanmukti*), with the Self his constant experience and the universe intact but no longer filled with suffering or misconceptions.[79]

At both the macrocosmic and microcosmic levels, Citi appears as a reflection (*vimarśana*) of Śiva's projected light. This relationship—and seeming separation—between light and reflection simultaneously produces a corresponding resonant vibration (*nāda*). In this way she is both a projection of light/form and an unfolding of sound.

This dyadic metaphor enables us to link the three images of Kuṇḍalinī as light's reflection, as an unfolding "serpent" coiled within the body, and as the currents of consciousness that assume different colors, shapes, and forms *with* her expression as resonance or sound heard both within and beyond oneself—as the sounds of Sanskrit (*mātṛkā-śakti*), as primordial sound absolute (*śabdabrahman*), as mantra, and as the guru's voice. Swami Chidvilasananda combines both light/form and sound metaphors in her own description of Kuṇḍalinī's nature:

> The Kundalini energy is finer than the finest. It appears as the sun and the moon and all the stars. It reveals itself as different sounds, different syllables, different objects, and different beings. Meditate on this energy which finally dissolves its own manifestation into the unmanifest. . . .
>
> As She gently moves in and around you, She sings to Herself. So listen to the sound She makes. Whatever you hear, every sound manifests from Her. As you become absorbed in the inner sound of the Shakti, you glide into meditation. Your breath is Her whisper. Your breath is Her song. Your breath is Her dance. To please the Shakti, to awaken Her within us, and to keep Her glory manifest in our being, we chant Her own song to Her—the sound *Om*.[80]

Swami Chidvilasananda makes clear that Kuṇḍalinī should neither be reduced to conceptual abstractions nor be removed from the experiences of our senses and bodies. While she is incomparable (*anuttara*) and beyond (*parā*), she is also the very life force and breath (*prāṇa*) that courses through our bodies and enlivens our minds. We may experience her as one of the three levels of being: mundane, subtle, or causal. To awaken Kuṇḍalinī then is to transform oneself from a being who merely lives *in* Kuṇḍalinī and *through* Kuṇḍalinī, to an aware and alive being who lives *as* Kuṇḍalinī and *by the grace* of Kuṇḍalinī.

Similarly, Swami Muktananda never fails to note that the same Kuṇḍalinī Śakti who creates the universe as consciousness, Citi, is the dynamic, ever-apparent life force ("outer Kuṇḍalinī") *and* the divinity who sleeps within everyone as his or her latent potential for Self-realization ("inner Kuṇḍalinī"). Citi Kuṇḍalinī is both ever-active *and* dormant until awakened from her slumber. Muktananda offers many examples of this simultaneity:

> A seeker who meditates on Kundalini in the *muladhara*, contemplating Her in Her eternal dormant form, which is symbolically represented as a serpent, considers Her to be the Mother as well as *maya*, knowledge, and the power of action.[81]

While her manifestation is constantly taking place at every level of being, one becomes a yogi "established in power" (*śaktiṣṭhā*) who sees her in her authentic nature (*svabhāvasthā*) as beyond all states and levels. This awareness is the result of awakening her through spiritual discipline (*sādhana*), that is, through *kuṇḍalinīyoga* effected by the guru's shaktipat.[82] Thus, bringing Kuṇḍalinī to recognition begins with a deeper appreciation of her as our most fundamental experience, as the breath, as the pulsation of the heart, as life itself. Swami Muktananda says:

> Understand at least this much, that everything is Chiti and the same Chiti is the Kundalini. . . . It is the same Chiti that makes you complete in yoga . . . .
>
> [A]s long as she is not activated in you, you are only half-alive. . . .
>
> People who believe in Kundalini say that Kundalini is based at the base of the spine, or in the head or somewhere else. However, the true understanding of Kundalini is to know that Kundalini exists at the rising and at the merging of the prana—wherever the prana merges and from wherever once again it arises. . . .
>
> The universal Consciousness, Bhairavi, Kundalini, Mahadevi, who is one with God, who has merged with God, who is God, has become this prana. Therefore, understand prana as universal Consciousness. Don't understand it as mere breath. It is through Her that everything functions.[83]

Kuṇḍalinī and Prāṇa: The Life Force and the Passage Through the Suṣumṇā

Here Swami Muktananda identifies Kuṇḍalinī with *prāṇa*, the life force within the breath which the ancient *Bṛhadāraṇyaka Upaniṣad* affirms is none other than the Self and the absolute.[84] In this sense, Kuṇḍalinī is not limited to its location in any particular place but rather is that which gives rise to the very notion of identity or place. *Prāṇa* in this sense is the source and origin of Being as it flows and moves through the breath and as the breath; it is another name for the absolute when it is experienced as one's Self. "When Shree Kundalini awakens within, She spreads throughout the body in the form of *prana,* and gives rise not only to inner sounds, but to many other divine experiences. . . . One may be overwhelmed with feelings of love and joy, and become ecstatic with divine bliss."[85]

However, Kuṇḍalinī is also described as that reality present in the moment between breaths, "at the rising and at the merging of the *prāṇa*—wherever the *prāṇa* merges and from wherever once again it arises." In this space or "middle" (*madhyam*), as the *Vijñānabhairava Tantra* calls it, the yogi can intuitively experience the point of convergence at which the energy of universal consciousness is both the eternal support of Being and the creative movement of Becoming.[86] The center point thus marks the time between moments, the interval between two thoughts, and the space between the breaths when the divine Śakti's activities of creation by expansion and contraction are simultaneously present. Following the breath thus becomes an exercise in which the yogi experiences the ascension and expansion of Śakti emerging from the perfect void of her union with Śiva, while simultaneously she descends to assume the forms of limited, embodied existence. (Swami Muktananda devotes an entire book, *I Am That,* to the description of this aspect of Kuṇḍalinī and to the practices associated with awakening Kuṇḍalinī through meditation on the breath and the mantra, *So'ham.*)

At the level of bodily awareness the yogi first follows the flow of the breath and perceptions, then rests in the moment between them, only at last to be freed from both, at which point consciousness alone remains as the pure experience of the Self.

Kṣemarāja in his *Pratyabhijñāhṛdayam* describes how consciousness contracts into the form of the life breath (*prāṇa*), thus opening a channel, piercing the center of the body, and traversing downward. At its resting point, the self-aware and self-delimiting Citi becomes the animate form of the body as so many thousands of channels (*nāḍī*), each of which is a conduit of the life-giving *śakti.*[87] Here at the base of the central channel or *suṣumṇānāḍī,* Citi turns upon itself, coiling as Kuṇḍalinī. It is from this point that Kuṇḍalinī is awakened. Swami Muktananda explains how Kuṇḍalinī is both pervading and "specially located":

> Although Kundalini pervades the human body, She has a special abode at the center of the body, in the muladhara cakra at the base of the spine. . . . The word *mūla* means "root," and *adhāra* means "support." According to the yogic scriptures, this root is three inches long, and within it the Shakti resides in a subtle form, coiled three and one-half times; this is why She is known as

Kundalini, "the coiled one." When She is awakened, She uncoils and begins to journey upwards toward the abode of Shiva in the *sahasrāra*.[88]

The subtle process of Kuṇḍalinī's descent and ascent within the body is mirrored physiologically by the activities of the breath. First descending with inhalation, she then reverses course; with exhalation the *prāṇa* flows upward, releasing Kuṇḍalinī who reverts to her original unbounded form.[89] Thus, the physical act of breathing functions as a mundane representation of the continuous, natural, and playful movement of Kuṇḍalinī. Commenting on this same verse from the *Pratyabhijñāhṛdayam*, Swami Muktananda describes how the macrocosmic act of the divine Śakti becomes the experience of both the mundane and subtle human bodies. His commentary is worth citing at length since, once again, he offers a summary of Kuṇḍalinī as both Goddess and energy of yogic discipline:

> Goddess Samvitti, the Goddess of universal consciousness, possessing infinite power and glory, is the true centre of this animate and inanimate universe. She dwells within all things, pervading them in subtle form. Without Her grace, no one can realise his real nature. She involves Herself, of Her own free will, in the sportful maze of Her own making, and manifests all the shapes and forms which fill the universe. Assuming prana and intellect, and all the other organs, and emanating thousands of nerves, She fashions the human body. The great Shakti pervades the body, particularly its central nerve, *sushumna,* which extends from the *sahasrar,* situated in the middle of the *brahmarandhra* in the brain, to the *muladhar* at the base of the spine. She supports both Brahman and pranashakti therein. All our thoughts, feelings and inspirations spring from the central nerve and subside in it. The mind arises from Brahman and vibrates into thoughts by the power of prana. One who lacks guru's grace is ignorant of these secrets.[90]

Here Swami Muktananda assumes the well-known physiology of the subtle body as it is described in virtually all the texts of *kuṇḍalinīyoga* tradition.[91] His focus, however, is on making connections between the manifestations of Kuṇḍalinī within the subtle body and the ways she is experienced physically, emotionally, mentally, and spiritually. He first draws attention to the subtle body's three major channels, the *iḍā* (left), *piṅgalā* (right), and *suṣumṇā* (center), which act as the conduits of the vital-force, and the *prāṇa* or *prāṇaśakti,* the life breath that supports Kuṇḍalinī. He pays special attention to the *suṣumṇā* since this is Kuṇḍalinī's chosen passage. He writes:

> And of these three, one is the most significant. That is *sushumna,* the *brahmanadi,* the Samvitti *nadi,* the *madhya nadi,* or the pathway of the great Kundalini. All nerves are supported by it. The various good and evil thoughts and feelings such as love, devotion, attachment and hatred appear from and disappear into it.[92]

The *suṣumṇānāḍī* here becomes a virtual synonym for the path of Siddha Yoga itself since all efforts and effects of spiritual discipline are contained within it. Thus, to enter onto the path of Siddha Yoga is to commence the inward journey of the "middle path," the journey of Kuṇḍalinī through the subtle body's centers from her initial unraveling in the *mūlādhāra* to her reunion with Śiva in the *sahasrāra*. Muktananda, however, also points to Kuṇḍalinī's presence throughout the subtle body and clearly identifies her awakening not only with the blossoming of the *sahasrāra* but as an opening of heart.[93] He writes:

> Kundalini has three basic locations: at the base of the spine, in the heart, and at the crown of the head. She is awakened at the base of the spine and is also activated in the heart, where She manifests as bliss.[94]

> Dwelling within the center of the heart, She shines with all the colors of the morning sun, and when She is awakened within us, we can see Her there, blazing in all Her effulgence.[95]

In any case, to concentrate on the path of the *suṣumṇā* is to go beyond simple worldliness and begin the "pilgrimage to liberation."

> Everyone's ida and pingala nadis are active, because when one inhales and exhales, the breath comes in and goes out through these nadis. However, most people are unaware of the sushumna nadi. . . . The sushumna controls all the other nadis. It extends in an unbroken line from the muladhara, where the dormant Kundalini lies coiled up, to the sahasrara, in the crown of the head, the seat of supreme Shiva. Within the sushumna is a subtle nadi called *chitrinī*, which is the channel for the movement of the Kundalini. . . .
>
> The unfolding of the central nadi is the pilgrimage to liberation, the path of Self-realization. If you have received Shakti from the Guru, then the central channel unfolds automatically.[96]

Swami Muktananda summarizes Kuṇḍalinī's journey:

> When the awakened Kundalini rises through the central channel, She pierces the six chakras, or spiritual centers . . . and finally brings about the *samādhi* state, the state of equality awareness, establishing the disciple permanently in the topmost spiritual center, the sahasrara, where he becomes one with the Lord Shiva. This manifestation of the Kundalini corresponds to raja yoga and culminates in the ultimate realization of God within oneself.[97]

To emphasize that Kuṇḍalinī acts as an intelligent and divine presence rather than as a "mechanism" simply "activated," Muktananda returns again and again to the guru's grace-bestowing power (*anugraha-śakti*) as the guiding initiation that directs divine unfolding and to Kuṇḍalinī's form as *citi-śakti.* Shaktipat is that indispensable beginning as well as the culminating reunion of Śakti with Śiva, of disciple with guru. As the seeker engages in various practices of Siddha Yoga—from meditation to *haṭhayoga* to chanting the divine names (*nāmasaṃkīrtana*)—the process of disciplining the *prāṇa* creates a natural, spontaneous, and practically effortless immersion into meditation. Though he is not reluctant to detail the intricacies of *kuṇḍalinīyoga,* including its relationship to the major channels, their extension into millions of *nāḍīs*, and *prāṇa*'s five particular functions as inhaling, exhaling, pervading, arising, and balancing (*prāṇa, apāna, vyāna, udāna,* and *samāna*), Swami Muktananda appears less interested in another elaboration of Kuṇḍalinī theory than in explaining the effects of Siddha Yoga practice.[98]

THE PRACTICE OF *KUṆḌALINĪYOGA* IN SIDDHA YOGA: THE FEATURES OF *MAHĀYOGA*

The Siddha Yoga gurus place *kuṇḍalinīyoga* practices within a larger context they call *mahāyoga* or the "great yoga." Swami Muktananda sees *mahāyoga* not only as a synthesis of virtually all other practices but more fundamentally in terms of the shaktipat guru's relationship with the divine Kuṇḍalinī.[99] He writes:

> Siddha Yoga is called Maha Yoga because it encompasses all other yogas. There are many kinds of yogas: hatha yoga, the practice of physical exercises; *bhakti* yoga, the path of love; *rāja* yoga, which is attained through meditation; mantra yoga; *laya* yoga; *jñāna* yoga and many others. When Kundalini is awakened, all these other yogas take place automatically. You don't have to make any effort to practice them; they come to you on their own.[100]

This statement should not be understood to mean that Swami Muktananda is discrediting the rigors of spiritual practice. Rather, since the shaktipat guru is essential to awakening Kuṇḍalinī, true spiritual attainment depends as much on the seeker's obtaining the guru's grace as it does on exercising self-effort. To put this in the language of nondualist Vedānta, one cannot effect the eternal, that is, the absolute must exist before it is realized as such. Knowledge "uncovers" the truth by removing the errors of misperception. The guru's grace is both his own direct experience (*anubhāva*), his own knowledge (*svajñāna*), and his ability to confer that knowledge on a disciple. Switching to the language of Kashmiri Śaivism, the concept of grace "guarantees" that one's efforts in sadhana do nothing to bring the absolute into being but rather initiate re-cognition (*pratyabhijñā*). In other words, one sees again, even if it seems like the first time, that which has always been true.

Establishing a relationship with Kuṇḍalinī that is beneficent, loving, constructive, natural, easy, and spontaneous is living in the guru's grace and what is meant by receiving it. Shaktipat, therefore, is the first element of *mahāyoga* and the first aspect of cultivating and awakening Kuṇḍalinī.

Kuṇḍalinī and Shaktipat

To map Kuṇḍalinī's movements is to follow the archetypal course of spiritual discipline which, according to the Siddha Yoga gurus, begins in earnest with shaktipat. As we consider the paradigmatic process, with its distinct set of actions and practices, we can as well notice the manifestations and experiences that appear differently in individuals. In this way, Kuṇḍalinī remains true to her nature: She is at once the same in everyone even as she appears uniquely in each individual.

One of the ways Swami Muktananda defined shaktipat was as Kuṇḍalinī's awakening by the grace of the guru. The guru's special gift, his grace, is precisely his intimacy with the divine Śakti which he offers in any number of ways:

> Now, what do we get from such a Guru? We get the inner shakti, the Kundalini Shakti or Chitishakti. How does he give us this shakti? By sight, by touch, by word, by grace.[101]

> Only one Shakti is transmitted in Shaktipat; however, people are of different capacities or temperaments. Each person receives Shaktipat according to his nature, his actions, and the accumulation of his sins and virtues. The Kundalini dwells in everyone; therefore, this energy can be awakened in everyone, but it depends entirely on one's faith, devotion, and desire for the awakening. The Guru gives Shakti to whomever takes it.[102]

Once shaktipat takes place, Kuṇḍalinī is set into motion, whether suddenly or gradually, according to her own will. The key to understanding the Siddha Yoga view is that the guru who confers shaktipat has experienced Kuṇḍalinī fully for himself. Part of the guru's experience is his assurance that his own ability "to hold the Śakti" within himself guarantees that all of the seeker's physical, emotional, and spiritual developments are part of the beneficent and loving expression of Kuṇḍalinī's cleansing revelation of herself. This is because the guru knows Kuṇḍalinī's nature as his own and as an utterly divine intelligence within us. Swami Muktananda describes it this way:

> Kundalini is all-knowing. She knows our past and our future, and She knows what is suited to us and what is not.
>
> Just as one experiences the movements of hatha yoga, other yogas also take place. Love arises, along with the ecstatic feeling of devotion which belongs to bhakti yoga. One attains spontaneous knowledge, as in jnana yoga, and the

> capacity for detachment in action, which belongs to karma yoga. You may hear inner sounds, perceive divine tastes and smells, or have visions of various lights, gods and goddesses, saints, holy rivers and mountains, and even distant worlds, as in laya yoga.[103]

Swami Chidvilasananda explains that the purification process initiated by shaktipat is no cause for fear, even if there are sensations of physical discomfort:

> . . . Sometimes this happens when the Kundalini is awakened. And if you have discomfort, do not worry about it. There's no need to be concerned. The awakened Shakti is the healing force.[104]

A distinctive feature of Siddha Yoga is that shaktipat experiences involving Kuṇḍalinī seem to occur before devotees have acquired the mystical vocabulary or much understanding of the normative tradition. In fact, experiences do not necessarily begin from any positive feelings about the guru whatsoever, though they typically involve the sensation of cleansing and transformation, as the example below suggests:

> . . . My idea of a Guru was that they would soak you for whatever they could get. Baba was sitting up front. Everyone was quiet. No one was talking to me. I was feeling very alone, very confused. I saw a woman wearing a sari. I figured that she was Indian and that she worked for Baba. I said, "Excuse me, do you work here?" She said, "Sort of." It turned out that she was Jewish and from Brooklyn, which was great because I'm Jewish from the Bronx. I felt we could communicate. I began to ask her all kinds of questions: Who is this Muktananda? Why does he wear such funny clothes? Why does he sit up front? Why are we sitting on the floor? Why do you have a red dot in the middle of your forehead? Why do we sing in a foreign language? What is this place? What's going on here? Why am I here? She tried to explain it all to me, and I tried to understand her. . . .
>
> Finally she said to me, "Would you like to meet Baba?" I said, "Sure." Just then Baba got up from his chair. The woman in the sari caught his eye, and Baba started walking in my direction. By this time I knew he was a holy man. I just knew it. As he approached me I thought to myself, "Oh my God, I'm about to meet a holy man. What should I say to him? How should I behave? What should I do?" A voice inside me said, "Bernie, just be humble." I thought, "Okay," but I realized I didn't know what it meant to be humble. Baba was getting closer and closer. I thought, "Well, humble is small." I kind of shrunk my body so I would be shorter than Baba. By now Baba was standing right beside me. I reached out my hand and said, "Hello, sir. How do you do?" With no hesitation, totally in command, Baba stepped right in front of me and looked me square in the eye. He put his hand on my shoulder and said, "hello," in a deep, powerfully resonant voice.

> When Baba put his hand on my shoulder my mind stopped. An incredible feeling of peace came over me. It started somewhere around my toes, or beyond my toes, and spread over my whole body. I stood there stunned, my mouth agape, staring into his eyes.
>
> . . . I went to pick up my kid and some of his friends at school. They wanted to play in the woods. They ran off and I ambled after them. It was a beautiful day, and I was just enjoying being with nature. Then, all of a sudden, I had this intense feeling in my chest, as though someone had struck it with a rock. I looked down, but there was no rock. The pain was right in the region of my heart. I thought that maybe I was having a heart attack. But I was breathing easily. As I breathed in I could feel a tremendously powerful energy in my body. It was moving in all directions at once. Every time I breathed in or breathed out I felt ecstatic. I had never had such a feeling in my life. I could feel, with each breath, this energy circulating all over my body. I looked down and I could literally see it going out of my toes and out of my fingertips. Then I could see the same energy emerging from the clouds and trees and rocks. I understood that everything in the universe is one energy. Nothing is different. I felt absolutely ecstatic. I started to laugh and laugh. I don't know how long I was standing there in that state. Suddenly I realized that what I was feeling was oneness with Baba. I felt that he was literally right there. I thought maybe he was hiding. I started to run through the woods and look behind the trees, saying, "Come out, Mr. Muktananda. Mr. Muktananda, sir, come out." I was running all over the place laughing. I was in heaven. It was the greatest experience of my life. I knew that I had latched onto something amazing.[105]

The shaktipat guru is indispensable because, as Swami Muktananda explains, Siddha Yoga is a path of grace *aided by but not solely determined by* self-effort. He writes:

> When Kundalini awakening takes place through grace, it will rise of its own accord and become established where it should be established. Kundalini will take care of Herself, for the Shakti is a conscious and all-knowing power. . . . If one has awakened the Kundalini through self-effort, it is very difficult to lead it upward, because right from the moment the Kundalini is awakened until the moment it finally merges in the sahasrara, the seeker has to depend on yogic practices. But when the Kundalini is awakened by the grace of the Guru, the grace itself will guide it in the correct manner. There is absolutely no danger in such a case.[106]

Swami Chidvilasananda explains the vital role shaktipat plays in Kuṇḍalinī's awakening:

> Shaktipat initiation, the awakening of the Kundalini Shakti, is the supreme act of the Master's grace. It is the lightning bolt that reveals the greatest treasure within. It is the ultimate gesture of compassion, the breath of the Abso-

lute that breaks the chains of endless death and rebirth and sets you free once and for all.[107]

The Siddha Yoga gurus distinguish Siddha Yoga from other types of spiritual discipline in which Kuṇḍalinī is treated as a technology or mechanism with the potential to go awry. More than a requirement for proper instruction or an exhortation to take a more reliable and therefore easier path, Swami Muktananda explains the Siddha Yoga path through this vital, organic, and divine relationship that links the guru and disciple to the personal experience of God. This is the core of what is meant by *mahāyoga*: that Kuṇḍalinī's awakening is directed by the guru's grace and that her awakening evokes the spontaneous gestures of burgeoning Self-realization.

The Siddha Yoga gurus teach that one of *mahāyoga*'s most important practices is the repetition (*japa*) of the divinely empowered mantra. Swami Muktananda writes that the mantra, as well as the ensuing upliftment that follows from resonating with the mantra, are but embodiments of Kuṇḍalinī:

> Kundalini, the universal Mother, encompasses all yogas. She is the form and essence of the mantra. When you receive the mantra through the Guru's grace, She is quickly awakened.
>
> The awakening of Kundalini—whose form is the mantra—and Her rejoicing are one and the same.[108]

Mantra is, like Kuṇḍalinī herself, both the divine's own form and the yogic instrument by which awakening occurs. Thus, the mantra enlivened (*caitanya*) through Shaktipat and received in initiation (*dīkṣā*) becomes another form of Citi Śakti, the repetition of whose own name draws her attention and awakens her from her own slumbers. In this sense, mantra repetition (*japa*) is the vehicle of awakening Kuṇḍalinī, even as it is the invocation of her divine essence as the form of one's own Self. Mantra becomes the key to meditation and can appear in any number of expressions, from silent contemplation to public chanting. In Siddha Yoga the science of mantra (*mantraśāstra*), like *kuṇḍalinīyoga*, is not a technical art whereby hosts of different divinities are invoked and called upon to create different yogic accomplishments (*siddhi*). Rather, mantras are all treated as singular forms of God. Even the lineage mantra, *Oṃ Namaḥ Śivāya,* is not a deity mantra properly speaking and therefore not a sectarian mantra which might be contrasted with mantras associated with other deities or teachings (*siddhānta*), such as *Oṃ Nārāyaṇāya Namaḥ* which is important to Viṣṇu-centered traditions. Instead, the Siddha Yoga gurus treat their lineage mantra, *Oṃ Namaḥ Śivāya,* as an invocation of one's own ultimate consciousness whose inner form is Kuṇḍalinī Śakti. Mantra is then the living impulse of the highest form of consciousness within the subtle body of every individual. In Siddha

Yoga there are no "sets" of mantra initiations or casts of deities associated with different levels of spiritual practice. Rather, there is a more direct and organic notion that when a mantra is filled with the guru's grace-bestowing power (*anugraha-śakti*), it is both an instrument and a form of the awakening divinity within.

In Siddha Yoga the gurus may offer initiation into several mantras, including *Guru Oṃ* and *So 'ham*, though the "mantra of the siddha lineage" is the root-mantra (*mūlamantra*) of Śiva: *Oṃ Namaḥ Śivāya*. Perhaps the distinctive feature of this initiation is that, like shaktipat, it happens on a wide scale, without any secretive trappings or discrimination on the basis of gender or religion or advancement, and is considered one of the true gifts of the siddha guru. Consistent with traditional views, the mantra becomes divine because it is transmitted through a guru who is Self-realized and whose authority is rooted in lineage connections. To put the matter of mantra initiation in more technical terms, the mantra is *caitanya*, or "filled with consciousness," and no longer *jaḍa*, or "inert." Of course, the mantra is none other than Kuṇḍalinī herself, since she is Citi Śakti or consciousness-power. It is not a mere representation of her, a "tool" or "technique."[109] Rather, the mantra is the living divinity's own pulsation. However, the mantra, like Kuṇḍalinī, "sleeps" until awakened: A mantra without the guru's empowering initiation is incapable of being used with total effectiveness. This understanding, entirely in keeping with the widespread traditions of *kuṇḍalinīyoga*, is clearly explained by Swami Muktananda:

> Worship the Chitishakti, who lives forever in your mind. Live your daily life always remembering this spiritual principle, which continually vibrates in each impulse of your mind.[110]

Here Muktananda refers to the so-called *ajapajapa*, the repetition that is no-repetition, that is, the continuous, no-longer-self-conscious reiteration of the divine sound as the pulsation of one's own inner being. The idea is subtle since the disciple's true spiritual path begins with shaktipat and so begins with grace. The gift of grace is cultivated and nurtured by discipline and committed practice, at which point, one's efforts are fulfilled again by grace which comes as the spontaneous effect of the Self's own divine luminosity. Thus mantras first willfully and self-consciously repeated are transformed by grace into self-generating and spontaneous pulsations of power by an unself-conscious but fully aware consciousness. Swami Muktananda continues:

> Everyone is filled with God in the form of Consciousness. . . . The mantra, since it is charged with the Shakti of Parashiva, the supreme Guru, is not a mantra in the ordinary sense, but a glorious, universal, secret, and divine power in which Parashiva and the Guru live as one. It is alive with Consciousness. It possesses the power of omniscience: *mantrah sarvajṇabalasalinah.* [111]

What disciples will experience through mantra *upāsana,* the bringing of the divinity "close by," as Swami Muktananda says, reflects his own direct experience of the guru-disciple relationship and the awakening of Kuṇḍalinī. There may or may not be a formal initiation from the guru, just as Kuṇḍalinī may act on her own accord. Swami Muktananda writes:

> A true Guru doesn't have to give initiation deliberately. Simply by spending some time with such a Guru or in the environment permeated by his Shakti, one can receive his initiation spontaneously.[112]

Devotees record experiences that match Muktananda's description:

> When Baba [Muktananda] visited Boston in 1974 a friend of mine stayed in the house where he was staying. After Baba and his staff left, my friend continued to live there. Not long after Baba's visit I went to see her. She asked me to write something down for her. I needed a hard surface on which to write, so she handed me a book. As it happened, the book was *American Tour, 1970,* a chronicle of Baba's first visit to the United States. After I wrote the note, I casually glanced through the book. All the while we were sitting in what had been Baba's bedroom, where he had recently been living and chanting and meditating and sleeping. My friend told me to take the book home and to read it. . . .
>
> *American Tour 1970* contains transcripts of various talks delivered by Baba. My reaction to his words was absolutely consistent from start to finish. I kept thinking, "No, this can't be true. No way. I can't prove it, but I know that none of this is true." I didn't want to believe any of it. And yet, I couldn't disprove what Baba was saying, and my own experience didn't contradict it, so his words lingered in my consciousness. In the back of my mind I was aware that a man had said these outlandish things that I couldn't disprove.
>
> Several years later my life had changed drastically. I had given up a good job, my marriage, my home, psychoanalysis, even my ingrained habit of smoking. All of the props of my identity had been stripped away. As I woke up one morning a powerful sensation seized me. My voice said, I'm tired of being negative. I'm tired of always seeing the least of all possible evils. I want something positive in my life. I want to see what is good, and I want to dedicate myself to it. . . .
>
> At that moment an image of Baba came into my mind. It wasn't as though I had kept thinking about him since reading his book; I hadn't. I had just tucked him away into a corner of my mind reserved for unresolved issues. I hadn't really dwelled on his words or contemplated them. When I saw Baba's image, I thought, I remember that man. I read his book. I remembered that Baba had said, "Through meditation, everything is transmitted." I thought, if he has anything he wants to let me know, anything to transmit, let him do it. I decided that I would meditate; that way I could pick up his message if in

fact he was sending one. I could find out whether his face appearing to me meant anything.

So I meditated, by which I mean that I sat up in bed and closed my eyes. Immediately, I saw Baba standing in front of me with a playful smile on his face, one finger pointing upward. He looked right at me and said: "I dare you to come to California and meet me." Startled, I opened my eyes. I was amazed. But I discounted the experience. After all, I hadn't really been meditating. When you meditate you have to sit in a formal posture and light a candle. I thought, Let me see if anything happens when I really meditate.

I went to a corner of my room and lit a candle. I sat on the floor, keeping my spine straight. I knew nothing whatsoever about meditation except what I had read years before in Baba's book. In fact, this was the first time that I had ever sat for meditation. I was thoroughly convinced that nothing was going to happen. Nonetheless, after I closed my eyes I was transported, like a mummy, with a grappling hook, the kind they used to hoist dead meat, lifting me from the ankles. I was one of a long series of dead bodies, all hanging upside down and wrapped in mummy-wrappings, moving as on a conveyor belt. Suddenly, I could see myself hanging in front of Baba. Although my back was turned to him, I could see in my vision exactly what he was doing. Baba's whole being was glistening. His clothes were an iridescent orange. Every time he moved the sunshine flashed off of him as though he were a mirror. His body and face were like nothing I had seen before, like balls of light. He was a perfect form, and perfectly himself.

He was wearing a scabbard slung around his waist, and he reached for it, wrapping his hand around the handle of a dagger which he withdrew. He touched the tip of the dagger to the base of my spine, and then, in one incredibly swift motion, drew it along my spine to the crown of my head. All of the mummy wrappings fell from my body. Then the vision ended.

At the time this experience was just a visual story to me. I knew nothing about the significance of the spine, about the subtle body and the chakras, about the Kuṇḍalinī, about Shaktipat. The scriptural aspects of what I had experienced were unknown to me. I knew nothing, but I knew inside that I had to meet this man. It made no sense at all in the context of my life and went against my instincts as a sober, East Coast professional, to hop on a plane at the urging of some bizarre meditative vision, and fly off to meet some seventy-year-old Indian saint. And yet that is exactly what I did.[113]

The authenticity of such a guru, however, is extremely important. It directly affects the seeker's relationship with the divine Kuṇḍalinī since the guru himself must have perfected his relationship to Kuṇḍalinī. This is likewise made explicit by Swami Muktananda:

Only that Guru can give Shaktipat who has received Shaktipat from his own Guru and whose Kundalini has fully unfolded, establishing him permanently in the place of perfection within, which is the source of the Shakti.[114]

This statement reveals a crucial aspect of Siddha Yoga's understanding of the relationship between grace and self-effort, posed in terms of Kuṇḍalinī's relationship with the guru and disciple. While Kuṇḍalinī is free to give to anyone, she is guided by the guru's grace-bestowing power (*anugraha-śakti*). The ability to accept this grace and develop its potential eventually requires the commitment and discipline of spiritual practices. In other words, self-effort without grace promises only limited results and grace left without self-effort is like a treasure squandered.

Meditation as Grace and Self-Effort

No practice or process is more important in Siddha Yoga than meditation. Viewed in light of shaktipat and the theology of Kuṇḍalinī, meditation is a natural and virtually spontaneous process by which the *sādhaka* is drawn inside toward his or her own deepest nature. The Siddha Yoga gurus suggest that meditation, while best accomplished under certain traditional circumstances of purity and silence, is not a "technique" so much as a spontaneous (*svecchā*) form of yoga in which Kuṇḍalinī Śakti begins her own process of Self-recognition. Meditation may occur spontaneously as well and carry over from different states of ordinary consciousness, that is, from waking to sleeping and into other more mystical states such as the *tandra*. The point is simply that meditation teaches the *sādhaka* meditation because the intelligent, free, and fully conscious Kuṇḍalinī is in her own process of awakening, initiated by the guru's shaktipat and propelled by the repetition of the mantra performed in contemplative awareness. Seen from this vantage point, meditation is more akin to removing the unnecessary and unwanted impediments to Kuṇḍalinī's progress than it is a "method," "practice," or "technique." The Siddha Yoga gurus naturally teach various methods of breath control (*prāṇāyāma*), posture (*āsana*), and instruction (*upadeśa*). These are, however, the aids of meditation and not meditation itself, which properly speaking is a spontaneous, natural, and instinctive movement toward the Self.

Meditation is best understood in the context of *kuṇḍalinīyoga*. Just as *kuṇḍalinīyoga* cannot be reduced to a mechanical process or a technique, meditation is not merely a way to sit quietly with one's eyes closed. Rather, "True meditation is remembering the Self in the midst of all activities."[115] Understood primarily in this light, meditation is not limited to any particular activity at all but rather is a state that should accompany every activity. To effect this state the seeker must calm the mind since "one's meditation has to be so deep that the waves of the mind become still," and yet this too is the work of Kuṇḍalinī awakened by shaktipat.[116] What at first appears to be only a matter of the individual's self-effort is shown instead to be an effect of the guru's divine grace. Thus while the guru commands that meditation requires the disciple to "perform every action with total concentration . . . without laziness . . . and great vigilance," it is also said that "through the grace of the Guru, one easily attains the state of meditation, which is filled with love and the welling up of great bliss."[117] Additionally, proceeding with sadhana is thought of as something of an art that requires the skill of constant reassessment and unfailing vigilance. Swami Chidvilasananda states:

> A true seeker is one who never slackens in his efforts. An effort, a practice, is not a mere exercise. It is the Lord Himself.
>
> When people ask, "Why must we perform the practices, why do *sadhana*?" the only answer is: The practices are the body of God. They are His visible form; they are vibrant with Shakti.
>
> If you hold on to this visible aspect of God, then you're able to receive the invisible aspect; you're able to experience the *atman*, the great Spirit.[118]

Without abandoning the rigorous demands of Patañjali's eight-limbs of yoga (*aṣṭāṅgayoga*), especially the practice of postures (*āsana*) and breathing (*prāṇāyāma*), or the relationship between *haṭhayoga* and Kuṇḍalinī's awakening, Siddha Yoga teaches meditation as both a practice-to-be-learned-and-cultivated and as a spontaneous-natural-condition-of-body-and-mind initiated by shaktipat and sustained and fulfilled by the guru's grace. To treat meditation solely in one fashion or the other would be to misconstrue the subtle relationship between self-effort and grace, both of which are necessary for the meditation that brings Self-realization. Swami Muktananda states clearly the purpose of meditation: "We meditate to attain our own Self, but in reality we attain that which we have already attained."[119] Thus, the demanding discipline and commitment required to advance in meditation reveals only our original nature, the primary indicator of that success being its presence in our ordinary lives, when we are "not" meditating. As Muktananda states, "In fact, meditation is not something separate from our daily existence, but a part of it."[120]

There is no accounting for how and why one will have a certain experience in meditation. Some Siddha Yoga practitioners report dramatic visions or highly altered states of consciousness, whereas others are aware only of subtle sensations of tranquility; and still others go for long periods with what appears to be nothing remarkable at all. Swami Muktananda continually advised steadfastness in practice in order to provide a solid foundation as a strong vehicle for the flow of *śakti*.

The Śaivite scriptures offer varying explanations for the unique path that the awakened Kuṇḍalinī takes in the life of an individual. Whereas some teachings point to the definitive role of Śiva's divine play, or *līlā*, in overseeing one's spiritual awakening, others state that it is the ripeness of one's own karma, that is, deeds and effort, that determines the intensity and direction of the unfolding of Kuṇḍalinī Śakti.[121] Siddha Yoga adopts this latter view, which is corroborated by the experiences of its practitioners.

> Everyone experiences meditation in his own way. It took me five years of seva to steady the mind enough to experience "spontaneous" meditation, but some people immediately enter into that state. My husband's first experience of meditating with Baba Muktananda revealed to him a vision of the chakras in his body, and he saw the golden light of the *sushumna nadi*, the central channel along which the chakras are strung. This light traveled from the base of his spine, through all the chakras, to the top of his head; there it became a crown of flames. He instantly realized he was the Absolute, he was one with God. My husband is a correctional officer who works at night at a local prison. After this first experience, he would sometimes find that during quiet times on his shift he was pulled into meditation and out of his body. He would float up around the ceiling. He could look down and see his body sitting in the chair at his post on death row. He had visions of Bhagawan Nityananda and experienced intense bliss. He saw that the intensity of the environment on death row did not have to have a negative character—it could be intense love. He had always seen the prisoners as human beings, as people worthy of respect, but now he could see that they too were graced. God's love is not confined to the walls of a temple or place of meditation.[122]

Those who honor and engage Kuṇḍalinī powerfully within themselves become immediately rooted in that meditation, which the Siddha Yoga gurus believe to be the direct means of Self-discovery. Meditation, with Kuṇḍalinī personally directing the spiritual unfoldment, inevitably entails a process of purification and a growing relationship with the divine. As previous karmas are rooted out, emotional and physical responses erupt into awareness to be cleansed, and the yogi entrusts the process to the guru's loving direction.

Kuṇḍalinī Creates Spontaneous Movements, or "Kriyās"

The process of spiritual cleansing of previous karmas is as old as yoga itself. In the great expansion of yoga theory that appears in texts centering on Kuṇḍalinī, this process receives a similar elaboration. In the *Śiva Saṃhitā*, for example, we have references to the spontaneous expulsions and expressions of Kuṇḍalinī as she purifies the subtle body, penetrates the knots (*grantha*), and continues her passage towards reunion with Śiva.[123] The effects of these penetrating movements of Kuṇḍalinī within the subtle body appear in the physical body as tremors, reactions, and movements, and in the emotions as a wide variety of feelings. They are, as it were, the outward forms of an inner process of purification and Self-awakening.

Siddha Yoga calls these spontaneous acts of yoga, often involving various postures, breathing, and powerful physical and emotional responses, *kriyās*, or "actions." They are, in fact, Kuṇḍalinī's self-revelations as she purges previous karmas and engages herself in divine play (*līlā*). The scriptural basis of the *kriyā* phenomenon is widespread. The process is like moving from the stillness of the hurricane's eye into its raging winds. Jñāneśvar provides the example closest to the view of Siddha Yoga:

> Then the signs of yogic experience appear outwardly in the body, and inwardly the mind stops functioning. Thought subsides, mental energy dies down, and the body and mind find rest. Hunger is forgotten and sleep disappears. Even the memory of them is lost; no trace is left. The downward moving vital force confined in the body turns back. Becoming compressed, it begins to expand. As it becomes more and more agitated, in the free space above, it rumbles and struggles against the solar plexus. When the struggle ceases, the whole body trembles to its very core. In this way the impurities of childhood are expelled. . . . The seeker should not allow himself to be frightened by these things. It reveals and removes diseases, and it stirs up the elements of earth and water. O Arjuna, the heat produced by the practice of this posture awakens the force called Kuṇḍalinī. . . . It is like a ring of lightning, folds of flaming fire, or a bar of pure gold.[124]

As shaktipat initiates the *kriyās*, Kuṇḍalinī begins her journey. Many *kriyās* are spoken of with great delight, as visions, sounds, and insights erupt spontaneously in meditation. When Kuṇḍalinī's movements create *kriyās* that seem distressing or difficult, Swami Muktananda assures disciples again and again that these reactions are nothing to worry about, since they are God's own ways working within us. The full range of emotions and human potentials for knowledge and experience are considered, linking Kuṇḍalinī to many tangible experiences. In speaking of the more enjoyable experiences, he says:

> Just as one experiences the movements of hatha yoga, other yogas also take place. Love arises, along with the ecstatic feeling of devotion which belongs to bhakti yoga. One attains spontaneous knowledge, as in jnana yoga, and the capacity for detachment in action, which belongs to karma yoga. You may hear inner sounds, perceive divine tastes and smells, or have visions of various lights, gods and goddesses, saints, holy rivers and mountains, and even distant worlds, as in laya yoga. . . . You may begin spontaneously to recite mantras in Sanskrit and other languages, to sing, to roar like a lion, hiss like a snake, chirp like a bird, or make various other sounds. You may be inspired to compose beautiful poetry. You develop a great interest in chanting, in repeating the name of God, and in reading the scriptures.[125]

While clearly everything that occurs may not be to the immediate delight of the yogi, Swami Muktananda believes that all such reactions and spontaneous feelings or insights are ultimately beneficial since they are guided by the guru and are manifestations of goddess Kuṇḍalinī. The following incident connects the guru's initiation with the effects of Kuṇḍalinī in the form of *kriyās*:

> I met Baba as a newspaper reporter, writing what I thought of as "a beginners' guide to meditation." He said a lot of things in the interview that I didn't understand, but one thing that was very clear to me I knew had to be wrong. Baba said that in meditation, people could go into *haṭhayoga* postures spontaneously. I had practiced *haṭhayoga* for a couple of years, and I had meditated, too, so I knew that these were two totally distinct occupations. I liked him, however, and I was inexplicably euphoric after this interview, so I ended up accepting his invitation to visit the house where he was staying in the mornings to meditate before I went to work. I did this the whole week Baba was in Honolulu. Nothing much seemed to happen until the last morning, in the last three minutes of the meditation, when my mind suddenly became quiet. For me this was a miracle. In this novel silence, I found myself looking around at a dark, inner spaciousness that I could actually feel and see. And then, like a curtain, this darkness opened, and behind it was a disk of energy, like the sun . . . except it was cool and inside me, and it radiated love.
>
> I changed most of my weekend plans, got up at two the next morning, and drove to a retreat Baba was giving in the country, getting there just in time for meditation. I slipped into a half-lotus [posture] in the back of the hall and waited for the inner sun to appear again. What happened is that my shoulders started to move—almost a shimmy—just slightly but enough so that I noticed. I stopped them. This was meditation, and I knew that meditation meant sitting still.
>
> Nothing seemed to be happening, and then I remember something Baba had said in the interview: "Whatever comes to you in meditation is a gift." I thought, "Well, maybe I blew it, maybe I shouldn't stop anything from happening. . . ."
>
> The shoulders started to shake again, just a little at first and then stronger and stronger, until my whole upper body was heaving back and forth, fast and strong, like someone had me by the shoulders and was shaking me. . . . The words that went through my mind were, ". . . It's shaking the shit out of me." It was clearly being done to me; it was nothing I would have thought to do to myself, nothing I had ever seen anyone else do.
>
> It went on for a while—I have no idea how long—and then I found myself somewhat collapsed and panting in what I thought was an aftermath. It was just the beginning of something else. My breath which was coming very fast didn't slow down; it got faster . . . and faster . . . and faster. And finally I realized with total astonishment that I was doing *bhastrika prāṇāyāma*, which I had

> been trying to do for the last three or four months in *haṭhayoga* class with no success at all. Now, suddenly here I was—spontaneously, in meditation!—doing this perfect bellows breathing, deep and rapid, and it was going on and on and on.
>
> When I got up from that meditation session, I felt as if pounds of pressure had been removed from my upper back. I had never realized it before, but as I walked out of the meditation hall I could feel that this was where I had been holding tension and that it was gone . . . it had literally been shaken out of me. I felt so light.
>
> And later, my *haṭhayoga* teacher explained that *bhastrika prāṇāyāma* is a great purification for the lungs. I had smoked cigarettes as if they were the key to life until just a few years before this, and for the first few months after I met Baba I did a lot of bhastrika. I always figured it was to finish cleaning the remaining nicotine drek from my lungs.
>
> About a week later I had another *haṭhayoga* meditation, though this one seemed to be more a shift in my awareness than a physical purification. It happened one evening when I was meditating at home. I found myself suddenly moving into the peacock pose, which is an *āsana* I had tried to do for fully six months without success. It's where the entire body weight is held on the forearms, with the hands locked, and the head and trunk and legs arched, like a "C" in the air. Well, I would always get to a certain point in this posture, and I would think, "I can't do it," and I would fall.
>
> This particular night, the energy moved me from seated meditation into the initial phases of the peacock again and again and again. Each time I would think, "I can't do it." Each time I would fall. And then, on maybe the fifth or sixth try, as I was about to pronounce my little statement of inadequacy, instead a voice inside me said, "You're NOT doing it." And I saw that was true—there was no way "I" was doing it. It was being done TO me. With that, I relaxed, and I watched as this exquisite inner energy, which had been moving me all evening long, took me all the way up until I was arched in the air in what I could feel was a perfect peacock . . . it was glorious. It was so exciting. It was like a statement of limitless potential. It was a gift.[126]

It is clear from Swami Muktananda's other writings that he does not mean that this explanation of the divine acting within abdicates the yogi from responsibility for his actions. Rather it provides a context through which to interpret the effects of Kuṇḍalinī and her encompassing role in the individual's complete experience of spiritual discipline.

The notion that a yogi may experience spontaneous movements, including gestures (*mudrā*), the recitation of sacred sounds or mantras, physical reactions, and inspired insights or knowledge is deeply rooted in the Indian tradition. Śaivism has always treated these reactions as more than simply primal emotions or "out-of-the-blue" insights, seeing instead the mysterious play of Kuṇḍalinī as innate and spontaneous. Behind the most basic claim that all oral and written canons are revelations (*śruti*) and recollections (*smṛti*) is a similar claim that the divine inspires and acts through the yogi or the seer.[127] Scriptures validate and provide important measures by which to assess the authenticity of one's reactions, perceptions, and insights but are themselves rooted in precisely the same notion of direct, personal experience (*anubhāva*). The best logic or repeated evidence is merely a confirmation of certain experiences.

Swami Muktananda's descriptions of his own experiences, especially the detailed accounts of his spiritual autobiography, *Play of Consciousness,* are not so much a paradigm that others will necessarily follow as they are a lucid description of one of the potentially infinite manifestations of divine Kuṇḍalinī Śakti. One of Siddha Yoga's distinctive features, indeed one of its practices, is to share one's own yogic experiences which, from the standpoint of the gurus, are similarly part of the process of Kuṇḍalinī's awakening. Rather than prescribe yogic experiences, the Siddha Yoga gurus explain the source, the process, and outcome of these experiences. Every individual's experiences of Kuṇḍalinī, therefore, are bound to differ according to his or her own karma and the intensity to which one devotes oneself to spiritual discipline. Kuṇḍalinī, like shaktipat, may be experienced in different degrees even as she manifests ultimately as the same divinity in all, conferring on everyone the same birthright to divine realization.[128] Indeed, Swami Chidvilasananda shares her own experiences with her devotees to provide inspiration in their sadhana. Recalling the remarkable period—less than one month—in which Swami Muktananda composed *Play of Consciousness,* she tells how the intense concentration of *śakti* affected her as a young devotee:

> Every day, whatever he had written was read aloud by one of his people. It was an incredible period of about twenty-four days. He spent hours and hours writing, and then for at least an hour someone would read out those pages. It was magical. The whole place had the *shakti* of the Blue Pearl [the light of the Ātman], and everywhere you walked, you would bump into Blue Pearls—so many blue dots. Until then, we didn't even know what the Blue Pearl was. And now you would just be walking through the corridor and there they were. You would go to sleep and there they were, not just one, but millions of them, hovering over you.
>
> I remember one night. It was eleven o'clock, and at that time we went to bed by nine. I began to have a vision of millions and millions of scintillating blue dots, and I knew what they were because I had heard about them during the day. Then, suddenly, they turned into a ball of brilliant light. They all became one huge ball of white light.
>
> I opened my eyes, and the whole room was lit up. I thought all the lights were on, because how can something that you see with your eyes closed still be there when you open them? When you have a dream and you open your eyes,

it goes away—it's not real. I was totally perplexed. I went to turn the lights off, but they were already off.

My roommate, who was an older lady, asked me what I was doing.

I said, "I'm turning off the lights."

She said, "The lights are not on!"

I said, "Yes, they are."

"Just go to sleep," she said.

I said, "I can't sleep while the lights are on."

She said, "Just go to sleep."

I tried to go to sleep but the whole room was lit up, and I could still see her sleeping. I said to her, "You know, this is really unusual."

She said, "What is happening?"

I said, "These blue dots have changed into a huge ball of white light and now the whole room is brilliant. I can't close my eyes because it's so bright. It is so bright that I can see you with the lights off."

She said, "You are hallucinating."

I said, "I don't think so."

She said, "You are hallucinating. You've been listening to Baba's book all day long. Just go to sleep." At that point I started having *kriyās,* so she got up and said, "Just cool down and go to sleep."

I said, "This light is making me have *kriyās*!"

This went on for two hours. . . .

The next day my roommate went to Baba. She didn't believe in any kind of experience or any kind of *kriyā,* and she told him, "Baba, you shouldn't have your book read in front of these teenagers because they hallucinate after hearing your experiences."

And Baba was so happy with it. He started laughing and laughing. He told me, "Meditate for three hours instead of one hour, so you will be able to digest what is happening to you. It is the power of the *shakti.*"[129]

The Emergence and Dissolution into the Divine Source

The experience of Kuṇḍalinī's climax of ascent and reunion with Śiva is variously described in traditional sources. In chapter six of *Jñāneśvarī,* her passages through the subtle body are described:

> Listen Arjuna! The element of earth is entirely consumed, and the element of water is dried up. When these two elements have been consumed, Kuṇḍalinī is fully satisfied and, pacified, remains close to the *sushumna.* The venom, which in its satisfaction it sends forth from its mouth, is the nectar which sustains vitality. This fire arises from within, but when it begins to cool down, both internally and externally the limbs regain the strength which they had lost. The *nadis* are closed off, the nine types of *prana* disappear, and the bodily functions cease. The *ida* and *pingala nadis* merge into the *sushumna,*

the three knots are loosened, and the six petals of the *svadhishthana chakra* open out. . . . [130]

Jñāneśvar continues to describe the activity of the subtle body as Kuṇḍalinī unfolds and notes as well—and at length—the effects on the physical body. He observes:

> . . . Beauty incarnates in the form of the body, covered by a veil of skin. . . . The beauty of the limbs looks like natural marble or the sprouting of seed jewels, as if the lovely hues of the evening sky were transferred to the body, or as if an image were fashioned from an inner radiance of the spirit. . . . [131]

The culmination of Kuṇḍalinī's journey is, as we noted, either at the pinnacle of the *sahasrāra* or in heart.[132] The "location" is not a physical matter but a subtle one, which Jñāneśvar reiterates is not limited to space or place and not fully within the grasp of words. Wherever the "location" may be, the final breakthrough brings the physical and subtle bodies into convergence and the dissolution of all "otherness" or alienation from the divine Kuṇḍalinī. It is invariably an experience of bliss that does not cease or oscillate and brings with it certain supra-normal powers. Jñāneśvar writes:

> The yogi can then see beyond all the oceans, hear the thoughts of the heavens, and read the mind of the ant. He rides the horses of the winds and walks on the surface of water, though his feet do not touch it. . . . Grasping the *prana* by the hand, ascending the stairway of the ether, Kuṇḍalinī enters the heart by the steps of the *sushumna nadi.* She is the Mother of the worlds, the glory of the empire of the soul, who gives shelter to the tender sprouts of the seed of the universe, The *lingam* of the formless Absolute, the vessel of Shiva, the Supreme Self, and the true source of *prana.* When the young Kuṇḍalinī enters the heart, the *chakra* there is awakened and sounds are heard. . . . A person must experience this to understand it. How can he imagine it? We cannot know what the source of this sound is. . . . In the innermost cavity of the heart, the divine Kuṇḍalinī lays out before Consciousness the feast of her own luster. . . . Upon entering the cave of the heart, it loses its separateness and is merged into the power dwelling within it. . . . The idea of accepting or rejecting a particular thought is now irrelevant. The subtle elements are clearly destroyed. "One body devours another." This is the secret teaching of the Nātha sect, but now Lord Vishnu has revealed it.[133]

As "one body devours another," the subtle body too dissolves (*laya*) in the culmination of Kuṇḍalinī's fullness. The image is stunning: Kuṇḍalinī's self-dissolution as a "separate energy" is her full "elongation," her awakening. Her awakening brings the yogi to Self-awakening and yet it too is a complete reversion to her original consciously vibrant but potential form: As one body devours another, so Kuṇḍalinī "the serpent-power" "swallows herself," with her own tail in her mouth, again to become one with Śiva, the divine conscious reality. The point is simply that the finale of her journey is ultimately not different from the origin. Kuṇḍalinī's journey "home," to reunite with Śiva, brings her to the same state in which she always existed; she is one with Śiva even as she appears to sleep and then awaken. The yogi is brought to the realization that Kuṇḍalinī's "sleeping" or "awakening" is only a matter of *his* experience of the divine; the divine experiences itself as ever the same throughout the process of unfolding and "re-folding," or "devouring." All the appearances and movements of Kuṇḍalinī as sleeping, waking, or devouring herself are but the yogi's dream. This dream is not unreal but, rather, as real as a dream is real to the one who experiences it as such. From the standpoint of Kuṇḍalinī's highest state, which is the siddha's state, the world is the loving gesture (*mudrā*) of her absolute freedom (*svatantra*) taking form (*rūpa*).

The Vision of the Blue Pearl: Kuṇḍalinī's Essence

Swami Muktananda's detailed experiences in *Play of Consciousness* effectively describe Kuṇḍalinī's passage and her reversion, within him, to her original state of bliss. Her progress is described as the passage of light, visions of planes of existence, and experiences of both the physical and subtle bodies:

> I kept seeing this divine flame, and as I contemplated it, other forms would appear within it, each form within the previous one: first the red aura, then the white flame, then the black light, and finally the Blue Pearl. As I passed through all these stages, moving ahead, my joy and ecstasy kept increasing.[134]

The Blue Pearl, or *nīlabindu*, is a name for the glowing blue light of consciousness that is radiant with the presence of the divine. Seeing it, one experiences the dissolution of all worldly differentiation into a single point. We should recall the discussion of Kuṇḍalinī in Kashmiri Śaivism as well as in Jñāneśvar to appreciate Swami Muktananda's descriptions of the final realization; these are steeped in the mystical language of *kuṇḍalinīyoga*:

> From within, Bhagawan Nityananda seemed to shake me, and then the rays of the red aura lit up the 72 millions *nāḍīs* and all the particles of blood. . . . With the Blue Pearl my meditation immediately became more intense. My gaze turned upward. The Blue *bindu* of my two eyes became so powerful that it drew out the Blue Person hidden within the *brahmarandhra* in the middle of the upper *sahasrāra* and placed Him before me. As I gazed at the tiny Blue Pearl, I saw it expand, spreading its radiance in all directions so that the whole sky and earth were illuminated by it. It was now no longer a Pearl but had become shining, blazing, infinite Light; the Light which the writers of scriptures and those who have realized the Truth have called the divine Light of Chiti. The Light pervaded everywhere in the form of the universe. I saw the earth being born and expanding from the Light of Consciousness, just as one

> can see smoke rising from a fire. I could actually see the world within this conscious Light, and the Light within the world, like threads in a piece of cloth, and cloth in the threads. Just as a seed becomes a tree, with branches, leaves, flowers, and fruit, so within Her own being Chiti becomes animals, birds, germs, insects, gods, demons, men, and women. I could see this radiance of Consciousness, resplendent and utterly beautiful, silently pulsing as supreme ecstasy within me, outside me, above me, below me. . . .
>
> Whenever I see anything, I see first the beautiful subtle rays of Consciousness, and then the thing itself. Wherever my mind happens to turn, I see the world in the midst of this shining mass of Light.[135]

In the final realization the awakening and complete unfolding of Kuṇḍalinī is the direct experience of God, guru, and one's own Self merging into their common essence. Yet, as Muktananda makes clear, the world of forms continues, though now encountered as an entirely different experience. Seeing the divine for oneself, as Jñāneśvar says, brings the ultimate transformation:

> The beauty of this yoga, this kingdom of contentment for which wisdom is essential, must be clearly seen by the mind through the practice of yoga. Seeing it, the seer becomes transformed into it. . . . With joy, they have easily entered the Eternal. Just as salt cannot be separated from water, in the same way, they attain union. Then in the palace of oneness with the Eternal, the world sees the festival of supreme bliss.[136]

The Siddha Yoga gurus see their mission as teaching the *siddhavidyā*, the science of perfection whereby one obtains this vision of the absolute, a vision of the Goddess Kuṇḍalinī. But they have shown as well that every effort to instruct and empower others toward this goal is the result of the guru's grace. In this way, Siddha Yoga is rooted in the exemplary lives of its own gurus and the transformation of their own mortal experience into the divine vision of the immortal Kuṇḍalinī.

Chapter Eight

Siddha Yoga as *Mahāyoga*
Encompassing All Other Yogas

S. P. Sabharathnam

AN OVERVIEW

Swami Muktananda in his spiritual autobiography, *Play of Consciousness,* consistently identified Siddha Yoga with the term *mahāyoga* (lit. "great yoga"). Throughout his writings, he used this term to convey what to him was a central distinguishing feature of the path of the guru's grace:

> Siddha Yoga is called Maha Yoga because it encompasses all other yogas. There are many kinds of yogas: hatha yoga, the practice of physical exercises; *bhakti* yoga, the path of love; *rāja* yoga, which is attained through meditation; mantra yoga; *laya* yoga; *jñāna* yoga and many others. When Kundalini is awakened, all these other yogas take place automatically. You don't have to make any effort to practice them; they come to you on their own.[1]

Siddha Yoga was defined by Swami Muktananda as the spontaneous inner process that begins once Kuṇḍalinī[2] has been awakened by a siddha guru. The awakened Kuṇḍalinī is, therefore, the very basis of Siddha Yoga sadhana (Sanskrit, *sādhana*). According to the Siddha Yoga gurus, the experiences of these seekers with awakened Kuṇḍalinī are subjective but not random or arbitrary. Instead, they coincide with descriptions of the classical yogas found in the tradition of the Śaiva Āgamas (a large set of religious texts honored and held sacred by worshipers of God as Śiva, who is believed to have revealed them for the benefit of the world), as well as in certain texts of the Vaiṣṇava Bhakti movements and in Krama and Śrīvidyā sources.[3] To Swami Muktananda, it was the fact that these spontaneous manifestations coincided with the experiences of the sages enshrined in the scriptures that validated their legitimacy as genuine yogic experiences. His description of Siddha Yoga as a form of "the great yoga" reflects this understanding; in *Play of Consciousness* he specifically equates *mahāyoga* with the spontaneous physical or subtle movements that may arise in a seeker after Kuṇḍalinī awakening. He writes:

> When the disciple is initiated, the Guru's Shakti enters him. As a tree exists in the form of a seed, so the Shakti exists in the form of the Guru, and entering the disciple, it induces many types of yogic movements. As the seeker, remembering his beloved Guru, sits for meditation, identifying himself with the Guru and repeating the Guru's mantra, then the Guru in the form of the mantra becomes active within him. These movements, or *kriyās*, are not meaningless or fruitless. It is the Guru's Shakti which works inside in the form of these kriyas, producing many different contortions of the body, many kinds of yogic postures, *prāṇāyāma*, dances, mantras, and *mudrās*. If anybody were to see these from the outside, they would look very strange and frightening, but the seeker is not afraid. He experiences from these movements a kind of intoxication, an ecstasy, a lightness of the limbs, a sturdiness of the body. Some of the kriyas are a part of *rāja* yoga, some of hatha yoga, some of mantra yoga, and some of *bhakti* yoga, for when the power of the Guru enters the disciple, all these yogas occur spontaneously according to the disciple's needs.
>
> When all four yogas come together to work within the disciple, this is called Siddha Yoga, or Maha Yoga.[4]

As the above statements demonstrate, when Swami Muktananda spoke of Siddha Yoga as a form of *mahāyoga*, he did not mean that it is a synthesis of different yogas, taking a few exercises from *haṭhayoga*, a few teachings from *rājayoga*, and so on. Rather, he used the term *mahāyoga* to indicate the wide range and scope of the spontaneous phenomena that he had observed arising in himself and disciples after the awakening of Kuṇḍalinī. He once said:

> It is only after the awakening that Maha Yoga (Siddha or Kundalini Yoga) begins. This yoga is called Maha Yoga or Supreme Yoga because it embraces all other yogas. It includes Jnana, Bhakti, Hatha and Laya Yoga, all of which come to the seeker automatically.[5]

Further, he said:

> All the classical yogas take place spontaneously in a seeker whose Kundalini is awakened. For this reason, it is said that Siddha Yoga encompasses all other yogas. For example, yogic postures, locks, and breathing techniques may occur spontaneously during meditation. . . . Just as hatha yoga occurs after the Kundalini is awakened, other yogas take place spontaneously as we need them. Love wells up within, as in *bhakti yoga*. Knowledge of the Self begins to arise on its own, as in *jnāna yoga*. We start to work selflessly in the world, as in *karma yoga*. . . . In meditation we may see inner lights or visions or hear inner sounds, as in *laya yoga*. We develop great interest in chanting, repeating the name of God, and reading the scriptures, as in *mantra yoga*. Ultimately, when the Kundalini rises to the topmost spiritual center, the

> *sahasrara,* we attain the *samādhi* state, the state of equality-awareness. This is the manifestation of *rāja yoga,* which culminates in the realization of God within.[6]

In short, *mahāyoga,* in the understanding of the Siddha Yoga gurus, is an umbrella principle, a term that describes what happens when the intelligent energy of Kuṇḍalinī, working within the seeker, spontaneously gives rise to certain forms of experience. Swami Muktananda held the view that only *later on* were these described, analyzed, and given quasi-independence in various texts.[7]

When Muktananda received shaktipat (Sanskrit, *śaktipāta*) from his guru—that is, when he received the initiation that awakens the Kuṇḍalinī—and he began experiencing these yogic movements, he had no background to understand them. As a traditional yogi, accustomed to relying on scriptural sources to authenticate his inner experience, he was greatly relieved when, at a moment of near despair, he discovered a scripture that described the experiences he was having.[8] From then on he sought out texts that could give him the intellectual clarification he needed in order to existentially assimilate his experience. He found them within the body of the Śaiva Āgamas as well as in modern yogic compilations like *Mahāyoga Vijñāna* and *Yoga Vāṇi,* which provided reliable definitions of the process he was experiencing.

Muktananda's dilemma and its resolution set a precedent in Siddha Yoga by which scriptural study became a means of delving more deeply into personal spiritual experience. In short, practitioners of modern-day Siddha Yoga are encouraged to study the scriptures, not in order to take up the practices described therein but because these texts serve as mirrors that reflect and clarify spiritual experience.

This chapter will examine texts of the long-established traditions of the Śaiva Āgamas, Upaniṣads, Purāṇas, and others. By looking at the ways in which these texts define yogic practice, we begin to understand how Muktananda himself used these texts to establish a vocabulary for his own experience and, therefore, for the experience of his devotees. Importantly, Swami Muktananda does not treat these sources as prescriptive. Rather, they provide descriptive analogies and explanatory terminologies to illuminate the experiences of Siddha Yoga seekers, locating experiences within traditional boundaries and giving a framework for understanding.

This chapter will also look at the variety of yogas subsumed under the heading *mahāyoga,* from their most physically oriented, exoteric features to their more subtle, esoteric, and internalized aspects. We will see how Muktananda's descriptions of *mahāyoga* have precedents in the scriptural traditions of India. We will also compare the descriptions in these texts with descriptions of experience by Swami Muktananda, Swami Chidvilasananda, and others, so that we can better discover which features of these traditions are echoed in contemporary Siddha Yoga.

LIBERATION AND YOGA IN THE ĀGAMIC TRADITION

The Āgamic tradition holds that the goal of human life is to be free from the state of being separate (*pṛthagbhāva*) from the divine source and to be permanently established in the state of total identity with Brahman. It describes this condition of oneness as *yogatva*, the state of "blissful union." In the Āgamic tradition, the spiritual disciplines and techniques that lead to that unified state of bliss are collectively known as "yoga." The *Yogaśikhā Upaniṣad* explains yoga as the means for neutralizing the complicated network of dualities that are responsible for the soul's bound state.[9] Yoga is, according to this text, a perfect technique for harmonizing the inner with the outer or the outer with the inner.[10] It is the means, when one is favored by the guru's grace, for harmonizing the limited micro-space of the individual body with the expansive, limitless macro-space of the absolute and, in turn, the micro-time of limitation with the macro-time that transcends temporal boundaries.

The Āgamic sources provide many disciplines such as physical exercise and posture (*āsana*), regulation of the breath (*prāṇāyāma*), centering of the mind (*dhāraṇā*), meditation (*dhyāna*), and so forth, in order to effect perfectly the harmonization of the interior with the exterior.

Some of these systems of yoga have been codified and given different names such as *haṭhayoga, mantrayoga, layayoga, rājayoga*, and so forth. All of these require a certain commitment and effort. The Āgamic text *Śivayogaratnāvalī*, for example, states that each one of these yogic systems has its significant technique that should be meticulously practiced and warns that a practitioner must expect to practice the technique for many years before it bears its fruit. However, numerous other sources such as the *Kūrma Purāṇa* and the *Vāyavīyasaṃhitā* speak specifically of a "supreme" (*para*) and "great" (*mahā*) yoga that includes within itself all of the above mentioned yogas, such as *haṭha, mantra*, and *laya* and state that this system is called *mahāyoga*.[11] More specifically, it is described as the yoga that arises from within as Kuṇḍalinī Śakti is awakened and kindled by the guru.[12]

These texts, like Swami Muktananda's own writings, make it clear that *mahāyoga* is considered the whole (*aṅgi*) and all other yogas such as *haṭhayoga, mantrayoga*, and so on are its parts or components (*aṅga*). As is stated in the *Yogaśikhā Upaniṣad*:

> There are *mantrayoga, layayoga, haṭhayoga* and *rājayoga* in order. When all these are coiled into and supported by one yoga, that is called *mahāyoga*.[13]

The *Yogasaṅgraha*, an important Āgamic text, enumerates five kinds of yoga: *mantrayoga, layayoga, haṭhayoga, rājayoga*, and *śivayoga*, the last one being the "accomplished" (*sādhya*) and the first four being the "means" of accomplishment (*sādhana*). From the descriptions in the text, *śivayoga* appears to be largely identical to the inner process that Swami Muktananda called "Siddha Yoga."

Just as the Āgamas claim that worship of Lord Śiva not only bestows its own intrinsic auspicious benefits but also those of worshiping all other deities,[14] even so the practice of *śivayoga* is said in these texts to grant spontaneously its own benefits as well as the benefits of all other yogas.

Based on the significance of its various aspects, this all-encompassing yoga is denoted by various names, which include but are not limited to: *sahajayoga, kuṇḍalinīmahāyoga, siddhamārga, siddhakṛpā, gurukṛpā, pantharājaḥ, kriyāyoga, pūrṇayoga, paraśivayoga, śāmbhavīyoga, citiyoga*, and *śaktipātayoga.* Swami Muktananda mentioned some of these in *Play of Consciousness*; he may have taken the name "Siddha Yoga" from the term used in the *Yogaśikhā Upaniṣad*, which he quotes in *Play of Consciousness*: "O Brahma, it is very difficult to achieve the state of beatitude through various paths. It can be achieved only through the Siddha Path (*siddhamārgeṇa*), and no other."[15]

In order to get a sense of the wide-ranging aspects of Siddha Yoga as *mahāyoga*, it is essential to understand the features of *haṭhayoga* and other yogas whose progressive features occur spontaneously in Siddha Yoga.

Haṭhayoga

Haṭha generally means "forcible," "voluntary," or "violent." "A practice that forcibly consumes the state of inertness and ignorance, which is the source of all defects and shortcomings, is known as *haṭhayoga*."[16] The term *haṭha* has been explained in two ways. According to the *Niśvāsa Kārikā Āgama, ha*, being the seed-letter exclusively related to Śiva, denotes the supreme and exalted state of *śivatva* (the state of actually experiencing oneself as Śiva, i.e., as all pervasive, omnipotent, formless, totally independent consciousness), and *ṭha* denotes the removal of the coverings or screening that shrouds the essential nature of the Self;[17] as such, *haṭhayoga* constitutes the supreme discipline that effects the manifestation of *śivatva* and the removal of the veiling. The *Yogaśikhā Upaniṣad* states that *ha* denotes sun and *ṭha* denotes moon; therefore, *haṭha* means the union of sun and moon, that is, the union of the complementary subtle breaths of *prāṇa* and *apāna*.[18]

More specifically, the discipline of *haṭhayoga* entails certain practices such as postures (*āsana*), locks (*bandha*), seals (*mudrā*), cleansing processes (*kriyā*),[19] and regulation of the breath (*prāṇāyāma*). In *haṭhayoga*, these various physical and mental exercises are practiced diligently, under the supervision of a master, for the purposes of purifying all the inner channels (*nāḍī*) and bringing about an even flow of *prāṇa*. When the flow of *prāṇa* is even, the mind, the inseparable associate of *prāṇa*, becomes still and at this stage the aspirant experiences equality consciousness and enters into the state of *samādhi*.

In classical *haṭhayoga*, an important purpose of doing these practices is to arouse Kuṇḍalinī Śakti.[20] However, in Siddha Yoga, the practitioner finds that the processes of *haṭhayoga* often occur spontaneously after Kuṇḍalinī has been awakened.

In the *Yogatattva Upaniṣad*, the progressive steps of *haṭhayoga* are presented in two separate groupings. The first grouping consists of the eight steps from *yama* to *samādhi* that are common to any yogic course:[21] *yama, niyama, āsana, prāṇāyāma, pratyāhāra, dhāraṇā, dhyāna,* and *samādhi*. The second set of steps of *haṭhayoga* includes the following progression: *mahāmudrā, mahābandha, mahāvedha, khecarī, jālandhara, uḍḍīyāna, mūlabandha, dīrghā, praṇava-saṃdhana, siddhānta-śravaṇa, vajrolī, amaroḷī* and *sahajolī*.[22] Here, each step in the progression is characterized by a specific yogic state, rather than a practice. It is the practices in the first list, however, that allow for the experiences of the second.

All yogic practices are centered on three principles—purification, concentration, and unification. In all its practices, *haṭhayoga* keeps these principles in view.

*Āsana*s are physical postures practiced to strengthen the body, purify the nerves, and develop one-pointedness of mind. To say that *āsana* is the habituating of the body to certain attitudes of immobility[23] is to reduce the applicational and pervasive nature of *āsana*. *Āsana* is more than habituation; it is tuning the body to the innate rhythmic movement of the inner śakti. In addition, the effects of *āsana* are not limited to the physical body, for they reach the subtle bodies as well. Nor could mental immobility be an effect of *āsana*: *Āsana*s help to arouse Kuṇḍalinī and to center the mind, and this state of one-pointedness of mind is by no means a state of mental immobility.

The *Gheraṇḍa Saṃhitā* prescribes eighty-four *āsana*s,[24] of which the following are considered to be most important: *padmāsana, svastikāsana, ardhacandrāsana, gomukhāsana, vīrāsana, yogāsana, paryaṅkāsana, prasāritāsana, sukhāsana,* and *bhadrāsana*. The Śaiva Āgamas provide lengthy directions for assuming these postures,[25] which are useful not only for physical well-being but also for meditation and *samādhi*. The *Yogasaṅgraha*, for example, states that *ardhacandrāsana* is helpful for meditative posture as it is specially beneficial for those with stiff knees.[26] Various Āgamas state that the *yogamudrāsana* not only tones up the visceral organs and the nervous system, reduces constipation, increases vitality, and helps the arousal of Kuṇḍalinī, it also furthers the attitude of surrender, the most important aspect of yogic practice. Likewise, they speak of *paścimottānāsana* (also known as *ugrāsana*) as capable of arousing Kuṇḍalinī and making the aspirant aware of subtle sounds.

Bandha, which literally means "lock," denotes various positions that are practiced along with *prāṇāyāma* breathing exercises to unite the two types of subtle breaths in the body, the *prāṇa* and the *apāna*. This is one of the traditional ways of awakening Kuṇḍalinī. Even though there are many *bandhas*, three are considered to be of vital importance—*mūla*, *uḍḍīyāna*, and *jālandhara*. *Mudrās* are *haṭhayoga* positions involving various physical organs (for instance, the tongue or the fingers); some *mudrās* help concentration, while others are said to remove diseases and disorders of the body. Some of the important *mudrās* explained in the discipline of *haṭhayoga* are *mahāmudrā*, *mahābandhamudrā*, *mahāvedhamudrā*, *nabhomudrā*, *khecarīmudrā*, *bhujaṅgiṇīmudrā*, *ṣaṇmukhīmudrā*, *śāmbhavīmudrā*, and *kākīmudrā*.

The role of *haṭhayoga* in Siddha Yoga is threefold. First, the basic attitude toward bodily discipline enfolded in the *haṭhayoga* texts is echoed in many statements of swamis Muktananda and Chidvilasananda on the respect, care, and discipline of the body, which they often describe in classical *haṭhayogic* language as a living temple of God. Secondly, since 1979, *haṭhayoga* has been an important adjunctive practice of the movement, and even before that, Swami Muktananda often taught *haṭhayoga* to selected disciples. *Haṭhayoga* classes are held daily at many Siddha Yoga ashrams. Gurumayi Chidvilasananda has personally taught *āsanas* and *prāṇāyāma* at Intensives, the programs where shaktipat is given in Siddha Yoga. Thirdly, as we said earlier, *haṭhayoga* is seen to take place as a spontaneous expression of the awakened Kuṇḍalinī—arising *without effort*, in the case of some aspirants, after shaktipat. The spontaneous performance of *haṭhayoga* postures, *bandhas*, and *mudrās* is called *kriyā* in the language of contemporary Siddha Yoga—a term that comes from such classical *haṭhayoga* texts as the *Yogaśikhā Upaniṣad*, as well as certain modern texts that state that when the awakened Kuṇḍalinī Śakti encounters the *bandhas*, there may occur gross (physical) or subtle (mental and emotional) purificatory movements.[27] The *Kulārṇava Tantra* also mentions the appearance of purificatory movements after shaktipat.[28] These movements, according to Swami Muktananda, purify the body and nervous system in order to enable the aspirant to endure the energy of higher states of consciousness.

The unique feature of Siddha Yoga, then, is the spontaneous occurrence of *kriyās*, which tune the physical body to bring it into harmony with the inner *śakti*. These movements are not practiced voluntarily, as are other yogic practices and movements. Says Swami Muktananda, "When the Kundalini Shakti is awakened, many different movements, or *kriyās*, take place in the gross body. These kriyas are not meaningless; they destroy sicknesses and purify the *nādīs*. . . . Usually, many different kriyas take place, continuing over a long period."[29] *Kriyās* are understood to make the body pure, well-proportioned, clean, and beautiful, giving it luster and radiance. They serve to remove the various imbalances that have settled in the body. During the occurrence of *kriyās*, the aspirant "may hop like a frog, spin, twist, run in circles, roll on the ground, slap his face, roll his head round and round, adopt different yogic postures. . . . He may make different sounds; he may roar like a lion or make other animal noises. . . . All these kriyas occur spontaneously during meditation."[30]

Swami Muktananda describes numerous instances in which he experienced spontaneous *haṭhayoga* postures. "Sometimes, my neck would roll my head around so vigorously that it would bend right below my shoulders so that I could see my back," Muktananda writes in *Play of Consciousness*. ". . . Sometimes as my neck rotated, my chin would get fixed in the jugular notch below the throat. This is a divine hatha yogic contraction or lock, which is called the *jālandhara bandha*. As this bandha took place there was another movement below—my anus would be automatically drawn in and then released."[31]

Swami Muktananda further describes in *Play of Consciousness* how *mūlabandha, uḍḍīyānabandha,* and *jālandharabandha* would often take place spontaneously when he sat in the lotus posture, and other Siddha Yoga students have reported the same phenomenon. In some texts, an *āsana* involving the three *bandhas—mūla, uḍḍīyāna,* and *jālandhara*—is called *vajrāsana*. In his commentary on the *Bhagavadgītā*, the Maharashtrian saint Jñāneśvar effectively explains how *vajrāsana* awakens the Kuṇḍalinī force:

> Then the signs of yogic experience appear outwardly in the body and inwardly the mind stops functioning. Thought subsides, mental energy dies down, and the body and mind find rest. Hunger is forgotten and sleep disappears. Even the memory of them is lost; no trace is left. The downward moving vital force confined in the body turns back. Becoming compressed, it begins to expand. As it becomes more and more agitated in the free space above, it rumbles and struggles against the solar plexus.
>
> When the struggle ceases, the whole body trembles in its very core. In this way the impurities of childhood are expelled. Instead of turning downward, it moves in the interior of the body and expels the bodily secretions. It releases the ocean of the bodily fluids, reduces the fat, and even draws the marrow out of the bones. It clears out arteries and loosens the limbs. The seeker should not allow himself to be frightened by these things. It reveals and removes diseases, and it stirs up elements of earth and water. The heat produced by the practice of this posture [*vajrāsana*] awakens the force called Kundalini.[32]

Masters of yogic science have stated that control over the subtle body is possible through mastering the *vajrolīmudrā* and *khecarīmudrā*,[33] both of which have been spontaneously experienced by practitioners of Siddha

Yoga. An aspirant on the path of yoga could make a nectarean fluid drop down from the *sahasrāra* to the nasal roof through the practice of *khecarīmudrā*, and by raising his tongue into the palatal cavity above the soft palate, he could taste that nectar. The fluid so tasted rejuvenates his whole body and vitalizes all the glands. He is established in youthfulness and he can digest even heavy poisons without being affected by them.[34]

In *Play of Consciousness*, Swami Muktananda describes at length his own experience of many of these *āsanas*, *mudrās*, and *bandhas*:

> . . . [T]he three *bandhas* came automatically. My heel locked itself against my anus, forcing it to contract. By this kriya, which is called *mūla* bandha, the *apāna* is drawn upward. It equalizes the upward-flowing movement of the *prāna* with the downward-flowing movement of apana, and through this destroys old age and sickness. . . .
>
> Simultaneously with this, my breath was expelled and my stomach drawn in, so that a small pit was formed. It felt as if air was being drawn up from the region below my navel. This kriya is called the *uddiyāna* bandha and is given much importance in the hatha yogic texts. It is even said in these texts that one can conquer death by it. It purifies the prana and the *nādīs*. When the nadis are purified, the gastric fire begins to blaze, and when the prana is purified, the mind stops wandering and becomes stable. After the uddiyana bandha, my chin was pressed down hard on my throat. This kriya is called the *jālandhara* bandha. It too is very important. Normally, the drops of nectar that trickle down from the *sahasrāra* are consumed by the fire of the sun in the navel *chakra*, but this bandha seals off its passage so that the fire can no longer burn the nectar to ashes. With its help, the *yogi's* mind soon becomes unconscious, which means that it attains stillness. . . . Sometimes I would put my hands on the ground, palms upward, put my head on them, and raise both legs straight up. I would remain steady for some time in this position. . . . Sometimes from this position my palms would be placed against the ground and I would push myself up on my arms, my head hanging down between them. This is known as the vajroli mudra, which gives sure control over the semen and prevents it from flowing downward by developing the power to retain it.[35]

Still later, he began to experience *khecarīmudrā*, where his tongue was drawn up into the pharynx, stretched far beyond its normal length; an inner voice told him that this was for the purpose of opening up the passageway to the *sahasrāra*, the spiritual center in the crown of the head.

Haṭhayoga discipline does not confine itself to the prescription of *āsanas*, *mudrās*, *bandhas*, and *prāṇāyāma* alone. It meticulously scans the entire spectrum of human life and speaks about other disciplines also. Thus the *Haṭhayogapradīpikā* states that the yogi should abandon feelings of fear, wrath, and idleness, and he should refrain from eating either too much or too little. It further instructs that excessive food, forced endeavors, frivolous talk, inadequate knowledge about the vows and restraints, association with unruly crowds, and unsteadiness—all these six spoil yogic practice. The aspirant's yogic practice is enriched and augmented by diligent effort, cleverness, courage, knowledge of the *tattvas*, certitude, and avoidance of unnecessary company.[36]

The Siddha Yoga gurus also teach the importance of maintaining discipline in eating, in speech, and in thought. One of Gurumayi Chidvilasananda's books, *The Yoga of Discipline*, contains many insights in common with *haṭhayoga* texts. For instance, she writes, "Most physical action occurs because of the influence of ego. The yogic scriptures say the reason your physical body cannot sit still is because of *ahaṃkāra*, or ego. As long as the ego is in control, the physical body cannot become still, no matter how much you try. Therefore, the sage talks about becoming detached from physical action. He doesn't tell you to put a stop to action, but rather to develop a new relationship with action, one that gives the great Self the upper hand."[37] Moreover, Siddha Yoga students have stated that after shaktipat, a natural attraction to discipline often arises spontaneously, as a kind of internal *kriyā*; one man said that after receiving shaktipat he found himself waking up at an hour when he would normally have gone to bed; while others have cited dramatic reorientation of their interests so that instead of finding pleasure in parties and restaurants, they begin to enjoy silence and yogic practice.

Even though the eight limbs of yoga are common to the various yogic courses, *haṭhayoga* texts explicate them elaborately, in minute detail. For example, they discuss four *avasthās*, or sequential stages: *ārambha, ghaṭa, paricaya*, and *niṣpatti*; three kinds of *prāṇāyāma*: *ujjāyī, sītkārī*, and *śītalī*; four kinds of *kumbhaka: sūrya, ujjāyī, śītalī*, and *bhastra*; and three kinds of focus: *antar, madhya*, and *bahiḥ*. *Haṭhayoga* texts also explain the subtleties of the wondrous threefold structure of the *suṣumṇānāḍī*, the "central channel": *vajra*, the outermost; *citriṇī*, the middle; and *viraja*, the innermost.[38] Also described is the system of *nāḍīs*, the "psychic channels" in the human body, to which Swami Muktananda often referred. In *Play of Consciousness*, he describes seeing these subtle channels in meditation:

> Sometimes [in meditation] I would see a beautiful, slender, silver-colored tube, standing like a pillar from the *mūlādhāra* to the throat. . . . Sometimes I would see a god in each chakra, and feel a slight pain there. Sometimes I would look right into my body at the nervous, circulatory, excretory, and digestive systems. The same multicolored light spread through all the nadis and illuminated them, so I could see them.[39]

Haṭhayoga texts like *Haṭhayogapradīpikā* describe the importance of purifying the *nāḍīs*, which are said to be channels for the flow of *prāṇa* in the subtle body; according to Muktananda, the main work of the awakened Kuṇḍalinī and the *kriyās* that ensue is to remove the blocks that keep *prāṇa* from flowing through the *nāḍīs*.

The *Yogasaṅgraha*, an Āgamic text, says *haṭhayoga* is the first step to enter into the higher yogas variously named in the texts as *rājayoga* and *śivayoga*.[40] The *Haṭhayogapradīpikā* states that it generally takes years from the commencement of the practice under the guidance of a guru to lead the Kuṇḍalinī to the *sahasrāra*, and that the appropriate *āsanas*, *bandhas*, and so forth should be chosen by the guru according to the physical features of the disciple.[41]

In the spontaneous *haṭhayoga* of Siddha Yoga, where the Kuṇḍalinī is identified with the guru who has aroused it, these *kriyās* are said to be guided by the intelligence of the awakened Kuṇḍalinī. In common with certain texts of the Śrīvidyā and Krama traditions, Swami Muktananda often stated that the movements performed spontaneously by the awakened energy are always appropriate and timely, whereas those that an aspirant performs on his own may not be what he needs.

Mantrayoga

Just as classical *haṭhayoga* requires practices for arousing the Kuṇḍalinī, even so in classical *mantrayoga* there is an emphasis on the practice of mantra repetition (*japa*) for leading the inner power, Kuṇḍalinī, to the highest and transcendental plane. Yoga practiced with the repetition of mantra is called *mantrayoga*, a system that also features *āsana*, *prāṇāyāma*, and *dhyāna*.

Mantrayoga is classically identified with *kuṇḍalinīyoga*; since Kuṇḍalinī is described in the Śaiva and Śākta texts as Śabda Brahman, the "supreme Self in the form of sound," all mantras are said to be her manifestations. Thus it is explained in the Āgamic texts that all mantras are charged with consciousness. Since Kuṇḍalinī and mantra are said to share the same essence, the *mantrayoga* texts claim that she is easily aroused by the repetition of mantra[42]—although it is said that only that disciple who is properly initiated into this yoga by the guru can gain success in making his inner *śakti* reach the crown-space (*sahasrāra*).[43] Initiation is said to activate the latent power in the mantras, which the *Tantrasadbhāva* says are "as ineffective as autumn [that is, rainless] clouds" without having been enlivened by the *śakti*.[44] In the Āgamic tradition, mantras that disciples receive from the guru are known as *śakti-samputita mantras*, literally, "mantras charged with the power of pure consciousness."

In Siddha Yoga, an empowered mantra is described as *caitanya*, "filled with awakened consciousness," and it is given to disciples as a major vehicle for initiation. When received from the guru, the initiation mantra—in

Siddha Yoga usually the *pañcākṣara* mantra *Oṃ Namaḥ Śivāya*—is considered to contain the guru's grace in its fullness.

A mantra is a sacred or mystic formula comprised of divinely charged syllables. Some mantras are the name of a deity; others are simply the arrangement of specific syllables that may or may not be associated with seed-letters (*bījākṣara*). There are various traditional etymologies for the word *mantra,* such as that given in the *Kulārṇava Tantra*: the syllable *man* is said to derive from the word *manana,* meaning "meditation" or "holding in the mind," while the syllable *tra* comes from *trayate,* meaning "it protects" or "it saves." The *Kulārṇava Tantra* says, "By meditation (*manana*) on the luminous deity who is of the form of Truth, it saves (*trayate*) from all fear, therefore it is called mantra."[45]

The Āgamic texts distinguish two types of mantras. One is known as *mūlamantra* (*mūla* meaning the "root" or "basic source"); this is directly related to the practice of yoga and the achievement of spiritual goals. The other is known as *sādhyamantra* or *kāmyamantra,* that is, "effective in gaining for the seeker worldly benefits and enjoyments." Although considered useful to ward off ritual pollution and evil forces, a *sādhyamantra* is not effective in yogic practice.

A *mūlamantra,* when associated with a deity, is said to be the form or body of that deity. The scriptures maintain that such a mantra is the manifested Śabda Brahman and that all of the letters of the Sanskrit alphabet, from *a* to *kṣa,* are charged with *kriyāśakti,* "active force," and conscious power. Each Sanskrit letter is said to be invested with a particular sound, color, effect, and animating power. Moreover, each letter of a mantra is said to constitute a part of the deity whose form is that mantra. In *mantrayoga,* the seeker identifies his body both externally and internally with the mantra in the same way that it constitutes the form of the deity. Thus the gross and subtle bodies are identified with the Self and the deity, through the vehicle of the mantra. Since "the guru dwells in the mantras in a living form,"[46] identity between the guru and the aspirant is also accomplished in *mantrayoga.* The *Sarvajñānottara Āgama* states that a soul who becomes totally and impeccably identified with the mantra is known as *mantrātma,* and is considered to have reached a state close to Lord Śiva.[47] Thus the practice of *mantrayoga* is meant to establish the seeker in the awareness of the unity of the seeker, mantra, deity, and the guru.[48] The continued practice of *mantrayoga* allows the seeker to merge the gross and subtle universes into pure consciousness within himself, thereby inducing the blissful state of *śivatva* or *śivo'ham bhāvana.*

The practice of *mantrayoga* enables the seeker to comprehend the power of letters, which permeates both the macrocosmic and microcosmic spheres; in Muktananda's words, "To understand the power of letters is to attain everything."

Swami Muktananda, whose technical contributions to the science of yoga are based essentially on his own extraordinary inner experiences, speaks of the importance of *mantrayoga,* which he considered the chief means to enter the thought-free state:

> There are two kinds of meditation: one is with *japa* and the other is without *japa. Japa* is mantra repetition. Mantra has great power and is very necessary. If you meditate with a mantra, you would become absorbed very quickly. However, in pure meditation there is absolutely no thought or object in the mind, not even the mantra. But you reach that state only through the mantra. As you repeat a mantra more and more, the mantra begins to disappear, and you get into a state in which you are aware of neither yourself nor God.[49]

The following mantras that appear in the Āgamas also appear in Siddha Yoga:

Oṃ Namaḥ Śivāya
the *mūlamantra* of the chosen deity (which in Siddha Yoga is *Oṃ Namaḥ Śivāya*)
prasādamantra (The mantra given by the guru; in Siddha Yoga this too is usually *Oṃ Namaḥ Śivāya.*)
praṇavamantra (*Oṃ*)
Śivo'ham
Haṃsa/So'ham

Oṃ in Siddha Yoga is rarely repeated silently on its own but is often chanted on special occasions as a way of becoming attuned to the resonant harmony that pervades body, speech, and mind.

It is *Oṃ Namaḥ Śivāya,* the *pañcākṣara* or "five-syllable" mantra, embellished with the syllable *Oṃ,* that is most central to the sadhana of siddha yogis. *Oṃ Namaḥ Śivāya* is the lineage mantra, the mantra of initiation, and the focal point of *japa* and meditation for most Siddha Yoga meditators. *Oṃ Namaḥ Śivāya* is chanted, repeated out loud and silently, and counted on *japamālas,* "hand rosaries," of Siddha Yoga devotees. Gurumayi Chidvilasananda has given initiation to more than three thousand people simultaneously with this mantra. It has been inscribed over the seat of the Siddha Yoga gurus.

The *pañcākṣara* evokes divine consciousness as one's own consciousness; Siddha Yoga gurus instruct their disciples to repeat it with the awareness of their own identity with the mantra. *Haṃsa* or *So 'ham* (the two are considered identical; the first meaning "I am That" or "I am He," the second meaning "That am I" or "He is I") also is presented as the natural mantra of the breath, which assists a meditator in discovering the Self by utilizing the sound of the breath to draw him into awareness of his identity with the absolute. According to the *Yogaśikhā Upaniṣad*, in a statement echoed by Swami Muktananda in his book *I Am That*:

> *Prana* is breathed out through *ha* and *prana* is breathed in through *sa*. This happens in all living beings, and this *Haṃsa* mantra is being repeated by all of them involuntarily. But when this mantra is repeated in reverse order as *So'ham*, after learning the exact process from the Guru, one experiences this process as Mantra Yoga, which is performed in relationship with the central *nadi*, the *susumna*.[50]

The *Makuṭa Āgama* describes the significance given to the *Haṃsa* mantra in the tradition:

> Lord Śiva presents himself in the heart-space essentially in the form of *Haṃsa*. *Haṃsa* is *Śakti*. *Haṃsa* is the essence of the *mahāvākyas* of the Vedas. *Haṃsa* manifests itself in the heart-space of all the deities and of all the beings. Nothing exists as different from *Haṃsa*. Nowhere is it seen that all the *tattvas* from *pṛthivī* to *Śiva*, all letters from *a* to *kṣa*, and all mantras designed by the *mātṛkās* could be different and distinct from *Haṃsa*.[51]

Swami Muktananda, in *I Am That*, claims a similar importance for this mantra. Basing his discussion on verse 24 of the *Vijñānabhairava*,[52] he writes:

> By understanding the mystery of *Hamsa*, you come to know the Self. . . . To understand these two syllables, *ham* and *sa*, as they really are is liberation. *Ham*, the sound that comes in with the inhalation, is Shiva, the pure I-consciousness, the inner Self. *Sa*, which goes out with the exhalation is Shakti, God's creative energy. . . . If you perceive this with true understanding, you realize the truth immediately.[53]

Only with the grace of the guru, Muktananda goes on to say, does *Haṃsa* reveal its mystery. For this reason, instruction in *Haṃsa* has traditionally been given at certain Siddha Yoga Intensives, where shaktipat is also bestowed, so that the power of shaktipat can make it possible for seekers to experience the subtle essence of the mantra.

Experientially in the field of yoga, there is no difference between the *Haṃsa* mantra and *So'ham* or *Śivo'ham* (I am Śiva). In *Play of Consciousness*, we read that this was the instruction that Bhagawan Nityananda gave to Swami Muktananda at the time of his initiation:

> "All mantras are one. . . . All are *Om*. *Om Namah Shivaya* should be *Shivo'ham*. *Shiva, Shiva* should be *Shivo'ham*. It should be repeated inside. Inside is better than outside. . . ."
>
> Gurudev had sat me next to him, and by giving me the highly charged mantra *Om Namah Shivāya*, by showing me the meaning of *Om*, and by uttering *Shivo'ham*, he had brought me to an awareness of oneness with Shiva. He had

> shown me the external practice of *Om Namah Shivāya,* the great five-letter mantra of salvation, and then spoken the word *Shivo'ham,* which is the form of the inner "I am Shiva" within the heart. In this way he gave me the undying message of Shiva, the immortal Lord. And by saying "All is *Om*" he gave me the insight that all is one Self.[54]

Although each of these mantras has its own stratagem and tradition, all mantras in Siddha Yoga are used in the same way. All aim at the recognition of the Self. Mantra in Siddha Yoga is seen both as the subtle *form* of the absolute and the primary means of *recognizing* the absolute. Muktananda writes in his book *Where Are You Going?*:

> As the influence of God's name penetrates the mind, the mind itself becomes the Name [*Kena Upaniṣad,* 1.59]; in other words, the mind becomes divine. Repetition of the Name of God causes a kind of earthquake in our inner consciousness. . . . At every moment, what we think is what we become. If the face of anger arises in the mind and we identify ourselves with it, we become filled with anger. In the same way, if we continually repeat the mantra with great love and interest, we will become absorbed in God. By its very nature the mantra has the ability to transform our awareness of ourselves as individuals into an awareness of ourselves as God.[55]

At the same time, since mantra in some way forms the key element in the transmission of *śakti,* it is the basis of the siddha guru's act of initiation. We have already seen how the lineage mantra was given to Swami Muktananda at his own initiation; filled with the guru's own *caitanya-śakti,* "awakened divine power," and the *śakti* of the lineage, the initiation mantra is considered by the siddha yogi as an indispensable tool in his practice.

According to the Āgamas, *mantrayoga* becomes fully effective only when the seeker becomes capable of experiencing the mantra in its most subtle state—the state characterized as *parā* and identified with the silence of absolute consciousness. To reach this state, the mantra repeater must transcend the earlier three levels of speech described in the Tantras and known as *vaikharī,* "articulated or gross speech"; *madhyamā,* "subtle sound" or "thought"; and *paśyantī,* "pre-articulate thought." *Parā,* "supreme speech" is the speech that has dissolved into its wordless source; it is equated with Kuṇḍalinī herself, and with the deepest states of meditation. The mantra scriptures describe how, as a seeker repeats his mantra, it gradually begins to resonate at deeper and deeper levels until finally sound merges into silence and the practitioner reaches the exalted state of absorption (*laya*) into the unified awareness.[56] In Siddha Yoga, this has been known to occur spontaneously through the power of the awakened *śakti,* which when activated can bring a mantra repeater to a state of complete absorption in an astonishingly brief time.

Layayoga

The term *layayoga* is used in the Āgamas to refer to the highest state of absorption into the absolute, as well as to describe certain techniques for achieving that absorption.[57] According to the *Yogaśikhā Upaniṣad,* on the attainment of union between the seeker's conscious Self (Ātman) and the absolute, *layayoga* dawns, the mind becomes absorbed in that state of unity, and the *prāṇa* acquires stability. "Laya," in short, is another name for the state of *samādhi.* According to the "map" of the higher stages of consciousness provided by the *Haṭhayogapradīpikā,* as Kuṇḍalinī rises up the *suṣumṇānāḍī* to the crown chakra, the yogi passes through various subtle stages known as *unmanī, manonmanī,* and so on.[58] *Laya* is identified with the stage known as the *manonmanī* state, literally, the state "beyond the mind." In Jñāneśvar's words, "This is the highest principle, without beginning and beyond measure, the beauty of the state beyond the mind, and the dawning of the experience of the soul's oneness with God."[59]

The *Yogaśikhā Upaniṣad* here describes *laya* as an inner state; *laya* is also a practice. Generally, a *layayoga* practitioner fosters the absorption of the mind into the Self by listening to the inner unstruck sounds.

By the evidence of *Play of Consciousness,* Swami Muktananda appears to have encountered the experience of *layayoga* at an advanced point in his sadhana. The *Yogaśikhā Upaniṣad* also attests that *layayoga* belongs to a subtle state of sadhana. That is because the yogi must be sufficiently indrawn to have contacted the subtle state in which he can hear the unstruck sounds (*anāhata*).

If, in an ordinary sense, sound is to be heard, at least two things must be struck together. The divine sounds, however, emanate within spontaneously and unceasingly, day in and day out, without anything being struck. Through the practice of yoga, the ears can be made receptive to the divine sounds, which are considered to be the absolute in the form of sound. The aspirant does this by keeping himself in the continued contemplation of the inner sounds (*nādānusandhāna*).

When the seeker, through meditation, enters that subtle state from which the unstruck sound originates, he begins to experience a series of melodies resembling the sounds of chiming bells, a flute, a drum, and so forth. The glowing effect of *layayoga* is the inner experience of the music of *anāhata-nāda,* the "sound of the unstruck (sound)." "Superior to this *nāda,* there is no mantra, and superior to the realized Self, which experiences this *nāda,* there is no deity"—thus the greatness of the experience of *nāda* is explained in the *Yogaśikhā Upaniṣad.*[60]

Both the Āgamic and Upaniṣadic texts enumerate ten unstruck and subtle sounds of Kuṇḍalinī. They are discussed in the *Haṃsa Upaniṣad* and the *Sarvajñānottara Āgama;* the latter text lists them in the following order:

a bell, a conch, the melodious *vīṇā*, cymbals, the flute, the *mṛdang*, the kettledrum, and thunder. This tallies with the experience of Swami Muktananda.[61] The blissful and beatific effects of hearing such divine and unstruck sounds are elucidated in great length in the *Haṃsa Upaniṣad*,[62] which instructs that the seeker should transcend the first nine sounds and listen to the tenth, the *meghanāda*, the sound of the thunder. Muktananda states: "When a yogi one-pointedly focuses his mind on the unstruck sound which resonates continuously, the true nature of supreme space, which is consciousness and luminosity, is revealed to him."[63]

It is said that the ultimate unstruck sound of thunder enables the seeker to realize the truth that *Oṃ* is self-existent (*svataḥsiddha*) and self-begotten (*svayambhū*). Swami Muktananda explains:

> After the nada of the kettledrum, I heard the final nada, which is called *meghanāda*, the sound of thunder. It is a most divine nada, the king of nada, the celestial cow which fulfills the wishes of yogis. When it is heard, the upper space trembles. For a few days the sadhaka is not himself because of this continuous thundering, for this is the nada that leads to *samādhi*, the goal of yoga. From within this nada, the yogi hears the chanting of *Om*. Then he learns that *Om* is self-begotten. It is not created by sages like the various mantras of different sects. No abbot composed it. It is self-existent. It arises by itself out of the upper spaces of the sahasrara.[64]

Continued and concentrated contemplation on the hearing of inner divine sounds is the most important phase of *layayoga*. Swami Muktananda writes of one of his experiences of *nāda*:

> My dear Siddha Students, when I heard the sounds of the flute in the sahasrara, I lost consciousness even of Tandraloka. I did not know where the inner Witness had gone. I had no idea where I was going or what was happening as I listened to the sweet music of the flute. . . . Sometimes I danced, sometimes I swayed, and sometimes I was drunk with love and lost in the divine nada. . . . I could observe the place from where sparks flew out of the divine light activated by the vibrations of the nada. All my senses were drawn towards it; even my tongue hurried towards it.[65]

Layayoga proceeds in two more phases, the phase of *ākāśa*, "space," and the phase of *tattvas*. In the space phase, *layayoga* enables the seeker to reach the final and absolute space known as *cidākāśa*. There are five spaces; the first four are to be "absorbed" and then transcended, and the fifth one is the final state and place of absorption. These spaces are: *paramākāśa, piṇḍākāśa, bhūtākāśa, mahākāśa*, and *cidākāśa*. The first space is absorbed in the second, the second space is absorbed in the third, and so on, until finally *cidākāśa* remains unabsorbed and undissolved.[66]

In the *tattvas* phase, all of the *tattvas* (principles of creation) beginning with *pṛthivī* (the earth) are transcended, and finally the seeker is established in the *bindu*, or *śivatattva* (the Śiva principle).[67]

Layayoga does not stop with the hearing of unstruck sounds. It causes the aspirant to perceive the visions of various lights, gods and goddesses, saints and siddhas, and holy rivers and mountains, and to experience divine tastes and smells.[68] Swami Muktananda and many subsequent siddha students have described such visions, fragrances and tastes, especially the vision of the tiny blue light known as the *nīlabindu*, or "Blue Pearl," which Muktananda (along with Jñāneśvar and Tukārām Mahārāj) described as the form of God within the human body.

Swami Muktananda describes his first vision of the blue light in this way:

> . . . [A] tiny, extremely brilliant dot shot out of my eyes with the speed of lightning and then went back in again. This is a secret, mysterious, and marvelous process. In an instant the tiny blue dot illuminated everything in every direction. . . . When I saw the Blue Pearl, the condition of my body and mind, and my way of understanding, began to change. I felt more and more delight in myself, and was filled with pure and noble feelings.[69]

This passage is notable in its description of the overall *effect* of seeing these visions through the agency of Kuṇḍalinī. As Muktananda repeatedly points out, authentic spiritual experiences and visions are not simply passing experiences, but help to effect positive changes in the character of the meditator. Although Siddha Yoga gurus caution seekers against regarding such visions as the *goal* of yoga, they value the *kriyās* and visions of *mahāyoga* both as signs of spiritual progress on the path of the awakened Kuṇḍalinī and for their purifying effect on the body, mind, and spirit.

Swami Muktananda also compares his experience of the blue light to the description given in the writings of Jñāneśvar:

> O seekers after the knowledge of perfection, the very eye of your eye, where the void comes to an end, the Blue Pearl, pure, sparkling, radiant, that which opens the center of repose when it arises, is the great place of the conscious Self. Look, my brother, this is the hidden secret of this experience. . . . Jnanadev says, "I saw this through the grace of my Sadguru Nivrittinath."[70]

Swami Muktananda, in his description in *Play of Consciousness* of the final stages of his spiritual journey, reveals what is in essence an experience of the goal of *layayoga*:

> As I gazed at the tiny Blue Pearl, I saw it expand, spreading its radiance in all directions so that the whole sky and earth were illuminated by it. It was now no longer a Pearl but had become shining, blazing, infinite Light; the Light which the writers of the scriptures and those who have realized the Truth have

> called the divine Light of Chiti. The Light pervaded everywhere in the form of the universe. I saw the earth being born and expanding from the Light of Consciousness, just as one can see smoke rising from a fire. I could actually see the world within this conscious Light and the Light within the world, like threads in a piece of cloth, and cloth in the threads. . . . In this condition the phenomenal world vanished and I saw only pure radiance. Just as one can see the infinite rays of the sun shimmering in all directions, so the blue light was sending out countless rays of divine radiance all about it. . . .
>
> [T]hen, in the midst of the spreading blue rays, . . . I saw my adored, my deity, Shri Nityananda. I looked again, and, instead, Lord Parashiva with his trident was standing there. . . . He was made solely of blue light. . . . As I watched, He changed, as Nityananda had changed, and now I could see Muktananda as I had seen him once before when I had had the vision of my own form. He too was within the blue light of Consciousness. . . . Then there was Shiva again, and after Shiva, Nityananda within the Blue. . . . How beautiful it was! Nityananda was standing in the midst of the shimmering radiance of pure Consciousness and then, as ice melts into water, as camphor evaporates into air, he merged into it. There was now just a mass of shining radiant Light with no name or form. Then all the rays bursting forth from the blue light contracted and returned into the Blue Pearl. . . . The Pearl went to the place from where it had come, merging into the sahasrara. Merging into the sahasrara, Muktananda lost his consciousness, memory, distinctions of inner and outer, and the awareness of himself. Here I have not revealed a supreme secret because Gurudev does not command me to do so, God does not wish it, and the Siddhas do not instruct me to write it.[71]

This experience of Swami Muktananda demonstrates many of the features of *laya,* absorption, including its final termination, beyond light and sound, in the totality of the absolute.

Rājayoga

There is a tradition that the name "*rājayoga*" derives from the fact that this path is considered the "royal" (*rāja*) or "sovereign" way to union. The root *rāj-* also connotes the idea of shining forth, or splendor. It is said that this discipline "shines forth" as the unfailing process leading to the ultimate realization of God within oneself, realization of oneness with Brahman.

Most of the scriptures associated with *rājayoga* expound upon the nature of its eight limbs (*aṅga*), which have caused this path to be called *aṣṭāṅgayoga,* "eight-limbed yoga." These are:

1) *yama*	practice of five moral restraints: nonviolence, abstention from untruth, abstention from stealing, noncovetousness, and abstention from sexual indulgence

2) *niyama*	practice of five observances: purity, contentment, austerity, study of scriptures, and surrender
3) *āsana*	postures
4) *prāṇāyāma*	regulation and restraint of breath
5) *pratyāhāra*	withdrawal of the mind from sense objects
6) *dhāraṇā*	concentration, fixing the mind on an object or place of contemplation
7) *dhyāna*	meditation
8) *samādhi*	complete absorption or identification with the object of meditation; meditative union with the absolute

It has already been stated that most systems of yoga make use of the eight limbs. However, the discipline of *rājayoga* pays particular attention to the last three aspects—*dhāraṇā, dhyāna* and *samādhi*. Indeed, some Āgamic scriptures and Upaniṣads speak of only six steps, as an advanced phase of *rājayoga*. For example, the *Raurava Āgama, Mataṅga Pārameśvara Āgama*, and the *Amṛtanāda Upaniṣad* enumerate the following six steps: *pratyāhāra, prāṇāyāma, tarka* (logic), *dhāraṇā, dhyāna*, and *samādhi*.[72]

According to the *Kiraṇa Āgama* and the *Dhyānabindu Upaniṣad*, the six steps are: *āsana, prāṇāyāma, pratyāhāra, dhāraṇā, dhyāna* and *samādhi*.[73]

While the *Maṇḍalabrāhmaṇa Upaniṣad* speaks of the eight subtle steps of yoga, the *Tejobindu Upaniṣad* speaks of fifteen.[74] Such variations and modifications have been fashioned only for the sake of aspirants at different levels of advancement or with different spiritual requirements. These variations, however, do not indicate anything contradictory in the processes related to *rājayoga*.

At the heart of *rājayoga* is the state of *samādhi*, or the state that transcends the mental functions, as is explained in the *Haṭhayogapradīpikā*:

> *Rājayoga, samādhi, unmanī, manonmanī, amaratva, śūnyāśūnya, parampada, amanaska, advaita, nirālamba, nirañjana, jīvanmukti, sahajāvasthā, turīya*—all mean one and the same state, that is the cessation of both mental functioning and action.[75]

Though as we have said before, the eight limbs from *yama* to *samādhi* are related not only to *rājayoga* but also to other yogas, there is a difference in the emphasis and in the state of *samādhi* as attained through each discipline:

Āsana and *prāṇāyāma* are the chief elements in *haṭhayoga*, and the *samādhi* state attained through *haṭhayoga* is characterized as *mahābodha*, the "attainment of profound knowledge."

Japa is the chief element in *mantrayoga*, and the *samādhi* state attained through *mantrayoga* is characterized as *mahābhāva*, "attainment of total identity or oneness."

Dhāraṇā is the chief element in *layayoga*, and the *samādhi* state attained through *layayoga* is known as *mahālaya*, "ultimate absorption."

Dhyāna is the chief element in *rājayoga*, and the *samādhi* state attained through *rājayoga* is known as *kaivalya*, "the state of single-pointedness."[76]

Each of the four yogas employs some methods of the other three, for which reason it is not necessary that all the four yogas be practiced step-by-step by a particular aspirant.

Other Yogas

In addition to the yogic systems presented above, it should be noted that other systems exist as well, whose complexity precludes their discussion here. Briefly, these include the following:

Bhaktiyoga is the "yoga of devotion," a path to union with the divine based on the continuous offering of love to God and the constant remembrance of the Lord expressed through song, dance, hymns, and so forth. The awakening of spontaneous devotional feelings, expressed as tears or as upsurges of love, bliss, and compassion, is widely documented in Siddha Yoga. Siddha Yoga gurus also emphasize many external aspects of traditional *bhaktiyoga*, such as chanting the divine names, ritual worship (*pūjā*), and other devotional practices, emphasizing all the while the goal of internal unity with the guru and the Lord. The divine names contain the power of the devotee's own higher Self; in rituals of worship, the devotee, objects of worship, and the Lord are all to be experienced as one reality.

Jñānayoga is the "yoga of knowledge," a spiritual path based on continuous contemplation, philosophical speculation, and self-inquiry. In *Play of Consciousness*, Swami Muktananda has documented his spontaneous experience of a process that he calls "the dawn of knowledge," in which the knowledge of the absolute came of itself. As he writes:

> In my meditation, the knowledge came by itself of that supreme Truth that is realized by the Vedantins through the Witness-consciousness, when the mind is in absolute stillness. I understood that Truth in which the most subtle intellect loses itself while probing it. . . . While man is awake, That which perceives the whole external world as *idam*, "this," as object, and yet remains aloof from

> and transcends the waking state; That which, when man is asleep and dreaming, does not sleep but remains awake, and with neither the mind nor the senses perceives the whole dream universe as "this,"; and when man is in the black depths of dreamless sleep where nothing is seen, That which remains as the illuminator and perceives this state of nothingness—I began to understand That as the unchanging Self, the supreme goal of meditation. . . . Under the dominion of ignorance man says, "I ate, I drank, I took, I gave," but the One who experiences all these things is the unmoving Witness, the inner Self—and that is God.[77]

Karmayoga is the "yoga of action," a spiritual path in which the aspirant performs actions without attachment to the fruits thereof, dedicating them to the Lord.[78] Siddha yogis practice *gurusevā*, "selfless service to the Master," in ashrams and centers as a way of learning nonattached action, and this is conceived as training in *karmayoga*.

The experiences expressed by Swami Muktananda in his *Play of Consciousness* and other works attest to the legitimacy of his claim that Siddha Yoga contains within itself all of the other yogas, and that it includes all other yogic disciplines and techniques.

Describing the effects that manifest in a seeker whose Kuṇḍalinī has been awakened through shaktipat, Muktananda writes:

> Love arises, along with the ecstatic feeling of devotion which belongs to bhakti yoga. One attains spontaneous knowledge, as in jnana yoga, and the capacity for detachment in action, which belongs to karma yoga. You may hear inner sounds, perceive divine tastes and smells, or have visions of various lights, gods and goddesses, saints, holy rivers and mountains, . . . [and] spontaneously [begin] to recite mantras in Sanskrit and other languages: to sing, to roar like a lion, hiss like a snake, chirp like a bird, or make various other sounds. You may be inspired to compose beautiful poetry. You develop a great interest in chanting, in repeating the name of God, and in reading the scriptures. These manifestations correspond to mantra yoga.
>
> When the awakened Kundalini rises . . . She pierces the six chakras . . . and finally brings about the *samādhi* state. . . . [T]his manifestation of the Kundalinī corresponds to raja yoga and culminates in the ultimate realization of God within oneself. In this way, Siddha Yoga is very easy, very natural. There are many paths through which you attain the final goal with great effort and difficulty, but in Siddha Yoga you attain it very naturally and spontaneously.[79]

Another yogi describes how at times a seeker "performs many exercises not found in any treatise on yoga; they are sometimes very intricate and difficult muscular exercises quite hard to be practiced otherwise."[80]

CONCLUSIONS

We have listed here only a few of the experiences—described by Swami Muktananda and others—that demonstrate how the elements of *mantra-yoga, layayoga, rājayoga,* and other yogic systems take place in Siddha Yoga spontaneously, and also how they are practiced purposefully by Siddha Yoga seekers to support the work of the unfolding Kuṇḍalinī. In reading the Āgamas in the light of Swami Muktananda's experiences, we have also seen how they contain descriptions of classical yogas and their effects that, as in the case of Muktananda, occurred spontaneously through the workings of Kuṇḍalinī. In this sense, we can say that the Āgamas seem to come alive through the descriptions in Swami Muktananda's and Swami Chidvilasananda's books. However, in looking at the relationship between the texts and the spontaneous expressions of the awakened Kuṇḍalinī described in Siddha Yoga, it is important to take note of several points.

First, when Swami Muktananda spoke of Siddha Yoga as *mahāyoga,* he was not claiming that Siddha Yoga is a syncretic phenomenon bringing together a number of different yogic traditions and techniques, nor was he attempting to associate himself with a specific tradition or set of doctrines (*siddhānta*). On the contrary, he turned to the Āgamas in order to find authoritative support for the experiences that arose from the awakened Kuṇḍalinī. Muktananda's basic grounding was always in the *experience* rather than in the texts. Starting from an experiential situation—his own powerful Kuṇḍalinī-based visions and yogic *kriyās*—he then turned to the Āgamas as a means of proof, or a means of knowing (*pramāṇa*). In the tradition, Āgama (meaning in this context the words of the scriptures believed to be divinely revealed) is considered primary among the means of knowing. So for Swami Muktananda, the fact that his experiences corresponded to the authoritative texts grounded them and gave them a certain authenticity in his own mind. Āgama is actually used by Swami Muktananda to provide the context of understanding rather than as a starting point for practice. Of course, the understanding was of crucial importance; in his autobiography, *Play of Consciousness,* he writes of how at a moment of despair, when he feared that his experiences were the result of a mental disturbance as a result of his sins, he found a book that explained them and located their source in Āgamic tradition. Finding the scriptural "proof" of the authenticity of the experiences changed his despair to relief. Nonetheless, the experience and its source in the awakened Kuṇḍalinī always came first, and then the authentication and understanding of it.

This represents, of course, a highly innovative use of Āgamic material; most teachers who point to these texts do so in the service of a particular doctrine. Swami Muktananda had no interest in promoting *mahāyoga* as a particular tradition or speaking as a representative of a presumed

"Mahāyoga Siddhānta." Moreover, at no point did he attempt to imitate the *prescriptions* in the texts, unlike those who locate themselves in a tradition such as *haṭhayoga*, who might take a text such as the *Haṭhayogapradīpikā* and attempt to reproduce the postures described in the text.

At all times, he was primarily interested in the experiential core about which these texts offer understanding, and Swami Chidvilasananda continues today to stress the primacy of experiential apprehension of truth. Although Muktananda expressed amazement and renewed gratitude to his guru when he discovered that in these scriptures he had been given a central key that allowed him to understand the mystical reality he was experiencing, he was never bound by the descriptions in the texts, since his eye was always on the mystical reality that lay within the descriptions. As he has often stated, the descriptions of the different yogas we have discussed in these pages only scratched the surface of the vast realm of experience that he perceived through the intelligent Kuṇḍalinī, whose expression these yogas were seen to be.

When we discuss Swami Muktananda's use of the term *mahāyoga*, then, we must remember that he used it neither to indicate a Siddhānta among other Siddhāntas, nor to indicate a mere agglomeration of different yogas such as *haṭhayoga* or *layayoga*. To Muktananda, the term *mahāyoga* described the effects of the living intelligent reality of Kuṇḍalinī, whom he saw expressing herself through experiences that could be described in terms of all these branches of yoga. *Mahāyoga*, then, was not only *mahā*, "great," because it was all-inclusive, it was "great" because it was the yoga generated and inspired by the Kuṇḍalinī energy—the energy of God. In this sense, *mahāyoga* for Muktananda is primarily a theological category. It is an expression of the sublime reality—the awakened Kuṇḍalinī—that stands behind all yogic traditions and gives them life. Just as the law of gravity simply describes a reality that we have all experienced and know to be true, the Āgamic descriptions of *mahāyoga* simply point to experiences that Swami Muktananda knew were real. We might compare his use of these texts to an experienced explorer, who stands in the country he knows well and uses a map to help his students understand the territory.

So in his use of the term *mahāyoga* and his reference to the scriptures of the Āgama, Muktananda was acting as siddhas have done throughout history. Standing in the experience of the Self, ultimately free of all traditions, the siddha nonetheless enlivens the tradition by relating it to living experience. Swami Muktananda did not simply seek to authenticate his experience by finding its confirmation in the texts of the Āgamas. He also validated the Āgamas themselves by proving that the experiences contained within them did not belong to an unrepeatable esoteric past, but are real and valid for today—through the workings of the marvelous Kuṇḍalinī.

Chapter Nine

THE ASHRAM
Life in the Abode of a Siddha

William K. Mahony

A PLACE OF PARADOX

Upon entering the grounds at Gurudev Siddha Peeth in Ganeshpuri, India, or at Shree Muktananda Ashram in South Fallsburg, New York, a visitor may well be struck by various contrasts between these rural Siddha Yoga retreat centers and their surroundings. The journey by road from Bombay to Ganeshpuri takes a traveler first through noisy, urban congestion and then through increasingly sparsely populated regions, dotted here and there by small villages, enclaves of huts formed from bamboo, mud, and straw. During the rainy season, the narrow road is covered by deep puddles and even at times may be washed out by the monsoon torrents, while during the hot summer months, the land here—in the words of an English professor from New York who first visited Gurudev Siddha Peeth in 1977—"sprawls in the dry heat as if it had been punched by a fist."[1] Entering the ashram's gates, one feels as if one has, in a sense, entered another world. Having made the long, dusty trip to the ashram, another writer noted that "as you enter the grounds from the suffocating Indian plain, you literally feel the temperature drop several degrees; it is as if someone turned on an air conditioner."[2] One steps first onto the cool marble floor of an outer courtyard dappled by the shade of a *parijāta* tree. The openness of the courtyard encourages cooling breezes that dance with wind chimes, the gentle, mellifluous tones of which envelop the quiet with a subtle richness. Farther inside the ashram grounds, one is embraced by waves of fragrance from innumerable flowering shrubs and trees; palm trees lean into open spaces as if they were sailing with a gentle wind. In the words of an early visitor to Gurudev Siddha Peeth, "A stroll around the Ashram was a breath-taking experience. I felt the Ashram garden was a veritable rendezvous of gods on earth!"[3]

To get to Shree Muktananda Ashram, the main Siddha Yoga ashram in the West, a visitor drives through quiet backcountry in the Catskill Moun-

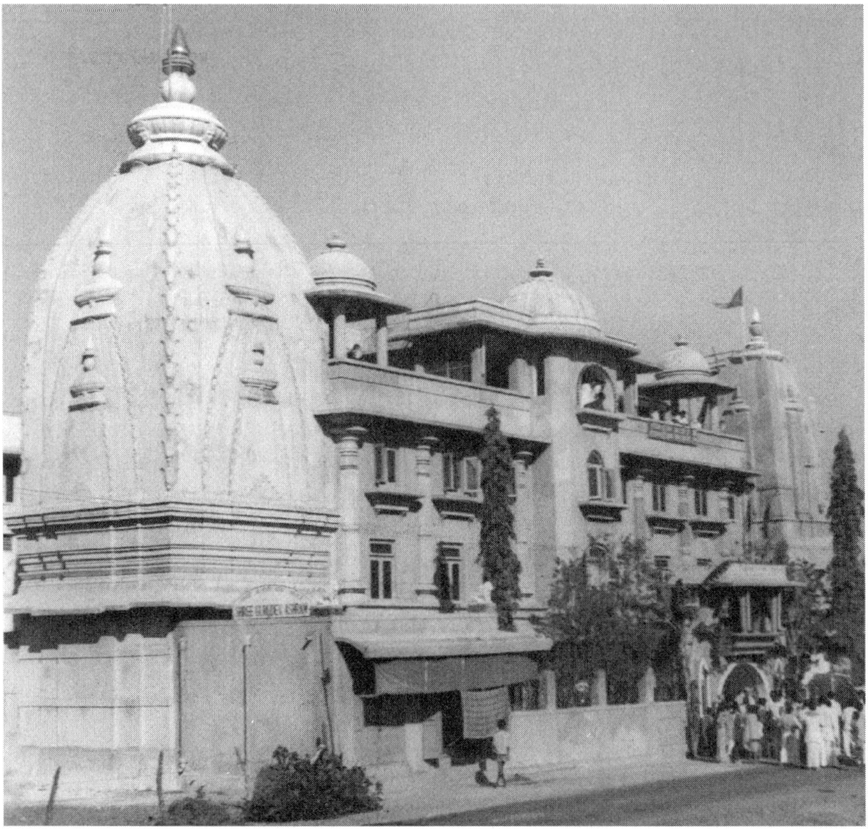

Figure 26. Gurudev Siddha Peeth, the Siddha Yoga ashram in Ganeshpuri, India, in the late 1970s

tains of upstate New York, where legend has Rip van Winkle walking the wooded hills. Passing through the small and now economically depressed town of South Fallsburg, the traveler turns a corner in the road and suddenly sees a large well-maintained white building, the architecture of which marks its earlier function as a vacation hotel. This is the central facility of the Shree Muktananda Ashram. Turning onto the grounds, the visitor notes that the entire area is immaculately kept. A stream tumbles playfully over small waterfalls and across the grounds as it makes its way past the white building and a striking glass-walled pavilion, which seems to float above the countryside. Swans and ducks glide silently across a large, landscaped reservoir known as Lake Nityananda. Walking across the grounds, one sees statues, or *mūrtis*, of various deities from the religious traditions of India: the celestial musicians Jaya and Vijaya guard the entrance from the street and the elephant-faced god, Gaṇeśa, is enthroned on the front lawn. It is a surprising sight: Hindu *mūrtis* in rural Sullivan County, New York.

Entering the grounds of both of these ashrams, the visitor is thus presented with a set of disjunctions or reversals of sorts. As we will see shortly, life within these ashrams also involves a set of paradoxes, emerging out of the fact that these are at once places of great calm and repose and also of remarkable and generative intensity. They are places where the serious student might experience a pervasive outer peace and yet also an inward fire, kindled and inflamed by his or her own intense spiritual discipline.

Perhaps these oppositions and paradoxes revolving around the unexpected eruption of the extraordinary into the ordinary are parallel in a sense to the structure of the contrast between what some theorists of religion call "the sacred" and "the profane."[4] A word or two regarding these terms, as they are used here, is in order. In this context, the two words do not describe particular places but rather characterize different ways of experiencing the world. So, for instance, "the profane" is not to be understood as referring to what is vulgar or contemptuous, but rather to a mode of existence that is marked by an unrelenting mundanity in which nothing seems to have any more true and lasting value than anything else. To live one's life from the perspective of the profane is to live a vague and undefined life in which nothing "stands out," as it were, and thus a life that leads one to feel unremarkable, unimportant and, finally, meaningless. "The sacred," on the other hand, refers to a mode of being or a way of seeing the world in which one experiences life as a revelation, or possible revelation, of transcendent truths and powers. To live a life from the perspective of the sacred is to experience the inherent dignity and meaning and value of life as a whole and, thus, of each and every person's life in particular, including one's own.

As modes of being, "the sacred" and "the profane" are thus in a structural opposition. One twentieth-century theorist of religious experience has argued that "the first possible definition of the sacred is that it is the opposite of the profane" and that a person "becomes aware of the sacred because it manifests itself, shows itself, as something wholly different from the profane."[5]

Perhaps the striking and unexpected presence of Gurudev Siddha Peeth and Shree Muktananda Ashram within their physical settings is structurally identical to the emergence, the surging forth, of the holy into the otherwise homogenous background of the mundane and ordinary.[6] If so, then perhaps these anomalous and paradoxical external places both represent and foster the inner transformations a seeker undergoes as he or she moves from a perception of life as untextured, diluted, frustrating, or even meaningless to a new or rejuvenated experience of what both Swami Muktananda and Swami Chidvilasananda hold to be the profound and pervasive sanctity of being.

Discussion in this chapter will involve further exploration into some of these apparent oppositions. We will see that the ashram is, indeed, a place both of peace and of fervent intensity and that this paradox is suggested by the very meaning of the word *ashram* (Sanskrit, *āśrama*). We will also note the way in which, throughout the history of Indian spirituality, life in an ashram ideally has stood in an opposition of sorts to life beyond its boundaries, and will point out some of the reasons this is believed necessarily to be so. Yet we will also see how both Swami Muktananda and Swami Chidvilasananda teach that the holiness-of-being devotees often report experiencing while in the ashram can, and should, be brought to mundane life outside of the ashram as well. The ashram, therefore, represents not a dam that separates the sacred from the profane but a bridge that links the two. Said differently, the ashram points out the existential distance between the sacred and the profane, and then dissolves that very difference. From the perspective of Siddha Yoga, all such distinctions evaporate when one comes to regard everything in the world as a stage for the play of divinity itself.

EMBODIMENT OF DIVINE ŚAKTI

Gurudev Siddha Peeth and Shree Muktananda Ashram are remarkably quiet and, in some ways, quite calm and still. Yet they also fairly shimmer with an invigorating intensity and energy. This conjunction of peacefulness and energetic fervor reflects a fundamental and even vital paradox that pervades everything that happens at the two ashrams. The professor of English described the silent intensity he experienced on his arrival at Gurudev Siddha Peeth:

> [Swami Muktananda] was just started on his morning walk when I came into the courtyard. He chuckled when he saw me, and took my hand. The court-

> yard felt like an aquarium, with flecks of sunlight cascading between the trees. It was so intensely quiet that for a moment I felt a pressure in my ears, as if I were indeed under water. The casualness of our meeting was like a meeting between old friends. Yet I couldn't help remembering [the] first time [I had met Muktananda in New York], two and a half years before, when my mind had opened into a shower of warm fiery pieces. That feeling of inner spaciousness had never entirely left me. It became palpable now in the brightness and calm of the courtyard.[7]

Yet quiet calmness was not the only quality this visitor encountered. Moments later, following Swami Muktananda on his walk, he noted, "Baba moved briskly through the ashram garden, striking off sparks of instruction to the manager, seemingly at every step, about irrigation channels, new tree plantings, what to feed the peacocks and deer."[8]

It is this very energy that built and continues to build the physical facilities and develop the grounds of the ashram, for it erects buildings, plants trees, and waters roses—and, clearly, part of the ashram's air of peacefulness derives from the beauty of the setting. At Gurudev Siddha Peeth, Muktananda and his followers have planted and cared for "beautiful and rare trees, such as the white coral, white swallow wort, white beech, white oleander, and chitrika," as well as "eleven varieties of champa, twelve varieties of chameli, twenty-two kinds of jasmine, forty kinds of roses, twenty kinds of Nilgiri eucalyptus, Japanese bamboos, Zanzibar plantains, eighteen varieties of coconuts, one hundred and eight varieties of mangoes":[9] the list of beautiful and visually refreshing plants goes on and on.

Swami Muktananda considered the beauty of an ashram and its grounds to be a matter of great consequence to the fulfillment of its spiritual purpose. This is true of an urban as well as a rural ashram. Shortly after arriving in the United States in December 1978, Muktananda inspected the facilities at the ashram he had founded in Oakland, California. "The ashram is beautiful," he said, and then he explained the importance of this beauty: "A place where you meditate, a place where you worship God, a place where you want to attain peace should be pure. It should look beautiful. The moment you sit there, your heart should open. The beauty, the purity, the clarity, the stillness of that place should be very pleasing to the heart."[10]

Yet the stillness and calm purity, the shimmering beauty of these ashrams comes only with immense effort. One of Swami Muktananda's earliest devotees, Venkappanna Shriyan, has described the care that Muktananda gave to the development of gardens around the three rooms given to him in 1954 by his own guru, Bhagawan Nityananda. (These three rooms came to serve as the nucleus of what was to become Gurudev Siddha Peeth.) Swami Muktananda and the half-dozen devotees who visited and lived with him in those early days would arise at two in the morning and carry water from the well in tin cans to water the garden. Muktananda had planted the bushes and trees himself, Venkappanna said, selecting the plants after great deliberation:

> He chose plants that had some medicinal qualities: mango trees, banana trees, coconut trees, and fragrant flowers like night-blooming jasmine and roses. These plants would create an atmosphere people could feel. The minute people walked into the ashram, they would calm down. Rather than focusing on their own problems, they would put their attention on the fragrance and the beauty of the plants. To this day, when you walk into the ashram garden, no matter what situation you come from, you forget all that; you just experience the joy of being in a beautiful place.[11]

The flowers and trees, the earth in which they are planted, indeed, every particle of dust in the ashram were for Swami Muktananda, and continue to be for Swami Chidvilasananda, a conduit for and revelation of the universal divine power that they feel sustains and gives life to the world as a whole. According to these teachers, this power is none other than universal consciousness itself, which, following Tantric Hindu spiritual tradition in general, they call "Chiti" (Sanskrit, *citi*: "consciousness") or "Shakti" (Sanskrit, *śakti*: "power"). While necessarily present everywhere, that universal power is said to be focused in various places, which then intensify and expand the possibility that people may experience it, like a lens both focuses and disperses light. Swami Muktananda used to say that this universal power, *citi-śakti*, is identical to the principal cause and propelling force behind a seeker's own inner transformation. He taught:

> Abodes of Siddhas, sacred places, and centers of pilgrimage are permeated by a divine power generated therein. It is the living, moving, talking power of God which, though established in its own glory, manifests itself by assuming a physical form for the sake of devotees. Those who live there permanently, stay for short periods, or even remember it with love, devotion, and reverence, are enveloped by this force. It enters all seekers, devotees, and visitors and works within, bestowing the highest reward on them.[12]

For Muktananda, the ashram was thus a physical embodiment of the power of God. Following Hindu tradition in general and Kashmiri Śaiva tradition in particular, Muktananda called *citi-śakti* the "divine force of universal Consciousness"; and, consistent with classical Hindu Tantric thought, he taught that *citi-śakti* is identical to "Kundalini Shakti" (Sanskrit, *kuṇḍalinī-śakti*), that is, to the power of transformation through which a human being moves closer to God. "Here [at the ashram] the radiant, blazing Chiti Shakti carries on her[13] sublime work," Muktananda wrote. "The ashram may appear to be an ordinary place to our physical eyes, but its every leaf, flower, fruit, tree, and creeper is pervaded by Kundalini Shakti."[14]

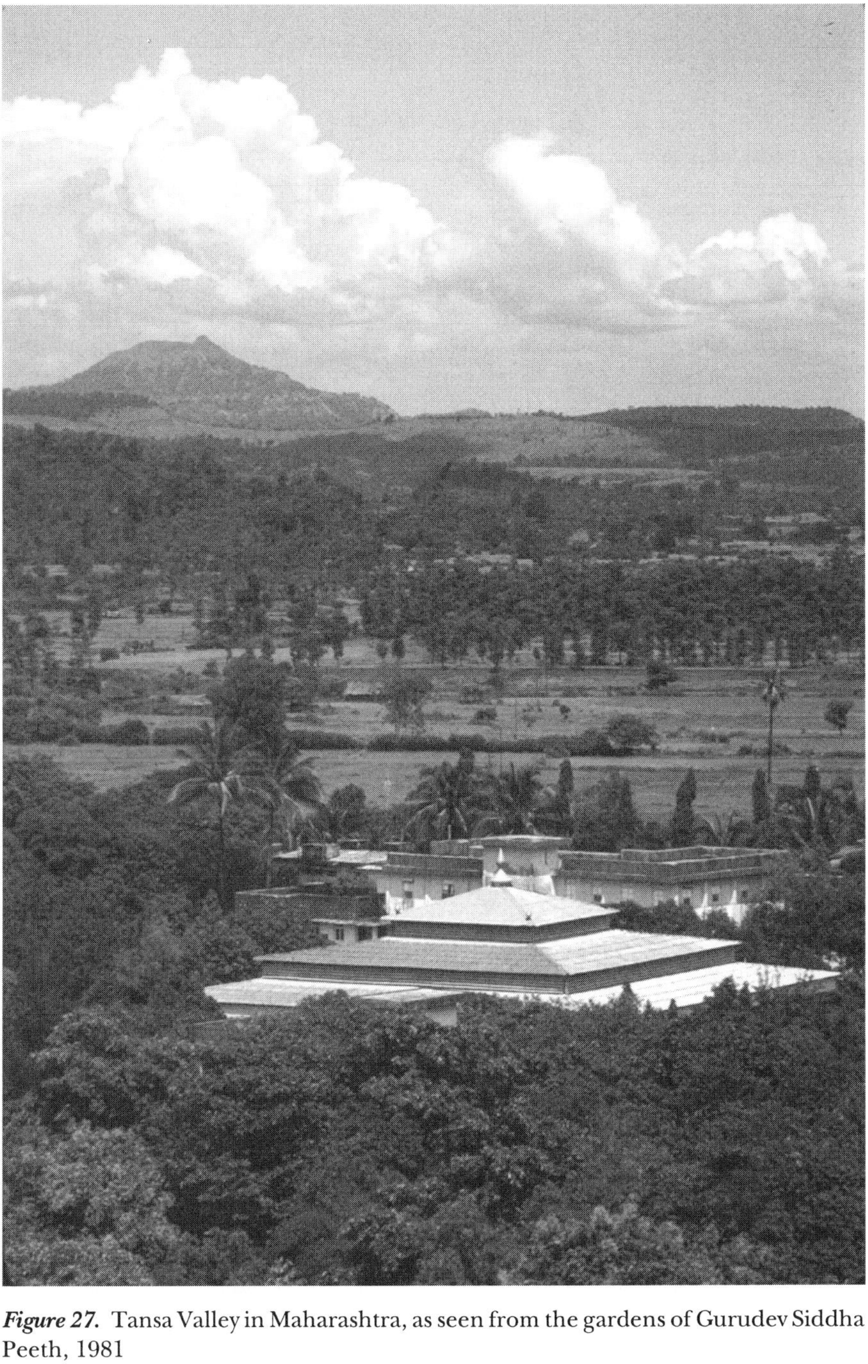

Figure 27. Tansa Valley in Maharashtra, as seen from the gardens of Gurudev Siddha Peeth, 1981

An embodiment of *śakti*, the ashram was indistinguishable from the siddha guru himself, who, Muktananda felt, expressed that same transformative force in his own personal being. According to Muktananda:

> The character of any place is constantly remolded by the actions of its inhabitants. Through interaction, the place and its inhabitants become adapted to each other. If a saint lives there, it becomes filled with the influence of that saint. Wherever a great saint dwells, he endows that place with the character of his profound inner state. In fact, each abode of a Siddha bears the impress of his unique state. His Shakti envelops the place—sporting, manifesting itself, and generating ever-new bliss which never dies. His abode is not a mere brick-and-mortar structure, but an incarnation of himself in flesh and blood. There is no distinction between a holy place and its presiding saint.[15]

A devotee has expressed a similar sentiment:

> The ashrams of Siddha Yoga, just like the Siddhas themselves, have their own particular way of manifesting. When you think about [Gurudev Siddha Peeth in] Ganeshpuri, for example, the senses and the mind rest on certain exquisite smells, sounds, tastes. You remember Baba's Samadhi Shrine, the gardens, the fragrant paths, the marble courtyard floor, the cool of the samadhi shrine, the rain on the roofs. [You remember] the mangoes, papayas and exotic plants, the sunrise and sunset on Tapovan Hill, the tranquility of Dakshin Kashi, the sound of the chants vibrating across the valleys, the superconscious energy as you walk inside the gate. You think of the bells and the chanting and the deep, deep ecstasy. You think of the village of Ganeshpuri and the great Siddhas who live there. It is India. It is Bhagawan Nityananda. It is Baba. It is thousands of years of concentrated worship and ritual and awareness of the presence of God. Ganeshpuri is magical and mysterious, unfathomable, thrilling. It is, as Baba used to exclaim, "shimmering Consciousness."[16]

If what Muktananda says is true—that there "is no distinction between a holy place and its presiding saint"—then at a deep level, the ashram *is* the guru.[17] Because of what Siddha Yoga holds to be the final identity of *citi-śakti, kuṇḍalinī-śakti*, and the guru himself, the ashram also therefore gives form to what is known as "Guru Shakti" (Sanskrit, *guru-śakti*), the transformative power of the teacher whose guidance allows the devotee to experience divinity in ever-deepening and increasingly intense ways. This graceful force is said to have many effects, one of which is to heighten one's experience of delight in life, one's sense of the newness of the moment that—again, paradoxically—also gives entry to a sense of abiding timelessness.

A Siddha Yoga monk described such an experience, which he had one day in Gurudev Siddha Peeth while overseeing the care of the *samādhi* shrine in which Swami Muktananda's body is interred. It was late afternoon, the time when the *ārati*, the ceremonial "waving of the lights," is performed in the ashram's temple before a life-size statue of Swami Muktananda's guru, Bhagawan Nityananda. The *ārati* in Indian tradition is the reverential circling of a small flame before a respected person or the image of a saint or deity. On this particular day, in what he described as the silent and "stupendously powerful" interval between cleaning the shrine and performing the *ārati*, the monk stood at one of the windows on the eastern wall:

> The light outside was brilliant with that very dramatic sunlight that comes at the end of the day, when the shadows are long and each form is seen in vivid detail. Someone was sluicing the small courtyard with a bucket of water, ready to wash the floor. Then someone else walked through with a basket of fruit from the kitchen, and someone else with baskets of flowers. It's hard to describe what I perceived. To my eyes, it looked like the most exquisite dance, perfectly choreographed, perfectly performed. I knew I was seeing people offering the activity of their physical bodies in service to the *śakti*, so that the *śakti* was moving through them. In my own state of heightened awareness, what might have looked at some other time like an ordinary action, could be seen for what it truly is: an act of worship.[18]

The very everydayness of this moment marks an important point: From the perspective of Siddha Yoga, cleaning a floor, serving the spiritual master, and worshiping God can be contained in a single action, if one's understanding of and attitude toward one's activities in general is undertaken as a celebration of the sacredness of being. It is to gain such a perspective and to act accordingly that devotees spend time in the ashram. The monk continued:

> The ashram is a place where one learns to serve God, to serve the *śakti*. The more you give yourself to the *śakti*, the more it moves through you, the more it makes you new and gives you knowledge. In this sacred space, even washing the courtyard is an act of worship.[19]

Swami Muktananda often spoke of the ashram as a repository of *citi-śakti*, *kuṇḍalinī-śakti*, and *guru-śakti*. As was noted earlier, he said that, "each abode of a Siddha bears the impress of his unique state. His Shakti envelops the place—sporting, manifesting itself, and generating ever-new bliss which never dies."[20] Again: "An Ashram is a place where God pervades completely. This doesn't mean that God does not pervade everywhere else. But you have to understand that every particle in the Ashram is filled with Chiti."[21] He told his disciples that in order to gain the highest good from their stay in the ashram, they needed to revere both the place and this power it contained. "The ashram is a great abode of the living God," he said. "This is the place where we attain peace of mind, and while staying here we should be fully aware that it is the very heart of God."[22]

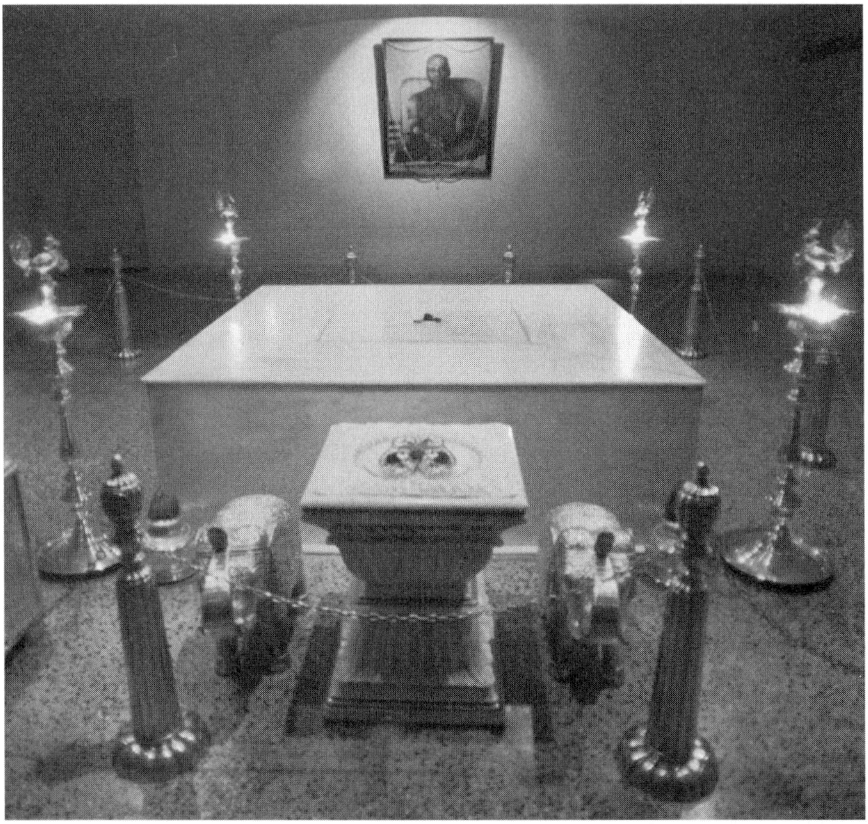

Figure 28. The Swami Muktananda Samadhi Shrine at Gurudev Siddha Peeth, 1996

A CENTER OF SPIRITUAL DISCIPLINE

The fact that this is a place where people "attain peace of mind" revolves around a paradox of spiritual life as it is understood by those who practice Siddha Yoga. Residents of Gurudev Siddha Peeth and Shree Muktananda Ashram note the peace they experience, yet they also often describe life in the ashram in terms connoting an intense inward burning of some sort. By this they generally refer to the nature of the *tapasya*, "austerity," they practice there. This word refers to the spiritual disciplines that foster *tapas*, a kind of inner, transformative, and creative "heat" or "fire" that is said to burn away psychological and spiritual impurities and thereby to cleanse the body, mind, and heart. Such *tapasya* can be difficult and, accordingly, anything but peaceful, because it challenges the ego's sense of self-importance, and the ego can put up a violent struggle to protect itself.

We return for a moment to the notion of the sacred and the profane. For our current purposes, these are not to be understood as objective *states* of being as much as subjective *modes* of being. To live in "the sacred" is to view life from a perspective that recognizes and affirms the possibility of a truly meaningful existence; "the sacred" is therefore not precisely a *thing* but rather a *way of seeing* things. As an anomalous abode of the sacred, the ashram points out the fundamental opposition between a sacred and a profane view of life. Life in the ashram thus induces in a seeker a form of what in Indian spiritual thought is called *viveka*, "discrimination." By the power and clarity of *viveka* one sees the difference between the real and the unreal, between the truly valuable and the merely attractive, between the good (*śreyas*) and the simply pleasant (*preyas*). Such *viveka* may be conscious or unconscious. In either case, it can at times bring a sense of anguish, for it may point out the ways in which one has not lived one's life in harmony with one's own inherent dignity of being. But the ashram also gives the genuine seeker a setting, a context, in which to engage and transform those inner forces, patterns of thought, and unconscious volitional tendencies (a loose translation of the yogic term *saṃskāra*)[23] that lead him or her to view the world from a profane perspective. The *saṃskāras* are deeply implanted in one's sense of "self" and of "other," and can be quite firm and unyielding. Nevertheless, they must be "burned out," as it were, if one is to be able to shift one's perspective toward the sacred.

This is why, following Indian tradition, Siddha Yoga masters hold that *tapasya* is important to a seeker's spiritual growth. Tradition holds that the inner fire enkindled by *tapasya* destroys one's *saṃskāras* and thereby frees one from the otherwise constant and recurrent cycle of existential disillusionment, doubt, and fear that those subliminal activators engender.

Many residents come to the ashram as a result of a deep yearning to know and experience God's presence in their lives. Swami Muktananda and

Swami Chidvilasananda have taught that this very yearning is itself an expression of the divine presence in the devotee's life. "Inner growth comes as a result of tapasya," Muktananda has said. "When your tapasya begins to bear fruit, you begin to grow inwardly. This separation from the Beloved is a very effective means to union with Him. The more acute the pangs of separation are, the sooner will a devotee be united with the Lord."[24] He also taught, "The more one follows the discipline of a sacred place, the higher will one rise, the more intense will be one's longing for God."[25] Swami Chidvilasananda has said that "the Truth is . . . attained by austerity. Austerity is called *tapasya. Tapasya* means burning in the fire of yoga. . . . When the individual soul is yearning for the supreme Soul, and the merging has not yet taken place, this is called *tapasya.* This struggle, this *tapasya,* is very good because it makes us attain the Truth."[26]

Speaking of life in the ashram, Swami Muktananda explained:

> Here, like the ancient seers, we are practicing intense tapasya, we are not wasting a single moment of our time. . . . Right from the moment you get up until the moment that you go to sleep something or other is taking place in the Ashram, and all the time you are being exposed to divine vibrations. . . .
>
> All the seekers here are performing such intense tapasya: they chant the *Guru Gita,* the *Vishnu Sahasranam, Shiva Mahimnah Stotra, arati,* and *dhuns* with such feeling, such purity and such devotion. Then they are working hard, putting in so much service to the guru. Some people are working in the garden, others sweeping the floors, still others are working in the office; yet others are doing some writing work. But that doesn't mean that one kind of work is superior to another. Whether you are writing or sweeping the floor, all your work is the same. What matters is the spirit behind it.
>
> So as time goes by, the Ashram atmosphere becomes more and more powerful and the seekers also become purer and purer. The seekers coming from abroad or coming from outside the Ashram, by living here for a certain period of time, begin to experience inner transformation. Here a *sadhaka* undergoes a complete change in the way he thinks, in the way he looks at different things, and he becomes divinised, as it were.[27]

Venkappanna Shriyan thought of his work in the garden as *tapasya,* and recalls that once, in the early days of the ashram, he was wondering aloud to some other devotees what he could possibly gain from all this effort. Later that day, he said, Swami Muktananda walked up to him looking like Rudra, the angry form of God. Muktananda asked:

> So, what are you going to get from coming to Baba? Nothing! Right? That's what you think? I have a whole ocean to give. Do you have the capacity to take it? Could you hold it? I have so much to give. You have to do tapasya, you have to do a lot of seva, you have to become strong—how else could you hold

> what I have to give? If I gave it to you now, you wouldn't be able to do anything tomorrow. And then it wouldn't stay with you. Only after you serve the Guru are you prepared to take what the Guru can give; only then can you contain it.[28]

Under the guru's guidance and direction, the ashram day is filled with spiritual practices and disciplines to help a seeker cultivate a deeper understanding of what are said to be sacred truths and a fuller experience of what is described as the presence of the divine in his or her life. Most of these disciplines have been practiced since the very earliest stages of religious life in India. Tradition regards such spiritual discipline as sadhana (Sanskrit, *sādhana:* "that which leads to completion"). One who practices sadhana is known as a *sādhaka.* Because a *sādhaka*'s movement toward spiritual maturity and freedom forces him or her to confront difficult psychological and other forms of resistance, such sadhana can at times be difficult—hence the importance of *tapasya.* Those who think that spiritual growth is easy are misinformed. In fact, sadhana must at times *necessarily* be difficult, for it involves the breaking of long-held and quite familiar, but nevertheless limiting and constricted, patterns of self-understanding. *Tapasya* purifies one's perspective of the world, dissolves one's sense of alienation from the divine, and thus brings about that experiential viewpoint we have called "the sacred." The flame of *tapasya* must always burn if one is to grow spiritually. But one is also to remember that the flame always burns upward.

Coming to the ashram allows one to see where one's spiritual discipline has wavered. Then, having discerned the difference between what one is and what one could be, one is given the place and opportunity to address one's weaknesses and augment one's strengths. The ashram gives a genuine spiritual seeker the opportunity to be a sadhu of sorts (Sanskrit, *sādhu*), that is to say, to be "one who is endeavoring toward the good" or to be "one who is working toward completion." In traditional India, a sadhu was one who renounced all ties to his family and occupation to live in austere simplicity in the forest. The genuine seeker who comes to a Siddha Yoga ashram is a modern sadhu, not because he or she has renounced responsibilities to the world (far from it), but rather because he or she is consciously and diligently performing sadhana. The modern-day sadhu's responsible behavior and spiritual discipline in the ashram—his or her "ashram dharma"—molds and shapes that sadhu's inner and outer life and leads him or her toward a life lived from the perspective of the sacred.

Perhaps mindful of the rather tawdry image that some false gurus and their retreat centers had garnered in the popular media in the late 1960s and following years, Swami Muktananda was firm in saying, "There is no place here for jokers or pretenders. A true seeker is interested only in sadhana, only in spiritual progress. He does not come to an Ashram for comfort or pleasure. In an Ashram he does not seek the kind of gratification that people seek in hotels or clubs or theatres or other modes of recreation and entertainment"; one who is looking only for sensual gratification "would find it very difficult to live here, because his primary interest is not sadhana."[29] He told his devotees, "In an ashram most of the time should be spent in meditation and contemplation of God. One should not fritter away one's precious time in a precious place on eating and drinking, sleeping, gossiping, and talking idly. . . . Otherwise, it will be no different from going . . . [anywhere] where one makes a lot of noise and comes back feeling empty, desiccated, and miserable."[30] Such discipline is said to allow one to express one's own inherent dignity and worth, the recognition of which Swami Muktananda taught is vital to the seeker's further and deeper experience of God. Furthermore, such discipline begins before one even steps onto the ashram grounds. "When entering an ashram," Muktananda taught, "one should be fully aware of one's true value. Enter it in a civilized, disciplined, calm, and humble manner. Let the mind be free from worldly burdens."[31]

Devotees who follow the ashram schedule find such lessons regarding the importance of respectful spiritual discipline embedded in the structure and patterns of their daily life. The schedule was instituted at Gurudev Siddha Peeth in 1966, and this same diurnal rhythm has been sustained with little variation in the intervening years. In the Introduction to Swami Muktananda's book, *Ashram Dharma*, a Siddha Yoga monk describes in detail the daily schedule when he first visited Gurudev Siddha Peeth in 1972:

> By 3:00 A.M. most of the ashramites had gotten up and walked past the courtyard to the bathrooms and our cold water bucket baths. [Rooms with adjoining baths and showers with heated water were built beginning in 1975.] By 3:30 almost the whole ashram was meditating in the Cave, as we called the meditation room under Baba's house, and also Dhyana Mandir, the area that is now Baba's Samadhi Shrine. Baba used to walk through Dhyana Mandir with a flashlight to check how we were meditating. Often he would transmit his own divine energy into a seeker by brushing the person's forehead or touching them between the eyebrows. People could feel the kundalini energy being awakened: they would have visions of inner light, or experience showers of love, or receive profound realizations. These early morning sessions of meditation would set the tone for the whole day. Those of us who lived in the ashram talked about our subtle experiences in the same way I remember once talking about news events or gossip. They were vital, they were real, they were the fabric of our lives—and, though these experiences of spirit weren't uncommon for us, they were always fresh.[32]

"The Cave," which Swami Muktananda called Chinmaya Guha ("the cave where one is absorbed in consciousness") was under his living quarters.

Dhyana Mandir ("the Meditation Temple") is now the Samadhi Shrine, where Swami Muktananda's body has been interred. Devotees also meditate in Turiya Mandir ("the Temple of the Absolute-beyond-Form") and in the Nityananda Mandir, the temple honoring Bhagawan Nityananda, both of which places they often describe as infused with these two teachers' powerful and loving presence.

> Chanting, which began long before dawn, was usually done in the Bhagawan Nityananda Temple. At 4:15 A.M. an *āratī* was performed to Bhagawan and we chanted mantras Baba himself had compiled from the scriptures in his Guru's honor. Then the *Guru Gītā* chant began at 5:30.[33]

The sonorous *Gurugītā*, the "Song of the Guru," is a 181-verse text that presents a dialogue between Śiva and his divine consort, Pārvatī, on the nature of the universal teacher and of the guru-disciple relationship. The *Gurugītā* recitation is considered the most important practice of the ashram day—Swami Muktananda described it as "the one indispensable text."[34]

> When Baba chanted with us, we had to keep perfect postures and remain completely still for the entire chant, which lasted an hour and a half. Only during the final *kīrtana, Shrī Krishna Govinda Hare Murare,* were we allowed to sway a bit. . . .
>
> The discipline had a great purpose: Baba was teaching us the power of *āsana* and *prāṇāyāma*, of controlling our posture and breath. With a still body and steady breath, one can tap into astonishing levels of inner bliss while chanting. Each morning as we sang the final *kīrtana,* we could look through the temple door or windows and watch the sun rising over the distant hills—a sublime moment in the day.[35]

Breakfast is served from 7:00 to 8:00. The ashram dining hall is named "Annapurna" in honor of the goddess of nourishing food, and the atmosphere is, as the monk wrote, "as sacred as that of the temple." He added:

> Baba always insisted that food be revered as God. The ashram meals were prepared with a great deal of attention and love, and they were eaten in silence. Baba wouldn't permit anyone to waste as much as a grain of rice.[36]

After breakfast all residents engage in various service projects: washing dishes, cutting vegetables for the day's meals, tending the gardens, preparing flower arrangements, distributing milk to local village schoolchildren, translating Sanskrit and other texts, maintaining and repairing the ashram's buildings, cleaning the temple—the list of such service is long and varied. This work is undertaken in the spirit of selfless service, seva (Sanskrit, *sevā),* and thus it is considered along with meditation and chanting to be an indispensable part of a seeker's disciplined spiritual practice.

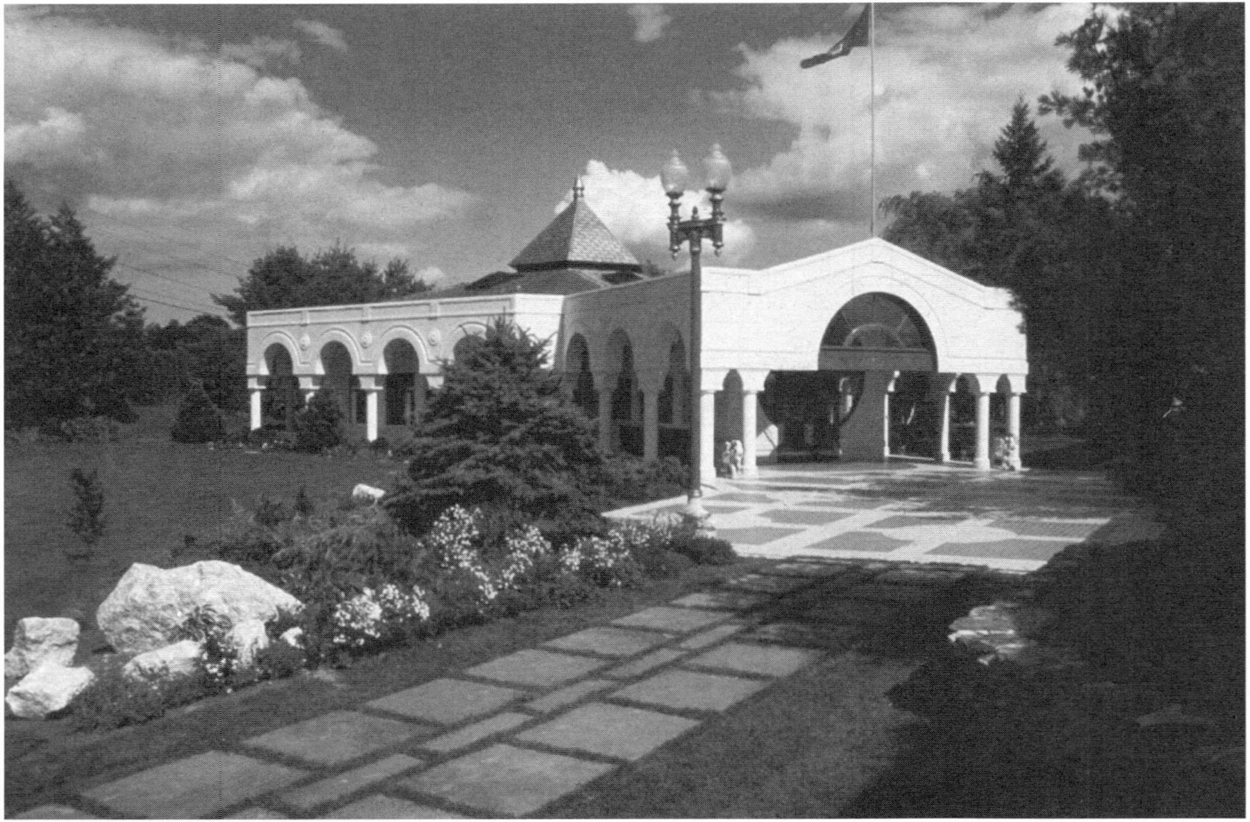

Figure 29. The Bhagawan Nityananda Temple at Shree Muktananda Ashram in South Fallsburg, New York, 1986

At 11:15 everyone is invited to sing the *Rudram*, a song to God in his awe-inspiring and fearful form, and at 11:50 the *Śiva Āratī*, a chant in which God is honored as the destroyer of all harmful forces such as ignorance and self-centeredness. Lunch is served from 12:00 to 1:00 P.M. The afternoon is dedicated to more seva.

There is another chant, the *Viṣṇusahasranāma* ("the Thousand Names of God as the Sustainer of the Universe"), in the Nityananda Temple at 2:00 P.M., and then at 6:00 P.M. there is a chant called the "Āratī"—the same mantras that are sung to Bhagawan Nityananda each morning. Following dinner at 6:45, the *Śiva Mahimna Stotra* ("Song to the Glory of Śiva") is sung at 7:45 in the courtyard, and the "*Śiva Āratī*" is sung again at 9:00 P.M. Most of the ashram residents go to sleep shortly thereafter, for the morning schedule begins again very soon.

The ashram day thus contains five hours of chanting. While it is rare that any one ashram resident will attend all of the scheduled chants during the day—for one thing, seva assignments often make this impossible—there is a conspicuous emphasis given to singing the divine name. In addition to the daily schedule, several times a year, often in association with important dates on the religious calendar, there is a *saptah*, an extended session of namasankirtana (Sanskrit, *nāmasaṃkīrtana*, the chanting of the names of God). The term *saptah* comes from the Sanskrit word for "seven" (*sapta*), referring to the seven-day period of time Swami Muktananda originally set for these sessions of continuous, day-and-night chanting. The term is now used in Siddha Yoga ashrams to refer to any extended time for chanting, an event that is greeted by residents with enormous enthusiasm. Once when asked about the relevance of chanting to the practice of Siddha Yoga, Swami Muktananda replied:

> Chanting plays the greatest part in this yoga; it is a magnet that draws the power of the Lord. Chanting makes meditation easy. The Kundalini Shakti within becomes very pleased with chanting. To discover how effective it is, you should chant. . . .
>
> It has enormous power. It not only purifies the heart but all seven constituents of the body. So chant continuously. Chanting will not only awaken your Kundalini and thus bring spontaneous meditation, but it will also fill you with peace.[37]

And there is much more offered in the ashram as well. Ashram residents may choose to practice together the various *āsana*s of traditional *haṭhayoga* under the guidance of trained teachers in order to loosen and strengthen their bodies so that they can meditate with more clarity and attention. They take formal classes taught by Siddha Yoga swamis or by lay scholars, some lasting several weeks, on the sacred texts and traditions that give expression to the teachings of the siddha gurus: the Upaniṣads, for example, and the *Yoga Sūtra* of Patañjali; Śaṅkarācārya's *Crest-Jewel of Discrimination*; the *Bhagavadgītā* and often its commentary the *Jñāneśvarī*; songs of the devotional poet-saints of western and northern India; important works from the tradition of Kashmir Śaivism such as the *Pratyabhijñāhṛdayam* and *Śiva Sūtra*—the list of such texts is long. Under Swami Chidvilasananda's guidance and inspiration, residents study these works closely and attentively, and do so in a manner that is academically responsible. But the purpose of such study is more than academic in nature. It is to assimilate these teachings as they progress in their individual spiritual growth. Swami Chidvilasananda once observed that in ancient times, students often studied the scriptures and the words of great beings in rustic circumstances, sitting outside under the trees. She said, "[I]n this ashram we try to maintain that simple tradition. Although there are buildings to accommodate all of us very well, yet we remember that the teachings of the great beings are not meant to be confined within concrete walls. The teachings of the great beings are meant to be practiced in our daily life."[38]

In many ways the most significant component of the instruction offered at the ashram comes in what is called "the Intensive," a program of usually two days—though it can be as short as one day or as long as a week—in which the core elements of Siddha Yoga are presented in a sharply focused manner. The participants hear sacred teachings and practice meditation, contemplation, chanting, and other forms of spiritual discipline. The Intensive was created by Swami Muktananda in 1974 on his second international tour as the vehicle for conveying in the West the existentially transforming initiation known as "shaktipat" (Sanskrit, *śaktipāta*). This is the powerful transmission of God's grace through the guru. Once Swami Muktananda described the Intensive as "an instantaneous way to embark on the spiritual path, as well as an easy way to deepen spiritual experience."[39]

At least once each year, ashram residents have the opportunity to watch as traditional brahmins perform various *pūjās*, ceremonies of worship, throughout the ashram in front of different iconographic images of various personalities and functions of the divine: Śiva as the Lord of the Dance, whose fluidly rhythmic movements create, sustain, and transform the universe while at the same time crushing the demon of forgetfulness whose power keeps the human spirit from remembering God's eternal grace; Durgā, the powerful and resolute goddess who destroys coldheartedness, ignorance, and evil; Gaṇeśa, who protects the world from harmful forces and removes obstructions from the spiritual path; there are many more. On special occasions, the brahmins also perform *havanas*, sacred rituals to the divine power of fire that is said to burn away impurities. And they periodically undertake the intricate and complicated offertory fire rituals known as *yajñas* in large open-air pavilions designed primarily for such functions, most of which last for several days at a time. These performances include the brahmins' precise and exact chanting of Vedic mantras for hours on end, many of which date to the second millennium B.C.E. According to Vedic tradition, such rites allow the human community, as represented by the priests and a chosen *yajamāna* couple, to offer praise and gifts of thanksgiving to the universal divine powers of life and regeneration and are undertaken for the welfare of the world as a whole. It is said that the vital essence of the different kinds of grains, flower petals, yogurt, clarified butter, and other gifts offered to the flame blazing in the fire pit rise with the column of ascending smoke high into the skies and heavens, whence its life-giving and restoring power spreads to all regions of the universe, both the material and subtle realms. Swami Chidvilasananda tells devotees to contemplate what she holds to be the deeper significance and implications of the *yajña*:

> According to the scriptures, humankind came into existence when the Lord performed a yajna, a fire sacrifice. He told His creatures, "This is the way to live. Whatever you do, offer it to God. Whatever actions you perform, offer them to the divine Will. Whatever you say, offer it to the fire, offer it to the Truth. As long as this offering exists, you will live a perfect life." For this to happen, the sacrifice must continue every moment, every hour of our life—not even for a second can we forget what our life is. Our whole life is yajna, our whole life is sacrifice.[40]

Residents of the ashram undertake their daily schedule and all that it includes whether or not the guru is in residence in the ashram at that time. Both Swami Muktananda and Swami Chidvilasananda have closely watched over and participated directly in all aspects of ashram life, and all the activities of the ashram reflect their teachings. A resident of the ashram is therefore like a student in ancient and classical India, whom tradition holds was to learn sacred teachings and be trained in religious disciplines while living in the *gurukula*, the "home of the spiritual master." Like their predecessors in the long history of India, swamis Muktananda and Chidvilasananda guide and teach through the power of their own example. Meditating as the guru meditates, chanting as the guru chants, chopping vegetables as the guru chops vegetables, listening to the guru's teachings, opening themselves to and caring for each other as the guru cares for all people, residents of the ashram are said to come closer to realizing the foundational dignity of existence and, thus, of what Siddha Yoga regards to be the God-given inner worth of all beings.

Such recognition, cultivated by the spiritual disciplines practiced at the ashram, is said to lead, in part, to a deep sense of the love that is held to be the foundation of the universe itself. Swami Muktananda taught his followers:

> It is your responsibility to preserve the Shakti that has been generated by chanting and meditation. If you start practicing truthfulness, silence, forgiveness and compassion, if you protect these divine virtues like a miser protects his money, you will soon accumulate a fortune of the true wealth, the inner riches. Always entertain pure and noble thoughts and never deprive yourself of inner or outer purity.
>
> You should try to understand the worth of the body you are living in. Man's worth is enormous and it is this realization which should govern your conduct and behaviour. Man can have dignity only if he lives a life of discipline and regularity. God has been very kind in providing us with such a beautiful world and bodies and minds with so many faculties. In order to pay off our debt to God, in order to obtain inner peace, we should remember God constantly. . . . It is necessary to start remembering Him from this very moment. While you are alive and strong and healthy you should be able to achieve inner quietude and *peace.* Remember that Lord Narayan dwells within you in His full glory, that you are divine. That knowledge can be attained if you know your true inner Self.[41]

IMPLICATIONS OF THE WORD *ĀŚRAMA*

Such is the ashram: first and foremost a place of intense religious discipline under the direct, comprehensive, and intimate guidance of the guru, it is also a place infused with serenity, quiet, and, in the case of Gurudev Siddha Peeth and the Shree Muktananda Ashram, of remarkable natural beauty.

These seemingly paradoxical qualities of an ashram—a center of fervent spiritual practice and yet also an abode of calm and peace—have been reflected in the various ways in which the word *ashram* has been defined and the way in which life in an ashram has been characterized. Both of these qualities of the ashram find expression in a notice written by the trustees of Gurudev Siddha Peeth and on display on a placard in the entry courtyard of that ashram:

> We welcome you all with great love and respect! This is an ashram, a place where shrama, fatigue, is destroyed. The ashram is not a tourist spot, a hotel or zoo. The ashram is for those who are interested in spirituality, in knowing the divine Self that dwells within. The ashram was founded by Swami Muktananda Paramahamsa in 1956, when his guru Bhagawan Nityananda gave him three little rooms on a small plot of land. Through the grace of his Guru and by his divine guidance, the ashram has become what it is today. The ashram is open to seekers who want to do sadhana and seva and want to attain peace. The ashram is for meditation and chanting.

The modern Indian word *ashram* comes from the Sanskrit *āśrama,* which consists of the word *śrama* joined by the prefix *ā-*. There is little debate regarding the essential definition of the noun *śrama* (which the trustees have spelled *shrama* in the passage above): it means "strenuous exertion" or "fervent activity." The word derives from the verbal root *śram-*, the meaning of which traditional Indian grammarians and lexicographers as well as modern linguists associate with both physical work and fatigue, on the one hand, and diligent spiritual discipline on the other.[42] Verses from the *Ṛgveda*, the earliest of Indian sacred texts (*ca.* 1500-1000 B.C.E.), use the term *śrama* and its derivatives both in a negative sense, suggesting weariness or exhaustion,[43] and in a more positive way, referring to strenuous or energetic activity that is undertaken to obtain a desired or desirable end.[44]

Indian tradition presents different perspectives regarding the meaning of the *ā-* appended to the noun *śrama* to form the word *āśrama.* According to one line of thought, the *ā-* here would be what Indian grammarians call the "expanded" or "swollen" form (*vṛddhi*) of the privative suffix *a-*, which negates the meaning of the word with which it is associated. If this were the case, then the word *āśrama* would be a place where there is "truly no *śrama,*" and thus it would be a place of calmness and peace. It seems that the trustees of Gurudev Siddha Peeth had this interpretation in mind when they wrote the welcoming statement quoted above. And this seems also to be the way the word has been used in a description of an *āśrama* appearing in the *Rāmāyaṇa* as a place that "destroys fatigue"[45] and in a passage from the *Mahābhārata* regarding an "*āśrama* which destroys fatigue and sorrow."[46]

It should be noted, however, that the ancient and classical Indian grammatical tradition represented by such systematizers as Pāṇini (sixth or fifth century B.C.E.) probably would not interpret the word in this way. According to Pāṇini's *Aṣṭādhyāyī,* likely the oldest extant grammar in the world, the *ā-* is not a *vṛddhi* form of the negative *a-* but rather the particle *ā-*,[47] which classical Sanskrit commentators generally feel serves to intensify the word with which it is associated.[48] This being the case, the word *āśrama* would refer to a place where there is a "great deal of *śrama*" and thus a place of strenuous activity and intense fervor. On the surface, this is of course just the opposite of the idea that an *āśrama* is a place of calm and peace.

To expand on this idea further, we might return for a moment to the meaning of the noun *śrama,* which in its earliest usage referred both to "toil" and to "diligent activity undertaken for a beneficial purpose." It is in the latter sense that Vedic texts dating to as early as the thirteenth to eighth centuries B.C.E. closely associate the word *śrama* with the work involved in the performance of the complicated offertory fire ritual (*yajña*),[49] as well as with diligent and reverential worship (*arcā* and other terms) and especially with the fervent, creative, and transformative heat (*tapas*) produced by intense practices of meditation and ascetic austerity. Some classical texts at times use the word *tapasya* to refer to practices that produce *tapas*[50] or to that which is associated with fervent religious asceticism in general[51]; others use the word *tapasya* as a nominal verb meaning to "undergo religious austerities."[52] A Vedic text dating to roughly the eighth century B.C.E. presents the idea that the universe in its entirety came about by means of the *śrama* and *tapas* of the god Prajāpati, the universal lord of creatures, who is said to have labored strenuously and heated himself up in his ascetic fervor:[53] The god's *śrama* and *tapas* first produced the primordial waters which, heated by his fervent activity, then formed foam, which became clay, which became sand, then stones, then the earth and its seasons and, finally, a young boy, who became the eight divine forms of the god of fire, Agni.[54] Another text, from the seventh to sixth centuries B.C.E., adds the element of the god's act of "worship" to this creative process:

> In the beginning there was nothing here, nothing whatsoever. Death covered all of this, or hunger; for hunger is death. He created the mind, thinking, "May I have a self." Then he moved about, worshiping. While he was worshiping, water was produced from him . . . . He wished, "May I again perform a sacrifice with a greater sacrifice." He toiled. He practiced austerity.[55]

In a variant of the ideas presented by these sacred narratives, another passage holds that human visionary seers themselves fashioned a meaningful world through the effective power of their *śrama* and *tapas*.[56] An Upaniṣad dating to roughly the fourth century B.C.E. states that when the seeker Bhṛgu approached his father for the knowledge of the absolute (Brahman), he was told over and over again to practice austerities and finally through that discipline came to see that Brahman is, in fact, deep and abiding bliss *(ānanda)*.[57] Another Upaniṣad of roughly the same time period recounts the way in which Śvetāśvatara came to experience Brahman through the transformative practice of *tapas* and with the grace of God.[58] A slightly later Upaniṣad notes the role *tapas* plays in the mind's movement toward the sublime: Such effort gives the mind the clarity (*sattva*) that allows it to know the soul.[59]

According to Tantric and Āgamic tradition, the practice of meditation and contemplation is to be accompanied in some way by an inward sacrifice of sorts (*antaryajña*) or by an offering to the inner fire (*antaragni*) which blazes within one's own being as the *prāṇa*, the warm breath of life. Outward expression of such an inward sacrifice took place in the performance of small ritual ceremonies in which one burned sacred offerings in one's own particular ceremonial flame. Classical Hindu works on religious life use the term *śrāmaṇaka*, which is related to the noun *śrama* and refers to the small fire a renunciant would light in his hermitage in order to perform such personal offertory rituals.[60] That such a fire plays a part in various contemplative traditions of India is supported by the fact that Buddhist as well as Hindu texts note the importance to the *āśrama* (Pali, *assama*) of the presence somewhere on its grounds of the sacred ritual fire,[61] a literal and symbolic expression of the transformative heat, the fervor that life in the *āśrama* engenders and requires.

The noun *śrama* thus in part connotes strenuous physical exertion associated with sacrifice, worship, and the practice of religious austerity. It is particularly in its association with the latter, *tapas,* that the related word *śramaṇa* came to refer to an ascetic who diligently practices such religious austerities. Buddhist and, to a lesser extent, Jain sources use the word *śramaṇa* (Pali, *samaṇa*)[62] to refer to a monk or a religious mendicant worthy of respect and support.[63] The earliest of the South Asian sacred texts describe such *śramaṇa*s as wearing little or no clothing (*vātaraśana*: "clothed by the wind") and associate them with the visionary seers (*ṛṣi*)[64] whose verses form the songs of the *Ṛgveda.* Hymns from the *Ṛgveda* suggest that such *ṛṣi*s lived in the forest, where they practiced the contemplation that brought them visions of the divine.[65] Those songs also describe *ṛṣi*s absorbed in *tapas* and note the power of such *tapas* in raising the lowest to the highest.[66] *Vātaraśana*s were associated with other types of ascetics: long-haired renunciants (*keśin*), for example, and quiet sages (*muni*), the latter of whom the great fourteenth-century commentator on the Veda, Sāyaṇa, described as "seers of the truth beyond the senses."[67] Like other ancient Indian ascetics, *keśin*s and *muni*s are reported to have lived in the forests, where they were said to commune ecstatically with the gods as they underwent their holy work.[68] The *Ṛgveda* also mentions ascetics known as *yati*s,[69] a word most likely derived from a verbal root *yat-*, meaning to "endeavor" and thus semantically similar to the meaning of *śrama*; it may also be connected with the root *yam-*, to "control," and thus related to *yama, niyama,* and other words that refer to physical self-control and moral self-discipline.

So an ashram, as we have suggested, may be understood to be either a place of peaceful calm or a place of diligent spiritual discipline. One might argue that these two functions and characteristics do not necessarily contradict each other, but instead in some important ways complement each other. For Indian religious traditions in general hold that it is more difficult to engage in productive spiritual discipline when one is distracted, enervated, and debilitated by an assaultive world than if one can, at least temporarily, live in an abode of peace far from the pressures and tensions of that world. Yet those who practice Siddha Yoga receive more than just a quiet place to visit from Gurudev Siddha Peeth, Shree Muktananda Ashram, and the other Siddha Yoga ashrams around the world. They receive a setting in which to practice under the guidance of a guru spiritual disciplines that are said to lead to their own experience of a deep and pervasive inner peace. Furthermore, it is that very peace itself that stands, in part, as the foundation on which the seeker then can engage productively in further and quite often difficult personal spiritual work (*sādhana*) and in selfless service to

God (*sevā*). Outward calm and inner peace ground spiritual fervor; spiritual fervor engenders inner peace and outward calm. In some ways, they are the same thing. This may be why the trustees of Gurudev Siddha Peeth say that the "ashram is open to seekers who want to do sadhana and seva and want to attain peace."

THE ASHRAM AS AN INDIAN RELIGIOUS INSTITUTION

Spiritual retreat centers of different types where seekers temporarily or for long periods of time forgo the pressures and demands of everyday life in order to cultivate spiritual growth have a long history in India. Historically such centers not only served as places of meditation and contemplation but also frequently were associated with the study of sacred texts and traditions as well as the practice of various physical disciplines and the performance of community-oriented service, such as performing sacred rituals. According to Indian thought in general, the goal of education is to train the mind and body not only to become receptacles for knowledge but also, more importantly, to become effective instruments of it. In ancient India, all forms of learning were considered means to *brahmavarcasa* ("the splendor of Brahman"), that is, to the liberating awareness and fulfilling embodiment of the absolute itself.

Why would this be so? According to much Indian thought, the mind is a purer and more powerful component of one's being than is the physical body and, accordingly, is closer in essence to the soul and thus to God. "Higher than the senses . . . is the mind," an Upaniṣad teaches, "and higher than the mind is the awakened intellect. Higher than the awakened intellect is the great [self]. Higher than the great [self] is the unmanifest. Higher than the unmanifest is the [supreme] Person. Higher than the Person there is nothing at all. That is the final goal; that is the highest course."[70] Indulgent and unthinking gratification of the physical body, therefore, can distract the mind and turn it from knowing its higher, sublime source. This distraction dilutes and weakens the power of the mind and thus prevents a person from knowing the soul.

The mind fulfills its function when it remains open to and in constant contact with the sublime, universal power of being, what thinkers aligned with the Sāṃkhya and the Yoga schools of philosophy call *prakṛti*, and what those belonging to various forms of Hindu Tantrism (including Kashmir Śaivism) call *śakti*. This vital energy infuses all physical things, giving them their very existence, but it is not dependent on them for its own existence. It is *svayambhū*, "self-originating," and thus autonomous and independent. Śaiva texts tend to link this active, universal power with the kindly auspiciousness of the divine: "More minute than the minute, in the midst [even] of confusion, the creator of all things, of many forms, the one embracer of the everything that is: by knowing him as benevolent [*śiva*], one gains peace forever."[71] The seeker therefore trains and disciplines the physical body in order to discipline the mind so that it can more fully and effectively serve as the foundation or base (*ādhāra*) upon which the universal divine energy can move and thrive. Prepared by such discipline, the *ādhāra* is better able to invite and withstand the full infusion of the *śakti*. A person who has completely and perfectly trained all of the denser physical, emotional, psychological, and spiritual components of his or her being thereby becomes one with the sublime *śakti* itself and is said in Tantric and other traditions to have become a *siddha*, a "completed" or "perfected" being.[72]

Indian tradition therefore holds the importance of physical and spiritual discipline to the cultivation of the mind and spirit. The long and influential tradition of Yoga, as taught by Patañjali (who lived either in the second century B.C.E. or the fifth century C.E.), has delineated some of the components of such discipline and has stated that without practicing these, a spiritual aspirant will not move further on the path to understanding. A student of Yoga is to practice five aspects of personal restraint (*yama*), characterized by being unwilling to do injury to living beings, telling the truth, not stealing, maintaining mental and physical purity, and turning away from envy (*ahiṃsā, satya, asteya, brahmacarya* and *aparigraha*, respectively).[73] So, too, such a seeker is to cultivate self-control (*niyama*) characterized by the practice of physical and mental hygiene, equanimity, austerity, reflective study of scriptures, and devotion to the Lord (*śauca, saṃtoṣa, tapas, svādhyāya,* and *īśvarapraṇidhāna*).[74]

Although these particular ten modes of self-discipline are enumerated specifically by the Yoga tradition, the essential values and intentions the list embodies pertain to Indian religious sensibilities as a whole. We might note here the importance of diligent and responsible practice to one's own physical, mental, and spiritual growth. Despite the significance placed on such self-effort, however, many traditional Indian perspectives place supreme emphasis on the importance of a teacher, a guru; for study by oneself is regarded as ultimately futile. One Upaniṣad, dating to roughly 400 B.C.E., maintains that "there is no access here without a teacher."[75]

A system such as this, in which spiritual growth, education, and personal service are so closely connected, necessarily places much emphasis on the need for a seeker to cultivate a style of life in which purification of the body and mind can take place. To live one's life in this way is to practice *brahmacarya* (the fourth of the disciplines pertaining to *yama*, as mentioned above), a word which means "to travel in the truth," in the sense of "to live constantly in the truth," and which carries the connotation of purity and thus of chastity. One who practices *brahmacarya* is a *brahmacārin*, a term often translated simply as "student" but which can justly be rendered as "seeker of the truth." In traditional India, the life of a true student was not easy, nor was it even possible for those lacking discipline and commitment to its practice. Sometimes the students had to prove to the teacher that they truly had such discipline and genuine interest in educational and spiritual growth. This is why a student in traditional India was sometimes also known as an *adhikārin,* "one who is entitled" to study with the teacher because he had displayed his commitment to the religious path as a whole.

Because "to live constantly in the truth" encompasses all aspects of life—in this case, everything from collecting wood for the household ritual fire to learning and singing sacred chants, undergoing diligent textual study, practicing disciplined meditation, learning the proper way to treat one's body, and gaining an understanding of how to treat one another—the *brahmacārin* or *adhikārin* was best able to learn effectively from the teacher if he lived in the guru's own home, that is, in the *gurukula.* Accordingly, the student was sometimes known as an *antevāsin,* that is, as "one who lives near" the teacher, who was himself sometimes known as the *kulapati,* or "master of the house." Sometimes the teacher's house was in the village or urban setting, but most often it was in the quiet forests (*araṇya, vana*) beyond the reach of the town or city, where the teacher and student could live, teaching and learning in the relative solitude and serenity much of Indian tradition holds to facilitate spiritual growth. It is likely that the Vedic lessons recorded in the Āraṇyakas, "Forest Teachings," dating to roughly 900-600 B.C.E. were first given by teachers to their students in such peaceful yet disciplined places of spiritual study. Various Purāṇic texts composed in the early centuries of the Common Era mention *gurukulas* in the homes of such teacher-sages as Dhaumya, Kaṇva, and Vālmīki.

It was here in the forest retreat where the teacher taught the student orally, repeating various mantras and other sacred lessons; it was here that the student reflected on the meaning of those lessons; and it was here that, using various contemplative techniques (*upāsanas*) that led to an intuitive realization of the absolute, the student meditated deeply on the insights to which such reflection had led. According to much Indian thought, such meditation is a more effective course in seeking to comprehend the truth in its fullness than is mere intellectual deliberation.

These three disciplines—hearing the teachings (*śravaṇa*), thinking about them (*manana*), and meditating (*dhyāna, nididhyāsana*) on the truth they reveal—have long been understood in India to lead to a knowledge of the absolute truth that undergirds and supports all things. Taken together, the practices encompassed by *yama* and *niyama* mentioned earlier, the silent repetition of mantra (*japa*), the performance of selfless service in honor of the teacher (*gurusevā*), and the disciplines of *śravaṇa, manana,* and *dhyāna* constituted, in part, the *śrama* or "diligent work" undertaken in the guru's *āśrama.*

Seekers of a variety of religious traditions practiced similar disciplines in centers that in at least some ways resembled ashrams. One thinks here of the various types of monastic institutions that have been part of the Indian legacy for 2,500 years and more. The historical origins of some of these types of monasteries can be traced to an ancient tradition in India by which some seekers of spiritual attainment would leave their own households and embrace a detached but liberating "homelessness." The Upaniṣads refer to such seekers as "travelers" (*caraka*) who spent their lives in constant search of truth and who spread lessons regarding that truth throughout the country. The *Bṛhadāraṇyaka Upaniṣad*, to pick just one example, recounts a teaching it attributes to the influential sage Yājñavalkya: "Having overcome the desire for progeny, for wealth, and for the various worlds, knowers of the absolute become wandering mendicants [*brāhmaṇāḥ . . . bhikṣācaryaṃ caranti*]."[76]

According to Buddhist traditions, the Buddha himself was one of such peripatetic seekers and teachers (Sanskrit, *parivrājaka*; Pali, *paribbājaka*: "wanderers") who had left the comfortable but for them spiritually distracting confines of village, town, and court to live in the outskirts and wildernesses beyond the urban precincts. Following his example, Buddhist mendicants (Sanskrit, *bhikṣu*; Pali, *bhikkhu*) would travel by foot across the expanses of India. During the rainy monsoon season these Buddhist wanderers would take up residence in small shelters or huts in the woods. Such rainy season retreats were known in the Buddhist community as *vassas*; the shelter itself was known as a *vihāra*. Over the years many of the *vihāras* grew in size and came to be built as permanent structures.[77] Eventually some of these *vihāras* developed from single shelters protecting solitary monks to larger facilities offering "bed and sitting accommodation" (*senāsena*) to a large number of such seekers. In time, colonies (*āvāsa*) of such *vihāras* and their supporting institutions arose in the forests of India.[78] The boundaries of an *āvāsa* were marked by natural objects such as a river or a mountain or a wooded grove. By the third or fourth centuries B.C.E., the Buddhist community had established a practice in which the various mendicants would gather in the *āvāsas* for the rainy season to help each other in their spiritual disciplines under the guidance and inspiration of an acknowledged master (Sanskrit, *śāstṛ*; Pali, *satthā*). Religious practices in these institutions stand as the foundation of the disciplined life in what came to be known as the Saṅgha, the Buddhist community as a whole.

Pali and later Sanskrit Buddhist texts often refer respectfully to a number of such monasteries, for example, at Jetavana, Ashokaram, and Kanchi. By the seventh century C.E., such practices had developed to the degree that they supported and infused the life of the immense Buddhist monastic university (*mahāvihāra*) at Nalanda, north of the ancient town of Rajagriha in what is now Bihar. According to journals kept by two great Chinese Buddhist pilgrims to India, Hsüan-tsang and I-ching, the *mahāvihāra* at Nalanda was home to several thousand Buddhist students and monks. Tibetan records note that another Buddhist center at Vikramashila in the northeast part of India under the direction of the great teacher (*ācārya*) Dīpaṅkara Śrījnāna (eleventh century C.E.) could be found on a hill near the Ganges, where that sacred river turned northwards.[79]

In a Buddhist text[80] dating to as early as the third or second century B.C.E., a description of a Hindu sage settling down with his students indicates that Buddhists in South Asia were aware of Brāhmaṇical Hindus who had established forest retreats similar to the Buddhist *vihāras*. True to their heritage, many of these had long been associated with education of the mind as well as cultivation of the spirit. In both the *Chāndogya* and the *Bṛhadāraṇyaka Upaniṣads* (ca. 700 B.C.E.),[81] for example, we hear of a *pariṣad,* a residential institute for advanced religious study and practice, to which the great philosopher-king Pravāhana Jaivali drove in his royal chariot every day so that he could sit in meditation and listen to the teachings presented there. Later texts were to hold that a *pariṣad* was to consist of at least ten students, and describes such a student as one who is "free from envy and pride . . . free from greed and from hypocrisy, arrogance, covetousness, delusions and anger [and who has] studied the Veda according to the prescribed method, together with its appendages."[82] A text dating to the fourth or fifth century C.E., includes references to a *maṭha* or "cloister" in which an ascetic teacher would accept and teach students. That the word *maṭha* appears in that text in the compound *vidyāmaṭha*[83] suggests that such a cloister was established for the purpose of teaching knowledge, *vidyā*; and that it similarly is joined to the word *āyatana,* "resting place, abode," to form the compound *maṭhāyatana*[84] indicates that such *maṭhas* were settled monastic or hermetic centers. At times, although not often, the word *maṭha* was used nearly synonymously with the term *dharmaśālā,* the latter referring to a temporary residence used by travelers, such as pilgrims en route to a holy site.[85] Historically, such *maṭhas* typically were located at some distance from urban centers or in small towns associated with temples. A *maṭha* was administered by a "self-possessed" leader (*svāmī,* thus "swami"), who watched over every detail and every function.[86] Such a director not only taught the students but also took care of the finances, supervised the construction of buildings, watched over the proper care of the gardens and animals, and so on. At the death of the head of the *maṭha,* authority over the cloister was transferred to a disciple the preceptor personally had chosen beforehand. That successor was installed and all property was transferred to his name.[87]

Perhaps the most well-known of such centers are the four *maṭhas* said to be founded by the great eighth-century Vedāntic thinker and teacher (*ācārya*), Śaṅkarācārya.[88] Said to have wandered the length and breadth of India, and seemingly impressed with the Buddhist *vihāras* that had taken hold in India by that time, Śaṅkara is remembered for the establishment of Hindu monasteries in the four extreme corners of the subcontinent: Joshi Matha at Badarinatha in the Himalaya mountains in the far northern part of the country, Shringeri Matha at Shringeri in the southern part, Sharada Matha at Dvaraka in the west, and Govardhana Matha in Puri in the east. When he founded each of these *maṭhas*, he also established the practice of ordaining especially devout and committed religious leaders into the celibate and renunciant life known as *sannyāsa*. Each *sannyāsin* was given the title "swami." He founded ten orders of such *sannyāsins*, including the Sārasvatī order into which Swami Muktananda himself was ordained as a young man twelve centuries later and therefore that order into which Swami Chidvilasananda and all other Siddha Yoga swamis have subsequently been initiated. Śaṅkara also established a lineage of teachers (a *guruparamparā*) through which the teachings would be transmitted from one generation to another through the power and example of the teacher's own learning and way of living.

THE ASHRAM IN INDIA'S LITERARY IMAGINATION

We have seen references in the preceding pages to spiritual disciplines practiced in quiet retreats in religious literature from India dating to as early as the latter part of the second millennium B.C.E. That they have been important elements of the imaginative as well as spiritual landscape in India throughout the many years since then is suggested by the fact that colorful and evocative depictions of mythic ashrams appear in the greatest and most influential works of classical Indian literature, as well as in explicitly religious and historical texts.

It is in Vālmīki's great epic the *Rāmāyaṇa*, for example, that we hear of the ashram where Lord Viṣṇu once lived. Vālmīki refers to it as a *siddha āśrama*, an "ashram of a perfected being." It "is known as the Ashram of the Perfected Being, for it was here that that great ascetic attained perfection."[89] Approaching it from a distance after traveling through a frightening wilderness, the hero Rāma notes, "I can see a dense mass of trees like a dark cloud over near that mountain." Turning to his companion, the visionary sage Viśvāmitra, Rāma asks, "What is it? I am very curious about it. It is lovely and quite charming, full of deer and adorned with all kinds of sweet-voiced birds. I gather from the pleasantness of the region, best of sages, that we have emerged from that terrifying forest. Tell me about it, holy one. Whose ashram is located here?"[90] Viśvāmitra responds that it was where Viṣṇu became incarnate as Vāmana the dwarf in order to trick the great demon Bali Vairocana, who had conquered all of the heavens, skies, and earthly realms that constitute the three worlds of the sacred universe.

Viśvāmitra then notes that since Viṣṇu "himself once dwelt here, this ashram allays all weariness."[91]

Also in the *Rāmāyaṇa* we read of the Dandaka Forest, entering which "Rāma, the self-disciplined and invincible prince, saw a circle of ashrams where ascetics dwelt. . . . [F]looded with brahmanical splendor, it was as luminous and blinding to the eye as the sun's circle in heaven." Vālmīki describes the ashram as a "a place of refuge for all creatures, its grounds were always kept immaculate. . . . Tall forest trees encircled it, holy trees that bore sweet fruit. It was a place of worship, of offerings and oblations, a holy place echoing with the sounds of *brahma,* the sacred *vedas.*" The poet continues:

> Wildflowers carpeted it, and there was a lotus pond filled with lotuses. Ancient sages were present there, temperate men who ate only roots and fruit, wore bark garments and black hides, and shone like fire or the sun. Supreme seers, holy men given to rigorous fasting, deepened its beauty. It resembled the abode of Brahmā; the sounds of *brahma,* the sacred *vedas,* echoed through it, and illustrious brahmans who knew the meaning of *brahma* deepened its beauty still further.[92]

Similar depictions of an ashram appear in a story which first appears in the great Indian epic, the *Mahābhārata* (fourth century B.C.E. to fourth century C.E.)[93] and which finds restatement in such works as the stirring and tender dramatic play many regard as the best single work of Indian literature of all time, *Abhijñānaśākuntala* ("The Recognition of Śakuntalā"), a love story by the great fifth-century C.E. Indian playwright and poet, Kālidāsa.

According to the epic version, King Duḥṣanta had set out on a hunting expedition accompanied by "hundreds of warriors carrying swords and lances, brandishing clubs and maces, wielding javelins and spears." Entering the forest, the king "wrought havoc, killing game of many kinds. Many families of tigers he laid low as they came within range of his arrows; he shot them with his shafts." He killed antelopes and deer and wild birds. Frightened and wounded elephants trampled many people. The forest became a place of death, "darkened by a monsoon of might and a downpour of arrows, its big game weeded by the king."[94]

Looking for more animals to kill, Duḥṣanta ventured farther into the forest when suddenly he came to "a vast wilderness that was dotted with holy hermitages, a joy to the heart and a feast for the eye." Here, the king noticed a "pleasantly cool and fragrant breeze that carried the pollen of flowers [and that] ran around the woods and accosted the trees as though to make love to them. Such was the woodland upon which the king gazed." Looking closer, he "saw an idyllic and heart-fetching hermitage, covered with all kinds of trees and alight with blazing [ritual] fires. Ascetics and anchorites peopled it and groups of hermits. Fire halls aplenty were scattered all over, and carpets of flowers." Seeing beasts of prey and gentle deer living in peace with each other, Duḥṣanta became "filled with the purest joy," for to him the place was "like another paradise of Indra"; it was a "hermitage that mirrored the world of Brahmā, echoing with the humming of bees and aswarm with all kinds of fowl." He heard brahmins "of boundless spirit" singing Vedic hymns, performing Vedic rituals, and "doing *pūjā* to the sanctuaries of the Gods." He learns that this is the ashram of the great yogi and teacher, Kaṇva Kāśyapa. Looking about him at "the great and sacred hermitage, protected by Kāśyapa's austerities and hallowed by the multitudes of its ascetics, he could not watch enough."

Struck by the ashram's powerful peacefulness, King Duḥṣanta decided to visit the *ṛṣi,* whom he described as "that dispassionate hermit of rich austerities" who was "surpassingly virtuous and who was of indescribable brilliance." Leaving behind weapons and royal regalia, he approached the ashram in humble dress in a manner befitting the simplicity and humility of the *ṛṣi* living there and out of respect for the residents of the ashram. Setting foot in the seer's "enchanted, holy" ashram, he "shed his hunger and thirst and became overjoyed."

In this epic version of the story, we see an explicit expression of the idea that life in an ashram is in many ways diametrically opposed to life in the world beyond its boundaries. Duḥṣanta's wanton arrogance in killing all of the animals in the forest characterizes life in a world driven by self-centeredness. Life in Kaṇva's ashram, on the other hand, is represented by images of religious discipline, peacefulness, and selfless activity. Impressed by and yearning to partake of that life, Duḥṣanta discards the weapons, takes off the royal clothing that marks his worldly might and authority, and enters the world of the ashram.

In Kālidāsa's *Abhijñānaśākuntala,* the king (whom the playwright calls Duṣyanta rather than Duḥṣanta) is perhaps a more refined young monarch. The action of the play begins with Duṣyanta out hunting in his woods, dressed in his finest regalia and accompanied by his charioteer. Seeing a single deer bounding away from him as if in flight, the king pulls the string on his bow tight and takes aim at the delicate animal. But, before he can loose his arrow, two ascetics (*tapasvin:* practitioners of *tapas*) jump out from the woods and stand between him and the deer. "This deer belongs to the ashram," one of them informs the king. "He should not be killed." They tell him to withdraw his weapon, which they say he should use to protect the weak rather than to injure the innocent. The king obeys.[95]

We see in this act of obeisance an expression of an important contrast: Duṣyanta's authority as king holds less sway over him than Kaṇva's authority as guru, represented here by the *tapasvins* who admonish Duṣyanta to put away the symbols of his royal prestige. We also note how deeply Kaṇva's teaching regarding ashram dharma has affected the residents, for the *tapasvins* resolutely continue to practice their religious disciplines even when the guru is physically absent from the ashram proper.

The ascetics tell Duṣyanta that they are collecting wood to burn in the ceremonial fires and point out to him the nearby ashram of Kaṇva, the patriarch of the sacred household (*kulapati*). Looking about himself, Duṣyanta sees some stones made slick with oil, water drops lining the pathways to nearby ponds, and deer who are not afraid of his presence. He realizes that he must indeed be near an ashram, for he infers that the stones have been used to open the nuts of the *ingudī* tree (the fruit of which was often strung into sacred necklaces worn by ascetics); the drops of water must have fallen off of the fringe of simple garments (which ascetics would have worn to perform their ritual ablutions); the deer are not afraid because they have never been threatened (since they live in an ashram, a place of peace and nonviolence). Attracted to the place, Duṣyanta takes off his royal ornaments, gives his bow to his charioteer, and approaches the ashram, which he describes as a "forest where austerities are practiced" (*tapovana*). He gives the reins of the chariot to his companion, for "there should be no distraction to the residents of the ashram." (By the way, Duṣyanta's Sanskrit is better when he speaks inside the ashram than when he is beyond its boundaries. We might say that the atmosphere in the ashram gives him a clarity of perception he lacks when outside.) Dressed in a humble manner, he turns towards the hermitage, noting as he does, "Peaceful is the site of this ashram."[96]

Soon after stepping into the ashram, Duṣyanta meets a delightful and pure young woman, Śakuntalā, and they immediately fall in love. They wish to wed, but—assuming that she must not be of the same warrior class as he—Duṣyanta worries that it would be an act of *adharma* for them to do so. But then he hears that she is actually the daughter of the great soldier-sage, Viśvāmitra, who was seduced from his own austerities by the celestial nymph, Menakā. Her parents had abandoned the young girl along the bank of the river when she was a baby, but the kind and compassionate Kaṇva found her and adopted her as his own, and she had lived ever since in the ashram. Her true parentage means that she is indeed of the *kṣatriya* class and thus able to be his wife. They marry according to what is known as the *gāndharva* rite, namely, through a mutual private affirmation of their loyalty and love. Act I ends with the report of a crazed elephant running wild nearby, threatening the peace of the forest. Heeding his responsibility to protect the people of his kingdom, Duṣyanta leaves the ashram so that he can take care of the threat. At his departure, he expresses his reverence for the ashram with one lyrical statement: "My body moves forward, but my restless heart runs backward, like the silk cloth of a banner carried against the wind."[97]

In Act II we see that Duṣyanta warns the soldiers that now accompany him to avoid distracting the residents of the ashram in any way, for "deep in ascetics' hearts, in those who are pre-eminent in peacefulness, there lies concealed a burning energy. They reveal this as if it were cool sun-jewels which are cool to the touch but which they emit when assailed by some external force."[98] We also see that Duṣyanta would like to do anything he could to stay in the vicinity of the ashram. His wish is fulfilled when two ascetics from Kaṇva's ashram ask him to protect the offertory rituals they must perform from the dangers presented by demons who were threatening them. The king is pleased to assume that responsibility.

In Act IV we see that Śakuntalā, filled with thoughts of her loved one, fails to welcome properly another visitor to the ashram, the foul-tempered Durvāsas. Angered by this apparent insult, Durvāsas inflicts a curse: Whoever is in Śakuntalā's thoughts at that very moment will not recognize her when he sees her again. Duṣyanta has had to leave the ashram and return to his kingdom at Hastinapura, not knowing that Śakuntalā had conceived a child. One of Śakuntalā's friends pleads with the curmudgeon to loosen the curse, which he does by saying that the spell will be broken if the king recognizes something from the ashram while he sits in his court at Hastinapura.

As Śakuntalā nears the end of her pregnancy, the sage Kaṇva blesses her and tells her that she must now leave the ashram to live with her husband, for she must fulfill her obligations as Duṣyanta's wife. Kālidāsa suggests here that the responsibility to others Śakuntalā learned in the ashram must now be taken to the world outside, for the ashram teaches the supreme importance of dharma itself. In touching language, Kālidāsa reports that all of the creatures of the ashram are sad to see Śakuntalā leave: The deer let fall the sweet *darbha* grass from their mouths; peacocks stop strutting and dancing; and vines drop their leaves, weeping. In describing them in this way, Kālidāsa implies that in the ashram there is a seamless relationship between the human and the natural world; the ashram thus embodies a harmonious cosmic unity of life.

Under Durvāsas's curse, Duṣyanta does not recognize his pregnant wife and orders her out of his court. Horrified, she tries to jog his memory by showing him a ring he had given her; but she is dismayed to find that the ring had slipped off her finger during the journey from the ashram to Hastinapura. Expelled from the city and lamenting her situation, she is visited by a celestial spirit, who carries her away. Duṣyanta is amazed at this incident and falls into a deep state of confusion as he ponders the identity of this mysterious and strangely familiar woman he does not recognize. He is further troubled by the fact that he has no son to whom to pass the royal responsibilities. Meanwhile, a fisherman who had found Śakuntalā's ring and been accused of its theft is brought to trial before the king. Recognizing the ring—and thereby something from the ashram—Duṣyanta is immediately released from the curse.

We might note here two ideas regarding this theme of forgetfulness and remembrance. First, because of the radical difference between life in an ashram and in the "outside" world, it is easy to forget what one has experienced in the ashram once one leaves. But, second, one can be reminded of the ashram by means that may be completely unexpected and, in this way, transport the experience of being in the ashram into one's daily life in the world.

Realizing he has lost his wife, the melancholy Duṣyanta tries to distract himself by accepting an invitation from Indra, king of the gods, to do battle with some demons who are annoying the celestials. Duṣyanta flies into combat in Indra's chariot. Returning from his successful mission, Duṣyanta sees from the vantage of the airborne chariot another ashram, that of the sage Mārīca. Entranced by the sight, he visits this ashram and encounters there a young boy who reminds him very much of himself and for whom he experiences an inexplicable love. Conversations with ashram residents slowly allow him to discover that the boy is of the Paurava clan (Duṣyanta's own, as well) and that his mother's name is Śakuntalā. When Śakuntalā herself appears, everything becomes clear to Duṣyanta: This is indeed his wife and his son.

The play ends with Mārīca's informing Duṣyanta that his son will grow up to be the most powerful king on earth. The boy is known now as Sarvadamana, "subduer of all," but since he will come to be the protector of all the world he will come to be known by the name Bharata, "protector." As Indians watching *Abhijñānaśākuntala* would know, Bharata was so great a leader that later generations of people in his kingdom came to be known as the Bhāratas, the "descendants of Bharata," and his name became the indigenous name of the land we now call India. The very title of the epic in which we find this story is the *Mahābhārata*, the "Great Bhārata," which means it is the sacred story of the people of that land.

We have lingered in the retelling of the story of Śakuntalā in order to make several points pertaining to the nature and function of the ashram and its relationship with the outside world, and because we wish to suggest that the function the ashram serves in this dramatic tale is similar in several ways to the function the ashram serves in the lives of the people who practice Siddha Yoga around the world today. We have already mentioned some of these perspectives: that the peaceful atmosphere in an ashram, where people find it easy to be nonviolent and humble, is in some ways the opposite of that found in the world in general, which tends to be filled with struggle and violence and arrogance (even Indra's heavenly world is tormented by demons); that in the ashram all people, even monarchs, are to live humbly and to treat all others with honor and respect; that all residents of the ashram are to live according to its rules; that the authority of the ashram's spiritual leader, even if he is temporarily absent, is more compelling than the authority of the most powerful leader in the secular world; that the ashram embodies a unity of being and thus provides an example of what the world could be like if people were to live their lives from such a seamless perspective; and that the world of sorrow and pain arises when one forgets the fulfillment that is found in a simple life of offering, such as that experienced in the ashram.

Some other conclusions regarding the ashram might justly be drawn from this story, as well. One is that the personal fulfillment found in living in the ashram is indistinguishable from that which comes to one who follows his or her moral obligation (dharma) to the world. Even though she has spent her life in the ashram, Śakuntalā must ultimately leave, for not only is she a wife and mother with all of the obligations these roles entail but also she is a *kṣatriya*, a member of the caste whose responsibility is to ensure that society be protected. Duṣyanta is in a similar position. This powerful king willingly surrenders his authority to Kaṇva while in the ashram, but eventually he must leave that sacred place to fulfill his responsibilities to his kingdom. This does not mean that Duṣyanta abandons the ashram or that he abnegates the authority of the head of the ashram. On the contrary, he yearns for his life in the ashram, as symbolized by his marriage to Śakuntalā; finally he comes to accept the importance of his royal dharma only when Mārīca himself, the head of an ashram, tells him that his son will grow up to be a righteous and powerful king.

In Kālidāsa's play, the ashram fundamentally resolves the apparent contradiction between the way life is and the way it ought to be. In the ashram all things are done according to the imperatives of dharma: Even the king must put down his weapons because he has improperly used them to injure rather than to protect; even the adopted daughter of the guru must perform her responsibilities as a *kṣatriya* wife and mother. Accordingly, in the ashram all things are the way they should be. The ashram is an ideal world and also a very real one, for it is here that people do live according to their dharma, the duties prescribed for them according to their role. The theme of forgetfulness seems significant here. Reminded of the ashram by the sight of his wife's ring, Duṣyanta's memory of this ideal life is restored. When one remembers the ashram, one remembers what life can be like when it is lived properly.

We might say that the opposition between the ashram and the outside world marks the difference between the sacred and the profane. In the ashram this opposition is acknowledged and then collapsed. In bringing Duṣyanta into the ashram, the *tapasvins* may be said to be bringing the profane into the sacred. Yet once in the ashram, Duṣyanta is transformed. Then the king, returning to his court, takes the ashram with him in the form of his own new outlook and in the persons of his wife and son. The transformative effect of the ashram thus spreads into the world. Indeed, without the ashram even the righteous protector of the Bhāratas themselves would not exist.

Brief reference to another work by Kālidāsa will make a similar point. In his long poem *Meghadūta,* "The Cloud Messenger," Kālidāsa describes the many sights a cloud sees as it passes over the mountains, rivers, lakes, and towns of the Indian terrain. The natural imagery here—a cloud that moves without effort or obstruction across what otherwise might stand as barriers—suggests that vision of the true nature of things is transmitted in a similar fashion. Such vision is flexible and yet constant, and its transmission can occur in the most natural of ways, for—like the cloud floating above the changing countryside below—the truth itself is a pure, untainted, primordial, and therefore timeless knowledge. As the cloud floats northward towards the sacred Himalaya mountains, it sees many ashrams populated by sages, sadhus, mendicants, monks and other religious seekers. The countryside is thus sanctified by the presence of these many ashrams. A reader of Kālidāsa's poem might note that while the many ashrams the cloud sees are located near rivers and mountains at some distance from busy cities, they are never completely isolated. This suggests the idea that even though the ashram may be removed from the pressures and concerns of the everyday world, it must not be inaccessible. The ashram thus serves as a *tīrtha,* a sacred "crossing place," or as a *setu,* a "bridge" or "dam," that both separates and links the sacred and the profane.

THE DISSOLUTION OF THE PROFANE INTO THE SACRED

Both Gurudev Siddha Peeth and Shree Muktananda Ashram serve as just that kind of special place that marks the apparent opposition between the sublime and the mundane and yet anchors and joins the power of the sublime to the everyday world itself. The power of a holy place can find expression in the simplest and purest of ways. One devotee has noted that he was inwardly moved simply by looking at the worn steps leading up to his dormitory room, when he arrived at Gurudev Siddha Peeth:

> Three years ago I had a chance to spend a month with Gurumayi at her Ashram in Ganeshpuri. It was my first time in Ganeshpuri and I was entranced by the beauty and power of the many sacred places in the Ashram. I was also amazed to find feelings of reverence even in the most humble settings. I particularly remember those feelings on the morning I arrived, when I was taking my bags up to my room in the Mukteshwar dormitory. The stone stairs were indented from the footsteps of the thousands of devotees who had walked

> them on their way to or from seva, a chant, meditation, or a darshan with Baba or Gurumayi. Those simple, worn steps glowed with the love of the devotees for the Guru. Every day of the month I spent in Ganeshpuri, whenever I saw those steps I felt inspired in my own sadhana. To this day, when I think of them, I feel uplifted.[99]

Gurudev Siddha Peeth is located between the small villages of Ganeshpuri and Vajreshwari, about 70 miles northeast of the bustling city of Bombay, in an ancient volcanic region near the base of Mandagni ("Fire Mountain") and near the banks of the Tejasa River (the name suggests that it is filled with *tejas*, "light"). Tradition holds that this area has been a great Shakti Peeth (Sanskrit, *śaktipīṭha*: "seat of divine power" or "seat of accomplished beings") since time immemorial. Lord Rāma's guru himself, Vasiṣṭha, is said to have performed great *yajñas* in this powerful place. Throughout history, ascetic Indian sages and saints have ventured through the thick jungles to come to this special area, which they are understood to have sanctified even more with the effect of their *tapasya*. The siddha guru Dattātreya and his followers are said to have stayed here some time in the long mythic past, as are many of the gurus in the Navanātha lineage of the great thirteenth-century Maharashtrian poet-saint Jñāneśvar. Also untold numbers of anonymous siddhas are believed to have meditated in their own private hermitages on the slopes of Mandagni and near the hot springs that bubble out of the ground along the bank of the Tejasa. Accordingly, the area came to be regarded not only as a *śaktipīṭha* but as a Siddha Peeth (Sanskrit, *siddhapīṭha*) as well.

The ashram received its name—originally Shree Gurudev Ashram and then changed in 1978 to Gurudev Siddha Peeth—from Swami Muktananda in honor of his own guru, Bhagawan Nityananda, to whom Muktananda devotedly referred as Gurudev, "divine teacher." A holy wanderer wearing nothing but a small loincloth, Nityananda had come to the area in the 1930s, from Kerala and Karnataka states in the south. A firm, austere, and yet deeply compassionate and loving man, Nityananda attracted followers from Bombay, indeed, from any place through which he had traveled. People found that his influence radically changed their lives. Many who had been moved or transformed by Nityananda would travel up the wild river valley to receive his darshan and to sit for a moment in his quiet presence. His followers would give him food and clothing as gifts, which he in turn immediately gave to the *ādivāsīs*, the "original people," of the area. Initially there were no roads in the jungle, but over the years a small footpath grew to become a muddy lane to accommodate the many pilgrims coming to see the reclusive sage. A small village arose to support those pilgrims. Since tradition holds that an ancient temple to Gaṇeśa lay buried under the area, the town came to be known as Ganeshpuri, the "city of Lord Gaṇeśa."

Swami Muktananda, himself an inveterate religious mendicant—he described himself as having "wheels for feet"—came to Ganeshpuri in the late 1940s to receive Nityananda's darshan.[100] Following his experience of shaktipat (Sanskrit, *śaktipāta*), Muktananda underwent intense sadhana in Chalisgaon, Yeola, and other places, during which time he would return to Ganeshpuri once or twice a year to visit Nityananda. When in the area, Muktananda tended to stay in a small temple dedicated to the goddess Vajreśvarī in a tiny village of the same name (Vajreshwari) about two miles from Ganeshpuri, from which he would walk to receive his guru's darshan. In roughly 1949, Nityananda asked some of his followers to build a three-room hut near a small temple to Gāvdevī, a local goddess, about a mile from Ganeshpuri, on the way to Vajreshwari. Muktananda continued to wander throughout India. Then, in 1952, Nityananda asked some of his followers to deliver a message to Muktananda. "Come and stay in the three rooms at Gavdev," he told the mendicant *sannyāsin*; "those are meant for you." Muktananda did stay in those rooms for about a year before yielding to the urge to wander again. At times nobody knew where he was.[101] Finally, in November of 1956, Nityananda sent another message to Muktananda. "Come back to Ganeshpuri and stay here," he said. Following these instructions, the itinerant sadhu returned.

Under Nityananda's direction, a trustee of the Bhimeshwar Mahadev Trust, which supported Nityananda's work, arranged to have a two-acre paddy field behind the hut filled and smoothed. Here, Muktananda began to plant a variety of flowers, shrubs, creepers, and trees. In the hot and dry summers, Muktananda watered the young plants with water he carried in jugs from the community well on an adjacent lot of land. He and a few workers built a fence around the rooms and the garden, forming a small compound.

Nityananda's devotees would pass by this small hut and its beautiful garden on their way to visit him at his own retreat near the Śiva temple in nearby Ganeshpuri. There, they would often find Swami Muktananda "tending the garden, pruning and watering and tying the flowering creepers into arches. He loved gardening and soon the visitors started to share this love with him and began bringing different plants and tools."[102] Other times they might see him sitting at the entrance to his small compound. Reports are that Muktananda invariably smiled warmly at each person and joined with them in conversation about the many practices, possibilities, issues, and problems of spiritual sadhana. He was fluent in Kannada, Marathi, and Hindi, and was well-read in the scriptures of Vedānta, Yoga, and Kashmir Śaivism, as well as with the devotional songs of the poet-saints of western and northern India. A skilled adept at *haṭhayoga*, he was also a superb nutritionist and herbalist, and was well-versed in the theory and applications of Āyurveda and other medicinal practices. Passersby found him to be an attractive, good-natured, highly accomplished, and yet humble and unpretentious yogi. An early disciple reports—

> [that he usually] would be sitting on a wooden box, clean-shaven head and face, wearing a *mālā* of large *rudraksha* beads, bare-chested with just an old *lungi* around his waist and wooden *paduka*[s] on his feet. His lustrous eyes, stirring voice and hearty laughter immediately struck the visitors, and nobody would have guessed that this healthy and well-built young sadhu was fifty years old.[103]

Soon three or four people began to stay with Muktananda, and others would visit for a few days at a time in his hermitage, which began to function more and more as a classic ashram. From the very beginning, Swami Muktananda made certain that Gurudev Siddha Peeth was a true ashram in the literal sense, namely, not only a calm and peaceful place that destroys fatigue but more importantly an intense and focused place where seekers diligently practice spiritual disciplines. "The entire ashram schedule—getting up early, meditating, chanting, working—should become a part of you," he told his followers in the early 1970s; "it should enter into your blood-stream and circulate throughout your entire body. You should begin to inwardly relish the chants, meditation, remembrance of the Lord, and the *Guru Gita*."[104] Writing in 1972 about her early years with Swami Muktananda, one disciple recalled:

> Those were days of wonderful peace. The homely, uncomplicated and rustic atmosphere of the compact little Ashram, its cool and fragrant air, the beautiful garden surrounded by fields and mountains all around, silent except for the rustle of the wind in the leaves and an occasional bird, and Swamiji's company—his inspiring and profound talks, sitting close to his loving presence—made it almost impossible for the devotees to tear themselves away and return to their everyday lives in the cities and towns.[105]

A young woman from Italy said this of her first stay at Gurudev Siddha Peeth in 1994:

> The first day I was in the ashram, I felt kind of negative about being there. I thought, "Maybe I won't stay here two whole months." I wasn't sure I could handle it: living in a dorm with twenty people, getting up early in the morning. The second day I went for a walk in the gardens, and then I started loving the ashram. It was so beautiful. I realized I didn't have to know how long I would stay; I could just take it all as it came.
>
> I spent a lot of time by myself, and that was very useful. I began to be very quiet. There was a lot of opportunity to be silent there: in the dining hall, you don't talk; at seva, you don't talk that much; when you chant, you don't talk. I began to have relationships with people that went much deeper than just

> words. I would see people I knew and we would smile at each other, without words, and there would be so much love flowing between us.
>
> As the days went by, I started feeling more and more in tune with the rhythm of the ashram: I went to the *Gurugītā* every morning, I did seva, I took courses. Mainly, I felt more inward. I started having feelings that I usually kept locked inside me. Sometimes it was ecstasy, sometimes depression, sometimes the flow of love between me and the Guru and other people, all held in the cradle of this beautiful, disciplined life.[106]

In 1970 Swami Muktananda built a veranda around his rooms so that his followers could sit in the shade while meditating. Other buildings and additions followed: Turiya Mandir was built along with a dining hall, a library, dormitories, sheds to house the growing number of ashram animals. More acres were added to the expanding gardens. The ashram continued to grow. A field was cleared so that brahmins could perform *yajñas* under temporary tents. Then, those tents were replaced by a permanent open-air pavilion designed to hold hundreds of people watching the performance of those ancient ceremonies. What began as a three-room hut grew to become Gurudev Siddha Peeth, an ashram that now stands like a well-kept university, with verdant gardens crossed by paved footpaths and dotted with buildings containing classrooms, vast auditoriums, dining facilities, dormitories, and other housing units.

Over the years, Nityananda had insisted that the legal title for the buildings and the land be transferred to Swami Muktananda's name. Reports are that Muktananda may have felt somewhat uncomfortable with this arrangement. An early Indian disciple put it this way:

> Swami Muktananda was however a *Sannyasi.* Ever since the age of fifteen he had travelled far and wide, from the lofty Himalayas in the North to the dark and rainy South, with only the *sannyasi*'s impedimenta, that is, the staff, *kamandalu* and saffron cloth; his head full of the scriptures, his strong heart full of the courage and strength of an enduring faith in God. . . . His spirit was that of a free traveller seeking the wide world for God. He rarely stayed in one place for long. Was the lion to be caged? Was the eagle to be chained?[107]

Accepting the responsibility given to him, Swami Muktananda oversaw the rapid growth of the ashram and attended personally to every detail to ensure that it was administered properly. After Nityananda's death in 1961, Muktananda established the Shree Gurudev Ashram Trust, which he registered under the Bombay Trust Act of 1950, and transferred his financial and legal authority to the trustees of that Trust. The *sannyāsin* who had temporarily owned property had given it all away again. Once more, he had nothing to own. The financial and legal affairs of Gurudev Siddha Peeth are still administered by that Trust.

Like Nityananda, Muktananda reached out to and cared for the *ādivāsīs* and other poor people of the area. With a medical van and supplies given to him by some of his followers, in 1978 Muktananda established a mobile hospital that has continued to bring free health care ever since to villagers in the surrounding valley. He also saw to it that several hundred sturdy houses were supplied to the *ādivāsīs* at cost (he felt that to give the houses to them outright might make them feel dependent and thus undignified) and that these houses were supplied with electricity, proper sewage, and clean drinking water. Such continuing seva projects and others stand as the prototypes for a number of other ongoing community health endeavors such as the establishment and running of regular eye camps in which skilled surgeons perform cataract surgery with intraocular lens implantations for local people who otherwise could not afford this, and a program in which free milk is distributed daily to hundreds of local village schoolchildren. These and other humanitarian projects have been and continue to be administered with Swami Chidvilasananda's blessings by an umbrella organization known as The PRASAD Project, and its Indian arm, PRASAD Chikitsa.

In 1975 Swami Muktananda established a second Siddha Yoga ashram in an impoverished inner-city neighborhood in Oakland, California. On the surface, the character of this ashram's rough physical environment was the opposite of Gurudev Siddha Peeth's truly sylvan and bucolic setting in Ganeshpuri. Muktananda seems however to have felt that it was an appropriate site for his ashram, for he expressed much enthusiasm for it and dedicated a great deal of energy to it. He insisted that life in the Oakland Ashram be as disciplined as that in Gurudev Siddha Peeth, and welcomed visitors from the surrounding neighborhood and cities to take part in the sadhana and seva practiced therein. The presence of the ashram soon began to have a transformative effect on the urban blight that surrounded it. Broken glass began to be swept off of the streets, flowers began to appear in neighboring yards, window sills on local houses smiled under fresh coats of paint. It seemed that the *śakti* of the ashram was moving through the neighborhood, cleansing and burnishing it, bringing it to its full beauty.[108]

Like Gurudev Siddha Peeth and Shree Muktananda Ashram (which was inaugurated in 1979), the Oakland Ashram continues to demonstrate the powerful quality of *ā-śrama* in both meanings of the word: It brings fulfillment and meaning to devotees' lives not only because it serves as a setting for their selfless service to the larger community but also because it gives them a focused context in which to pursue their own diligent spiritual work on themselves. Speaking of time she spent in the Oakland Ashram, a devotee has said:

> In the 1970s the Oakland Ashram was established in a run-down neighborhood, riddled with the suffering of disrupted social, economic, and family

> structures. The Ashram community was creating a vegetable garden in one of the vacant lots which had been paved in broken glass and discarded automobile parts. Once, when I was spending time there, I had the seva of weeding and tending to the rows of carrots. The sun was bright and the earth, which had been prepared by the ashramites, smelled fertile and was filled with mantra. I spent the day squatting among the green heads of the carrots, tending, weeding, pulling, and chanting. That evening during the program, as we chanted and then closed our eyes to meditate, the green leafy carrot heads began to appear before me; then they opened up into a magnificent shower of light, widening and widening, wave after wave like an enormous display of fireworks, filling the sky of my inner vision. The light kept coming and bursting in ecstatic showers and I became completely absorbed in the playful ecstasy. Where had it come from, this extraordinary experience described in the rhapsodies of the great mystics? I hadn't been looking for it. I had simply spent the day weeding a garden carved from the concrete of Oakland, California. But for several years I had been living in the ashram of a Siddha and following the practices he prescribed. It was by the grace of his power and knowledge, and the strength and support of the ashram life, that the vision of my own ecstatic light had been given to me.[109]

Between 1976 and 1981, Swami Muktananda established other Siddha Yoga ashrams in New York City, New Delhi, Melbourne, Boston, Sydney, and Mexico City. In 1975 he established the Siddha Yoga Dham Associates (SYDA) Foundation, originally based in Oakland, to serve as the legal name and as the financial trust that would support his work. In 1979 the SYDA Foundation purchased and began extensive renovations on the former Gilbert Hotel in South Fallsburg in the Catskill Mountains of New York. Here, Swami Muktananda established the international offices that administered Siddha Yoga programs around the world. This was also to become Shree Nityananda Ashram and, accordingly, a place of intense spiritual discipline and selfless service. A former ballroom was converted to a large meditation room. Swami Muktananda planned and oversaw the construction of a beautiful temple honoring Bhagawan Nityananda. In 1983 another former hotel nearby, the Windsor, was converted to more dormitory and office space. In 1985 construction began on an immense open-air pavilion known as the Shakti Mandap, where *smārta yajña*s are performed around fires blazing in a ceremonial pit. The grounds were planted with many varieties of flowers, shrubs, and trees. Quiet walkways and trails were built in the neighboring forests leading up to an expansive hilltop known as Mount Kailas and to a large dormitory and residential complex a half-mile distant known as Atma Nidhi ("treasure of the soul"), the former Brickman Hotel, which the SYDA Foundation purchased and renovated in 1986. Legal and financial management was administered by the SYDA Foundation itself. This arrangement continues today.

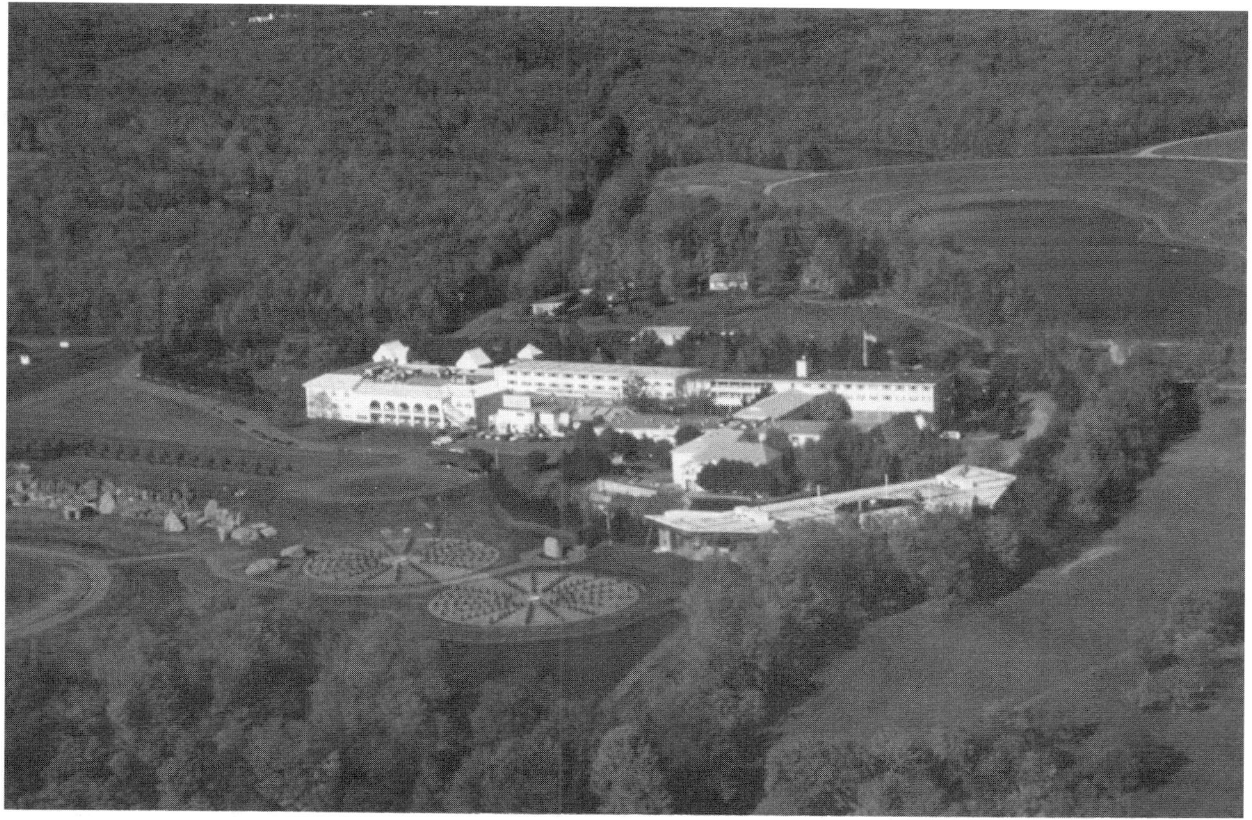

Figure 30. An aerial view of Anugraha, the oldest facility at Shree Muktananda Ashram, October 1996

After Swami Muktananda's death in 1982, Swami Chidvilasananda changed the name of Shree Nityananda Ashram to Shree Muktananda Ashram. Her devotees regard the Shree Muktananda Ashram as a genuine *siddhapīṭha* filled with the grace and transformative power of the universal *śakti* that is so evident to them at Gurudev Siddha Peeth. Life in both Gurudev Siddha Peeth and Shree Muktananda Ashram, first under Swami Muktananda's and now under Swami Chidvilasananda's direction, is similar in many ways to that of an ancient Indian *gurukula*; when they are in these ashrams, students are in the "guru's house." Under the guru's personal guidance, *sādhakas* practice the many different components of spiritual discipline and study many subjects pertaining to that discipline. Such discipline leads to the devotee's fuller recognition and celebration of his or her own inner dignity.

The innate divinity of one's very being: This is a central message Swami Muktananda and now Swami Chidvilasananda have taught over and over again. Life in these teachers' ashrams reflects the importance they place on their devotees' experience and subsequent responsible expression of such inner worth. The entire sum of such expressions constitutes a distinct "ashram culture," which has its own history and *raison d'être.* In the 1960s and early 1970s Swami Muktananda attracted a good number of vagabond and itinerant spiritual seekers from the West, some of whom had rejected what they may have felt were stultifying social norms regulating dress and personal hygiene. He accepted them, encouraged them, and treated them with honor and dignity, just as he did people from all economic strata of India and other Asian societies. He did insist, however, on cleanliness. Everyone in the ashram was to bathe every day, and their clothes were to be modest and clean—the latter not always being an easy task in the hot dusty climate of Indian summers or in the virtually continuous rain of the monsoon. In 1975, while in his ashram in Oakland, Muktananda began to teach that one's way of dressing reflects the respect one feels for oneself and for others, and that sometimes the ego is just as strong in its assertion to dress in a slovenly manner as it is to dress well. After that, women devotees slowly but noticeably started wearing skirts and dresses and putting on small amounts of makeup. Men began trimming their beards or shaving them off entirely. Muktananda did not specifically instruct his followers to do so, but he reminded them to respect the Self as it appears within others as well as within oneself.[110]

The Siddha Yoga "ashram culture" reflects the importance of self-respect in many other ways, for ashram dharma in general expresses this value and fosters its cultivation. Both Swami Muktananda and Swami Chidvilasananda have insisted, for example, that devotees are not to go into financial debt in order to live in the ashram, for to go into debt in this way does not show respect for one's responsibilities to oneself and others. Similarly, the music that is performed during formal programs at the ashram is expertly played; it, too, reflects the respect the musicians have for themselves, their fellow devotees, and their guru. The various halls and pavilions are kept immaculately clean, as are the grounds and gardens. Siddha Yoga's monthly magazine, *Darshan*, is an attractive and well-edited publication. People are expected to clean the area in which they ate before leaving the dining table and to make their bed every morning before the *Gurugītā* chant. Bedrooms and bathing areas are to be kept clean. Muktananda and Chidvilasananda have insisted that there be no material waste at their ashrams; even note paper is recycled.

For a period of some years in the late 1980s and early 1990s the atmosphere at both Gurudev Siddha Peeth and at Shree Muktananda Ashram changed somewhat. More and more people wished to visit these two ashrams, which were coming to be even more widely known for their peaceful beauty and openness to guests. However, ashram residents spent more and more time administering to these visitors—preparing their food, cleaning their dishes, tending to their housing needs—and consequently less and less time on their own sadhanas. They did so willingly, but Swami Chidvilasananda and the two ashrams' Executive Management Councils came to see that the ashrams were beginning to serve more as traditional *dharmaśālās* (temporary rest stations for a large number of pilgrims on a pilgrimage elsewhere) than as autonomous spiritual centers in which students not only performed seva but intensely practiced the contemplative aspects of sadhana. Accordingly, in 1994, Swami Chidvilasananda began to shift the mood at the ashrams back to the more traditional *gurukula* model. Since then, ashram residents have been more like traditional Indian *antevāsins*, *śiṣyas*, and *adhikārins* who demonstrate their seriousness in pursuing their sadhana under the tutelage of the guru. The result is that once again the atmosphere at both ashrams is remarkably peaceful and quiet and yet filled with the fervent energy of spiritual discipline.

Due to their responsibilities elsewhere, some people may be able to stay at Gurudev Siddha Peeth or Shree Muktananda Ashram for just a few days at a time. On the other hand, some people have lived in these ashrams for years. Once there, each individual seeker's personal experiences of an ashram will of course be different in some ways. But it is fair to say that no matter how long they stay, many find it difficult to leave when they must. Perhaps they feel like King Duṣyanta, as we may recall, when he was called from Kaṇva's ashram to take care of his obligations as king. Duṣyanta said, "My body moves forward, but my restless heart runs backward, like the silk cloth of a banner carried against the wind."[111] Perhaps those seekers might feel somewhat better if they remember, like Duṣyanta when he saw the ring, that the special time in the ashram can always be recalled in the memory in unexpected, transforming, and supremely fulfilling ways. Remembering it,

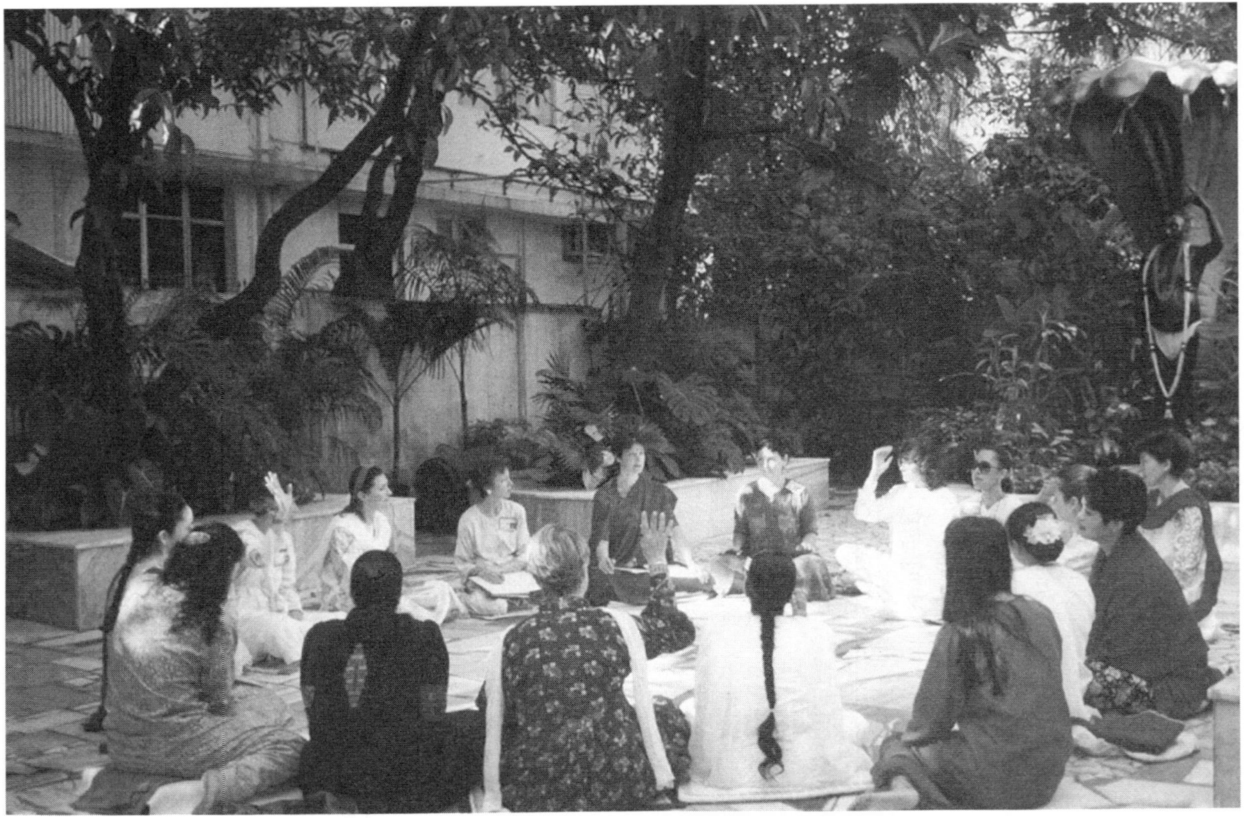

Figure 31. A scriptural discussion group in the courtyard at Gurudev Siddha Peeth

they can keep the spirit of the ashram with them wherever they are. As both Duṣyanta and Śakuntalā found out, it was in the ashram that they learned more fully just what their true dharma in the larger world was. Because of their experience *in* the ashram, Duṣyanta and Śakuntalā could see their true worth as people who must by necessity live *outside* of the ashram. Similarly, life in Gurudev Siddha Peeth or Shree Muktananda Ashram can allow a modern-day Duṣyanta or Śakuntalā to see that a truly meaningful life is one in which a person sees his or her own inner Self as filled with inherent dignity and worth, no matter where he or she lives. Might we rephrase this to say that the ashram allows one to see all of one's life from the perspective of "the sacred"?

In collapsing the distinction between the sacred and the profane by enveloping all within the sacred, the ashram thus demystifies itself. It becomes an open door to the very sanctity of what otherwise might be experienced as mundane. After a month in Gurudev Siddha Peeth, following the daily discipline of chanting, meditating, and offering *gurusevā*, the English professor we mentioned at the beginning of this chapter wrote:

> It occurred to me that I had never been in a less mysterious place, and that my journey had come full circle. The hot bright days, the simple decor of the meditation halls, the immaculate gardens with their temples and statues and their groves of fruit trees, were the setting for an exercise in self-knowledge that was not alien or occult, but simply human. If there was a mystery here, it was in myself; if there was a "secret," I was it. As for Baba, his power lay precisely in his lack of mystery. If he was a wizard, he was a wizard of the ordinary, and that was the mystery.
>
> The feeling of inner spaciousness that settled over me when I sat to meditate, and the moments of absorption when the inner and outer spaces no longer seemed quite so separate, as if a membrane of self-definition had suddenly become porous and the currents of life were mingling freely through it, these were not Indian or Eastern experiences; they were simply ways of being human. In a certain sense I was not in India at all, certainly not in some exotic ritual setting. I was in myself, or, alternatively, I was in the world.[112]

Part of sadhana necessarily involves the seeker's diligent willingness to continue practicing at home or anywhere else the spiritual disciplines he or she has undertaken in the ashram. Doing this, the *sādhaka* will come to regard all places as the ashram; for, as we suggested earlier, while at first it establishes an opposition between the sacred and the mundane, the ashram itself finally dissolves that distinction. Speaking to an American devotee who was leaving Gurudev Siddha Peeth, Swami Muktananda had this to say:

> When you return to the States you should follow the same schedule. There also, you should work for seven to eight hours every day wherever you can find

> work, in an office or elsewhere. Then you should meditate a little every day with a calm mind. Live a regular life, and if you do that you will always live in the Ashram. The Ashram is not just this that you see; the entire cosmos is an Ashram. This attitude will be good for you.[113]

According to Muktananda's vision, there is ultimately no place that is not an ashram for those who work diligently at spiritual discipline. These practices, taught by the many siddhas in the long history of Indian spirituality, lead finally to the transforming and liberating experience of the divine: meditation, prayer, selfless service, chanting the names of God, studying the sacred texts, treating each other compassionately and without violence, cultivating mental and physical health. "Continue to cleanse yourself by *tapasya* with full eagerness," Swami Muktananda has said.[114] The teachings of Siddha Yoga maintain that to practice these disciplines is to honor the divine Self, which is the ground of all being and which accordingly dwells within the heart of all creatures, including one's own.

Such honor can be expressed in any place at any time. Siddha gurus have taught that such *tapasya* leads to a radical change in the way one lives and perceives one's life in general, a shift that allows one to experience love burning deep within one's own being. According to those teachers, that love is timeless and yet ever-new, and to experience it sets the heart free. Swami Chidvilasananda has said:

> This life-transformation is not just in the way you think; it is not just a transformation in the way you fold your clothes or drive your car or go to sleep. It is an absolute transformation. It makes you feel . . . as if you have a new self. Tapasya allows us to become new once again. There is such bliss in the newness of our own being, such ecstasy in newly experiencing the love that has been inside us all along.[115]

Siddha Yoga holds that to honor the divine is also to live in love with God, a state of being which Swami Chidvilasananda describes as the purpose of meditation itself: "The goal of meditation," she says, "is nothing but living constantly in the supreme love for God."[116] One need not be in the physical ashram to cultivate and experience this inward love and to express it outwardly in the form of selfless service to others. As Swami Muktananda has said:

> [O]nce you have lived in the ashram, once you have recognized your own Self, then you can live anywhere you want, and still be happy. Wherever you go, consider that place the ashram. Consider the entire world the ashram. No matter where you go, keep your actions very clean and clear, and your heart very pure.[117]

Appendix 1
Siddha Yoga Publications

The Siddha Yoga teachings have been widely disseminated in books written by Swami Muktananda and Swami Chidvilasananda and in periodicals published by Siddha Yoga ashrams and by SYDA Foundation. The list below, which gives the title and first date of publication, includes some of Swami Muktananda's earliest writings, which were in pamphlet form, and the date of English translations for books first published in Hindi or Gujarati. It does not attempt to document exhaustively the translation of the various works into additional languages. Siddha Yoga books now appear in fifteen languages, including Chinese, Polish, and Russian, as well as Indian languages such as Marathi and Tamil.

Swami Muktananda

Guru Darshan (Hindi) (Later published as "Guru-premamrit," a chapter in *Light on the Path*)	1959
Adesh (Hindi) ("Commandments"; English translation, 1963)	1962
Paramartha Prakash (Hindi) ("Light on the Path")	1967
Light that Leadeth: *Extracts from the Writings of Swami Muktananda*	1968
Bhagawan Nityananda (Hindi) (English translation, 1972)	1968
Ashram Darshan (Hindi) (English translation, *Ashram Dharma,* 1975; published in Hindi as *Ashram Dharma,* 1982)	1968
Lalleshwari (Hindi) *Rendered by Swami Muktananda* (English translation, 1981)	1968
Swadhyaya Yoga (Hindi)	1968

Mukteshwari, Part I (Hindi) (English translation, 1972)	1969
So'ham Japa (Hindi) (English translation, 1972)	1969
Yoga Upasana (Hindi)	1970
Chitshakti Vilas (Hindi)	1970
Guru (First English translation, abridged)	1971
Light on the Path (English translation) (With an additional essay)	1972
Chitshakti Vilas (English, unabridged) (Republished as *Play of Consciousness*, 1974)	1972
Paramartha Katha Prasang: (Gujarati) *Spiritual Conversations with Swami Muktananda* (English translation, 1981)	1972
Mukteshwari, Part II (Hindi) (English translation, 1973)	1973
Gems from Ganeshpuri	1973
Satsang with Baba, Vol. 1 (Questions and Answers)	1974
Getting Rid of What You Haven't Got	1974
Siddha Meditation	1975
I Love You	1975
Satsang with Baba, Vol. 2	1976
Selected Essays	1976
What Is an Intensive?	1976
A Book for the Mind	1976
Satsang with Baba, Vol. 3	1977
Satsang with Baba, Vol. 4	1978

Satsang with Baba, Vol. 5	1978
In the Company of a Siddha	1978
God Is with You	1978
I Am That	1978
Play of Consciousness (Retranslation of *Chitshakti Vilas*)	1978
I Welcome You All with Love	1978
To Know the Knower	1979
Kundalini: The Secret of Life	1979
Meditate (Chapter by Swami Chidvilasananda added in 1991)	1980
Reflections of the Self	1980
Kundalini Stavah	1980
Secret of the Siddhas	1980
The Perfect Relationship	1980
The Self Is Already Attained	1981
Does Death Really Exist?	1981
Where Are You Going? A Guide to the Spiritual Journey	1981
The Mystery of the Mind	1981
The Glory of the Guru	1983
I Have Become Alive	1985
From the Finite to the Infinite (Questions and Answers, 2 Vols.)	1989
Bhagawan Nityananda of Ganeshpuri (New material added to *Bhagawan Nityananda*)	1996

Swami Chidvilasananda

Kindle My Heart	1989
Ashes at My Guru's Feet	1990
Siddha Yoga Diksha (Hindi)	1991
My Lord Loves a Pure Heart: The Yoga of Divine Virtues	1994
Inner Treasures	1995
The Yoga of Discipline	1996
The Magic of the Heart: Reflections on Divine Love	1996

Books of Contemplations

Everything Happens for the Best	1993
Blaze the Trail of Equipoise	1995
Resonate with Stillness: Daily Contemplations from the Words of Swami Muktananda, Swami Chidvilasananda	1995
Be Filled with Enthusiasm and Sing God's Glory	1996

Texts for Scriptural Recitation

Swadhyaya Sudha (Hindi) (English translation, 1972, retranslated and issued as *The Nectar of Chanting*, 1975)	1968
Vishnu Sahasranama	1972
Shree Rudram	1978
Shree Guru Gita As sung in the ashrams of Swami Muktananda. (With Devanagari and English translation)	1981
Kundalini Stavah, Bhaja Govinda	1986
The Power of Chanting	1990
Arati	1996

Books Commemorating Tours

Swami Muktananda in Australia	1971
American Tour 1970	1974
Sadgurunath Maharaj ki Jay	1975
Baba's Shakti	1976
Muktananda Thanks You	1976
Dhyana Chakra	1976
Transformation: On Tour with Gurumayi Chidvilasanda, Vol. 1	1985
Transformation: On Tour with Gurumayi Chidvilasanda, Vol. 2	1986
Transformation: On Tour with Gurumayi Chidvilasanda, Vol. 3	1987
We Have Met Before: On Tour with Gurumayi Chidvilasananda	1996

Siddha Yoga Periodicals

Guruvani ("Words of the Guru")
Published annually on Guru Purnima (July) between 1964 and 1982. Until 1971 the first several articles in each issue were published in Hindi. With Vol. 6, the title changed to *Shree Gurudev-Vani.*

Siddha Vani
An annual published by Siddha Yoga Dham New Delhi from 1970 to 1981.

Shree Gurudev Ashram Newsletter (later, *Siddha Yoga*)
Published monthly. It was published as *Shree Gurudev Ashram Newsletter* from December 1971 through February 1979, as *Gurudev Siddha Peeth Newsletter* from March 1979 through January 1981, and as *Siddha Yoga* from February 1981 through January 1984.

Ashram Patrika (Hindi)
A monthly publication of Shree Gurudev Ashram (or, after 1978, Gurudev Siddha Peeth), which began with a double issue in January-February 1972. The final issue was December 1985.

Siddha Path
Began as *The Siddha Path* in August 1975. It was published monthly through No. 15 (October-November 1976), when it merged with *Baba* Magazine. It was then called

Muktananda: The Siddha Path until August 1978, when it was named, once again, *The Siddha Path.* In January 1980 it became *Siddha Path.* The last issue was September 1986.

Baba
Three issues, published in 1976.

Baba Company
Initially a quarterly that began publication with the Autumn 1977 issue. In 1981, it became bimonthly; the final issue was No. 17 (July-August 1981).

Meditate
A quarterly publication, in newspaper format, published during Swami Muktananda's third world tour (1979–82).

Siddha Yoga (Gujarati)
Published monthly by Gurudev Siddha Peeth. The first issue was a double issue appearing in January-February 1984. In January 1990, *Siddha Yoga* was redesigned to become a sister magazine to the Hindi-language *Neeleshwari.* The final issue was published in August 1992.

On Tour with Gurumayi
This periodical, which reports the events around the Guru, has taken different forms and names over the years. It first appeared in the spring of 1984 as *On Tour,* a tabloid published four times a year. From April 1987 to February 1989, "On Tour with Gurumayi" was a monthly feature in *Darshan* magazine. In March 1989, it became a supplement to the magazine, and over the next five years the name changed several times, ending with *The Siddha Path: News of Siddha Yoga Around the World.* Beginning in April 1994, *The Siddha Path* newsletter has been distributed by facsimile transmission to Siddha Yoga centers and ashrams worldwide ten to twenty times a year, depending on the need.

Young Yogi
A magazine for children, published from July 1984 to September 1986 as a supplement to *Siddha Path.*

Neeleshwari (Hindi)
The current Hindi-language magazine, published by Gurudev Siddha Peeth. The first issue was March 1987.

Darshan
The current magazine of SYDA Foundation. The first issue was April 1987; it has been published monthly, with annual double-issues during the first several years of publication.

Appendix 2
Swami Muktananda's Three World Tours

Below are the itineraries of the three tours of the West undertaken by Swami Muktananda as he set the foundation for Siddha Yoga as a worldwide movement. This information is included here for the purposes of historical documentation and the establishment of a chronological perspective for Swami Durgananda's account of the history of Siddha Yoga. Please note that often when he stayed for some length of time in a particular city, Swami Muktananda would take day trips to nearby locations to give programs and satsangs; these have not been listed. Overnight stays and the weekend meditation retreats that were a feature of the first tour, and the early months of the second tour, are mentioned, but the dates are not listed. Swami Chidvilasananda has toured nearly every year since 1983, and so a full itinerary of the Siddha Yoga gurus would be prohibitively long.

First World Tour (August 21—November 29, 1970)

August	21	Bombay
		Delhi
	22	Rome
	24	Geneva, Switzerland
		Lausanne, Switzerland
	27	St. Genis Laval, France
	29	Paris
	31	London
September	3	New York (During his New York stay, Muktananda held retreats every weekend in September at Big Indian in the Catskill Mountains.)
October	1	Boston
	2	New York
	3	Dallas, Texas
	8	Houston, Texas
	9	Los Angeles
	14	Big Sur, California
	15	Oakland, California
	19	Salt Lake City, Utah
		Logan, Utah

	23	Oakland, California (with a retreat in the Santa Cruz Mountains)
	30	Los Angeles (with a retreat in the San Bernadino Mountains)
November	3	Honolulu, Hawaii
	9	Melbourne, Australia
	25	Singapore
	28	Madras
	29	Bombay

Second World Tour (February 26, 1974—October 9, 1976)

1974

February	26	Ganeshpuri, India
		Bombay
		Singapore
March	1	Perth, Australia
	8	Melbourne
	29	St. Helens, Tasmania
April	2	Sydney
	12	Honolulu, Hawaii
	13	Piedmont, California (with three retreats in La Honda)
May	30	Pasadena, California (with three retreats in Calabassas and Los Angeles)
July	1	Piedmont, California (with a retreat in La Honda)
	11	Portland, Oregon
	15	Seattle, Washington (with a retreat in Olympia)
	22	Piedmont (with a retreat in La Honda)
	30	Honolulu, Hawaii (with retreats near Kaneohe, Oahu, and in Makawao, Maui)
August	8	Piedmont, California
	9	Denver, Colorado (with a retreat in Evergreen, two retreats in Elbert, and the first Intensive in Aspen on August 27–30)

September	2	Oklahoma City, Oklahoma (with a retreat in Pink)
	9	Chicago
	13	Indianapolis, Indiana
	17	Chicago (with a retreat in Round Lake)
	23	Ann Arbor, Michigan (with retreats in Jackson and Ortonville)
October	6	New York (with a retreat in Silver Lake)
November	21	Washington, D.C.
December	1	New York
	5	Columbus, Ohio
	9	New York
	20	Boston
	22	Atlanta, Georgia (with two retreats in Mountain City)

1975

January	13	Gainesville, Florida (with a retreat in Ocala)
	20	Miami
February	3	Los Angeles (with an Intensive at La Honda and a retreat in Calabassas)
	19	San Diego, California
	24	Los Angeles (with a retreat in Calabassas)
March	3	Honolulu, Hawaii
	10	Wailuku, Maui
	17	Honolulu
April	1	Oklahoma City (with a retreat at Lake Texoma)
	7	Houston, Texas
	14	Dallas, Texas (with a retreat in Midlothian)
	21	Albuquerque, New Mexico

	28	Oakland (with a retreat in La Honda)
July	6	Lawton, Oklahoma (for the Kiowa Society Celebration)
	7	Oakland
August	15	Arcata, California
September	3	Oakland

1976

March	28	South Fallsburg, New York
August	29	Chobham, Surrey, England
September	6	Munich, Germany
	13	Bern, Switzerland
	19	Massabielle, France
October	6	London
	9	Bombay
		Ganeshpuri, India

Third World Tour (August 18, 1978–October 21, 1981)

1978

August	18	Ganeshpuri
		Bombay
	19	Singapore
	20	Melbourne, Australia
October	23	Sydney
	28	Tokyo, Japan
		Honolulu, Hawaii
December	15	Oakland, California

1979

April	29	South Fallsburg, New York

November	1	Boston
	20	Miami, Florida

1980

May	3	Boston
	25	South Fallsburg
October	14	Santa Monica, California

1981

April	30	South Fallsburg
October	21	Ganeshpuri, India

Appendix 3
Siddha Yoga Courses and Intensives Held During the Year 1994

In the dissemination of the Siddha Yoga teachings, a curriculum has been set in place for Siddha Yoga ashrams and meditation centers around the world. Below is the curriculum of courses and Intensives offered during 1994 in Shree Muktananda Ashram in South Fallsburg, New York, and Gurudev Siddha Peeth in Ganeshpuri, India, as well as in other Siddha Yoga ashrams and centers. The year 1994 was chosen arbitrarily, for the sake of example; courses and Intensives offered in other years cover other topics. The courses vary in length from a half-day to a week or longer, and some of the study groups meet once or twice weekly for a period of several months. Most Intensives are two days in length.

The courses that are most consistently offered are those listed as "foundational courses." These courses give instruction in the core Siddha Yoga practices—meditation, *haṭhayoga*, chanting, *gurusevā*—and an opportunity to examine the basic issues that arise on the spiritual path. "Blue Pearl" courses, named for the inner light described by Swami Muktananda and others as one of the highest visions of meditation, offer advanced instruction in meditation, with a focus on uninterrupted practice. Most of these foundational courses are offered several times a year in ashrams and periodically in centers. There is also a full schedule of music courses with instruction in the instruments that accompany chanting.

The topics of "elective courses"—which are taught by Siddha Yoga swamis, teachers, or visiting university professors—change each year. Some of these courses, however, are offered the following year as "video courses" in other ashrams and centers.

"Study groups" focus on a particular scriptural text, often combining lectures with discussion groups.

Several Intensives each year are transmitted to other ashrams and centers by live audio or satellite hookup, and some of the Intensives are also offered the next year as "video Intensives." The video courses and Intensives below were held in a variety of locations; in most cases the list includes only a representation of the cities involved.

Additionally, Siddha Yoga swamis and teachers sometimes go on tours, offering courses in centers in many parts of the world.

Appendix 3

Foundational Courses

Meditation

Learn to Meditate

Siddha Meditation I
Meditation: Laying the Foundation

Siddha Yoga Meditation II
Mastering the Mind: The Yoga Sutras of Patanjali

Siddha Yoga Meditation III
Spanda: The Secret of Dynamic Meditation

Blue Pearl I
The Light of Consciousness

Blue Pearl II
Entering the Highest Inner Realms

Blue Pearl III
The World of the Thousand-Petaled Lotus

Blue Pearl IV
The Guru's Form: The Mystery of Yoga

Spiritual Philosophy and Practice

The Radiant Path: The Inner Journey

The Philosophical Traditions of Siddha Yoga

The Path of the Siddhas

The Dharma of Shaktipat

Haṭhayoga

Asana, Insight, and Transformation

How to Strengthen Your Meditation Posture

The Standing Poses

Hatha Yoga Level I
Establishing Your Practice

Hatha Yoga Level II
Steadfast in the Experience

Service

Guruseva Awareness
Nectar of Service Workshop, Levels I & II

Shree Muktananda Ashram

Elective Courses

How Am I Doing in My Sadhana?

Contemplation: The Inner Wisdom

Siddhas, Saints, and Sages

Contemplating the Guru Gita

Bhagawan Nityananda Course

The Nectar of Self-Awareness:
The Profound Practices of Kashmir Shaivism

The World Is a Play of Consciousness:
The Life and Teachings of Baba Muktananda

How Can I See God Through the Ups and Downs of Daily Life?

Kundalini Course

The Practice of Relaxation

How Can I Attain Shivadrishti?:
The Way the Lord Perceives the Universe

The Mantra Experience

The Samadhi Course:
Let Your Knowledge Turn Into Light

Study Group

When Will I Ever Be Free?
(*Vivekacūḍāmaṇi*, "The Crest-Jewel of Discrimination")

Intensives

Faith and Doubt: The Battle at the Gates of Love
(Audio broadcast in Shree Muktananda Ashram)

Awake! Rejoice! Life Is a Gift!
(Audio broadcast in Shree Muktananda Ashram)

I Am the Self Seated in the Heart of All Beings

Peace Follows Renunciation

May All the Divine Powers Make Our Two Hearts One

Everything Happens for the Best: Change Yourself!
(Audio broadcast to North and South America)

Shaktipat: The Great Awakening
(For beginners; held four times during the summer retreat)

Getting Rid of What You Haven't Got

Who Is My Guru?
(Audio broadcast to North and South America)

The Seeds of Destiny and the Fruit of Self-Effort

How Does Everything Happen for the Best?

The Light of a Thousand Suns
(Audio broadcast to North and South America)

The Bliss of Freedom: Muktananda

Siddha Yoga Meditation New Year's Intensive 1995
(Global broadcast)

Intensives on Video

Truth and Beauty: The Nature of One's Own Self

Compassion and Contentment: The Conscious Practice of Kindness

Spiritual Practice: The Delight of the Soul

Gurudev Siddha Peeth

Elective Courses

Contemplation Course

Ganeshpuri: Land of Yoga

Poet-Saints of Maharashtra

Be with Baba

Fearlessness Course

How to Face Death

Gratitude Course

Sadhana Course

The Kundalini Course

Upanishad Course

Brihadaranyaka Upanishad

Training for Teachers

Siddha Yoga Meditation Course Training

Study Groups

Katha Upanishad

Retreat

Five-Day Ganeshpuri Retreat

Intensives

Faith and Doubt:
The Battle at the Gates of Divine Love

Become Shiva by Worshiping Shiva:
Enter into the Heart of Shiva

A Life of Service:
Living for the Love of God

Siddha Yoga: The Path of Devotion

Everything Happens for the Best:
Change Yourself

The Great Power Dwells in the Guru's Command

Fullness of the Heart Invokes the Power of Protection

Getting Rid of What You Haven't Got

Muktananda—the Bliss of Freedom

May I Praise You with Every Breath

New Year's Intensive

Video Intensives and Courses Around the World

One-day Intensives

A New Beginning
Sydney, Busselton, and Port Douglas, Australia; Vienna, Austria; Biel, Switzerland; Heidelberg, Germany; Honolulu; Tokyo; Mexico City

Meditation: Entering the Kingdom of the Heart
Stockholm; Cincinnati, Ohio; Mexico City and San Jeronimo, Mexico

Eternal Bond of Love
Melbourne, Busselton, and Gold Coast, Australia; Edmundton, Canada; Munich, Germany; Rosario, Argentina; Santa Cruz, California

Two-day Intensives

The Turning Point
Paris; Munich; Puerto Rico; Anchorage, Alaska; Guadaloupe; Martinique; Curacao; Tokyo; Tahiti

Everything Happens for the Best
Held in 17 cities, including: Tournai, Belgium; Ariccia and Cordovado, Italy; Jerez, Spain

Awake! Rejoice! Life Is a Gift!
Adelaide and Melbourne, Australia; Tokyo; Wellington, New Zealand; Zurich, Switzerland; Honolulu

Faith and Doubt:
The Battle at the Gates of Divine Love
Held in 21 cities, including: Lyon and Montpellier, France; Hong Kong; Vicenza, Italy; Manila, Philippines; Las Palmas and Valladolid, Spain

Immerse Yourself in Baba's Ecstasy
Held in 32 cities, including: Fort Lauderdale, Florida; Rio de Janeiro and Sao Paulo, Brazil; Frankfurt, Germany; Guadalajara, Mexico; ChristChurch, New Zealand; Caracas, Venezuela

Courses on Video

"Be with Baba"
Held in 67 cities in 16 countries

The Bhagawan Nityananda Course
Held in 35 cities in 9 countries

Count Your Blessings with a Heart Full of Gratitude
Held in 58 cities in 13 countries

Courses Taught by Swamis or Teachers of Siddha Yoga

Fear Not, Have Faith:
A Course on Fearlessness, the Protection of a Seeker
Held in Philadelphia, Honolulu, and Portland, USA; Vancouver, Canada; Mexico City and Guadalajara, Mexico; Brisbane, Australia; Rio de Janeiro, Brazil

Pilgrimage to the Infinite I
Held in Canberra, Australia; New York, Ann Arbor, Oakland, Seattle, and Baltimore, USA; Mexico City, Mexico

The Practice of Relaxation: Body and Mind
Held in 25 cities in 8 countries

Notes

Foreword

1. Mircea Eliade, *Yoga: Immortality and Freedom,* trans., Willard R. Trask (Princeton/Bollingen Series LVI: Princeton University Press, 1969), p. 111.

2. Eliade, *Yoga: Immortality and Freedom,* p. 79.

Introduction

1. For more on the Greeks' accounts of ancient India see A. L. Basham, *The Wonder That Was India* (New York: Grove Press, 1977). Dozens of other scholarly works on this subject are also available.

2. In the contemporary West, the suspicions of insincerity and charlatanism are most frequently, I think, associated with stories of financial malfeasance or other abuses. In India, yogis are more likely feared or avoided because of their reputations for using their powers capriciously or to manipulate the vulnerable.

3. Wayne Proudfoot offers an important distinction in the study of religious experiences when he contrasts the methods of descriptive and explanatory reduction. In descriptive reductions the experiential claims are dismissed as untrue on the basis of the scholar's privileged knowledge or on scientific or historical grounds. To put this matter succinctly, what people say about themselves is false precisely for the reasons that they give. For example, a person who claims that "Zen is not a form of Buddhism" has this experience denied by the scholar who believes that Zen is, in fact, a Buddhist phenomenon. To submit the same statement to the principle of explanatory reduction the scholar must take the claim seriously as the true experience of the person making the statement. The scholar then asks, "What does this person mean when they report their experience that Zen is not Buddhism?" In explanatory reduction what people say about themselves is true but perhaps for different reasons than the ones they offer as *their own* explanations (that is, if they offer any explanations at all). This book uses the principle of explanatory reduction not to dismiss people's experiences but to cast them in a new light of understanding. See Wayne Proudfoot, *Religious Experience* (Berkeley: University of California Press, 1985).

4. See *The Bhagavadgītā in the Mahābhārata,* text and translation by J. A. B. Van Buitenen (Chicago and London: University of Chicago Press, 1981), pp. 17ff.

5. Swami Chidvilasananda, *The Yoga of Discipline* (South Fallsburg, New York: SYDA Foundation, 1996), p. 25.

6. *The Bhagavadgītā in the Mahabharata,* p. 18.

7. *The Yoga of Discipline,* p. 49.

8. The "one guru" or *ekaguru* concept does not *always* mean that an individual has but one spiritual guru, though this too is part of many traditions. Rather, it means that one needs to distinguish the one true yearning or quest for personal transformation and Self-realization from the other arts and sciences that enrich human life. While these endeavors may also be part of a person's spiritual discipline (*sādhana*), the one guru is that person (or in some cases, persons) who has the spiritual goal as his first and last agenda. The supposition of yoga traditions that include the *ekaguru* concept is that spiritual awakening and fulfillment is the *summum bonum* of human life and the very reason for having been born.

9. These requirements are described in some detail in Swami Durgananda's chapter entitled "To See the World Full of Saints: The History of Siddha Yoga as a Contemporary Movement."

10. Cf., Keshav Ramchandra Joshi, *Jnaneshwari Siddha Yoga Darshan* (Poona, India: Siddha Yoga Prakashan, 1978), written as a dissertation at the University of Poona.

11. Perhaps one of the confusing issues in the works of Swami Muktananda is that he seems to use *Siddha Yoga* in both senses, that is, as a generic term to describe the much larger phenomenon of the yoga of perfected beings and as a specific term designating his lineage transmission and teachings. It is this latter sense that is most significant since it effectively narrows the meaning and association of "Siddha Yoga" to Muktananda's lineage and his spiritual intentionality. There is every reason to believe from careful study of Swami Muktananda's works that it was his intention to use "Siddha Yoga" as a proper noun and that he indeed succeeded in creating this explicit association with his lineage. Scholars and others might still discuss the "yoga of the siddhas" in more general terms, though it seems clear that "Siddha Yoga" has now become a given name, a "sectarian name" as it were, that refers to Muktananda's spiritual intentionality (*saṅkalpa*) and his designated lineage (including the rules and criteria of succession that he set forth).

12. Certainly many of the teachings and texts that Swami Muktananda used belong to the larger Vedic and Hindu-inspired traditions. In this way it would be no more possible to define Siddha Yoga through its particular canon than it would be to use the Bible to designate only *one form* of Christianity. The Bible, like the texts of Siddha Yoga, belongs to more than one group, movement, or theological school. However, the particular intention and use of these texts, their distinctive interpretation *as a complete canon* enables us to distinguish a particular Siddha Yoga view, one that Swami Muktananda set into motion and which continues now through the work of Swami Chidvilasananda. For more on the canon of Siddha Yoga and the particular ways we might think about Siddha Yoga's scriptural resources in relation to the guru's intentionality, see the article on this subject in this volume.

13. The image and the spiritual qualities associated with the guru and the yogi are nearly as ancient as India itself. Most of the textual sources, however, for the forms of yoga the Siddha Yoga gurus draw from emerge in written forms between the seventh and sixteenth centuries. See the chapter "The Canons of Siddha Yoga: The Body of Scripture and the Form of the Guru" for a review of these sources.

14. Some scholars, including those who study the yoga of the siddhas, have been quite careful *not* to use the term *siddhayoga* in their studies precisely because they wish to include *more* than lineage of Swami Muktananda and his legacy of teach-

ings. One might see, for example, David Gordon White's *The Alchemical Body* (Chicago: University of Chicago Press, 1996). In this remarkable study of siddha lore, White does not use the compound *siddhayoga* and spares his readers any confusion between "the yoga of siddhas" and the spiritual movement of Swami Muktananda lineage known as "Siddha Yoga."

15. This claim is effectively no different than that of the Pope or the Dalai Lama who have an ultimate authority as to what is and is not accepted as the teachings of their respective "churches." Any Roman Catholic or Yellow Hat Tibetan Buddhist can say this or that about the teachings and practices of the "church," but this does not make it the "church's" view or an authorized teaching as such.

16. One important resource for understanding these boundaries and intentions is the Constitution of Siddha Yoga which Swami Muktananda composed in 1961 and which stands today as a clear statement of his principles, values, and the rules detailing such matters as the grounds for lineage succession. Part of what can be construed from this document are the legitimate claims of the continuance of Swami Muktananda's Siddha Yoga as such. In other words, Muktananda left clear directions concerning the gurus' *right* to teach, to interpret, and to extend the name "Siddha Yoga" as part of his lineage's spiritual intentionality. More about the history of Siddha Yoga can be found in this volume in Part I, written by Swami Durgananda.

17. Bhagawan Nityananda's life and legend is well-outlined in Swami Durgananda's "To See the World Full of Saints: The History of Siddha Yoga as a Contemporary Movement," while Paul E. Muller-Ortega offers some important clarifications regarding the so-called "born siddha" (*janmasiddha, saṃsiddhika siddha*) phenomenon in "The Siddha: Paradoxical Exemplar of Indian Spirituality."

18. Swami Muktananda, *Secret of the Siddhas* (South Fallsburg, New York: SYDA Foundation, 1994), p. 2.

19. *Secret of the Siddhas,* p. 2 (verse 9).

20. *Secret of the Siddhas,* pp. 1–6 (verses 1, 30, 36).

21. For a classic example of perennialism, see Aldous Huxley, *The Perennial Philosophy* (New York: Harper and Row Publishers, Inc., 1944, reprint edition 1970).

22. *Secret of the Siddhas,* p. 7 (verse 44).

23. In *Reflections of the Self* (South Fallsburg, New York: SYDA Foundation, 1993), a book in which he delineates the attitudes and behaviors that support spiritual work, Swami Muktananda writes (pp.62–63, verses 207–208):

> Awake early.
> After rising, meditate on your chosen deity.
> Eat and sleep punctually.
> Perform all your work with discipline.
>
> With great vigilance, observe good conduct.
> Be careful to bathe and to cleanse your body.
> By mastering asanas and mudras,
> bring your body, senses, and mind under your control.

24. *Secret of the Siddhas,* p. 5 (verse 24).

25. *Secret of the Siddhas,* p. 5 (verse 28).

26. *Secret of the Siddhas,* p. 5.

27. We should note that Swami Chidvilasananda has made similar statements. She has said, for instance, "Siddha Yoga is not a religion but a way of life" (unpublished transcript, December 15, 1985). Also, "This is why Siddha Yoga is not a religion. Most people think of a religion as a set of rules enforced by a god who punishes you for every mistake. It is a very limited understanding. In Siddha Yoga this is why we always say, open your mind, open your heart, open your inner world. Siddha Yoga is the inner journey to the heart." (Unpublished transcript, March 8, 1991).

28. *Secret of the Siddhas,* p. 2 (verses 7–9).

29. *Secret of the Siddhas,* pp. 2–3 (verse 10).

30. *Secret of the Siddhas,* p. 3 (verse 16).

31. We might apply two of the better known definitions of religion to Siddha Yoga to test our own claim that Swami Muktananda's statement that Siddha Yoga is not a religion does not mean that Siddha Yoga fails to conform to criteria that scholars have used to define religions. Seen from this vantage point, Muktananda's statement is a *religious statement* offered from within the contexts of his distinctive religious world view.

For a sociological definition of religion, we can turn to the classic formulation of Émile Durkheim in his *The Elemental Forms of the Religious Life.* Here religion is defined by the community's collective understanding of the distinction between sacred and profane, not as categories of existents or things but rather as modes of interaction.

Melford Spiro offers another definition, one equally rooted in observable criteria and yet more theologically focused. His definition centers on the cultural postulation principle of the relationship between human beings and what he calls superhuman beings.

32. *Secret of the Siddhas,* p. 1.

33. *Secret of the Siddhas,* p. 8.

34. This distinction of Left and Right Currents is generally one associated with so-called "Tantric" traditions. The word *tantra* (and related forms) is perhaps even more loaded and misunderstood than *guru* or *yoga.* (For a detailed study of this problem see Douglas Renfrew Brooks, *The Secret of the Three Cities: An Introduction to Hindu Śākta Tantrism* (Chicago: University of Chicago Press, 1990). Siddha Yoga, as we shall come to understand in the following essays, is what Indological scholarship calls a "*guruvāda,*" or a guru-based tradition, and has much in common with Tantric traditions and the particularly useful distinction of Right and Left Currents as it is spelled out here. More subtle distinctions from within the Indian mystical traditions are also considered in subsequent chapters; for example, Siddha Yoga's deep interest in Kashmiri Śaivism and the work of Abhinavagupta does not mean that Siddha Yoga belongs to the Trika school or Kaula tradition [Cf., Paul E. Muller-Ortega, *The Triadic Heart of Śiva, Kaula Tantricism of Abhinavagupta in the Non-Dual Śaivism of Kashmir* (Albany: State University of New York Press, 1989)].

35. Clearly in consonance with the traditions of Kashmiri Śaivism, Siddha Yoga maintains the theological position known as *svātantryavāda,* the doctrine of absolute or pure freedom.

36. The implicit criticism of the Left-Current is that their demonstrations of countering norms is not an expression of the boundary-less siddha but rather a simple boundary-breaking act that creates the very notions of boundary, compli-

ance, and defiance.

37. For the details of this situation and the reasons why Muktananda assumes this position, see Swami Durgananda's "To See the World Full of Saints: The History of Siddha Yoga as a Contemporary Movement."

38. *Secret of the Siddhas,* p. 53.

39. *Secret of the Siddhas,* p. 62.

40. *The Yoga of Discipline,* p. 103. This entire text has as one of its primary themes the subject of discipline, freedom, and an exemplary life as part of the siddha's own state.

41. *Resonate with Stillness: Daily Contemplations from the Words of Swami Muktananda, Swami Chidvilasananda* (South Fallsburg, New York: SYDA Foundation, 1995), July 10.

42. *The Yoga of Discipline,* pp. 31, 47.

43. *The Yoga of Discipline,* p. 33.

44. *The Yoga of Discipline,* p. 59.

45. In contrast to strict Śaṅkara-inspired Advaita or nondualist Vedānta, which eschews all forms, Siddha Yoga takes a view more akin to the Tantra-inspired traditions of Kashmiri Śaivism and the devotional traditions of the Bhaktas and *nirguṇi* (formless school) Sants. For more about these various traditions and resources, see the article on the canons of Siddha Yoga.

46. *The Yoga of Discipline,* p. 59.

47. See the works of Rabinow, Clifford, Sax, and Brooks as cited in the Bibliography.

48. Clifford Geertz, *Works and Lives, The Anthropologist as Author* (Stanford, California: Stanford University Press, 1988), pp. 4–5.

49. Especially important are the works of William Scott Green and Jacob Neusner, both scholars of Judaism and particularly of Rabbinic Judaism. Green and Neusner have argued that the rabbi is the key to understanding what the canon is and how it has been made sacred. See William Scott Green, "The Otherness Within," in E. Frerichs and J. Neusner, eds., *To See Ourselves as Others See Us : Christians, Jews, and "Others" in Late Antiquity* (Atlanta, Georgia: Scholars Press, 1985), and Jacob Neusner, *Midrash in Context: Exegesis in Formative Judaism* (Atlanta, Georgia: Scholars Press, 1988).

PART I. HISTORY

Chapter 1. To See the World Full of Saints

1. Swami Muktananda, *In the Company of a Siddha* (South Fallsburg, New York: SYDA Foundation, 1985), pp. 7, 36.

2. Swami Muktananda, *Secret of the Siddhas* (South Fallsburg, New York: SYDA Foundation, 1994), p. 2 (verse 9).

3. See the chapter entitled "Shaktipat: The Initiatory Descent of Power," by Paul E. Muller-Ortega, in this collection.

4. From Swami Vishnu Tirtha Maharaj, *Devatma Shakti* (Delhi, India: Swami Shivom Tirth, 1974), p. 77.

5. *In the Company of a Siddha,* p. 4.

6. *Resonate with Stillness: Daily Contemplations from the Words of Swami Muktananda, Swami Chidvilasananda* (South Fallsburg, New York: SYDA Foundation, 1995), April 5.

7. See Paul E. Muller-Ortega's articles in this volume, "Shaktipat" and "The Siddha: Paradoxical Exemplar of Indian Spirituality," for further explanations of the siddha's relationship to the process of shaktipat.

8. Swami Muktananda, *Play of Consciousness* (South Fallsburg, New York: SYDA Foundation, 1994), p. 5.

9. For a description of Siddha Yoga's definition of liberation, see Muller-Ortega's "The Siddha" in this collection.

10. Interview with Gangubai Bhopi, 1989. Much of the information on events prior to 1970 has been gained from interviews by Siddha Yoga archivists with the following people: C. N. Bagve, Gangubai Bhopi, Murlidar Dhoot, Rajgiri Gosavi, Prya & Deepa Gowramma, Yashpal Jain, Harenbhai Jokhakar, Gopal Karkera, Sri Koshandhashiti, B. D. Nagpal, Captain C. P. K. Nair, Sharada Patel, S. Ramachandran, Babu Rao Pahelvan, Swami Sevananda, Bhau Shastri Vaijapurkar, Sushila Shenoy, Babu Shetty, Shri Kaup Shetty, Vasu Shetty, Venkappanna Shriyan, Pratima Shukla, Nirmala Thakkar, Prahjiwanda Thakkar, Indutai Thia, Paraji Triambake, Prajna Trivedi, Pratap Yande. Discussion in the first two sections of this chapter draws on these various sources.

11. Swami Muktananda, *Bhagawan Nityananda of Ganeshpuri* (South Fallsburg, New York: SYDA Foundation, 1996), p. 15.

12. The Sanskrit word *avadhūta* is derived from the verbal root *dhū-*, meaning: 1) "to shake, move, cause to tremble," 2) "to discard, reject," 3) "humiliated," or 4) "unsurpassed." An *avadhūta* could be described as one who has "surpassed" bodily needs or desires; has "shaken" the attachment to the world; has "discarded" false identification and "rejected" what is false; is often "humiliated" or "despised" by the unknowing; and is given to teaching in ways that "surpass" the ordinary and overcome the obvious, sometimes through "insults." The *avadhūta* has "contempt" for death, having "attacked" and "overcome" it. A Sanskrit hymn sung in Siddha Yoga ashrams contains several verses that point to the qualities tradition ascribes to the *avadhūta*:

Nirmamaṃ nirahaṅkāraṃ
sama-loṣṭāśma-kāñcanam/
Sama-duḥkha-sukhaṃ dhīraṃ
hyavadhūtaṃ namāmyaham//

Free of possessiveness, free of egoism, regarding as the same a clod, a stone, and gold, even-minded in happiness and sorrow, all-enduring—to that *avadhūt*, indeed, I bow. (verse 3)

Nāhaṃ deho na me deho
jīvo nāham ahaṃ hi cit/

> *Evaṃ vijñāya santuṣṭaṃ*
> *hyavadhūtaṃ namāmyaham//*
>
> "I am not the body, nor the body mine; I am not a bound soul, for I am consciousness." Thus reflecting, he is content—to that *avadhūt,* indeed, I bow. (verse 5)
>
> *Jñānāgni-dagdha-karmāṇaṃ*
> *kāma-saṅkalpa-varjitam/*
> *Heyopādeya-hīnaṃ taṃ*
> *hyavadhūtaṃ namāmyaham//*
>
> His deeds burned up by the fire of realization, purged of desire and ambition, free of the need to accept or reject—to that *avadhūt,* indeed, I bow. (verse 7)

"*Śrī Avadhūta Stotram,* Hymn Praising the Avadhūt," from *The Nectar of Chanting* (South Fallsburg, New York: SYDA Foundation, 1983), pp. 58–59).

13. See Swami Muktananda, *Bhagawan Nityananda of Ganeshpuri,* p. 7.

14. See Muller-Ortega's article "The Siddha" for the relationship between the siddha, the "accomplished" or realized yogi, and *siddhis,* "supernatural powers."

15. The circumstances of Bhagawan Nityananda's early years were verified by Swami Anantananda in 1995 interviews with Ishwara Iyer's relatives and neighbors and with others in the town of Qualandi.

16. See Swami Muktananda, *Bhagawan Nityananda of Ganeshpuri:*

> My Guru also had a Guru. His name was Ishwara Iyer. My Baba stayed in his house and he would wash the dishes and scrub the floor. Ishwara Iyer was a great yogi who had practiced austerities. He was an enlightened Siddha Guru. (p. 76).

17. *Bhagawan Nityananda of Ganeshpuri,* p. 5.

18. Interview with Vasu Shetty, October 1994.

19. Statements here and in the following two paragraphs are from an interview with Sushila Shenoy, March 9, 1994.

20. *Bhagawan Nityananda of Ganeshpuri,* p. 7.

21. *Bhagawan Nityananda of Ganeshpuri,* p. 8.

22. Interview with Vasu Shetty, October 1994.

23. Interview with Ani, 1997, author's notes.

24. Interview with Gopal Karkera, November 28, 1994.

25. Interview with Gopal Karkera, November 28, 1994.

26. Swami Muktananda, "Truly Know Others," *Darshan* No. 56 (November 1991), p. 44.

27. Incident recounted in *Where Are You Going? A Guide to the Spiritual Journey* (South Fallsburg, New York: SYDA Foundation, 1994), pp. 25–26.

28. Swami Muktananda, *Meditate* (Albany: State University of New York Press, 1991), p. 15.

29. Swami Muktananda, *From the Finite to the Infinite* (South Fallsburg, New York:

SYDA Foundation, 1994), pp. 227–29 and p. 71.

30. *Play of Consciousness*, p. 68.

31. Interview with Vasu Shetty, October 1994.

32. Interview with Vasu Shetty, October 1994.

33. See *From the Finite to the Infinite*, p. 41.

34. Interview with Babu Shetty, April 25, 1982.

35. Interview with Vasu Shetty, October 1994.

36. V. K. Sethi, *Kabir: The Weaver of God's Name* (Amritsar: Radha Soami Satsang Beas, 1984), p. 652.

37. Interview with Babu Shetty, 1983.

38. See chapter 2 of the *Avadhūtagītā* and the *Śrīmadbhāgavatam* 11.11.10–17.

39. *Bhagawan Nityananda of Ganeshpuri*, p. 85.

40. Swami Venkatesananda, *Sivananda Yoga: A Series of Talks by Swami Venkatesananda to the Students of the Yoga-Vedanta Forest Academy* (Sivanandanagar, India: Divine Life Society, 1980), p. 32.

41. Interview with Gopal Karkera, November 28, 1994.

42. Interview with Vasu Shetty, October 1994.

43. See *Play of Consciousness*, p. xxvii, and *From the Finite to the Infinite*, p. 478, for an account of his mother's influence.

44. See *A Search for the Self* (pp. 9–10) by Swami Prajnananda, first published by Shree Gurudev Ashram, Ganeshpuri, India, in 1969. Swami Prajnananda, who died in 1994, was a professor of Sanskrit at Bharatiya Vidya Bhavan College in Bombay before coming to live in Swami Muktananda's ashram, and she was the editor of most of Swami Muktananda's early publications.

45. *From the Finite to the Infinite*, p. 478.

46. *Bhagawan Nityananda of Ganeshpuri*, p. 79.

47. *From the Finite to the Infinite*, p. 33.

48. Swami Muktananda, "What Is Greater Than the Self?" *Siddha Path* (September 1980), p. 16.

49. Swami Muktananda, *Satsang with Baba*, Vol. 3 (Oakland, California: SYDA Foundation, 1977), p. 91.

50. *Bhagavadgītā* 4.34.

51. See "The Self: A Vedāntic Foundation for the Revelation of the Absolute" by William K. Mahony in this collection.

52. *From the Finite to the Infinite*, p. 12.

53. This synopsis of Swami Muktananda's years of wandering is drawn from the previously cited *A Search for the Self* by Swami Prajnananda.

54. *From the Finite to the Infinite*, p. 12.

55. Swami Muktananda, *Satsang with Baba*, Vol. 2 (Ganeshpuri, India: SYDA Foundation, 1976), p. 111.

56. Interview with Babu Rao Pahelvan, June 6, 1989.

57. Interview with Babu Rao Pahelvan, "The Early Days," *Darshan* No. 18–19 (October 1988), p. 9.

58. *Bhagawan Nityananda of Ganeshpuri*, p. 79.

59. Swami Muktananda often said that though Zipruanna lived on a garbage heap, his skin gave off a sweet fragrance, this in itself being evidence of the purity he had attained through yoga. See *Satsang with Baba*, Vol. 3, p. 274.

60. See *Bhagawan Nityananda of Ganeshpuri*, p. 80
61. *Bhagawan Nityananda of Ganeshpuri*, p. 81.
62. Swami Muktananda, *I Have Become Alive* (South Fallsburg, New York: SYDA Foundation, 1992), pp. 26–27.
63. See *From the Finite to the Infinite*, p. 459.
64. *Bhagawan Nityananda of Ganeshpuri*, p. 85.
65. *Secret of the Siddhas*, p. 68
66. Swami Muktananda, "The Nature of the Guru," *Baba Company* (Midsummer 1980), p. 8.
67. *Play of Consciousness*, p. 72.
68. Bhagawan Nityananda, speaking in *Play of Consciousness*, p. 73.
69. *From the Finite to the Infinite*, p. 48.
70. *Play of Consciousness*, p. 77.
71. *Play of Consciousness*, p. 77.
72. *Tantrāloka* 1.44, as cited by Debabrata SenSharma in *The Philosophy of Sādhana* (Albany: State University of New York Press, 1990), p. 83.
73. *In the Company of a Siddha* p. 14.
74. *Play of Consciousness*, pp. 85–86.
75. For further discussion of this name and its significance for Siddha Yoga, see "Siddha Yoga as *Mahāyoga*: Encompassing All Other Yogas," by S. P. Sabharathnam, in this collection.
76. *Tantrāloka* 1.41, as quoted by SenSharma in *The Philosophy of Sādhana*, pp. 82–83.
77. *Play of Consciousness*, p. 106.
78. *Play of Consciousness*, p. 109.
79. *Play of Consciousness*, pp. 91–92.
80. In Swami Muktananda's description of *nīlabindu* in *Play of Consciousness*, he quotes the Maharashtrian poet-saints Jñāneśvar and Tukārām. Jñāneśvar writes:

dolānchī pāhā dolā shūnyāchā shevata
nīla bindū nīta lakhalakhīta
visāvo āle pātale chaitanya tethe
pāhe pā nirūte anubhave
pārvatīlāgi ādīnāthe dāvile
jñānadevā phāvale nivrittikripā

> O seekers after the knowledge of perfection, the very eye of your eye, where the void comes to an end, the Blue Pearl, pure, sparkling, radiant, that which opens the center of repose when it arises, is the great place of the conscious Self. Look, my brother, this is the hidden secret of this experience. This is what Parashiva, the primal Lord, told Parvati. Jnanadev says, "I saw this through the grace of my Sadguru Nivrittinath." (pp. 166–67.)

Tukārām writes:

tilā evadhe bāndhūni ghara
āta rāhe vishvambhara
tilā ituke bindule
tene tribhuvana kondātale

hariharāchyā mūrti
bindulyāta yetī jātī
tukā mhane he bindule
tene tribhuvana kondātale

[Muktananda writes,] Tukaram Maharaj says in this verse that God, the nourisher of the universe, lives in a house as tiny as a sesame seed. He is called the nourisher because He sustains the whole universe. The Lord of the universe, the supreme Self of all living beings, the power of *prāna*, who is known inwardly through the higher intuition by yogis, devotees, and jnanis, who is the treasure-house of omniscience, has made His dwelling place a house as small as a sesame seed. Just as a huge spreading tree grows from a tiny seed, the nourisher of all, who manifests Himself in an infinity of forms, shapes, and sizes, has a tiny seed for a house. The tiny seed is the source of the huge tree, the tree is contained in the seed, but the seed has a separate existence as a seed. One seed can grow into a tree, and the tree gives birth to countless seeds that are essentially the same as the first; in the same way, the *bindu*, the divine seed, can manifest in endless ways and forms and yet preserve its original identity. The Lord who lives in the bindu never loses His integrity nor His original power. His greatness and glory remain complete and unchanging." (p. 159.)

The *bindu* appears in the center of the Śrī Yantra diagram, and is mentioned in various Tantras. See *Sammohana Tantra, Bhūta-śuddhi Tantra* (quoted by Sir John Woodroffe, *The Serpent Power* (New York: Dover Publications, Inc. 1974), p. 423, and *Sat Chakra Nirupana*, and *Todala Tantra* (Woodroffe, *The Serpent Power*, pp. 428–30).

81. *Play of Consciousness*, p. 207.
82. *Spandakārikā* 3.1.
83. Interview with Rajgiri Gosavi, 1990.
84. Interview with Indutai Thia, 1990.
85. Interview with Shri Kaup Shetty, November 6, 1994.
86. Swami Muktananda, from an unpublished transcript, August 30, 1975.
87. Interview with Venkappanna Shriyan, 1992.
88. *A Search for the Self*, p. 60.
89. Reprinted in *Where Are You Going?* pp. 145–146.
90. Swami Muktananda used to tell the story of a South Indian saint who passed the lineage *śakti* on to his successor by spitting into his hand. Until that time, none of the saint's disciples had even been aware of the successor's existence.

In traditional accounts, the preeminent guru of the Vīraśaiva tradition of Hinduism, Allamaprabhu, received both his initiation and his empowerment as a guru in a private encounter with his guru, Animiṣayya. According to the account given by A. K. Ramanujan in the introduction to his translation of the Vīraśaiva poets, *Speaking of Śiva*, (Penguin Books, London: 1973, p. 144), Allama met his guru in a cave. Animiṣayya handed Allama a *śivaliṅga*, and in that moment, Animiṣayya's life abruptly ended. In that moment of transference, Allama was enlightened, and was subsequently recognized as a guru by his contemporary Vīraśaivas, including Basavanna, Akkamahādevī, and Cennabasava.

Thomas Hoover in *The Zen Experience* (New American Library, New York: 1980, p. 125) relates that the Zen master Huai-hai designated a certain Huang-po as his "successor in Dharma, via a famous transmission exchange in which Huang-po finally demonstrates wordless communication." According to the story, one day Huai-hai asked Huang-po, "Where have you been?" The answer was that he had been at the foot of the Ta-hsiung Mountain picking mushrooms. Huai-hai continued, "Have you seen any tigers?" Huang-po immediately roared like a tiger. Huai-hai picked up an axe as if to chop the tiger. Huang-po suddenly slapped Huai-hai's face. Huai-hai laughed heartily, and then returned to his temple and said to the assembly, "At the foot of the Ta-hsiung Mountain there is a tiger. You people should watch out. I have already been bitten today." Hoover notes that this enigmatic utterance by Huai-hai has been taken by many to signify that Huang-po was being acknowledged as successor.

For yet another example, Heinrich Dumoulin, in *A History of Zen Buddhism* (tr. By Paul Peachey, Beacon Press, Boston: 1963, p. 82), writes of the famous transmission from the fifth Patriarch, Hung-jen, to the sixth, Hui-neng. Hui-neng was an illiterate peasant lad who challenged Hung-jen's chief disciple by offering a brilliant solution to a koan. Afterwards, the master secretly called Hui-neng to his room and conferred the patriarchal insignia on him. Then, fearing the envy of the chief disciple, he ordered Hui-neng to flee south, where he founded the southern school of Chinese Zen.

Often in siddha lineages, the evidence that the lineage has been passed on to a particular person is recognized when the recipient exhibits signs of spiritual power. For example, in the Radha Soami tradition, a story is told that when guru Har Krishnan died, he did not name his successor, but only said that he would be found in a certain village. As a result, a number of disciples claimed to be the successor. According to the story, the true successor was discovered only when a devotee, saved in a shipwreck through his prayers to the former guru, offered *dakṣiṇa* to all the claimants in gratitude. Only the true successor understood the reason for the offering, and thus he was recognized by the devotees as his guru's true heir. Though this story is probably hagiographical, the fact that it has gained popular currency indicates how commonly gurus have been being recognized by demonstrating that they have received the *śakti* of the previous guru. (See Huzur Maharaj Sawan Singh, *Tales of the Mystic East*, published by Radha Soami Satsang Beas, Punjab, India, 1983, p. 235.)

91. *Kulārṇava Tantra* 13.99–101 and 107–108, as cited by Ram Kumar Rai, *Kulārṇava Tantra* (Varanasi, India: Prachya Prakashan, 1983), pp. 256–57.

92. Swami Muktananda, *Satsang with Baba*, Vol. 1 (Ganeshpuri, India: SYDA Foundation, 1974), pp. 327–28.

93. "Report from Ganeshpuri," *Siddha Path* (September 1978), p. 22.

94. *Play of Consciousness*, p. 251.

95. Swami Muktananda's remarks to the second annual meeting of the Ashram Council on April 26, 1964, as recounted in *Paramartha Katha Prasang*, pp. 104–105.

96. Swami Muktananda, quoted by Ma Durgananda in "The Whole World Is Home," *Siddha Path* (October-November 1981), p. 13.

97. Conversation with Pratap Yande, author's notes, January 1989.

98. Interview with Venkappanna Shriyan, October 14, 1996.

99. See Kulārṇava Tantra, which councils a disciple to "use even his own wealth only after offering it to the Guru." *Kulārṇava Tantra*, 12.76, as translated by Ram Kumar Rai, p. 233. See also the *Gurugītā*, verse 27, which states, "A disciple should

offer a seat, a bed, clothing, ornaments, a vehicle, and other things that will please the Guru."

100. *Play of Consciousness*, pp. 260–61.

101. Interview with Nirmala Thakkar, 1990.

102. B. N. Nanda, "Glimpses of Ganeshpuri," *Guruvani* (1967), pp. 23–24.

103. R. N. Marwah, "My Second Birth," *Swami Muktananda Paramahamsa: 60th Birthday Commemoration Volume*, (1968), p. 75.

104. Gita Obel, "Muktananda's Joy," *Swami Muktananda Paramahamsa: 60th Birthday Commemoration Volume*, (1968), p. 62.

105. "A Unique Blend," *Swami Muktananda Paramahamsa: 60th Birthday Commemoration Volume*, (1968), p. 46.

106. Siddha Yoga Experience Archives.

107. *Play of Consciousness*, p. 15.

108. Interview with Swami Sevananda, March 31, 1988.

109. B. P. Dalal, "Experience at Ganeshpuri," *Guruvani* (1964), pp. 27–28.

110. Author's notes.

111. Swami Nirmalananda, "The Guru Makes You Full of Life," *Siddha Yoga* (May 1, 1982), pp. 23–26.

112. Swami Muktananda, *Ashram Dharma* (South Fallsburg, New York: SYDA Foundation, 1995), pp. 4–5.

113. M. P. Pandit, from a lecture given in Miami Siddha Yoga Dham, March 1980, author's notes.

114. *From the Finite to the Infinite*, p. 139.

115. *The Nectar of Chanting*, p. x.

116. Dattātreya is considered to be a form of God-as-the-guru. His iconographic form is that of a yogi, and he is considered to contain the three forms of the Hindu Godhead—Brahmā, Viṣṇu, and Śiva—within himself. Legend has it that Dattātreya periodically incarnates as a human guru; several lineages of Maharashtrian saints are reputedly descended from one or another of his incarnations. Swami Samarth of Akalkot was popularly supposed to have been an incarnation of Dattātreya.

117. Interview with Swami Shantananda, January 10, 1995.

118. Interview with Swami Sevananda, September 24, 1996.

119. *I Have Become Alive*, p. 78.

120. "Editorial: Ashram Discipline," *Shree Gurudev-Vani* (1969), p. xi.

121. Interview with Carol Friend, September 25, 1996.

122. Interview with Helen Argent, September 19, 1996.

123. Swami Prajnananda, "Discovering the Guru," *Gurudev-Vani* (1981), p. 12.

124. Author's notes.

125. Interview with Venkappanna Shriyan, January 22, 1993.

126. Malti, (Swami Chidvilasananda), "Growing up with Baba, Part One," *Siddha Path* (February 1982), p. 12.

127. Swami Chidvilasananda, "The Truth Is I Am," *Darshan* No. 20 (November 1988), pp. 61–62.

128. Malti, "Devotion to You," *Siddha Path* (April 1980), p. 4.

129. This and the next three extracts are from Malti's article, "Growing up with Baba, Part Two," *Siddha Path* (March 1982), pp. 16–17.

130. Conversation with Shyama Shivastava, author's notes (1981).

131. Interview with Venkappanna Shriyan, December 28, 1995.

132. Interview with Murlidhar Dhoot, August 1987.

133. This and the two extracts following are from "Growing with Baba, Part II," p. 18.

134. Author's notes.

135. Swami Muktananda, *Selected Essays* (South Fallsburg, New York: SYDA Foundation, 1995), p. 44.

136. Here Swami Muktananda is consistent with his view of this power as the universal Goddess. For more on this see subject, "Kuṇḍalinī: Awakening the Divinity Within" by Douglas Renfrew Brooks and Constantina Rhodes Bailly.

137. *Play of Consciousness,* p. xxviii.

138. See Peter Washington, *Madam Blavatsky's Baboon* (New York: Schocken Books, 1985), for a detailed, though unsympathetic, account of some of these movements.

139. Interview with Venkappanna Shriyan, 1990.

140. Yogananda, "Baba Abroad," *Shree Gurudev-Vani* (July 1971), p. 24.

141. Swami Muktananda, quoted by Yogananda in "Baba Abroad," *Shree Gurudev-Vani,* p. 24.

142. This and the extract following are from an interview with Don Harrison, August 18, 1995.

143. Interview with Swami Sevananda, January 28, 1988.

144. Ram Dass, "Meeting Babaji," *Shree Gurudev-Vani* (July 1971), p. 33.

145. Interview with Don Harrison, August 18, 1995.

146. Interview with Ron Brent, February 22, 1993.

147. This and all statements and quotes regarding Ram Dass's relationship with Swami Muktananda come from "Meeting Babaji," *Shree Gurudev-Vani* (July 1971), pp. 31–33.

148. Ram Dass, "Meeting Babaji," *Shree Gurudev-Vani,* p. 33.

149. Interview with Steven Auerbach, October 1992.

150. Interview with Don Harrison, August 19, 1995.

151. Interview with Steven Auerbach, October 1992.

152. *Swami Muktananda Paramahamsa in Australia,* p. 27.

153. Ram Dass, "Meeting Babaji," *Shree Gurudev-Vani,* p. 33.

154. Interview with Gauri Hubert, author's notes.

155. Swami Muktananda, "Dhyana Chakra Pravartana," *Dhyana Chakra* (February 26, 1974), p. 8.

156. Interview with Swami Sevananda, January 27, 1988.

157. From a sharing at the Oakland Siddha Meditation Ashram, May 1988.

158. Interview with Swami Sevananda, March 31, 1988.

159. Interview with Swami Maheshananda, September 19, 1996.

160. Interview with Peggy Bendet, December 16, 1994.

161. Interview with Mac Littlefield, January 1996.

162. Siddha Yoga Experience Archives.

163. See "Siddha Yoga as *Mahāyoga*: Encompassing All Other Yogas," by S. P. Sabharathnam, for a further explanation of the significance of these yogic movements.

164. Kathleen Riordan Speeth, "The Guru in the Context of Western Psychotherapy," *Shree Gurudev-Vani* (1975), p. 33.

165. Paul Zweig, "Shaktipat," *Gurudev-Vani* (1975), pp. 62–63.

166. One of his favorite spiritual passages was the verse from the *Taittirīya Upaniṣad* (3.6.1) that says:

> *ānando brahmati vyajānāt /*
> *anandādd hy eva kalvimāni //*
> *bhūtānijayante ānandena /*
> *jatāni jīvantijanandam prayantyabhisaṃiśanti //*
>
> For truly, beings here are born from bliss;
> when born, they live in bliss;
> and into bliss, when departing, they enter.

The translation is from Sarvepalli Radhakrishnan, *The Principal Upaniṣads* (London: George Allen & Unwin, Ltd., 1978), p. 557.

167. Author's notes.

168. Author's notes.

169. Speeth, "The Guru in the Context of Western Psychotherapy," *Shree Gurudev-Vani*, p. 33.

170. "Letter from Melbourne," *Siddha Path* (November 1978), p. 4.

171. This and the extract following are from an interview with Penny Clyne, September 23, 1996.

172. Swami Muktananda, *Kundalini: The Secret of Life* (South Fallsburg, New York: SYDA Foundation, 1994), p. 25.

173. Swami Muktananda, "The Guru Principle," *Darshan* No. 75 (June 1993), p. 20.

174. Interview with Philip Goff, March 1992.

175. From a talk by Swami Ishwarananda, July 1985.

176. Interview with Swami Sevananda, March 31, 1988.

177. Interview with Swami Sevananda, September 24, 1996.

178. "Letter from Miami," *Siddha Path* (May 1980), p. 3.

179. Interview with D. R. (Ram) Butler, September 17, 1996.

180. Interview with Carolyn Zeiger, September 25, 1996.

181. Interview with David Pierce, 1994.

182. Interview with Norman Monson, October 2, 1995.

183. Interview with Peter Sitkin, July 14, 1995.

184. Interview with Karen Shiarella, September 18, 1996.

185. Swami Umeshananda, from a talk given in July 1991.

186. Interview with Harold Ferrar, August 18, 1996.

187. Interview with Swami Shantananda, January 1995.

188. Barbara Hamilton, quoted in George Franklin's "A Harvest of Grace: Baba Muktananda's Third World Tour," *Darshan* No. 30–31 (September–October 1989), p. 85.

189. Author's notes.

190. Interview with Mercedes Stewart, April 15, 1994.

191. Interview with Helen Argent, September 19, 1996.
192. "A Harvest of Grace," *Darshan* No. 30–31, pp. 83–84.
193. From a meeting with the SYDA Foundation staff members, 1987, author's notes.
194. Interview with Peggy Bendet, December 16, 1994.
195. Interview with Swami Maheshananda, September 19, 1996.
196. Interview with Swami Shantananda, June 1995.
197. Swami Muktananda, *Muktananda Thanks You* (Oakland, California: SYDA Foundation, 1976), p. 2.
198. Interview with Swami Sevananda, January 27, 1988.
199. Interview with Swami Maheshananda, September 19, 1996.
200. In 1996, there were twenty-five swamis in Siddha Yoga, five of them women.
201. Interview with Swami Shantananda, "A Monk's Dharma," *Darshan* No. 15 (July 1988), p. 43.
202. Interview with Swami Shantananda, June 1995.
203. Swami Muktananda, quoted in the "Report from Ganeshpuri," *Siddha Path* (June-July 1977), p. 7.
204. Interview with Swami Sevananda, March 31, 1988.
205. See "The Siddha" by Muller-Ortega.
206. Swami Muktananda, quoted by Werner Erhard in an interview with the author.
207. Statements in this and the next paragraph are from an interview with Swami Shantananda, June 1995.
208. Interview with Swami Sevananda, September 1996.
209. From an interview with Swami Chidvilasananda, "To Experience the Inner Love," *Shree Gurudev-Vani* (1982), p.20.
210. *Where Are You Going?* p. 125.
211. "The Whole World Is Home," *Siddha Path* (October-November 1981), p. 6.
212. See "The Guru-Disciple Relationship: The Context for Transformation" by William Mahony for more on the criteria for gurus and disciples.
213. Swami Muktananda, speaking in a press interview in Honolulu on July 30, 1974 (unpublished transcript).
214. *From the Finite to the Infinite*, p. 53.
215. The ashram in South Fallsburg, New York, was renamed Shree Muktananda Ashram in 1983 by Swami Chidvilasananda.
216. Malti, "The Guru Is the Means," *Siddha Path* (March 1980), p. 10.
217. Barbara Hamilton, quoted in George Franklin's "A Harvest of Grace," *Darshan* No. 30–31, p. 85.
218. Jaideva Singh, *Śiva Sūtras: The Yoga of Supreme Identity* (Delhi: Motilal Banarsidass, 1979), p. lix, translation of *sūtra* 1.17.
219. Swami Chidvilasananda, from an unpublished transcript, September 9, 1985.
220. Interview with Barbara Hamilton, 1990.
221. Swami Chidvilasananda, *Ashes at My Guru's Feet* (South Fallsburg, New York: SYDA Foundation, 1990), p. 28.
222. *Selected Essays*, p. 138.

223. "Interview," *Siddha Path* (June-July 1982), p. 14.

224. "The Whole World Is Home," *Siddha Path* (October-November 1981), p. 13.

225. "Silence Is a Sadhana: A Letter from South Fallsburg," *Siddha Path* (August 1981), p. 8.

226. For a concise history of these events, see Gene Thursby, "Swami Muktananda and the Seat of Power" in *When Prophets Die: The Postcharismatic Fate of New Religious Movements*, edited by Timothy Miller (Albany: State University of New York Press, 1991), pp. 125–129.

227. The history of religious and spiritual movements is laden with incidents of complicated succession processes. Lise Vail, in a series of interviews for a doctoral dissertation, "Renunciation, Love, and Power in Hindu Monastic Life" (University of Pennsylvania, 1987), discussed issues of lineage-succession with the current *jagadguru* of the Vīraśaiva Tontadarya Maṭh in northern Karnataka, Siddhalinga Swami. The maṭh historian, Siddhalingayya Hosamath, in an interview on July 17, 1978, described how the four sublineages (*samaya*) of Virakta swamis (Tontadarya *jagadgurus* belonging to one of these) began in the seventeenth century. Rachoti Swami had three important disciples, all of whom wanted to succeed him. When Rachoti named another disciple to his seat, the three left the *maṭha* and formed their own *maṭhas*, with their disciples subsequently forming separate lineages. On another occasion, Siddhalinga Swami described a court battle that was currently running over the succession in Shivananda Maṭha in Gadag, "for which there [were] three claimants: the swami in Nandishwara Maṭha; Atmananda, the son of the former Swami Shivananda who had been . . . married before he became a *sannyāsi*; and Dr. Medleri, a medical doctor. . . ."

Oral history documents the events that occurred when the eighth *jagadguru* of the Tontadarya lineage, Kaudi Mahanta Swami, attempted to install a young boy named Aralalimath as heir to his seat. The swami's other disciples became so enraged that they allegedly plotted to kill the boy, who escaped through a warning from his guru in a dream, and subsequently proved his fitness for the seat by demonstrating miraculous powers (pp. 137–38). *In many such cases, the fitness for the seat is proved by the successful performance of the functions of the guru.*

In the history of Buddhism, there are several reported cases in which the more spiritually qualified successor is required to prove himself through a series of subtle tests. See *A History of Zen Buddhism* by Heinrich Dumoulin, SJ, translated by Paul Peachey (Boston: Beacon Press, 1963), pp. 82–83; *The Zen Experience* by Thomas Hoover (New York and Scarborough, Ontario: New American Library, 1980), p. 163.

Within the history of the papacy, and indeed the Catholic Church in general, there are numerous instances of prelates and bishops being deposed for improper conduct. See Kenneth Pennington, *Pope and Bishops: The Papal Monarchy in the Twelfth and Thirteenth Centuries* (University of Pennsylvania Press, 1984) p. 125; and *The Papacy* by Bernhard Schimmelpfennig, translated by James Sievert (New York: Columbia University Press, 1992), p. 55 and pp. 195–97.

In a sense, the retirement of Swami Nityananda could be classified as a type of monastic reform, similar to reforms carried out throughout the history of the Christian churches. (See *Western Civilizations: Their History and Their Culture*, by Edward

McNall Burns, Robert E. Lerner, and Standish Meacham, 10th Edition, London, 1984, pp. 326–27.) For an account of a rather dramatic instance of reform in Tibetan Buddhist history, see the report on the deposing of the sixth Dalai Lama in *The Buddhist Religion: A Historical Introduction* by Richard H. Robinson and Willard L. Johnson (Belmont, California: Wadsworth Publishing Company, 1982), pp. 144–45.

228. Author's notes.

229. For example, in 1981, while leading a group of people in describing their experiences at one of Swami Muktananda's Intensives, Nityananda said, "It's been three years now that I've been taking these Intensives and meditating at all these four meditation sessions. For the first time today, though, I think I had a spiritual experience." He then went on to describe an inner vision, which ended when someone sitting next to him tapped him on the knee. "What I figured out was that I wasn't ready to hold the experience longer, for more than a few seconds." (From an unpublished transcript, March 14, 1981, Shree Muktananda Ashram Historical Archives.)

230. Swami Muktananda, from an unpublished transcript, July 18, 1981.

231. Interview with Swami Shantananda,

232. Interview with Helen Argent, September 19, 1996.

233. Literally, the perfect or complete "I," or the awareness of completeness. In Kashmiri Shaivism, this term refers to the experience that one's "I," or true Self, contains the universe. Swami Chidvilasananda is describing the experience of losing the ordinary ego or I-sense.

234. *Ashes at My Guru's Feet*, pp. 30–32.

235. *Ashes at My Guru's Feet*, p. 33.

236. "Pattabhishek," *Siddha Path* (June-July 1982), pp. 32–35.

237. From the unpublished transcript of an interview with Swami Chidvilasananda by Eugene Callender, October 19, 1982.

238. This and the statement following are taken from an interview with Swami Sevananda, October 14, 1982.

239. From a talk given in an Intensive in honor of Swami Muktananda's *mahāsamādhi* anniversary, October 1, 1995.

240. Interview with David Kempton, September 17, 1996.

241. Siddha Yoga Experience Archives.

242. Interview with Swami Shantananda, January 10, 1995.

243. Interview with John Greig, August 14, 1996.

244. In his "Swami Muktananda and the Seat of Power," published in *When Prophets Die*, Thursby traced the departure of three monks who "previously held secondary but prominent leadership roles within the movement." (p. 180)

245. In "Swami Muktananda and the Seat of Power," Gene Thursby wrote that factions form in "many Indian movements that have a Guru at their center" during the succession of power. Thursby cited a similar pattern in the Radhasoami movement in north India. (pp. 180–81)

246. Interview with Janet Dobrovolny, 1996.

247. The name came from an *abhaṅga*, a devotional song by the Maharashtrian poet-saint Tukadhyadas which has the refrain "Avadali Gurumayi." In Marathi, *gurumāyi* means "guru-mother," although a closely related Sanskrit word, *gurumayi*, means "one who is filled with the guru."

248. Author's notes.

249. Talk by Swami Ishwarananda, July 1991.

250. Author's notes.

251. The remarks here and in the next several paragraphs are from an interview with Robert Kemter, September 24, 1996.

252. Swami Chidvilasananda, from an unpublished transcript, December 24, 1984.

253. Interview with Mary Adams, September 1996.

254. Swami Chidvilasananda, from an unpublished transcript, March 3, 1985.

255. Interview with Swami Ishwarananda, 1996.

256. Interview with Rebecca Pratt, March 1995.

257. Shree Muktananda Ashram Audio Archives.

258. Interview with Swami Shantananda, November 1985.

259. In part, his Intensive speech read, "Baba's will made me a Guru, and it is Baba's will that I retire from the seat after three years. . . . I am undergoing scriptural ceremonies so that I may be dharmically released from my responsibilities as Guru and my vows of *sannyāsa,* in order to eliminate any trace of identification with my former role. . . . Now, Gurumayi is the only living Guru of Siddha Yoga. She always had, she has, and she always will have Baba's Shakti. . . . In South Fallsburg this past summer I asked Gurumayi to accept me as her disciple and she agreed. (November 3, 1985)

260. Author's notes, from Swami Chidvilasananda's final remarks in an Intensive, November 3, 1985.

261. In his speech at the investiture ceremony, he said, "During the time that I sat on the chair I did experience Baba's Shakti and power working through me and Gurumayi's Shakti supporting me in doing Baba's work. Those who received experiences during that time should understand where those experiences came from. It was not me. It was the power of Baba's command, the Gurushakti." (November 10, 1985)

262. Thursby, "Swami Muktananda and the Seat of Power," *When Prophets Die,* pp. 176–77. In this monograph, Thursby goes on to note that Muktananda set standards supporting an orderly transfer of allegiance from Muktananda to his successors and that, after three years, one of the successors resigned because he had not upheld these standards. Thursby adds that once Nityananda had disqualified himself, "Siddha Yoga subsequently deleted him from its history in order to maintain the traditional emphasis on the unbroken continuity of lineage." (pp. 179–80) Thursby notes that the succession of authority in Siddha Yoga seems typical of a general pattern that occurs in many Indian movements. He quotes Lawrence Babb's study of the Radhasoami movement, another guru-centered tradition:

> With the passing of each generation there are new disciples and splits, and the branching lines of descent show every sign of continuing to ramify as long as the movement exists.
>
> But from the inside, the history of the movement . . . appears not as branching lines but as one line. Because there can only be one sant satguru at a time, the other lines of spiritual "descent" are not really lines of descent at all. (From Lawrence A. Babb's *Redemptive Encounters: Three Modern Styles in the Hindu Tradition,* published in Berkeley, University of California Press, 1986, p. 30.)

Siddha Yoga recognized Gurumayi as the sole guru in the ceremony of 1985—thus reaffirming the single line of descent to which Lawrence Babb refers.

263. A copy of this decision is on file in Gurudev Siddha Peeth Archives.
264. Author's notes.
265. Interview with Swami Ishwarananda, January 1995.
266. Interview with Swami Shantananda, 1996.
267. Tour Archives, 1995–96, report from the month of January.
268. Linda Johnsen, *Daughters of the Goddess*, p. 81.
269. Swami Chidvilasananda's statements in this paragraph are from unpublished transcripts, November 28, 1987; June 21, 1986; and July 25, 1987.
270. Talk by Swami Umeshananda, July 1987.
271. Interview with Swami Anantananda, September 25, 1996.
272. Author's notes.
273. Swami Chidvilasananda, *Inner Treasures* (South Fallsburg, New York: SYDA Foundation, 1995), p. 22.
274. Author's notes.
275. Interview with Swami Ishwarananda, January 1995.
276. Author's notes.
277. This and the statement in the next paragraph are from an interview with Penny Clyne, September 23, 1996.
278. Author's notes.
279. Author's notes.
280. Interview with Edward De Bellevue, November 26, 1995.
281. Interview with Martin Brost, June 1996.
282. Interview with Renato Rezende, September 19, 1996.
283. Tour Archives, 1995–96 Tour, month of March.
284. Author's notes.
285. Interview with Elsa Cross, June 12, 1996.
286. Author's notes.
287. Poem posted for a time in the dishroom in Shree Muktananda Ashram.
288. Interview with Alexandra Gonsalez, 1996.
289. *From the Finite to the Infinite*, p. 424.
290. Tony Greco, "More Than You Remember Being," *Darshan* No. 35 (February 1990), p. 69.
291. *We Have Met Before: On Tour with Gurumayi Chidvilasananda* (South Fallsburg, New York: SYDA Foundation, 1996), p. 41.
292. Interview with Shubhada Vora, 1993.
293. From a talk by Catherine Parrish, June 23, 1996.
294. Interview with Martin Brost, June 1996.
295. From an unpublished transcript, March 26, 1995.
296. Interview with Swami Gitananda, 1996.
297. Conversation with John Grimes, author's notes.
298. Siddha Yoga Experience Archives.
299. Author's notes.
300. From a talk by Swami Ishwarananda, August 6, 1994.
301. Swami Chidvilasananda, *Transformation: On Tour with Gurumayi*, Vol. I, p. 109.

302. Author's notes.

303. Interview with Carmen Soria, June 5, 1996.

304. Interview with Françoise Lexa, June 7, 1996.

305. Interview with Catherine Parrish, January 23, 1996.

306. The PRASAD Project works with people in a way that is local, personal, and specific. For example, a vehicle from Gurudev Siddha Peeth makes a daily milk run to local schools, where this milk is often the only significant daily source of protein for the children—and devotees come along to play with the children and learn their ways. In 1989, the ashram adopted a local village so primitive that its name, "Usgaon," simply means "that village." Volunteers (mostly devotees) helped to plant shade trees and stock a local lake with hundreds of thousands of baby fish—enabling local fishermen to pursue their subsistence-level trade more successfully. PRASAD's other development projects in the area have included drilling new deep wells and reconstructing and covering old wells to provide clean drinking water year-round, reforesting depleted local hillsides, and assisting villagers in roofing their huts. PRASAD offers college scholarships to the top students in local high schools, and academic awards in the lower grades, and in 1996 was finalizing plans for a permanent hospital in the valley.

Another major project of PRASAD in India is the operation of highly successful eye camps. Twenty-one million people in India suffer vision impairment from cataracts; and over ten million of them are blind. For villagers whose families live on the economic edge, blindness often means an early death, since it places an enormous burden on subsistence-level families to support a non-contributing family member. Eye camps are a common means of providing cataract surgery for the poor; what is uncommon about Netraprakash is the quality of care.

In the four Netraprakash eye camps, Western eye surgeons working in partnership with doctors from the Aravind Eye Clinic in Madurai have performed cataract operations on nearly three thousand patients, implanting intraocular lenses, as well as housing and feeding them and providing free transportation to and from their villages. The camps have also offered free eye examinations, vision screening, vitamins, ophthalmic medication, and free glasses to nearly forty thousand more.

Netraprakash was the first eye camp in the world to provide free intraocular lenses to all cataract patients. When the cataract-clouded natural lens is removed surgically, its function must be replaced, either by a pair of thick glasses (the usual option in camps worldwide) or by an artificial lens implant (the standard operating procedure in private surgeries and in developed countries). The intraocular lens not only gives better vision but also does away with the need for the thick glasses, which in the harsh conditions of village life are usually lost or broken within a year of the surgery.

307. Swami Muktananda, *Getting Rid of What You Haven't Got* (South Fallsburg, New York: SYDA Foundation, 1974), p. 35.

308. Interview with Diego Santiago, "Opened Up," *Darshan* No. 82 (February 1994), p. 49.

309. Alan Gompers, "You Are Great!" *Darshan* No. 56, p. 31.

310. Tom Toomey, "History of the Prison Project," a thesis in the Siddha Yoga Experience Archives, October 1, 1993.

311. *Daughters of the Goddess*, p. 77–78. For a discussion of the Goddess, see "Kuṇḍalinī: Awakening the Divinity Within" by Douglas Refrew Brooks and

Constantina Rhodes Bailly.

312. Swami Chidvilasananda, *Enthusiasm* (South Fallsburg, New York: SYDA Foundation, 1997), pp. XXX.

313. Author's notes.

314. Tour Archives, 1995–96, report from the month of December.

315. Marilyn Goldin, *Siddha Path Newsletter* (December 12, 1995).

316. Author's notes.

317. Author's notes.

318. Tour Archives, 1995–96, month of December.

PART II. THEOLOGY

Chapter 2. The Siddha

1. See Mircea Eliade, *Yoga: Immortality and Freedom,* translated by William R. Trask (New York: Harcourt, Brace and World, 1959), for numerous examples.

2. David White's recent study is really the first major advance in the scholarly study of the siddha traditions specifically. David G. White, *The Alchemical Body* (Chicago: University of Chicago Press, 1996).

3. Monier-Williams' Sanskrit dictionary lists meanings for two-thirds of a column. Among these are: accomplished, fulfilled, effected, gained, acquired; one who has attained the highest object; perfected, become perfected, beatified; endowed with supernatural faculties; sacred, holy, divine, illustrious; established, settled, proved. A Siddha or semi-divine being of great purity and perfection and said to possess the eight supernatural faculties; any inspired sage or prophet or seer; any holy personage or great saint; any great adept in magic or one who has acquired supernatural powers. From p. 1215, *A Sanskrit-English Dictionary,* Monier-Williams (Delhi: Motilal Banarsidass, first Indian edition 1970).

4. Swami Muktananda, *From the Finite to the Infinite* (South Fallsburg, New York: SYDA Foundation, 1994), pp. 56–57.

5. For a discussion of the *ātman,* the "Self," see William K. Mahony's chapter "The Self: A Vedāntic Foundation for the Revelation of the Absolute," in this collection.

6. *From the Finite to the Infinite,* p. 57.

7. Swami Muktananda, *Satsang with Baba,* Vol. 1 (Oakland, California: SYDA Foundation, 1974), p. 173.

8. The literature on Ramakrishna is quite large. An excellent starting place is Christopher Isherwood, *Ramakrishna and His Disciples* (New York: Simon and Schuster, 1970).

9. A comprehensive study of this engaging and paradoxical figure is to be found in Antonio Rigopoulos, *The Life and Teachings of Sai Baba of Shirdi* (Albany: State University of New York Press, 1993).

10. Swami Muktananda, *Secret of the Siddhas* (South Fallsburg, New York: SYDA Foundation, 1994), p. 31 (verse 145).

11. Swami Muktananda, *Light on the Path* (South Fallsburg, New York: SYDA Foundation, 1994), p. 74.

12. *Secret of the Siddhas*, p. 31–32 (verse 146).

13. It is clear that the Datta *sampradāya* in Maharashtra, including Akalkot Maharaj (whom he spoke of many times), had a strong influence on Muktananda.

14. *Secret of the Siddhas*, 33–34 (verses 153, 154).

15. June McDaniel, *The Madness of Saints: Ecstatic Religion in Bengal* (Chicago: the University of Chicago Press, 1989).

16. *Secret of the Siddhas*, p. 51 (verse 200).

17. *Secret of the Siddhas*, pp. 25–26 (verse 124).

18. Swami Muktananda, "What Is Greater Than The Self," *Siddha Path* (September 1980), p. 16.

19. *Secret of the Siddhas*, p. 26 (verse 125).

20. *Secret of the Siddhas*, p. 26 (verse 126).

21. *Secret of the Siddhas*, p. 26 (verse 127).

22. Swami Muktananda, *Play of Consciousness* (South Fallsburg, New York: SYDA Foundation, 1994), p. 20.

23. *Secret of the Siddhas*, pp. 59–60 (verse 220).

24. David White demonstrates this historically in his *Alchemical Body*, Chapter 4.

25. For detailed historical information see Paul E. Muller-Ortega, *The Triadic Heart of Śiva* (Albany: State University of New York Press, 1989).

26. For a rendering of this important Tamil text into English see *Thirumandiram, A Classic of Yoga and Tantra by Siddhar Thirumoolar*, English translation and notes by B. Natarajan, edited by M. Govindan (Montreal: Babaji's Kriya Yoga Publications, Inc., 1993).

27. For more information on the Maheśvara Siddhas, see V. V. Ramana Sastri, "The Doctrinal Culture and Tradition of the Siddhas," *The Cultural Heritage of India* (Calcutta: The Ramakrishna Mission Institute of Culture, 1978), p. 305.

28. See A. K. Ramanujan, *Speaking of Śiva* (London: Penguin Books, 1973).

29. White's *Alchemical Body* is the most complete treatment of the Nāthas.

30. See White, *Alchemical Body*, for more on the alchemical traditions of India.

31. See Mark Dyczkowski, *The Canon of the Śaivāgama and the Kubjikā Tantras of the Western Kaula Tradition* (Albany: State University of New York Press, 1988).

32. For more information on this topic, see R. D. Ranade, *Mysticism in India: The Poet-Saints of Maharashtra* (Albany: State University of New York Press, 1983).

33. On the Buddhist siddhas see S. Dasgupta, *Obscure Religious Cults* (Calcutta: Firma KLM private, 1976).

34. White in *Alchemical Body* has tried quite admirably.

35. *Yoga Sūtra* 3.32; 3.51 and commentary.

36. Though much later, echoes of this usage of the notion of *siddhas* may still be present for example in the devotional text of the *Gurugītā* (86, 173) where the *siddhas* are mentioned in the context of gods, *gandharvas*, *pitṛs* and *yakṣas*, and are described as still seeking liberation.

37. See White's *Alchemical Body* for an expansion of this notion.

38. One reference to this classification as applied to gurus is to be found in the ca. fourteenth-century text *Kulārṇava Tantra* (6.63 ff.).

39. In this regard, it might be noted that for Swami Muktananda, the "deity" of Siddha Yoga is the siddha guru, that is to say, his guru, Bhagawan Nityananda. During his life, Swami Muktananda oversaw the building of two temples to his guru, one

at the Gurudev Siddha Peeth in Ganeshpuri, India, and the other at Shree Muktananda Ashram in South Fallsburg. It is also important that the morning chant in these two ashrams (and in other ashrams worldwide) was changed by Swami Muktananda in early 1970 from a recitation of the *Bhagavadgītā* to a recitation of the *Gurugītā,* a text with important connections to the siddha lineage and which exalts the worship of the guru.

40. White, *Alchemical Body,* p. 11.

41. Mircea Eliade, *Yoga: Immortality and Freedom* (New York: Bollingen Foundation Inc., 1975), p. 304.

42. *Jñāneśvarī* 18.1729–39, from Swami Kripananda's *Jnaneshwar's Gita: A Rendering of the Jnaneshwari* (Albany: State University of New York Press, 1989), p. 349.

43. For more on the historical problems surrounding Matsyendranātha and Gorakṣanātha see White, *Alchemical Body.*

44. Swami Kripananda, *Jnaneshwar's Gita: A Rendering of the Jnaneshwari* (Albany: State University of New York Press, 1989), p. vi.

45. A rendering of the poems of Kabir was done by Rabindranath Tagore, *Songs of Kabir* (New York: Samuel Weiser, 1974). See also Linda Hess and Shukdev Singh, *The Bījak of Kabir* (Delhi: Motilal Banarsidass, 1986), and Charlotte Vaudeville, *A Weaver Named Kabir: Selected Verses* (Oxford: Oxford University Press, 1993).

46. See Ramanujan, *Speaking of Śiva.*

47. He is said to have stayed in a place in Vajreshwari which had a small Dattātreya temple close to it. There is a large image of Dattātreya installed in the Ganeshpuri Ashram.

48. *Play of Consciousness,* p. 223.

49. *Play of Consciousness,* p. 223.

50. Keith Dowman, trans., *Masters of Enchantment: The Lives and Legends of the Mahasiddhas* (Rochester, Vermont: Inner Traditions International, Ltd., 1988), p. 14.

51. Swami Muktananda, *Satsang with Baba,* Vol. 3 (Oakland, California: SYDA Foundation, 1977), p. 240.

52. Swami Muktananda, *Satsang with Baba,* Vol. 5 (Ganeshpuri, India: SYDA Foundation, 1978), p. 128.

53. There is always an ambiguity in these terms between their usage to designate one who has achieved the highest goals of a path and one who is yet striving to do so. This ambiguity extends to the term *siddha,* although Swami Muktananda often distinguishes between it and "Siddha students," for example.

54. *From the Finite to the Infinite,* p. 62.

55. *Tantrāloka,* Chapter 4.

56. Swami Muktananda, *Selected Essays* (South Fallsburg, New York: SYDA Foundation, 1995), p. 110.

57. The literature on perennialism is quite large. A classic example of its argument is presented by Aldous Huxley in his *The Perennial Philosophy* (New York: Harper & Row, Publishers, Inc., 1970).

58. Swami Muktananda, *Paramartha Katha Prasang* (Ganeshpuri, India: Gurudev Siddha Peeth, 1981), p. 313.

59. *Paramartha Katha Prasang,* pp. 313–14.

60. Swami Muktananda, "The Way of the Siddhas," *Shree Gurudev-Vani* (1973), p. 68.

61. *Paramartha Katha Prasang*, p. 314.
62. *Paramartha Katha Prasang*, p. 314.
63. *Paramartha Katha Prasang*, p. 314.
64. *Play of Consciousness*, p. 186.
65. *Secret of the Siddhas*, pp. 65–66 (verse 230).
66. Swami Muktananda, *The Perfect Relationship* (South Fallsburg, New York: SYDA Foundation, 1985), pp. 16–17.
67. *Secret of the Siddhas*, p. 2 (verse 8).
68. Actually, there are sometimes many more "levels" of knowledge, but we are simplifying here for the sake of clarity. On these matters, Ninian Smart, *Doctrine and Argument in Indian Philosophy* (London: George Allen and Unwin, Ltd., 1969) and Karl Potter, *Presuppositions of India's Philosophies* (Westport, Connecticut: Greenwood Press, 1976) are both very instructive.
69. *Secret of the Siddhas*, pp. 51–52 (verse 201).
70. *Light on the Path*, p. 61.
71. *Secret of the Siddhas*, p. 51 (verse 200).
72. *Secret of the Siddhas*, p. 53 (verse 205).
73. The third *pada* of the *Yoga Sūtra* is devoted to an enumeration of these *vibhūtis* or supernatural, yogic attainments.
74. The *Śiva Saṃhitā*, the *Haṭhayogapradīpikā*, and the *Gheraṇḍa Saṃhitā* can be consulted usefully for later versions of these yogic attainments.
75. This distinction is exemplified in the texts in a variety of ways. In the *Parātriṃśikā-vivaraṇa* of Abhinavagupta, for example, there is the distinction between the *khecarī-siddhi* which is equivalent to what is here called the supreme *siddhi*, and the *kaulika-siddhi* which may be interpreted in terms of this secondary *siddhi*.
76. *From the Finite to the Infinite*, p. 317.
77. *Tantrāloka* 13.285:

purāṇe'pi ca tasyaiva prasādād bhaktir iṣyate/
yayā yānti parāṃ siddhiṃ tadbhāvagatamānasāḥ//

a translation of which would be:

> Indeed, in the *Purāṇa* [it is said]:
> By his grace alone does devotion arise. It is by such devotion that those whose minds are deeply steeped in the feeling of love for God reach the supreme accomplishment.

78. *Secret of the Siddhas*, p. 66 (verse 231).
79. For a detailed discussion on shaktipat, see Paul E. Muller-Ortega's article (Chapter 6) in this collection.
80. *Secret of the Siddhas*, p. 53 (verse 206).
81. *Light on the Path*, p. 67.
82. For further details, see Gerald J. Larson, *Classical Sāṃkhya: An Interpretation of Its History and Meaning* (Delhi: Motilal Banarsidass, 1979).
83. On the Upaniṣads, a useful translation is Robert Hume, *The Thirteen Principal Upanishads* (New Delhi: Oxford University Press, 1995). Also useful are Sarvepalli Radhakrishnan, *The Principal Upaniṣads* (New York: Humanities Press, Inc., 1975) and Patrick Olivelle, *Upaniṣads* (Oxford: Oxford University Press, 1996).
84. See for example the excellent study by David Haberman, *Acting As a Way of*

Salvation (New York: Oxford University Press, 1988).

85. See for example the works of Edward Conze on early Buddhism. His *Buddhist Thought in India* (London: George Allen & Unwin, 1983), though highly technical, traces the details of the evolution of this idea.

86. See Padmanabh Jaini, *The Jaina Path of Purification* (Berkeley: University of California Press, 1979).

87. *Secret of the Siddhas,* p. 57 (verse 217).

88. See the very useful collection of articles on this topic edited by Andrew Fort and Patricia Mumme, *Living Liberation In Indian Thought* (Albany: State University of New York Press, 1996).

89. *Play of Consciousness,* p. 223.

90. *Play of Consciousness,* pp. 169–70.

91. "Editorial," *Siddha Path* (March 1979), p. 3.

92. Swami Chidvilasananda, "God in His Creation," *Darshan* No. 53 (August 1991), p. 42.

93. *Parātrīśikā-laghuvṛtti,* commentary on *ślokas* 11–16.

94. See Eliade, *Yoga: Immortality and Freedom,* for a discussion of the "enstatic" as opposed to the truly "ecstatic" mysticism here being considered.

95. *Play of Consciousness,* p. 296.

96. *Play of Consciousness,* p. 205.

97. One of the clearest technical descriptions of this entire process is to be found in Abhinavagupta's *Parātrīśikā-laghuvṛtti.*

98. *Play of Consciousness,* p. 227.

99. *Play of Consciousness,* pp. 228–29.

100. *Play of Consciousness,* p. 229.

101. See *Śiva Sūtra* 3.13.

102. *Play of Consciousness,* pp. 230–31.

103. *Play of Consciousness,* p. 229.

104. *Play of Consciousness,* p. 231.

105. *Secret of the Siddhas,* p. 27 (verses 128, 129).

106. *Śiva Sūtra* 3, 27.

107. *Secret of the Siddhas,* p. 27 (verse 129).

108. Swami Chidvilasananda, *Inner Treasures* (South Fallsburg, New York: SYDA Foundation, 1995), p. 20.

Chapter 3. The Guru-Disciple Relationship

1. See *Atharvaveda* 11.5. For a relevant verse from this hymn, see page 261.

2. See *Chāndogya Upaniṣad* 8.7–12.

3. *Rāmāyaṇa* 2.1.24, 2.4.22, 4.54.4.

4. Swami Muktananda, *Secret of the Siddhas* (Gurudev Siddha Peeth, Ganeshpuri, India: SYDA Foundation, 1994), p. 59 (verse 220).

5. Swami Muktananda, *Play of Consciousness* (South Fallsburg, New York: SYDA Foundation, 1994), p. 59.

6. Swami Muktananda, *Where Are You Going? A Guide to the Spiritual Journey* (South Fallsburg, New York: SYDA Foundation, 1994), p. 125.

7. On the Vedic and Vedāntic texture to the Siddha Yoga notion of the "Self"

see the chapter "The Self: A Vedāntic Foundation for the Revelation of the Absolute," elsewhere in this collection.

8. *Brahma Upaniṣad* 16–17.

9. *Kena Upaniṣad* 1.3.

10. *Kaṭha Upaniṣad* 2.8–9.

11. See *Chāndogya Upaniṣad* 6.14.1–2.

12. *Ṛgveda* 10.32.7.

13. *Secret of the Siddhas,* p. 68 (verse 236).

14. For further discussion regarding the idea that the universal Self is of the nature of love, see William K. Mahony, "The Self: A Vedāntic Foundation for the Revelation of the Absolute," elsewhere in this collection.

15. *Secret of the Siddhas,* p. 61 (verse 223).

16. *Secret of the Siddhas,* pp. 61–62 (verse 224).

17. *Secret of the Siddhas,* p. 68 (verse 236).

18. The different types listed here are *preraka, sūcaka, vācaka, darśaka, śikṣaka,* and *bodhaka,* respectively. See *Kulārṇava Tantra* 13.128.

19. *Kulārṇava Tantra* 13.128.

20. *Kulārṇava Tantra* 13.129.

21. For a more extensive discussion on this subtle inner terrain, see the chapter by Douglas Renfrew Brooks and Constantina Rhodes Bailly, "Kuṇḍalinī: Awakening the Divinity Within," in this collection.

22. *Śiva Sūtra Vimarśinī* 2.6.

23. Swami Muktananda, *From the Finite to the Infinite* (South Fallsburg, New York: SYDA Foundation, 1994), p. 365.

24. *Kulārṇava Tantra* 13.51–52. The phrase "physical form of the guru" translates *sākṣāt gururūpa.*

25. *Yoginī Tantra,* Chapter 1. Reference and text in Arthur Avalon, *Tantra of the Great Liberation [Mahānirvāṇa Tantra]* (London: Luzac and Co., 1913; reprint edition, New York: Dover Publications, 1972), p. lxxi.

26. *Jñāneśvarī* 12.172, commenting on *Bhagavadgītā* 12.16. This and all subsequent passages from *Jñāneśvarī* are from Swami Kripananda's *Jnaneshwar's Gita: A Rendering of the Jnaneshwari* (Albany: State University of New York Press, 1989).

27. *Jñāneśvarī* 12.173.

28. "Report from Ganeshpuri," *Siddha Path* (March 1978), p. 10.

29. Various Tantric traditions regard what is described as the spiritual energy residing within each and every person as the goddess Kuṇḍalinī, the inward presence of *citi-śakti,* the supremely powerful consciousness that fashions, supports, and enlivens all things in the universe. Regarding Kuṇḍalinī, see note 46, below.

30. *Play of Consciousness,* p. 18.

31. Swami Chidvilasananda, from an unpublished transcript, July 14, 1995, morning, Shree Muktananda Ashram, South Fallsburg, New York.

32. July 14, 1995 transcript.

33. July 14, 1995 transcript.

34. July 14, 1995 transcript.

35. Swami Chidvilasananda, *Ashes at My Guru's Feet* (South Fallsburg, New York: SYDA Foundation, 1990), p. 7.

36. See *Bṛhadāraṇyaka Upaniṣad* 4.6.1.

37. *Yoga Sūtra* 1.26: *pūrveṣāmapi guruḥ kālenānavacchedāt.*

38. Drawing perhaps on the *Mahāyoga Vijñāna,* a recent compilation of various Sanskrit texts, Swami Muktananda has said that "the Siddha Yoga lineage originated with Parashiva and was passed on to Lord Narayana, who assumed the form of a yogi and taught Siddha Yoga to all the sages. After this, the great sage Bhagawan Sanatkumara gave the wisdom of this sublime yoga to Samvarta, the best among sages. The great yogi Sanandanda granted it to the sage Pulaha, and he in turn gave it to the sage Gautama. The sage Angiras gave it to the seer Bharadwaja, the knower of the Vedas. The Siddha Kapilamuni, the king of yogis, conferred the same knowledge on the yogi Jaigishavya as well as on Panchashikhacharya." Muktananda also refers to an account in the *Kūrma Purāṇa* (2.11) which purports to trace the lineage of those ancient sages teaching what he calls "Siddha Yoga." See *The Perfect Relationship,* pp. 16–17.

39. "Letter from South Fallsburg," *Siddha Path* (June-July 1981), p. 10.

40. *Vivekacūḍāmaṇi* 3.

41. Swami Muktananda, *Light on the Path* (South Fallsburg, New York: SYDA Foundation, 1994), p. 41.

42. *The Nectar of Chanting* (Ganeshpuri, India: SYDA Foundation, 1983), p. xiv.

43. Swami Muktananda, *Mukteshwari* (South Fallsburg, New York: SYDA Foundation, 1995), p. 190 (verses 600, 601).

44. The literal meanings of the English words *disciple* and *discipline* are relevant to the discussion at hand. They may derive from the Latin *disciplus,* "pupil," which itself comes from *dis-capere,* "to grasp." To be a disciple or to be disciplined is in this sense both to "grab hold of" a teaching or teacher as well as to be "grabbed by" that guiding force. If they do in fact derive from *disciplus,* the words *disciple* and *discipline* are thus distantly related through the Indo-European *kap-* ("grab") to the words *captive* and *captivate.* Used in this sense, we may say that a disciple is "captivated" by the teachings of his or her teacher. Alternatively, *disciple* and *discipline* may derive from the Latin *discere,* "to learn." If so, they are distantly related not only to such words as *doctrine,* but also to *decent* and *dignity.* Accordingly, to be a disciple and to lead the life of a spiritual disciple leads to a life of inner as well as outer decency and dignity. For similar discussion, see William K. Mahony, "Spiritual Discipline," in *The Encyclopedia of Religion,* edited by Mircea Eliade, *et al.* (New York: Macmillan and The Free Press, 1987), Vol. 14, pp. 19–29.

45. For discussion of the three *malas,* see Paul E. Muller-Ortega's chapter, "Shaktipat: The Initiatory Descent of Power," elsewhere in this book.

46. For more on Siddha Yoga and Kuṇḍalinī, see the chapter by Douglas Renfrew Brooks and Constantina Rhodes Bailly, "Kuṇḍalinī: Awakening the Divinity Within," elsewhere in this collection.

47. See Paul E. Muller-Ortega's chapter, "The Siddha: Paradoxical Exemplar of Indian Spirituality," elsewhere in this book.

48. For a discussion of shaktipat, see Paul E. Muller-Ortega's chapter on the topic elsewhere in this collection.

49. *Resonate with Stillness: Daily Contemplations from the Words of Swami Muktananda, Swami Chidvilasananda* (South Fallsburg, New York: SYDA Foundation, 1995), April 8.

50. For an historical review of Siddha Yoga, based on biographical accounts

and narratives of these three teachers, see Swami Durgananda's "To See the World Full of Saints: The History of Siddha Yoga as a Contemporary Movement." Bhagawan Nityananda's guru is sometimes identified as Ishwar Iyer, a south Indian brahmin with whom Nityananda lived as a child. Many devotees regarded Nityananda as a *janma-siddha,* that is, as "one who is born a perfected being" and therefore as one who was initiated into the lineage of siddha gurus by a teacher in another lifetime. (For more on this type of siddha, see Paul E. Muller-Ortega's, "The Siddha: Paradoxical Exemplar of Indian Spirituality" elsewhere in this collection.)

51. Swami Muktananda used this very phrase for the title of his book *The Perfect Relationship: The Guru and the Disciple* (South Fallsburg, New York: SYDA Foundation, 1985).

52. *The Perfect Relationship,* p. 2.

53. Swami Chidvilasananda, *Transformation: On Tour With Gurumayi Chidvilasananda,* Vol. 3 (South Fallsburg, New York: SYDA Foundation, 1987), p. 177.

54. Swami Chidvilasananda, "You Must Trust Yourself," *Darshan* No. 52 (July 1991), p. 53.

55. *From the Finite to the Infinite,* p. 47.

56. *From the Finite to the Infinite,* p. 364.

57. See *Ṛgveda* 1.147.4. The context here is of the seer Dīrghatamas's fear that another seer will use the power of his visionary knowledge for evil purposes. Addressing the god of fire, Agni, Dīrghatamas asks that such a wayward seer's intentions bring him distress, and that "may this, [Dīrghatamas's] powerful verbal expression of weighty force return to him" [*mantro guruḥ punar astu so asmai*].

58. *Muṇḍaka Upaniṣad* 2.1.12.

59. See *Chāndogya Upaniṣad* 4.10.1–4.15.6.

60. *Chāndogya Upaniṣad* 4.14.1. "But only one who moves in the Way can tell you the Way" translates *ācārya tu te gatiṃ vakteti.*

61. See Pāṇini's *Aṣṭādhyāyī* 3.4.68.

62. *Aṣṭādhyāyī* 3.2.109.

63. See the *Aṣṭādhyāyī* 2.1.65. For further discussion, see V. S. Agrawala, *India as Known to Pāṇini,* Second Edition (Varanasi: Prithivi Prakashan, 1963), pp. 283–84.

64. See *Aṣṭādhyāyī* 4.2.84.

65. See the *Aṣṭādhyāyī* 2.1.65.

66. Reference in Agrawala, *Indian as Known to Pāṇini,* p. 282.

67. For a fuller discussion of the place of such retreats in the spiritual life of India and in Siddha Yoga, see William K. Mahony "The Ashram: Life in the Abode of a Siddha" elsewhere in this collection.

68. *Aṣṭādhyāyī* 1.3.57, 3.2.108.

69. *Aṣṭādhyāyī* 3.4.68.

70. *Aṣṭādhyāyī* 4.3.77.

71. *Atharvaveda* 11.5.3.

72. *Śatapatha Brāhmaṇa* 11.3.3.6.

73. *Ashes at My Guru's Feet,* p. 61.

74. Swami Chidvilasananda, *Inner Treasures* (South Fallsburg, New York: SYDA Foundation, 1995), pp. 35–36.

75. *Resonate with Stillness,* May 12.

76. *Vivekacūḍāmaṇi* 37-38.

77. *Gurugītā* 1-3.

78. *Bhaktivijaya* 7.26-33, translated here by Justin E. Abbott and N. R. Godbole in *Stories of Indian Saints*, reprint edition (Delhi: Motilal Banarsidass, 1982), pp. 109–11.

79. From the public domain, translated here by Viju Kulkarni.

80. See *The Perfect Relationship*, pp. 80–81.

81. Swami Chidvilasananda, "Live in the Realm of Great Experiences," *Darshan* No. 62–63 (May–June 1992), p. 90.

82. *Manu Smṛti* 2.69–249. For a translation, see *The Laws of Manu*, translated by Georg Bühler (Oxford: Oxford University Press, 1886; reprint edition, New Delhi: Motilal Banarsidass, 1979), pp. 42–74.

83. See, for example, Bühler, *The Laws of Manu*, p. 59 (2.159–161).

84. *Muṇḍaka Upaniṣad* 1.2.13. The phrase "imperishable Self" translates *akṣaram puruṣam*.

85. *Upadeśasāhasrī* 4–5.

86. *Vivekacūḍāmaṇi* 8–9, 13–15.

87. *Vivekacūḍāmaṇi* 17.

88. *Vivekacūḍāmaṇi* 18.

89. *Vivekacūḍāmaṇi* 19.

90. *Vivekacūḍāmaṇi* 20.

91. *Vivekacūḍāmaṇi* 21.

92. *Vivekacūḍāmaṇi* 22–26.

93. *Vivekacūḍāmaṇi* 27.

94. *Vivekacūḍāmaṇi* 28–30.

95. *Vivekacūḍāmaṇi* 31–32.

96. *Vivekacūḍāmaṇi* 33–34.

97. *Vivekacūḍāmaṇi* 42.

98. *Kulārṇava Tantra* 13.23–30.

99. *Kulārṇava Tantra* 13.31–50. This translation shortens a longer passage in the original text.

100. *Śiva Saṃhitā* 3.12–14, 18–19.

101. See, for example, *Jñāneśvarī* 13.184–860, on *Bhagavadgītā* 13.8–12.

102. These virtues serve as the topic for a series of talks Swami Chidvilasananda gave in 1993 and which have been published in book form as *My Lord Loves a Pure Heart: The Yoga of Divine Virtues* (South Fallsburg, New York: SYDA Foundation, 1994).

103. For more on the *Bhagavadgītā*'s teachings regarding selfless service to God, see William K. Mahony, "The Self: A Vedāntic Foundation for the Revelation of the Absolute," in this collection.

104. *Bhagavadgītā*: 18.23. See also *My Lord Loves a Pure Heart*, p. 122.

105. *My Lord Loves a Pure Heart* p. 122, quoting *Bhagavadgītā* 18.23 and *Jñāneśvarī* 18.585–87.

106. Swami Chidvilasananda, *Kindle My Heart*, Vol. I (South Fallsburg, New York: SYDA Foundation, 1989), p. 153.

107. *Kindle My Heart*, Vol. I (1989 edition), p. 154.

108. See *Muṇḍaka Upaniṣad* 2.1.12, also quoted above.

109. *Vivekacūḍāmaṇi* 34–35.
110. *Śiva Saṃhitā* 12–14.
111. *Jñāneśvarī* 13.414–23.
112. *From the Finite to the Infinite,* p. 297.
113. Swami Muktananda, *Sadgurunath Maharaj ki Jay* (New York: SYDA Foundation, 1975), p. 155.
114. *From the Finite to the Infinite,* p. 53.
115. Swami Muktananda, *Satsang with Baba,* Vol. 2 (Oakland, California: SYDA Foundation, 1976), p. 13.
116. *Where Are You Going?* p. 132.
117. *From the Finite to the Infinite,* p. 297.
118. *Taittirīya Upaniṣad* 1.3.3. "Older form" and "younger form" translate *pūrvarūpa* and *uttararūpa,* which might more literally be rendered "former form" and "latter form."
119. Swami Muktananda, *I Have Become Alive* (South Fallsburg, New York: SYDA Foundation, 1992), p. 28.
120. *From the Finite to the Infinite,* p. 239.
121. *The Perfect Relationship* p. 32.
122. Translated here by Mark S. G. Dyczkowski in *The Aphorisms of Śiva: The Śiva Sūtra with Bhāskara's Commentary, the Vārttika* (Albany: State University of New York Press, 1992), p. 81.
123. See the chapter on the Self elsewhere in this collection.
124. From the public domain, translated here by Viju Kulkarni.
125. *Where Are You Going?* pp. 140–41.
126. *Where Are You Going?* p. 141.
127. Ram Butler, "No One Else Can Do It," *Darshan* No. 44 (November 1990), p. 67.
128. Quoted in Swami Chidvilasananda, *Kindle My Heart,* Vol. I (1989 edition), p. 146.
129. *Jñāneśvarī* 18.1557–59.
130. *Amṛtānubhāv* 2.1–5, with the translation from *The Nectar of Self-Awareness* (South Fallsburg, New York: SYDA Foundation, 1979).
131. *Kindle My Heart,* Vol. I (1989 edition), p. 147.
132. Namely, the *Kaṭha, Īśā,* and *Śvetāśvatara Upaniṣads* from the Vedāntic Period as well as the many Śaiva, Vaiṣṇava and Śākta Upaniṣads of the later Classical Period.
133. *Śvetāśvatara Upaniṣad* 6.23.
134. *Vivekacūḍāmaṇi* 46, paraphrasing *Kaivalya Upaniṣad* 1.2.
135. *Vivekacūḍāmaṇi* 25.
136. *Vivekacūḍāmaṇi* 31-32.
137. *Bhagavadgītā* 10.18.
138. *Bhagavadgītā* 7.2, *Jñāneśvarī* 7.2.
139. *Bhagavadgītā* 18.73.
140. *Jñāneśvarī* 18.1553–55.
141. *Jñāneśvarī* 18.1560.
142. *Bhagavadgītā* 18.55.
143. *Jñāneśvarī* 18.1221–2.

144. *Jñāneśvarī* 18.1219.

145. See *Nārada Bhakti Sūtra* 2–3. The phrases "transcendent love" and "nectarean ambrosia" translate *paramapremarūpa* and *amṛtasvarūpa*, respectively.

146. *Nārada Bhakti Sūtra* 6.

147. *Nārada Bhakti Sūtra* 15–18. The relevant terms here are *pūjā, kathā,* and *ātmaratyavirodha.*

148. *Nārada Bhakti Sūtra* 19.

149. *Nārada Bhakti Sūtra* 33.

150. *Nārada Bhakti Sūtra* 67.

151. *Nārada Bhakti Sūtra* 68–69.

152. *Nārada Bhakti Sūtra* 58.

153. See *Nārada Bhakti Sūtra* 56–57: "Devotion directed to an object with characteristics is of three kinds, according to the quality of its physical nature. . . . [But] each preceding one leads to a better succeeding one for the sake of the good [*śreyas*]."

154. *Nārada Bhakti Sūtra* 38–41.

155. *Nārada Bhakti Sūtra* 19.

156. See *Nārada Bhakti Sūtra* 7–10.

157. *Bhagavadgītā* 4.34.

158. *Jñāneśvarī* 4.164–66.

159. *Jñāneśvarī* 16.1–2.

160. Compare *Gurugītā* 23: "The syllable *gu* is darkness, and the syllable *ru* is said to be light. There is no doubt that the Guru is indeed the supreme knowledge that swallows [the darkness] of ignorance."

161. *Kulārṇava Tantra* 17.7–9, translated here by Ram Kumar Rai (Varanasi: Prachya Prakashan, 1983), p. 328.

162. *The Nectar of Chanting,* "Āratī: Morning and Evening Prayer," pp. 129–30 (verses 3, 4).

163. See *The Nectar of Chanting,* p. xiii. For a discussion of the *Gurugītā* as an element of the canon of Siddha Yoga, see Douglas Brooks's "The Canons of Siddha Yoga: The Body of Scripture and the Form of the Guru," elsewhere in this collection.

164. *Gurugītā* 23. As a text, the *Gurugītā* shares some of its language, imagery, and ideas regarding the nature of the guru and of the guru-disciple relationship with a number of other works. This is why, for example, verse 23 sounds so similar to *Kulārṇava Tantra* (17.7–9), quoted above.

165. *The Perfect Relationship* p. 1.

166. *Śvetāśvatara Upaniṣad* 1.15–16.

167. *Sāyaṃprātaḥ kī āratī,* verse 23. See *Svādhyāya Sudhā,* Twelfth Edition (Ganeshpuri, India: Gurudev Siddha Peeth, 1994), p. 118. See also *The Nectar of Chanting,* p. 137.

168. *Satsang with Baba,* Vol. 2, p. 97.

169. For a brief summary of various Hindu perspectives regarding the relationship between God and the soul, see William K. Mahony, "The Self: A Vedāntic Foundation for the Revelation of the Absolute," Chapter 5 in this collection.

170. *Īśā Upaniṣad* 1.1.

171. Swami Muktananda, from an unpublished transcript, March 20, 1978.

172. *From the Finite to the Infinite,* p. 274.

173. Swami Muktananda, *Satsang with Baba*, Vol. 5 (Oakland, California: SYDA Foundation, 1978), p. 138.

174. *Amṛtānubhāv* 2.54–56, 2.61, 2.66–68, with the translation from *The Nectar of Self-Awareness*, pp. 15–16.

175. Swami Chidvilasananda, "Love and Nothing Else," *Darshan* No. 24 (March 1989), p. 88.

176. Swami Muktananda, *Selected Essays* (South Fallsburg, New York: SYDA Foundation, 1995), p. 51.

177. *From the Finite to the Infinite*, p. 62.

178. The original story appears in the Indian national epic, the *Mahābhārata*. See J. A. B. van Buitenen, *The Mahābhārata*, Book One: "The Book of the Beginning" (Chicago: University of Chicago Press, 1973), pp. 270–73.

179. Swami Muktananda, *Satsang with Baba*, Vol. 4 (Ganeshpuri, India: SYDA Foundation, 1978), p. 259–60.

180. *Satsang with Baba*, Vol. 4, p. 260. For other accounts of this story, see also Swami Durgananda, "Report from Ganeshpuri," *Siddha Path* (March 1978), p. 8; *Satsang with Baba*, Vol. 1 (Oakland, California: SYDA Foundation, 1974), pp. 184, 219; *Satsang with Baba*, Vol. 3 (Oakland, California: SYDA Foundation, 1977), pp. 152, 325; *Where Are You Going?* pp. 78–80.

181. *From the Finite to the Infinite*, p. 288.

182. *Play of Consciousness*, p. 58. The phrase *dhyānamūlam gurormūrtiḥ* appears in *Kulārṇava Tantra* 12.13 and in *Gurugītā* 76.

183. Translated in *Play of Consciousness*, pp. 63–64.

184. Translated in *Play of Consciousness*, p. 64.

185. *Selected Essays*, p. 51. Compare *Gurugītā* 38: "Salutations to Śrī Guru, who illumines this [world] but whom the mind cannot illumine. [He also illumines] the waking, dreaming, and deep sleep states."

186. *From the Finite to the Infinite*, p. 59.

187. *Jñāneśvarī* 15.1–8.

188. *Sadgurunath Maharaj ki Jay*, p. 104.

189. *Gurugītā* 57–58.

190. *From the Finite to the Infinite*, p. 307.

191. *Sadgurunath Maharaj ki Jay*, pp. 116–117.

192. *Kulārṇava Tantra* 12.13. See also *Gurugītā* 76.

193. *From the Finite to the Infinite*, pp. 62–63.

194. *Śrī Guru Pāduka-Pañcakam* ("Five Stanzas on the Sandals of Śrī Guru"), verses 2 and 5, in *The Nectar of Chanting*, pp. 4–5.

195. *From the Finite to the Infinite*, p. 275.

196. *From the Finite to the Infinite*, p. 285.

197. *Gurugītā* 62.

198. *Where Are You Going?* p. 127.

199. *Kulārṇava Tantra* 12.24.

200. *The Perfect Relationship*, p. 160.

201. *Kulārṇava Tantra* 13.52.

202. *Kulārṇava Tantra* 12.32.

203. Kṣemarāja, *Śiva Sūtra Vimarśinī* 2.6.

204. Kṣemarāja, *Śiva Sūtra Vimarśinī* 2.6, also quoted above. See also Swami

Muktananda's reference to this statement in *Where Are You Going?* p. 127 and in *The Perfect Relationship* p. 25.

205. *Jñāneśvarī* 12.1.
206. *The Perfect Relationship*, p. 25.
207. *The Perfect Relationship*, p. 160.
208. *From the Finite to the Infinite*, p. 59.
209. *Jñāneśvarī* 14.1–2.
210. *Gurugītā* 32.
211. *Gurugītā* 80.
212. *Gurugītā* 82.
213. *Gurugītā* 77, 90.
214. Swami Chidvilasananda, "Transform Your Vision," *Darshan* No. 82 (January 1994), pp. 41–42.
215. Siddha Yoga Experience Archives.

Chapter 4. The Canons of Siddha Yoga

1. Jacob Neusner has argued that the rabbis provided the canonical authority of Judaism rather than the text of the Torah. This provocative and ingenious notion has also been researched by William Scott Green. In the case of Hinduism, we have a similar notion expressed in the tradition of Śrīvidyā. [See Douglas Renfrew Brooks, *Auspicious Wisdom, The Texts and Traditions of Śrīvidyā Śākta Tantrism in South India* (Albany: State University of New York Press, 1992)]. It is my contention that Siddha Yoga's understanding of the guru follows a similar pattern.
2. This may strike us as peculiar since we may have the belief that all Christians have the "same" Bible as their canonical authority. However, this is not the case. There are subtle variations and choices made even with respect to this basic resource. Further, the Bible is not the only canonical resource for many Christians. Siddha traditions are, in this way, directly comparable.
3. In this sense "Siddha Yoga" is a proper noun used to specify that distinctive lineage and canon as defined by the gurus of this lineage. Presumably future Siddha Yoga gurus will continue to develop the canon and its interpretation. The selection of the next guru is in the hands of Swami Chidvilasananda.
4. Other lineages or gurus may borrow another's teachings, sometimes giving proper attribution and sometimes trespassing on words or interpretations.
5. This is not to say that all the texts or genres that have been mentioned are important to all siddha gurus. Rather, we note here the importance of the relationship between the inclusive canon and the lineage canon. Just as all lineage canons are unique, not all notions of the inclusive canon are identical.
6. Siddha Yoga is not unique in this respect. For example, the institutional Śāṅkara traditions similarly adopt many *smārta* beliefs without engaging in the formal canonical rejection of Tantric teachings, which they too affirm selectively.
7. Swami Muktananda, *Secret of the Siddhas* (South Fallsburg, New York: SYDA Foundation, 1994), p. 5 (verse 29).
8. *Secret of the Siddhas*, p. 2 (verses 8, 30).
9. *Secret of the Siddhas*, pp. 7, 2–3 (verses 45, 10).
10. *Secret of the Siddhas*, pp. 1, 2 (verses 1, 8).

11. Swami Chidvilasananda, *Kindle My Heart,* Vol. I (South Fallsburg, New York: SYDA Foundation, 1989), p. 16.

12. See Teun Goudriaan, and Sanjukta Gupta, *The History of Hindu Tantric and Śākta Literature* (Wiesbaden: Otto Harrassowitz, 1981).

13. Any number of contemporary scholarly sources will elaborate this point. See works by André Padoux, Teun Goudriaan, Agehananda Bharati, V. V. Dvivedi, Sanjukta Gupta, or Douglas Renfrew Brooks.

14. See *The Nectar of Chanting* (South Fallsburg, New York: SYDA Foundation, 1983), p. xxiii.

15. Like many other comparable texts, such as the *Lalitāsahasranāma,* which is said to appear in the *Brahmāṇḍa Purāṇa,* the *Gurugītā* does not, in fact, appear in either of these texts as part of any ordinary edition. Rather, it is a case of attribution in which the purpose is to align a text so that it achieves a certain recognition and set of associations.

16. The six *darśanas,* or "viewpoints," are traditionally organized in pairs: Logic and Ontology (Nyāya and Vaiśeṣika), Enumeration and Yoga (Sāṃkhya and Yoga), and Earlier Analysis Ritual and Later Analysis Philosophy (Pūrva Mīmāṃsā and Uttara Mīmāṃsā/Vedānta). Each *darśana* has a root text composed in the style of aphorisms (*sūtra*) and a wealth of commentarial traditions that follow which link as well as distinguish them from one another. Not strictly sectarian traditions of worship but rather ways of viewing the world for analytical purposes, the six *darśanas* form the common philosophical core of classical Hinduism.

17. Swami Chidvilasananda, *My Lord Loves a Pure Heart* (South Fallsburg, New York: SYDA Foundation, 1994), p. 12.

18. While Advaita Vedānta has historically been a *smārta* tradition, supporting an ascetic tradition institutionalized by the Śaṅkarācārya lineages and orders, the nondualist Śaivism of Kashmir is clearly Tantric in its ethos. These are complex lines to draw: Śrīvidyā Tantrism, for example, has a long association with the Śāṅkara traditions of south India while many Kashmiri Śaivite writers were undoubtedly *smārta*-following brahmins.

19. We might compare the Siddha Yoga gurus to the eighteenth Bhāskararāya, whose own brand of Śrīvidyā draws from Vedānta, Kashmiri Śaivism, and the lore of siddhas. The point is simply that this synthetic approach to these historically distinguishable traditions is not idiosyncratic to Siddha Yoga.

20. Careful reading of Swami Muktananda's works may suggest his own interpretive preferences but this is not the same as becoming an active participant in the polemic.

21. *Secret of the Siddhas,* p. 35 (verses 158–160).

22. We can, of course, distinguish the schools and movements within Kashmiri Śaivism—Trika, Kaula, Pratyabhijñā, Spanda, Krama, etc.— though this is not at issue in Siddha Yoga.

23. Though all are considered siddhas, scholars usually distinguish the devotees (*bhakta*) from the saints (*sant*) by their deeply theistic orientation and their emphasis on *saguṇa brahman* or the absolute-with-qualities. In contrast, the saints are noted for their emphatic nondualism and emphasis on *nirguna brahman* or the absolute-without-qualities.

24. An important reason for this is that the south Indian Śaivas are largely dual-

ists in thought and/or strictly sectarian in their approach to devotional theology.

25. Abhinavagupta, for example, clearly sees the importance of devotion, disinterested action, and knowledge but ranks knowledge as the final liberative force when it is accompanied by the grace of God expressed in devotion. See his comments on chapters 2 and 3 of the *Bhagavadgītā.*

26. *My Lord Loves a Pure Heart,* p. 50.

27. That Swami Muktananda had his shaktipat experience on the exact day and year of Indian independence has created a special place in his work for Gandhi, though it is not the political figure but rather the ethical and spiritual one who seems to have been foremost in his mind.

28. There is lore attributed to Bhagawan Nityananda by others outside Siddha Yoga, such as M. U. Hatengdi and Swami Chetanananda's *Nitya Sutras: The Revelations of Nityananda from the Chidakash Gita* (Cambridge, Massachusetts: Rudra Press, 1985).

29. See note 28.

30. For a complete list of writings and dates see appendix 1.

31. Sometimes the "essence" or the "meaning" of a text is in its performance as a ritual or in its memorization for the purposes of recitation. Certainly not all "meaning" entails exegesis or interpretation. Rather, the point is that a text or a value is taken to heart and then expressed in one way or another.

32. A living master may occasionally suggest that the guru lives in the hearts of disciples but is no longer physically alive. This sense is, however, not the primary meaning nor the one that I think best describes what is vital to understanding the *guruvāda* tradition.

33. I have deliberately excluded the Tibetan tradition of the lama (or guru) as the fourth refuge and do not mean to overgeneralize the case. Rather, I am speaking here primarily about the views of the Pāli canon.

34. Buddhist Tantrics, in contrast, fall more squarely within the *guruvāda* traditions and ultimately treat texts as extensions of the guru's own body. In Tibetan traditions, the guru (Tibetan, *blama*) is the fourth refuge, on a par with the Buddha, dharma, and *saṅgha.*

35. There are, of course, guru-centered Buddhist traditions. One can point particularly to Tantric and Zen traditions for such examples.

36. Arguably, all spiritual traditions have some stake in similar matters. The Reformation of Western Christianity, for example, dealt with comparable issues of authority and interpretation. What is the relationship between the preacher and the preached? How can (or should) these two be distinguished? What is the relationship between traditional understandings and practices and the scriptures themselves?

37. *Secret of the Siddhas,* p. 62 (verse 226).

38. Fundamentally, the veracity of a siddha guru's experiential claim to authority is something that disciples affirm not only in their guru but within themselves. The guru's state of consciousness, however, has its own effects and verifying power. Traditional texts that describe the siddha's state offer descriptions of the guru and the guru-disciple relationship that create means by which true gurus (*sadguru*) can be distinguished from pretenders, charlatans, or those who would adopt the title without having met the criteria of qualification (*adhikāra*) and attainment (*siddha*).

With the potential for false or unqualified gurus to abuse the power invested in the living master, it is little wonder that the guru becomes the major topic of textual study and oral explication. In siddha traditions, the guru is always at the center of the canon as the topic and the interpreter.

39. *Gurugītā* 168. Cf. *Paraśurāmakalpa Sūtra* for the Śākta notion of *ekagurūpāsti*.

40. *Tantrāloka* 35-40a, quoted from Mark S.G. Dyczkowski, *The Aphorisms of Śiva* (Albany: State University of New York Press, 1992), p. 191.

41. *Svacchanda Tantra* 4.313:

yatra yatra mano' yati jñeyam tatraiva cintayet/
calitvā yasyate kutra sarvaṃ śivamayaṃ yataḥ//

42. *Śrīkularatnamāla* is quoted in Kṣemarāja's *Vimarśinī* on *Śiva Sūtra* 3.43.

43. *Śiva Sūtra* 2.6.

44. *Tantrāloka,* 15.38–39, reads in its entirety:

tatrādau śivatāpattisvātantryāveśa eva yaḥ/
sa eva hi guruḥ kāryastataho'sau dīkṣaṇe kṣamaḥ//

45. *Tantrāloka* 4.42ab, 4.45cd:

abhiṣikthaḥ svasaṃvittdevībhirdīkṣitaśca saḥ/
sarvaśāstrārthavettṛtvamakasmāccāsya jāyate//

46. Swami Muktananda, *The Perfect Relationship* (South Fallsburg, New York: SYDA Foundation, 1985), p. 15.

47. *The Perfect Relationship,* pp. 2–3.

48. *The Perfect Relationship,* p. 11.

49. *Kulārṇava Tantra* 13.54:

manuṣycarmaṇābaddhaḥ sākṣāt paraśivaḥ svayam/
sācchiṣyānugrahārthāya gūḍham paryaṭati kṣitau//

50. Cf. Mark S. G. Dyczkowski, *The Stanzas on Vibration* (Albany: State University of New York Press, 1992), Chapter 11.

51. Quoted from Dyczkowski, *The Stanzas on Vibration,* p. 175.

52. *The Perfect Relationship,* p. 10.

53. See Dyczkowski, *The Stanzas on Vibration,* p. 106.

54. *The Perfect Relationship,* p. 25.

55. Swami Muktananda, from an unpublished transcript, November 15, 1976.

56. *The Perfect Relationship,* p. 67.

57. *Gurugītā* 7–8.

58. Similarly, Govinda, the historically silent teacher of the prolific Vedāntin Śaṅkara, provides yet another example of the interpretation of the guru's command and of the possibilities for development within a lineage. One would have expected Śaṅkara to name at least some of his guru's compositions had he written any.

59. Swami Muktananda, *Paramartha Katha Prasang: Spiritual Conversations with Swami Muktananda* (Ganeshpuri, India: Gurudev Siddha Peeth, 1981), pp. 36–37.

60. *My Lord Loves a Pure Heart,* p. 26.

61. *Tantrāloka* 4.77cd, 78ab:

yataḥ śāstrakramāttajjnaguruprajñānuśilanāt//
ātmaprayiyatam jñānaṃ pūrṇatvādbhairavāyate//

62. Quoted from Dyczkowski's *The Stanzas on Vibration*, p. 189. The quotation is *Tantrāloka* (4.179b–180a) and reads:

kramasya niyamaḥ kvacit kramābhāvānna yugapattadabhāvātkramo'pi na/
kramākramakathātītam samvittattvaṃ sunirmalam/
tadasyāḥ samvido devyā yatra kvāpi pravartanam//

63. See Dyczkowski's *The Stanzas on Vibration*, p. 107.
64. See Dyczkowski's *The Stanzas on Vibration*, p. 175.
65. Swami Muktananda, quoting *Jñāneśvarī* 18.1470–75 in *The Perfect Relationship*, pp. 188–89.
66. *The Perfect Relationship*, p. 189.
67. Though many traditions of Bhakti and Tantra claim that spiritual *adhikāra*, "qualification," should not be caste- or gender-prejudiced, this is hardly reason to think of them as socially revolutionary. As it has been shown elsewhere, such counter-orthodox claims of inclusion are often used to reinforce the status quo rather than discredit or subvert social prerogatives. In this sense, Muktananda's egalitarianism is all the more remarkable. Cf. Douglas Renfrew Brooks, "Encountering the Hindu 'Other': Tantrism and the Brahmans of South India," *Journal of the American Academy of Religion*, LX/3, pp. 405–36.
68. The three *pramāṇas* are *pratyakṣa* ("sense perception"), *anumāna* ("inference"), and *śabda* ("scripture" or "revelation"). Though *śabda* in Vedāntic terms means the revelation of the Veda (*śruti*), for Abhinavagupta and Muktananda the "word" (the literal the meaning of *śabda*) can apply equally to the guru's pronouncements and interpretations. This is, at least partially, a result of their Śaivite view that Śiva is the author of revelation and that the guru is none other than Śiva. See *Īśvarapratyabhijñāvivṛtivimarśinī* for a more detailed discussion of Abhinavagupta's understanding of the *pramāṇas*.
69. One might further identify the synchronic truth with the experience of the guru within, that is, with the ever-present guru that appears in meditation. Likewise, the diachronic truth of the guru is the physical being, whether living or enshrined.
70. For a brief and accurate summary of the *upāya* theory in Kashmiri Śaivism see the Introduction in Constantina Rhodes Bailly, *Shaiva Devotional Songs of Kashmir* (Albany: State University of New York Press, 1990).
71. See Dyczkowski, *The Stanzas on Vibration*, pp. 106-108.
72. Swami Muktananda, *Satsang with Baba*, Vol. 4 (Oakland, California: SYDA Foundation, 1978), p. 200.
73. *Bhagavadgītā* 11.48.
74. *The Perfect Relationship*, p. 189.
75. *The Perfect Relationship*, p. 73.
76. *My Lord Loves a Pure Heart*, p. 20.
77. Swami Kripananda, *Jnaneshwar's Gita: A Rendering of the Jnaneshwari* (Albany: State University of New York Press, 1989), 13.823–824, 830–831, 835, p. 208.
78. *Jnaneshwar's Gita* 13.836–839, pp. 208–9.

79. *The Perfect Relationship*, p. 64.

80. *Secret of the Siddhas*, p. 135 (verse 335).

81. *The Perfect Relationship*, p. 77.

82. Swami Muktananda, *Bhagawan Nityananda of Ganeshpuri* (South Fallsburg, New York: SYDA Foundation, 1996), p. 65.

83. Swami Muktananda, *Play of Consciousness* (South Fallsburg, New York: SYDA Foundation, 1994), pp. 22–23.

84. *The Perfect Relationship*, p. 73.

85. *Play of Consciousness*, p. 68.

86. *Bhagawan Nityananda of Ganeshpuri*, pp. 38–39.

87. Swami Chidvilasananda, *Ashes at My Guru's Feet* (South Fallsburg, New York: SYDA Foundation, 1990), p. 44.

88. See *My Lord Loves a Pure Heart* and several essays in *Kindle My Heart*, Vols. I and II (1989 edition), especially "A Clean Heart Reflects the Light of God."

89. *Secret of the Siddhas*, p. 85 (verse 271).

90. *My Lord Loves a Pure Heart*, p. 20.

91. *Secret of the Siddhas*, pp. 5–6 (verse 31).

92. *Secret of the Siddhas*, p. 6 (verse 34).

93. *My Lord Loves a Pure Heart*, p. 20.

94. *Secret of the Siddhas*, p. 123 (verse 323).

95. *My Lord Loves a Pure Heart*, pp. 20–21.

96. *Secret of the Siddhas*, p. 122 (verse 322).

97. *My Lord Loves a Pure Heart*, pp. 23–24.

98. *Secret of the Siddhas*, pp. 7–8 (verse 46).

99. *The Perfect Relationship*, pp. 11, 14.

100. *My Lord Loves a Pure Heart*, p. 22.

101. *Secret of the Siddhas*, p. 123 (verse 323).

102. *Secret of the Siddhas*, p. 39 (verse 174).

103. *Play of Consciousness*, p. 27.

104. *My Lord Loves a Pure Heart*, p. 24.

105. *Secret of the Siddhas*, p. 31 (verse 145).

106. *Play of Consciousness*, pp. 230–31.

107. *Secret of the Siddhas*, p. 32 (verse 146).

108. *Play of Consciousness*, p. 123.

109. *My Lord Loves a Pure Heart*, p. 52.

110. Swami Muktananda, *From the Finite to the Infinite* (South Fallsburg, New York: SYDA Foundation, 1994), p. 314.

111. *From the Finite to the Infinite*, p. 371.

112. *The Perfect Relationship*, p. 2.

113. For example, the *Kulārṇava Tantra* seems to endorse unambiguously the so-called *pañcamakāra* or "five m-words," which include intoxicants, nonvegetarian food, and ritual sex. Swami Muktananda is explicit in his rejection of such behaviors. In his *Secret of the Siddhas* (p. 5, verse 25) he writes: "Siddha Yoga avoids all intoxicants, including marijuana, opium, cocaine, hashish, and other drugs. They corrupt the mind, destroy the intellect, and trouble one's life."

114. It is fair to say that most Siddha Yoga devotees, unfamiliar with the details and breadth of the literature from which Swami Muktananda draws, would likely be

astonished to learn that many of the texts he quotes include passages entirely foreign to their understandings of moral life (*dharma*) and spiritual discipline (*sādhana*).

115. *Play of Consciousness*, p. 232.

116. *From the Finite to the Infinite*, pp. 321–22.

117. *From the Finite to the Infinite*, p. 239.

118. *From the Finite to the Infinite*, pp. 364–65.

119. *Play of Consciousness*, p. 21.

120. *Play of Consciousness*, p. 22.

121. *Play of Consciousness*, p. 33. Also see Zipruanna's comments to Swami Muktananda on p. 122.

122. *Play of Consciousness*, pp. 254, 257.

123. See the Constitution of the Siddha Yoga Foundation (printed in part in Part I of this volume, "To See the World Full of Saints: The History of Siddha Yoga as a Contemporary Movement") which states Swami Muktananda's vision of lineage leadership. His assertion that the Siddha Yoga guru must be a lifelong celibate who becomes a formal renunciant is unambiguous. Any deviation from that condition would formally disqualify a person, even if that person had already assumed the position of lineage leadership.

124. One can surmise two important implications from Swami Muktananda's views about the leadership of the Siddha Yoga lineage. First, the prerequisite of lifelong celibacy guarantees the integrity of the gurus' relationship with disciples. Any transgression on the part of future leaders would vitiate the possibility of leadership. Second, because sexual abstinence is characteristic of a shaktipat guru and Swami Muktananda places such a high value on the guru's example, the requirement of *sannyāsa* removes any shard of doubt concerning the appropriate relationship between guru and disciples. In other words, the outer relationship mirrors the spiritual ideal of love without lust.

125. *Secret of the Siddhas*, p. 5 (verse 228). For an example of a householder siddha who also happened to be a woman see the story of the Maharashtrian yogini Sākhubāī retold in *Secret of the Siddhas*, pp. 46–47 (verse 186).

126. *Play of Consciousness*, pp. 254–55.

127. *Play of Consciousness*, p. 256.

128. *My Lord Loves a Pure Heart*, pp. 31–32.

129. *Secret of the Siddhas*, p. 5 (verse 29).

130. *Play of Consciousness*, p. 257.

131. In his spiritual autobiography, *Play of Consciousness*, Swami Muktananda narrates in some detail his own process of self-transformation, including the very frank discussion of his own sufferings from dualism and desire. (p. 102)

132. *From the Finite to the Infinite*, pp. 309–310.

133. Krishna's remark in the *Bhagavadgītā*, 2.20 ff., is an example of this effort to put understanding before dogmatism. We might also consider the entire mode of understanding Hindu law found in the *Manusmṛti*. Here Manu the Law-Giver, though seemingly prescriptive and at times dogmatic, is more inclined to offer multiple opinions and a variety of contextual understandings. Rather than expressing indecision it is more likely a reflection of Manu's view that context and circumstance demand a deeper contemplation of truth.

134. *Secret of the Siddhas*, p. 15 (verse 81).

135. Swami Muktananda says in *Secret of the Siddhas* (p. 3, verse 12), "In Siddha Yoga we attain the knowledge of our birthright."

136. *The Perfect Relationship*, p. 58.

137. *The Perfect Relationship*, p. 64.

138. *Secret of the Siddhas*, p. 143 (verse 342).

139. *The Perfect Relationship*, pp. 58–59.

140. *Secret of the Siddhas*, p. 54 (verse 209).

141. *The Perfect Relationship*, p. 63. Quoting from the scriptures without citation is a common practice among traditionalist Indian writers.

142. *Secret of the Siddhas*, p. 128 (verse 329).

143. *Play of Consciousness*, p. 257.

144. *Īśvarapratyabhijñāvimarśinī* 2.59.

145. See Dyczkowski's *The Stanzas on Vibration*, p. 200 and note 139.

Chapter 5. The Self

1. See Swami Muktananda, *Meditate* (Albany: State University of New York Press, 1991), p. 41. This teaching appears with slight variations in several of Swami Muktananda's and Swami Chidvilasananda's works. See, for example, Chidvilasananda's reference to Muktananda's words—"Honor your own Self. Meditate on your own Self. Worship your own Self. Kneel to your own Self. Understand your own Self. Your God dwells within you as you"—in *Resonate with Stillness: Daily Contemplations from the Words of Swami Muktananda, Swami Chidvilasananda* (South Fallsburg, New York: SYDA Foundation, 1995), January 5.

2. Swami Chidvilasananda, *Kindle My Heart* (South Fallsburg, New York: SYDA Foundation, 1996), p. 185.

3. See *Qur'ān* 59.24 (which refers to God as al-Bāri'), 13.16 (al-Khāliq), 3.2 (al-Qayyum), 4.85 (al-Muqīṭ), 5.117 (ash-Shahīd).

4. The rather tentative phrasing here reflects the fact that the word *Hinduism* does not represent an indigenous Indian category but rather reflects the legacy of non-Indian hegemony and colonialism on the subcontinent. The term *hindu* derives from the word *indus*, meaning, simply, "that which flows" and thus the origin of the name for the Indus River, which flows into the Arabian Sea having drained the western Himalayas and much of what is now Pakistan. The Achaemenid Persians called the Indus River the Hindu, while the Greeks called it the Indos. Arabs came to call the region drained by the Indus River "al-Hind" and referred to the people who lived in al-Hind as *hindi*. Primarily for the purpose of determining taxation, Muslim rulers then came to use the term *hindu* as a way to group in a single category the many non-Muslims living in al-Hind. European colonialists used the word in a similar way (usually spelling it *hindoo*), namely, to refer to anything Indian which was neither European nor Muslim. The word was thus originally a political, economic, and cultural term with no real reference to any particular religious tradition or community, for there were any number of such traditions practiced in al-Hind, some of which were quite different from each other. It would be as if all of the various religions practiced by all of the people living in the area drained by the Mississippi River were to be labeled "Mississippism."

5. *Qur'ān* 50.16.

6. See for example, *Qur'ān* 57.3.

7. For reasons implied in Note 4 (above), there are many forms of what has come to be called "Hinduism." Siddha Yoga does not share the same values, ideas, and practices with all of these different philosophies, traditions, and perspectives. For example, it has little in common with the Cārvāka and Lokāyata philosophical stances. These are classical Indian schools of thought based on the idea that the world known through the senses is the only truly knowable world; accordingly, they are thoroughly materialistic world views that reject both the idea of any transcendental being and the notion of a soul. For another example, Siddha Yoga would not identify with the more visceral forms of "Hindu" sacerdotal sensibilities undergirding various regional Indian traditions in which, for example, a water buffalo or a goat is slaughtered as part of a ritual offering. For yet another example, Siddha Yoga is not to be identified with any particular political party or movement in India that draws on Hindu nationalist sentiments. For a consideration of the "canon" of Siddha Yoga as a religious movement, see Douglas Renfrew Brooks's "The Canons of Siddha Yoga: The Body of Scripture and the Form of the Guru" elsewhere in this collection.

8. For a text that uses the term *jinissai jiko* in this sense, see *Shōbōgenzō: Yuibutsu Yobutsu* ("Only the Buddha Together with the Buddha") by Dōgen Zenji (1200–1253), the founder of Sōtō Zen in Japan. For a discussion of Dōgen's teachings regarding the all-encompassing Self, see Kōshō Uchiyama, *Opening the Hand of Thought,* translated by Shōhaku Okomura and Tom Wright (New York: Penguin Arkana, 1993), pp. 8–13, 107–48, and *passim.*

9. These terms include not only *shinnyo, jissō,* and *nyonyo* (all of which are Japanese equivalents of the Sanskrit *tathatā*: "Suchness") and *nyoraizō* (Sanskrit, *tathāgatagarbha*: "womb of Suchness"), but also *busshō* (Sanskrit *buddhatā*: "Buddha-nature"), *yuishin* (Sanskrit, *cittamātra*: "Mind-Only" or "Mind-Source"), *isshin* (Sanskrit, *svacittamātra*: "One-Mind"). See also Uchiyama, *Opening the Hand of Thought,* p. 102n.

10. *Resonate with Stillness,* January 5.

11. *Meditate,* p. 14.

12. *Bhagavadgītā* 13.1.

13. *Meditate,* pp. 14–15.

14. *Meditate,* p. 15.

15. See Swami Muktananda, *From the Finite to the Infinite* (South Fallsburg, New York: SYDA Foundation, 1994), pp. 22–23.

16. Swami Muktananda, "To Know the Knower," *Siddha Path* (March 1981), p. 16.

17. Swami Muktananda, *Sadgurunath Maharaj ki Jay* (New York: SYDA Foundation, 1975), p. 125.

18. Swami Muktananda, *Reflections of the Self* (South Fallsburg: SYDA Foundation, 1993), p. 60 (Part I, verse 280).

19. All quotations in this paragraph come from Swami Muktananda, *Where Are You Going? A Guide to the Spiritual Journey* (South Fallsburg, New York: SYDA Foundation, 1994), pp. 27–28.

20. Swami Chidvilasananda, "Go Deep Within Yourself," *Darshan* No. 57 (December 1991), p. 43.

21. Swami Chidvilasananda, "See the Same Self in All," *Darshan* No. 106 (January 1996), p. 45.

22. *Resonate with Stillness,* December 26.

23. Swami Chidvilasananda, "The Supreme Self Is Changeless, Unborn, Ancient," *Darshan* No. 56 (November 1991), p. 58.

24. "The Supreme Self Is Changeless, Unborn, Ancient," *Darshan* No. 56, p. 59.

25. Swami Muktananda, *Bhagawan Nityananda of Ganeshpuri* (South Fallsburg, New York: SYDA Foundation, 1996), p. 25.

26. *Sadgurunath Maharaj ki Jay,* p. 16.

27. "The Supreme Self Is Changeless, Unborn, Ancient," *Darshan* No. 56, p. 58.

28. Swami Chidvilasananda, "Four Means of Recognizing the Self," *Darshan* No. 79 (October 1993), p. 28.

29. "Four Means of Recognizing the Self," *Darshan* No. 79, p. 28.

30. *Reflections of the Self,* p. 143 (Part II, verse 203).

31. *Sadgurunath Maharaj ki Jay,* p. 37.

32. See *Bhagavadgītā* 13.2. See also *Meditate,* p. 15.

33. *Meditate,* p. 25, quoting *Bṛhadāraṇyaka Upaniṣad* 3.7.20 and *Kena Upaniṣad* 1.5.

34. *Meditate,* p. 15. See also *Ātmabodha* (popularly attributed to Śaṅkarācārya), verse 36.

35. "See the Same Self in All," *Darshan* No. 106, p. 43.

36. *Sadgurunath Maharaj ki Jay,* p. 37.

37. *Reflections of the Self,* pp. 14–15 (Part I, verses 64, 66).

38. *Where Are You Going?* p. 260.

39. *Where Are You Going?* p. 26.

40. *Resonate with Stillness,* December 21.

41. *Reflections of the Self,* p. 140 (Part II, verse 194).

42. Swami Chidvilasananda, *Inner Treasures* (South Fallsburg, New York: SYDA Foundation, 1995), p. 28.

43. *Meditate,* p. 23.

44. *Meditate,* p. 23.

45. *Meditate,* p. 22.

46. *Meditate,* pp. 22–23.

47. *Meditate,* p. 23.

48. *Where Are You Going?* p. 26.

49. *Meditate,* p. 13.

50. *Inner Treasures,* p. 19. In reading such assertions we need to remember that because the Self is not limited or defined by personal characteristics, such "happiness" and "joy" of which swamis Muktananda and Chidvilasananda speak are not associated with the gratification of sense desires or the fulfillment of personal needs. According to these spiritual teachers, one's true being is of the nature of unconditional happiness. The Self therefore requires nothing to be happy, for it already is happy. It does not need gratification. Siddha Yoga as taught by Muktananda cannot therefore be associated with any quasi-religious and pseudo-religious movement that advocates "self-actualization or "self-fulfillment" centered on egocentric or idiosyncratic self-gratification.

51. "Four Means of Recognizing the Self," *Darshan* No. 79, p. 26.

52. Swami Chidvilasananda, *My Lord Loves a Pure Heart: The Yoga of Divine Virtues* (South Fallsburg, New York: SYDA Foundation, 1994), p. 107.

53. See *From the Finite to the Infinite*, pp. 25–26.

54. Swami Muktananda, *Play of Consciousness* (South Fallsburg, New York: SYDA Foundation, 1994), p. 266.

55. *Play of Consciousness*, p. 266.

56. Swami Muktananda, quoting verse 51 of Nārada's *Bhakti Sūtra* in *Play of Consciousness*, p. 168.

57. Swami Muktananda, *Secret of the Siddhas* (South Fallsburg, New York: SYDA Foundation, 1994), p. 39 (verse 172).

58. *Reflections of the Self*, p. 15 (Part I, verse 65).

59. *Inner Treasures*, p. 51. Each of these four statements forms what is known as a "great teaching" (*mahāvākya*) of the Vedānta. The instruction *prajñānam brahma* appears in the *Aitareya Upaniṣad* 3.1.3; *ayam ātmā brahma* in the *Māṇḍūkya Upaniṣad* 2.7; *tat tvam asi* in the *Chāndogya Upaniṣad* 6.8.7 (and elsewhere); and *aham brahmāsmi* in the *Bṛhadāraṇyaka Upaniṣad* 1.4.10. The *Aitareya Upaniṣad, Māṇḍūkya Upaniṣad, Chāndogya Upaniṣad,* and *Bṛhadāraṇyaka Upaniṣad* are parts of the *Ṛgveda, Atharvaveda, Sāmaveda,* and *Yajurveda,* respectively.

60. For a discussion of the various religious texts and traditions on which Siddha Yoga draws, see Douglas Renfrew Brooks's, "The Canons of Siddha Yoga: The Body of Scripture and the Form of the Guru," and S. P. Sabharathnam, "Siddha Yoga as *Mahāyoga*: Encompassing All Other Yogas," elsewhere in this collection.

61. For example, Muktananda dedicates an entire chapter to Vedānta in a book that otherwise presents Kashmir Śaiva teachings: see *Secret of the Siddhas*, pp. 167–75.

62. See *Śiva Sūtra* 1.1: *caitanyamātmā* "The Self is consciousness."

63. *Śvetāśvatara Upaniṣad* 1.15.

64. *Kaṭha Upaniṣad* 3.5.

65. Śaivism is the set of religious ideas and practices based on the worship of God as Śiva; Śāktism refers to the related tradition that reveres the divine as Śakti, the divine universal power identified as the Goddess.

66. See *Aparokṣānubhūti* 2.

67. *Reflections of the Self*, p. 20 (Part I, verse 89).

68. *Reflections of the Self*, pp. 152, 160 (Part II, verses 235, 267).

69. Swami Muktananda, *Satsang with Baba*, Vol. 5 (Oakland, California: SYDA Foundation, 1978), p. 322.

70. *Ṛgveda* 1.52.7.

71. See *Ṛgveda* 1.93.6.

72. *Atharvaveda* 12.1.29.

73. *Atharvaveda* 12.1.1.

74. *Atharvaveda* 10.8.33, 37.

75. *Ṛgveda* 10.25.2.

76. *Atharvaveda* 10.8.1–2, 6, 12, 24.

77. *Atharvaveda* 10.8.25.

78. *Atharvaveda* 10.8.27–28.

79. This line is reminiscent of a well-known Vedic verse (see for example *Śatapatha Brāhmaṇa* 14.8.1 and *Bṛhadāraṇyaka Upaniṣad* 5.1) with which swamis

Muktananda and Chidvilasananda have taught Siddha Yoga students to conclude the singing of the *Gurugītā* and other devotional songs: *pūrṇam adaḥ pūrṇam idam pūrṇāt pūrṇam udacyate pūrṇasya pūrṇam ādāya pūrṇam evāvaśiṣyate.*

80. *Atharvaveda* 10.8.29, 31–32.

81. *Ṛgveda* 1.164.46.

82. *Bṛhadāraṇyaka Upaniṣad* 3.9.1–11.

83. *Kauṣītaki-Brāhmaṇa Upaniṣad* 3.2.

84. *Kauṣītaki Brāhmaṇa Upaniṣad* 3.2. The verses "When we speak, the breaths of life speak" and following are actually a paraphrase. A literal translation would more properly read, "When speech speaks, all of the vital breaths speak after it," and so on.

85. *Muṇḍaka Upaniṣad* 2.2.10. See also *Kaṭha Upaniṣad* 5.15 and *Śvetāśvatara Upaniṣad* 6.14.

86. See *Brahma Sūtra* 1.3.22.

87. See *Kaṭha Upaniṣad* 2.5.

88. See *Chāndogya Upaniṣad* 6.8.6.

89. *Chāndogya Upaniṣad* 4.10.5.

90. *Taittirīya Upaniṣad* 2.1.1.

91. *Taittirīya Upaniṣad* 3.1.1.

92. *Taittirīya Upaniṣad* 3.1–6.

93. See *Chāndogya Upaniṣad* 7.1.1–5.

94. See *Chāndogya Upaniṣad* 7.2–23.

95. *Brahmabindu Upaniṣad* 12–14. The *Brahmabindu Upaniṣad* is sometimes known as the *Amṛtabindu Upaniṣad.* The image of the identity of the space within a jar to represent the individual soul and its identity with the universal Self is repeated in a number of Vedāntic texts. A classic example appears in the *Gauḍapāda Kārikā* by the Advaita Vedāntin philosopher Gauḍapāda (fifth to sixth century). In the third book of that work, Gauḍapāda notes that the relationship of the apparent individual to the Self is equivalent to that between the empty space within a pot (*ghaṭākāśa*) and the space outside a pot (*ākāśa*). The two appear to be different from each other, although in fact they are exactly the same thing. He maintains therefore that the apparent multiplicity of beings in the world is actually a misunderstood unity (*advaita*) of being.

96. *Vivekacūḍāmaṇi* 347–48.

97. *Meditate,* p. 15.

98. That is, *at-* and *ap-*, respectively. See Yāska's *Nirukta* 3.15.

99. *Pāṇinīya Dhātupāṭha* 1.38.

100. Śaṅkarācārya, *Aitareya Upaniṣad Bhāṣya* 1.1. Reference in Sarvepalli Radhakrishnan, *The Principal Upaniṣads,* reprint edition (London: George Allen & Unwin; New York, Humanities Press, 1978), p. 73 n. 2.

101. For etymological discussions, see Paul Deussen, "Ātman," in *The Encyclopedia of Religion and Ethics,* edited by James Hastings (New York: Charles Scribner's Sons, 1924), Vol. 2, p. 195; Baldev Raj Sharma, *The Concept of Ātman in the Principal Upaniṣads* (New Delhi: Dinesh Publications, 1972), pp. 11–13.

102. See, for example, *Ṛgveda* 7.87.2.

103. See, for example, *Atharvaveda* 1.18.3, 3.29.8, 5.1.7, 5.6.11, 7.57.1, 11.1.3, 11.5.22, 12.3.54.

104. Compare Radhakrishnan: "Ātman is the principle of man's life, the soul that pervades his being, his breath, *prāṇa*, his intellect, *prajña*, and transcends them. Ātman is what remains when everything that is not the self is eliminated." See Radhakrishnan, *The Principal Upaniṣads*, p. 73.
105. Radhakrishnan, *The Principal Upaniṣads*, pp. 73–74.
106. Radhakrishnan, *The Principal Upaniṣads*, p. 74.
107. See *Aitareya Upaniṣad* 1.3.11–12.
108. See *Taittirīya Upaniṣad* 2.2.1, 2.5.1.
109. *Bṛhadāraṇyaka Upaniṣad* 2.4.3–4.
110. *Bṛhadāraṇyaka Upaniṣad* 2.4.5.
111. See *Bṛhadāraṇyaka Upaniṣad* 3.9.26, 4.2.4, 4.4.22, 4.5.15.
112. See *Chāndogya Upaniṣad* 8.12.2.
113. See *Māṇḍūkya Upaniṣad* 2–7.
114. *Māṇḍūkya Upaniṣad* 7.
115. *Māṇḍūkya Upaniṣad* 12.
116. See *Maitrī Upaniṣad* 6.19 and 7.11; *Bṛhadāraṇyaka Upaniṣad* 5.14.3–7.
117. *Māṇḍūkya Upaniṣad* 7 and 12.
118. *Chāndogya Upaniṣad* 6.12.1–3.
119. See *Taittirīya Upaniṣad* 2.2–5.
120. *Maitrī Upaniṣad* 2.7.
121. *Maitrī Upaniṣad* 3.1–2.
122. *Bṛhadāraṇyaka Upaniṣad* 4.5.7.
123. *Kaṭha Upaniṣad* 4.1–2.
124. *Māṇḍūkya Upaniṣad* 2.
125. *Muṇḍaka Upaniṣad* 2.2.9 and 3.1.7. The phrase "abiding in the cave of the heart translates *nihitam guhāyām*, more literally perhaps "placed in the secret place." But the word *guhā* also refers more figuratively both to the heart and to a cave, thus the current translation, "in the cave of the heart."
126. On Svayambhū Ātman, see *Kaṭha Upaniṣad* 4.1.
127. On Svayambhū Brahman, see, for example, *Śatapatha Brāhmaṇa* 10.6.5.9.
128. *Vivekacūḍāmaṇi* 225–26.
129. *Vivekacūḍāmaṇi* 223.
130. See *Aitareya Upaniṣad* 1.3.12.
131. *Aitareya Upaniṣad* 1.3.14.
132. *Kena Upaniṣad* 1.1.
133. *Kena Upaniṣad* 1.3.
134. *Kena Upaniṣad* 5–7.
135. *Bṛhadāraṇyaka Upaniṣad* 3.4.1–2.
136. We see occasional mention of the entry of the universal Being into the individual being by means of the top of the head. In a Vedāntic assertion that foreshadows later Tantric teachings, the *Aitareya Upaniṣad* 1.3.11–12 holds, for example, that the universal Creator enters "through the opening at the very end of the head [*sīman*]." According to Tantric thought, this is the place of the *sahasrāra-cakra*, the "thousand-petalled lotus" shimmering at the highest level of consciousness. Similarly, the *Taittirīya Upaniṣad* 1.6.1 teaches that "this space that is within the heart: therein is the immortal and resplendent Person," and that such a divine presence enters by means of the "hair at the top of the skull." The image here is plainly similar

to that presented in later centuries by those traditions of Tantra that center on the worship of the divine as the goddess Kuṇḍalinī and which include the practice of *kuṇḍalinīyoga.* (For a discussion of Kuṇḍalinī and Siddha Yoga, see the essay on this subject by Douglas Renfrew Brooks and Constantina Rhodes Bailly elsewhere in this collection.) Texts that do not mention the soul's entry point still maintain that the divine Self lives in the heart. The *Muṇḍaka Upaniṣad* 2.2.5–6, for example, urges the seeker to—

> Know him alone as the One Self:
> He on whom heaven, earth and sky are woven,
> as are the mind and the vital breaths.
> Dismiss all other [mistaken] lessons.
> This is the bridge to immortality.
> Where the arteries of the body are gathered together
> like spokes at the center of a wheel:
> there, within it [the Ātman] becomes manifold.

137. *Chāndogya Upaniṣad* 8.1.1.
138. *Chāndogya Upaniṣad* 8.1.3.
139. *Chāndogya Upaniṣad* 8.1.5.
140. *Chāndogya Upaniṣad* 8.3.4.
141. *Bṛhadāraṇyaka Upaniṣad* 2.5.14–15.
142. *Śvetāśvatara Upaniṣad* 3.7.
143. *Śvetāśvatara Upaniṣad* 4.1–2.
144. *Śvetāśvatara Upaniṣad* 4.11; 4.14–16.

145. Such Śaiva Upaniṣads include the *Akṣamālaka, Atharvaśikhā, Atharvaśira, Kālāgnirudra, Kaivalya, Gaṇapati, Dakṣiṇāmūrti, Pañcabrahma, Bṛhajjābāla, Bhasmajābāla, Rudrahṛdaya, Rudrākṣabālā,* and *Śarobha.*

146. Vaiṣṇava Upaniṣads include the *Anyakta, Kalisaṃtaraṇa, Kṛṣṇa, Garuḍa, Gopālapūrvatāpanīya, Gopālottaratāpanīya, Tripāddvibhūtimahānārāyaṇa, Dattātreya, Nṛsiṃhapūrvatāpanīya, Nṛsiṃhottaratāpanīya, Rāmapūrvatāpanīya, Rāmottaratāpanīya, Vāsudeva,* and *Hayagrīva.*

147. The Śākta Upaniṣads include the *Tripurā, Tripurātāpanīya, Tripurārahasya, Sarasvatīrahasya, Saubhāgyalakṣmī, Bhāvanā, Bahvṛcā, Devī,* and *Sītā.*

148. *Tripurā Upaniṣad* 1.6.10, translated by Douglas Renfrew Brooks, *The Secret of the Three Cities* (Chicago: University of Chicago Press, 1990), pp. 151, 164, 174.

149. *Bahvṛcā Upaniṣad* 5–8. The reference to the "Three Cities" reflects a Tantric idea that the absolute assumes triadic form and function as it devolves from primordial unity. For example, it becomes will (*icchā*), action (*kriyā*), and knowledge (*jñāna*); creator, creation, and the process of creativity; and the knower, the object of knowledge, and the process of knowing. There are other triadic formulations as well. For a discussion of this theme, see *The Secret of the Three Cities,* p. 97, and references in the Index, *s.v.* "Tripurā."

150. *Śvetāśvatara Upaniṣad* 2.14–15.

151. The phrase *satyaṃ jñānam anantam brahma* ("Brahman is truth, knowledge, and infinity") in this, an early Upaniṣad, predates what was to become a well-known Vedāntic description of Brahman as *sat-cit-ānanda*: "being, consciousness, and bliss." Some later Upaniṣads were to make use of the latter formula. See for

example *Nṛsiṃhottaratāpanī Upaniṣad* 4.3: "This Ātman, the highest Brahman . . . shines forth . . . filled with being, consciousness and bliss," and 7.2: "This whole world consists of Brahman, which consists of truth, consciousness and bliss." See also *Rāmapūrvatāpanī Upaniṣad* 92.

152. *Taittirīya Upaniṣad* 2.1.

153. *Varāha Upaniṣad* 2.45–47.

154. *Śvetāśvatara Upaniṣad* 2.8–10.

155. The Siddha Yoga gurus pronounce this sacred syllable as *oṃ*.

156. For an analysis of the twelve components of the *praṇava* (a form of *nāda*, the universal "tone" or "sound"), see *Nādabindu Upaniṣad* 6–18.

157. *Kṣurikā Upaniṣad* 3–4b.

158. *Yogaśikhā Upaniṣad* 2–3. See Paul Deussen, *Sixty Upaniṣads of the Veda*, translated by V. M. Bedekar and G. B. Palsule (Delhi, India: Motilal Banarsidass, 1987), p. 610.

159. *Kaṭha Upaniṣad* 2.20.

160. *Śvetāśvatara Upaniṣad* 3.20.

161. *Yogatattva Upaniṣad* 68–71.

162. *Bhagavadgītā* 18.61.

163. *Bhagavadgītā* 15.17.

164. *Bhagavadgītā* 15.15.

165. *Bhagavadgītā* 7.7.

166. *Bhagavadgītā* 10.39.

167. *Bhagavadgītā* 4.35.

168. *Bhagavadgītā* 6.29.

169. *Bhagavadgītā* 13.28.

170. *Bhagavadgītā* 6.29–30.

171. See *Bhagavadgītā* 5.18.

172. See *Bhagavadgītā* 6.9.

173. *Bhagavadgītā* 6.31–32.

174. *Bhagavadgītā* 5.25.

175. *Bhagavadgītā* 3.35; 18.47.

176. *Bhagavadgītā* 18.55.

177. *Bhagavadgītā* 18.58.

178. *Bhagavadgītā* 12.20.

179. *Secret of the Siddhas*, p. 169 (verse 374).

180. *Secret of the Siddhas*, p. 167 (verse 374).

181. *Secret of the Siddhas*, p. 172 (verse 376), quoting *Bhagavadgītā* 13.15.

182. *Secret of the Siddhas*, p. 172 (verse 376).

183. *Secret of the Siddhas*, pp. 167–68 (verse 374).

184. *Secret of the Siddhas*, p. 168 (verse 373).

185. *Secret of the Siddhas*, p. 169 (verse 374).

186. *Secret of the Siddhas*, p. 169 (verse 374).

187. *Secret of the Siddhas*, p. 172 (verse 376).

188. *Secret of the Siddhas*, pp. 173–74 (verse 377).

189. *Secret of the Siddhas*, p. 173 (verse 377).

190. *Secret of the Siddhas*, pp. 174–75 (verse 378).

191. *Secret of the Siddhas*, p. 174 (verse 377).

192. *Secret of the Siddhas*, p. 174 (verse 377), quoting *Bhagavadgītā* 13.28.

193. Swami Chidvilasananda, "See the Same Self in All," *Darshan* No. 106, p. 43.

194. *Resonate with Stillness*, December 27.

195. *Resonate with Stillness*, January 5.

196. For an extended discussion of this event from the perspective of Siddha Yoga, see Paul E. Muller-Ortega's essay, "Shaktipat: The Initiatory Descent of Power," elsewhere in this collection.

197. Swami Muktananda, *I Have Become Alive* (South Fallsburg, New York: SYDA Foundation, 1995), p. 50.

198. For various possible answers to this question from the perspective of Siddha Yoga, see the section "Who Is the Guru?" in the chapter by William K. Mahony, "The Guru-Disciple Relationship: The Context for Transformation," elsewhere in this collection.

199. *Gurugītā* 51, 71, 75, 90. See *The Nectar of Chanting* (South Fallsburg: SYDA Foundation, 1984), pp. 20, 26, 27, 31.

200. See Swami Muktananda, *The Perfect Relationship* (South Fallsburg, New York: SYDA Foundation, 1985), p. 1.

201. *Sāyaṃprataḥ kī āratī*, verse 23. See *Svādhyāya Sudhā*, Twelfth Edition (Ganeshpuri: Gurudev Siddha Peeth, 1994), p. 118. See "Āratī: Morning and Evening Prayer," *The Nectar of Chanting*, p. 137.

202. See *Kaṭha Upaniṣad* 2.22 and *Muṇḍaka Upaniṣad* 3.2.3:

> This Ātman is not gained by means of instruction
> nor by the intellect, nor by much hearing.
> He is to be gained only by the one whom He [the Self] chooses.
> To such a person the Self reveals his own nature.

203. *Secret of the Siddhas*, p. 175 (verse 379).

204. For a discussion of Kuṇḍalinī, see the chapter by Douglas Renfrew Brooks and Constantina Rhodes Bailly elsewhere in this collection.

205. Swami Chidvilasananda, "More Power than the Atom Bomb," *Siddha Path* (June 1984), p. 19.

206. Swami Chidvilasananda, "Knowledge Has to Be Practiced," *Darshan* No. 92 (November 1994), p. 42.

207. "Knowledge Has to Be Practiced," *Darshan* No. 92, p. 41.

208. Swami Chidvilasananda, "Siddha Gita: Song of the Siddhas," Part I, *Siddha Path* (July 1984), p. 34.

209. Swami Chidvilasananda, *Kindle My Heart*, Vol. I (New York: Prentice Hall Press, 1989), p. 23.

210. See *Muṇḍaka Upaniṣad* 3.1.5.

211. *Resonate with Stillness*, June 5.

212. *Meditate*, p. 15.

213. *Meditate*, p. 16.

214. Swami Chidvilasananda, "A Torch on the Path to the Highest Attainment," *Darshan* No. 3 (June 1987), p. 71.

215. *Play of Consciousness*, p. 267.

216. *Play of Consciousness*, p. 267.

217. Swami Chidvilasananda, "This Precious Gift," *Darshan* No. 23 (February 1989), p. 89.

218. Swami Chidvilasananda, "Polish the Mind Again and Again," *Darshan* No. 28 (July 1989), pp. 53, 55.

219. *Play of Consciousness*, p. 280.

220. *Play of Consciousness*, p. 281.

221. *My Lord Loves a Pure Heart*, p. 85.

222. *My Lord Loves a Pure Heart*, p. 85.

223. *My Lord Loves a Pure Heart*, p. 88.

224. *My Lord Loves a Pure Heart*, p. 85.

225. *My Lord Loves a Pure Heart*, p. 85.

226. *My Lord Loves a Pure Heart*, p. 85.

227. *Reflections of the Self*, pp. 114–15 (Part II, verses 107, 108, 111).

228. *Play of Consciousness*, p. 43.

229. Quoted by Swami Chidvilasananda in *Inner Treasures*, p. 17.

230. *Reflections of the Self*, p. 115 (Part II, verse 109).

231. *Reflections of the Self*, p. 114 (Part II, verse 104).

232. Swami Chidvilasananda, "Give Your Blessings to Others," *Darshan* No. 21 (December 1988), p. 74.

233. *Play of Consciousness*, p. 281.

234. *Play of Consciousness*, p. 280.

235. *Play of Consciousness*, p. 280.

Chapter 6. Shaktipat

1. There occur references to shaktipat in the early *Tirumantiram* in the south, and in the Āgamic and Tantric literature of the Śaivism of Kashmir.

2. Though shaktipat is often spoken of as constituting the highest essence of initiation, it should be noted that the domains of shaktipat and of initiation are at least conceptually differentiable. Certainly, not all initiations grant shaktipat. Moreover, shaktipat as the grace of the Lord need not necessarily occur in the strict context of a ritual of initiation. The discussions and divergences on this theological point are quite old. See, for example, Richard Davis, *Ritual in an Oscillating Universe* (Princeton, New Jersey: Princeton University Press, 1991), p. 90, n. 6.

3. See, for example, Mukund Rām Shāstrī, ed., *The Tantrasāra of Abhinavagupta* (Srinagar: The Research Department, Jammu and Kashmir States, 1918), p. 3, n. 8.

dīyate jñānasadbhāvaḥ
kṣīyate paśuvāsana

4. See, for example, the reference in verse 110 of the medieval devotional work *Śrī Gurugītā*. In Sanskrit:

guroḥ kṛpāprasādena ātmarāmaṃ nirīkṣayet /
anena gurumārgeṇa svātmajñānaṃ pravartate / /

The English translation in *The Nectar of Chanting* (South Fallsburg, New York: SYDA Foundation, 1983), p. 37, is as follows:

One should perceive the inner Self through the gift of the Guru's grace.
By this path of the Guru, knowledge of one's Self arises.

5. Swami Muktananda, *Light on the Path* (South Fallsburg, New York: SYDA Foundation, 1994), p. 12.

6. From Swami Chidvilasananda's preface to Peter Hayes's book, *The Supreme Adventure* (New York: Dell Publishing Group, Inc., 1988), p. xiii.

7. A classic reference is found in the *Kulārṇava Tantra* (14.34). Initiation is of three kinds: initiation by touch (*sparśa*), initiation by sight (*dṛksaṃjña*), and initiation by thought (*mānasa*)—all these three are done without rituals and without exertion.

8. Swami Muktananda, *Sadgurunath Maharaj ki Jay* (New York: SYDA Foundation, 1975), p. 106.

9. Swami Chidvilasananda, in *Transformation: On Tour with Gurumayi Chidvilasananda,* Vol. 3 (South Fallsburg, New York: SYDA Foundation, 1987), pp. 44–45.

10. For more information about the effects of the awakened *kuṇḍalinī* that follows from shaktipat, see "Kuṇḍalinī: Awakening the Divinity Within" by Douglas Renfrew Brooks and Constantina Rhodes Bailly, chapter 7 in this collection.

11. Interview with Pratap Yande, March 25, 1989.

12. Swami Muktananda, *Where Are You Going? A Guide to the Spiritual Journey* (South Fallsburg, New York: SYDA Foundation, 1994), pp. 60–61.

13. For a wider context concerning Swami Muktananda's "meditation revolution," see Swami Durgananda's "To See the World Full of Saints: The History of Siddha Yoga as a Contemporary Movement" in this collection.

14. Siddha Yoga Experience Archives.

15. Annick Baud, 1993, Siddha Yoga Experience Archives.

16. The sacred thread ceremony of the brahmanical tradition comes to mind.

17. See, for example, Abhinavagupta's discussion in the *Tantrāloka* (*āhnikas* 15–21) of the various kind of *dīkṣā.* For more details, see Alexis Sanderson, "Śaivism and the Tantric Traditions," *The World's Religions,* edited by Stewart Sutherland, et al. (London: Routledge, 1988), 692 ff. Also see Richard H. Davis, *Ritual in an Oscillating Universe: Worshipping Śiva in Medieval India* (Princeton, New Jersey: Princeton University Press, 1991).

18. See for example Alexis Sanderson's article cited in the previous note.

19. *Tantrāloka* 23.33–36:

hṛccakrādutthitā sūkṣmā śaśisphaṭikasaṃnibhā/
lekhākārā nādarūpā praśāntā cakrapaṅktigā//

dvādaśānte nirūḍhā sā sauṣumne tripathāntare/
tatra hṛccakramāpūrya japenmantram jvalatprabham//

cakṣurlomādirandhraughavahajjvālaurvasaṃnibham/
yāvacchāntaśikhākīrṇaṃ viśvājyapravilāpakam//

tadājyadhārāsaṃtṛptamānābhikuharāntaram/
evaṃ mantrā mokṣadāḥ syurdīptā buddhaḥ sunirmalāḥ//

20. Swami Muktananda, *Secret of the Siddhas* (South Fallsburg, New York: SYDA Foundation, 1994), pp. 65–66 (verses 230, 231).

21. *Resonate with Stillness: Daily Contemplations from the Words of Swami Muktananda, Swami Chidvilasananda* (South Fallsburg, New York: SYDA Foundation, 1995), April 7 and 8.

22. Although he does not use the term *shaktipat* but rather the expression "divine initiation" (*dīvya-dīkṣā*), it becomes clear later on that that is precisely what takes place.

23. See Swami Muktananda, *Play of Consciousness* (South Fallsburg, New York: SYDA Foundation, 1994), pp. 71–79.

24. *Play of Consciousness*, p. 72.

25. *Play of Consciousness*, p. 72.

26. Swami Muktananda, "Intensive Talk," *Siddha Path* (December 1980), p. 5.

27. *Light on the Path*, p. 13.

28. *Light on the Path*, p. 13.

29. *Play of Consciousness*, p. 91.

30. *Play of Consciousness*, p. 97.

31. Swami Prajnananda, *A Search for the Self: The Story of Swami Muktananda* (India: Gurudev Siddha Peeth, 1979), p. 42.

32. *Play of Consciousness*, pp. 114–15.

33. *Play of Consciousness*, p. 116.

34. From a Western perspective, the usage of the term *Śiva* in this context clearly parallels some Western notions of God. It is also important to mention that in India terms such as *Rāma* and *Kṛṣṇa* are used in the same way to name the absolute consciousness.

35. *Light on the Path*, pp. 13–14.

36. *Light on the Path*, p. 14.

37. *Light on the Path*, p. 14.

38. *Resonate with Stillness*, April 5.

39. Interview with Swami Durgananda, 1995.

40. *Light on the Path*, p. 15.

41. *Light on the Path*, p. 15.

42. *Resonate with Stillness*, June 21.

43. *Light on the Path*, p. 15.

44. *Light on the Path*, pp. 18–19.

45. *Tantrāloka* 13.103–104:

devaḥ svatantraścidrūpaḥ prakāśātmā svabhāvataḥ/
rūpapracchādanakrīḍāyogād aṇuranekakaḥ//

sa svayaṃ kalpitākāravikalpātmakakarmabhiḥ/
badhnātyātmānam eveha svātantryād iti varṇitam//

svātantryamahimaivāyaṃ devasya yadasau punaḥ/
svaṃ rūpaṃ pariśuddhaṃ satspṛśatyapyaṇutāmayaḥ//

46. *Tantrāloka* 13.116b–117a:

tena śuddha svaprakāśaḥ śiva ekātra kāraṇam/
sa ca svācchandyamātrena tāratamyaprakāśakaḥ//

47. For further details on Abhinavagupta's schema on the levels of intensity of shaktipat, see *Tantrāloka* 13.129 ff.

48. *Parātrīśikālaghuvṛtti*, comment on *śloka* 10:

etat bījaṃ yo labhate sa lābhakāla eva na paśuḥ; yato'smin labdhe etat tasya hṛdayaṃ jāyate. etad hṛdayataiva bhairavatam. atha rudrayoginīyāmalena yāvan na jātaḥ kṛtaśaktipātalakṣaṇasvarūponmīlanaḥ tāvad etad hṛdayaṃ kathaṃ asyonmīlati.

49. Jaideva Singh, *Pratyabhijñāhṛdayam: The Secret of Self-Recognition* (Delhi: Motilal Banarsidass, 1980), pp. 73–74.

50. Kṣemarāja's comment on *Śiva Sūtra* 2.6.

51. *Kulārṇava Tantra* 14.38:

śaktipātanusāreṇa śiṣyo'nugrahamati/
yatra śaktir na patati tatra siddir na jāyate//

52. Discussions of the three *malas* are to be found in Abhinavagupta's works, especially the *Paramārthasāra*, the *Tantrasāra*, and the *Tantrāloka*.

53. See Debabrata SenSharma, *The Philosophy of Sadhana* (Albany, New York: State University of New York Press, 1990), for a very useful treatment of the issues surrounding the three *malas* and other aspects of Śaivite technicalia.

54. *Kulārṇava Tantra* 13.53–63; *Kulārṇava Tantra* translation by Ram Kumar Rai (Varanasi: Prachya Prakashan, 1983).

55. Swami Muktananda, *From the Finite to the Infinite* (South Fallsburg, New York: SYDA Foundation, 1994), p. 113.

56. Swami Muktananda, from an unpublished transcript, April 19, 1978.

57. Swami Muktananda, from an unpublished transcript, September 22, 1979.

58. *Tantrāloka* 13.110b–112a:

īśvarasya ca yā svātmatirodhitsā nimittatām//

sābhyeti karmamalayor ato'nādivyavasthitiḥ/
tirodhiḥ pūrṇarūpasyāpūrṇatvaṃ tacca pūraṇam//

prati bhinnena bhāvena/
spṛhato lolikā malaḥ//

59. *Tantrāloka* 13.112b–113a:

viśuddhasvaprakāśatmaśivarūpatayā vinā/
na kiṃcid yujyate tena heturatra maheśvaraḥ//

60. *Tantrāloka* 13.113b–116a:

itthaṃ sṛṣṭisthitidhvaṃsatraye māyāmapekṣate//

kṛtyai malaṃ tathā karma śivecchaiveti susthitam/
yattu kasmiṃścana śivaḥ svena rūpeṇa bhāsate//

tatrasya nāṇuge tāvadapekṣye malakarmaṇī/
aṇusvarūpatāhānau tadgataṃ hetutām katham//

vrajenmāyānapekṣatvamata evopapādayet//

61. For a clear and comprehensive explication of the transforming effect of shaktipat, see Swami Kripananda, *The Sacred Power: A Seeker's Guide to Kundalini* (South Fallsburg, New York: SYDA Foundation, 1995), particularly "The Unfolding" and "The Chakras," pp. 55–109. As was mentioned earlier, the scope of Swami Muktananda's introduction of shaktipat to the West is described in Swami Durgananda's "To See the World Full of Saints: Siddha Yoga as a Contemporary Movement" in Part I of this collection.

62. Swami Chidvilasananda, from an unpublished transcript, August 14, 1985.

63. There is no adequate means of quantifying the subtle experiences that can come when shaktipat has been received. Even if a recipient experiences nothing at all, the impact of shaktipat is the same. For a lucid account of the life changes and opening to love that can occur without any other experiential indication of shaktipat, see Robert Kemter's "The Quickening Force" in *Darshan* No. 52 (July 1991), pp. 6–12.

64. *Resonate with Stillness,* April 9.

Chapter 7. Kuṇḍalinī

1. Swami Muktananda, *Kundalini: The Secret of Life* (South Fallsburg, New York: SYDA Foundation, 1994), p. 3.

2. Historically speaking, *kuṇḍalinīyoga* is most clearly associated with the Tantric tradition, though this label can be misleading unless we understand Tantra as permeating virtually all aspects of Indian spirituality. See Douglas Renfrew Brooks's *The Secret of the Three Cities: An Introduction to Hindu Śākta Tantrism* (Chicago: University of Chicago Press, 1990), for a detailed examination of Tantra's influence on the wide scope of Indian thought and practice.

3. Swami Muktananda, *Play of Consciousness* (South Fallsburg, New York: SYDA Foundation, 1994), p. xxvii.

4. Swami Muktananda, *Mukteshwari* (South Fallsburg, New York: SYDA Foundation, 1995), p. 37 (verse 105).

5. *Resonate with Stillness: Daily Contemplations from the Words of Swami Muktananda, Swami Chidvilasananda* (South Fallsburg, New York: SYDA Foundation, 1995), April 3.

6. An oft-repeated instruction of Swami Muktananda and his signature teaching is "Meditate on your own Self. Kneel to your own Self. Honour and worship your own inner Being. Chant the mantra always going on within you. God dwells within you as you." [Swami Muktananda, *American Tour 1970* (Piedmont, California: Shree Gurudev Siddha Yoga Ashram, 1974), p. 2.]

7. There is nothing particularly idiosyncratic about Siddha Yoga's view on this matter, as the article on shaktipat in this volume demonstrates.

8. *Play of Consciousness,* p. 43.

9. For a discussion of the origin of the Kuṇḍalinī concept in its literary form,

see David Gordon White, *The Alchemical Body* (Chicago: University of Chicago Press, 1996). Here White argues for the initial appearance of the term *kuṇḍalinī* in the *Kaulanirṇaya Tantra* and mentions arguments suggesting an earlier presentation in the *Manthānabhairava Tantra.* In vernacular literatures, we find Kuṇḍalinī in the work of the sixth-century Tamil siddha Tirumūlar in his *Tirumantiram.*

10. Rather than reiterate this basic subtle body physiology in depth, we refer the reader to a standard resource that maps out these models. For a discussion of the *cakras*, see Jean Varenne, *Yoga and the Hindu Tradition* (Chicago: University of Chicago Press, 1976).

11. See Bhāskararāya's *Varivasyārahasya,* for example, for a fairly standard exposition of this later elaboration. S. Subrahmaṇya Śāstri, ed. and trans., *Varivasyārahasya by Bhāskararāya with His Auto-Commentary Entitled Parimala,* 3rd edition (Madras: Adyar Library, 1968). (Adyar Library Series, 28).

12. See Jean Varenne, *Yoga and the Hindu Tradition,* chapter 11, for a discussion of the subtle body.

13. Swami Muktananda, *Kundalini Stavah* (Ganeshpuri, India: Gurudev Siddha Peeth, 1980), p. 5.

14. For a detailed discussion, see Lillian Silburn, *Kuṇḍalinī: Energy of the Depths* (Albany: State University of New York Press, 1988).

15. *Pratyabhijñāhṛdayam, sūtra* 1, reads in its entirety: "Consciousness of her own free will is the cause which brings about the universe" (*citiḥ svatantrā viśvasiddhi-hetuḥ*).

16. Swami Muktananda, *From the Finite to the Infinite* (South Fallsburg, New York: SYDA Foundation, 1994), p. 239.

17. See *Spandakārikā* 18–19 and the corresponding commentaries in Mark S. G. Dyczkowski's *The Stanzas on Vibration* (Albany, New York: State University of New York Press, 1992), pp. 96–100, 156–57, 221–23.

18. With regard to *Spandakārikā* 1, see the commentary of Kṣemarāja entitled *Spandasaṃdoha* for an elaboration of the description of the "homogeneous unity," or *sāmarasya* of the undifferentiated divinity. (Dyczkowski's *The Stanzas on Vibration,* pp. 62–72).

19. Peter Mann, Siddha Yoga Experience Archives.

20. The reader should consult both the articles on shaktipat and on the siddha in this volume for further details regarding the historical development of these concepts and their interpretation by the Siddha Yoga gurus.

21. *Kundalini,* p. 15.

22. *Kundalini,* p. 16.

23. *Śiva Sūtra* 3.8–10.

24. *Bhagavadgītā* 2.69.

25. Harold Ferrar, "The Cosmic Key," *Shree Gurudev-Vani* (1980), p. 78.

26. *Bhagavadgītā* 3.23; 3.26b.

27. For a synopsis of this myth, see Cornelia Dimmitt and J. A. B. Van Buitenen, eds. and trans., *Classical Hindu Mythology* (Philadelphia: Temple University Press, 1978).

28. See Sudhir Kakar's *Shamans, Mystics, and Doctors: A Psychological Inquiry into India and Its Healing Traditions* (Chicago: University of Chicago Press, 1990).

29. We do *not* mean to suggest that the erotic and sexual imagery associated

with *kuṇḍalinīyoga* is mere allegory or is unimportant. Neither do we see the need to "rehabilitate" the Tantras of the Left in which blatantly erotic and sexual imagery and practices are described and endorsed. Instead, we merely wish to point out that the Yogic traditions do not universally endorse morally questionable or antinomian behaviors, inside or outside of ritual, even as they use or express themselves universally in and through erotic imagery and symbolism.

30. To offer one comparison, the Śrīvidyā traditions of Goddess worship in South India retain erotic imagery—since *no one abandons it*—but are, in large part, similarly disinterested in eroticism or sexually explicit meanings. See Douglas Renfrew Brooks's *Auspicious Wisdom* (Albany: State University of New York Press, 1992) and forthcoming work, *Ascending Sumeru: The Worlds of South Indian Tantrics in the Tradition of Auspicious Wisdom.*

31. For a detailed study of the Right/Left distinction see Douglas Renfrew Brooks's *The Secret of the Three Cities: An Introduction to Hindu Śākta Tantrism.*

32. *Kundalini Stavah,* p. 20.

33. Swami Chidvilasananda, from an unpublished transcript, April, 13, 1991.

34. Swami Chidvilasananda, *Kindle My Heart* (South Fallsburg, New York: SYDA Foundation, 1996), p. 197.

35. *Play of Consciousness,* p. 39.

36. *Play of Consciousness,* p. 126.

37. *Kundalini Stavah,* pp. 32–33.

38. Swami Chidvilasananda, from an unpublished transcript, May 14, 1989.

39. *Play of Consciousness,* p. xxvi.

40. From Swami Chidvilasananda's "Introduction" to Swami Muktananda, *I Am That* (Ganeshpuri, India: Gurudev Siddha Peeth, 1983), p. xxiii.

41. *Play of Consciousness,* p. 16.

42. *Kundalini Stavah,* p. 14.

43. *Play of Consciousness,* p. 29.

44. *Kundalini Stavah,* p. 16.

45. Swami Muktananda, *Secret of the Siddhas* (South Fallsburg, New York: SYDA Foundation, 1994), p. 11 (verses 65, 67).

46. *Secret of the Siddhas,* p. 16 (verse 84).

47. Swami Muktananda affirms this teaching by writing a commentary on the *Kuṇḍalinī Stavaḥ,* "Verses in Praise of Kuṇḍalinī," in the most traditional manner, glossing each word of the text and then offering an insight into its deeper meanings. This particular resource complements Muktananda's experiential teachings and his other extensive elaborations. Only the subjects of the guru and the nature of the Self receive a comparable volume of reflection.

48. The phenomenon we call Kashmiri Śaivism is, in fact, a number of doctrinally distinct schools (*siddhānta/mata*), movements (*ācāra*), and modes of worship (*upāsana*).

49. *Kundalini,* pp. 4–5.

50. *Kindle My Heart* (1996 edition), p. 221.

51. Jñāneśvar is claimed by many sects, including the Nātha *sampradāya* and the cult of Viṭṭhala in Pandharpur. Clearly, the *Jñāneśvarī*'s point of reference is Kṛṣṇa.

52. For example, Patañjali's dualistic vision which forever separates matter (*prakṛti*) from spirit (*puruṣa*) is rejected by the nondualist Kashmiri Śaivites and

Siddha Yoga gurus. However, a vast array of his teachings on ethics, discipline, posture, breathing, and bodily movement is not only incorporated but simply assumed as a kind of prerequisite to *kuṇḍalinīyoga*.

53. Swami Muktananda is hardly unique in his use of Vedānta sources and concepts to elaborate the subject of Kuṇḍalinī. One need only compare him to Bhāskararāya, the great Śākta writer who stands in the center of the southern tradition of Śrīvidyā which carries on the legacy of Kashmiri Śaivism and draws freely from Vedānta.

54. *Kundalini Stavah*, p. 30.

55. Swami Muktananda, *Satsang with Baba*, Vol. 2 (Oakland, California: SYDA Foundation, 1976), pp. 13–14.

56. *Kindle My Heart* (1996 edition), p. 231.

57. *The Nectar of Chanting* (South Fallsburg, New York: SYDA Foundation, 1978), p. 21 (*Gurugītā* 53).

58. One might further consider the interest of the Siddha Yoga gurus in living a physically healthy and active life, including their discussion of food, healing, and the practices of yoga that contribute to this larger concern for well-being. However, in this particular context such considerations are beyond our purview.

It is noteworthy in another way that Abhinavagupta, for example, seems little interested in the subtle body physiology that involves the discussion of the *cakras* so common to the later sources of the Nātha yogis, including Gorakṣanātha's classic *Amaraughaśāsana*, and such fundamental texts of *haṭhayoga* tradition such as the *Haṭhayogapradīpikā* and the *Ṣaṭcakranirūpaṇa*. While Abhinavagupta certainly predates the composition of these texts, it seems evident that the basic thrust of this ideology, as well as the elements of practice, were in full blossom in the Tantras and Āgamas with which he was so familiar.

Further, the Siddha Yoga gurus' interest in Vedānta is not merely philosophical. See the article by William K. Mahony, "The Self: A Vedāntic Foundation for the Revelation of the Absolute," in this volume for further details regarding the incorporation of Vedāntic ideas and methods in Siddha Yoga practice.

59. For a detailed academic study of the Nātha siddhas and the traditions of Indian alchemy, see White's *The Alchemical Body*.

60. The Siddha Yoga gurus reject the notion that bodily immortality is immortality. Once when asked about a yogi's immortality, Swami Muktananda replied: "A yogi is called a conqueror of death because before his physical death, he dies at least once in meditation. He becomes emancipated. Every yogi passes through a stage of intense fear of death. Through that he lives forever and becomes stabilized in the immortal state. After that experience in meditation, he becomes absolutely fearless. Then even when he leaves his body he does not experience death. Only the spectators think he has died." This passage is from Swami Muktananda's *Satsang with Baba*, Vol. 1, (Oakland, California: SYDA Foundation, 1974), p. 87.

61. Swami Chidvilasananda, *Transformation: On Tour with Gurumayi Chidvilasananda*, Vol. 2 (South Fallsburg, New York: SYDA Foundation, 1986), p. 173. Swami Chidvilasananda, "One Day It Will Just Happen," *Darshan* No. 61 (April 1992), p. 47.

62. See *Play of Consciousness*, pp. 39–40.

63. Siddha Yoga Experience Archives. For further discussion of the Kuṇḍalinī

as experienced by Siddha Yoga students, see Swami Kripananda, *The Sacred Power: A Seeker's Guide to Kundalini* (South Fallsburg, New York: SYDA Foundation, 1995).

64. *Kundalini Stavah*, p. 18.

65. In his *Bodhapañcadaśikā*, "Fifteen Verses on Awakening," Abhinavagupta writes, "Śakti and Śakti's Abiding Forms never seek to exclude each other, for their identities are as inseparable as heat is to fire."

66. These are the three traditional features that define a *yajña*. See Fritz Staal's *Agni: The Vedic Ritual of the Fire Altar*, 2 Vols. (Fremont, California: Jain Publishing Co., 1983) for a detailed description in these terms.

67. *Bhagavadgītā* 4.24.

68. Dyczkowski, *The Stanzas on Vibration*, p. 62.

69. *Kundalini*, p. 28.

70. Swami Muktananda reiterates the scriptural view that *nāśivam vidyate kva cit*, that is, "Nothing exists that is not Śiva." The attribution of this statement to *Svacchanda Tantra* is unattested.

71. We should note that Śaṅkara never describes the absolute as inexplicable; rather it is the later Vācaspati Miśra who makes this point. The Siddha Yoga gurus seem to prefer the Kashmiri Śaivite perspective outlined here.

72. These impurities, or *malas*, which are generally divided into three forms, are discussed more fully in the articles on shaktipat and the siddha.

73. *Kundalini Stavah*, pp. 24–25.

74. Swami Chidvilasananda, "Shaktipat: Like a Ring of Lightning," *Darshan* No. 59 (February 1992), p. 47.

75. Swami Chidvilasananda, "Creating a Body of Light," *Darshan* No. 41–42 (September 1990), p. 164.

76. Quoted from Dyczkowski's *The Stanzas on Vibration*, p. 189.

77. *Kundalini*, p. 5.

78. *Kundalini*, p. 7.

79. See Dyczkowski's *The Stanzas on Vibration*, pp. 250–51.

80. "Creating a Body of Light," *Darshan* No. 41–42, pp. 164–65.

81. *Kundalini Stavah*, p. 22.

82. Dyczkowski, *The Stanzas on Vibration*, p. 213.

83. "Report from Ganeshpuri," *Siddha Path* (September 1978) p. 12; "Shakti—The Universal Energy," *Siddha Path* (August 1980), p. 4; "Editorial," *Siddha Path* (August 1978) pp. 4–6.

84. *Bṛhadāraṇyaka Upaniṣad* 4.4.8.

85. *Kundalini Stavah*, pp. 29–30.

86. *Vijñānabhairava Tantra* 61.

87. *Pratyabhijñāhṛdayam* 17.

88. *Kundalini*, p. 9.

89. While we have no comparable references to this activity of Kuṇḍalinī in the words of the Siddha Yoga gurus, this description outlines patterns and images that pervade the discussion of Kuṇḍalinī in other sources. See Dyczkowski's *The Stanzas on Vibration*, p. 251.

90. Swami Muktananda, *Siddha Meditation* (Ganeshpuri, India: Gurudev Siddha Peeth, 1982), p. 77.

91. See, for example, the *Haṭhayogapradīpikā*, *Ṣaṭcakranirūpaṇa*, and compa-

rable modern sources such as Swami Shankar Purushottam Tirtha's *Yoga Vani* (Varanasi, India: Ayurveda Holistic Center Press, 1992) and Swami Vishnu Tirtha Maharaj's *Devatma Shakti* (Delhi: Swami Shivom Tirth, 1974).

92. *Siddha Meditation,* p. 78.

93. It seems that Swami Muktananda is here referring to the three types of Kuṇḍalinī, rather than to the opening of the heart per se. It was Muktananda's consistent position that Kuṇḍalinī's ultimate union with Śiva (Self-realization) occurs in the *sahasrāra.* On the twin metaphors and images of the blossoming thousand-petaled lotus and the emergent heart see Paul Eduardo Muller-Ortega's *The Triadic Heart of Śiva: Kaula Tantricism of Abhinavagupta in the Non-Dual Shaivism of Kashmir* (Albany: State University of New York Press, 1989).

94. *Secret of the Siddhas,* p. 9 (verse 53).

95. *Kundalini,* p. 3.

96. *Kundalini,* pp. 21–23.

97. *Kundalini,* p. 20.

98. See *Play of Consciousness,* pp. 32–33.

99. On the notion of developing a distinctive identity by a series of characteristics rather than in terms of a single feature see the discussion of polythetic classification in Brooks, *The Secret of the Three Cities.*

100. *Kundalini,* p. 18.

101. *Kundalini,* p. 16.

102. Swami Muktananda, *Sadgurunath Maharaj ki Jay* (New York: SYDA Foundation, 1975), p. 196; *Kundalini,* p. 16.

103. *Kundalini,* p. 19.

104. Swami Chidvilasananda, "Shaktipat: Like a Ring of Lightning," *Darshan* No. 59, p. 49.

105. Bernard Clyne, Siddha Yoga Experience Archives.

106. *Kundalini,* p. 25.

107. Swami Chidvilasananda, "One Day It Will Just Happen," *Darshan,* No. 61, p. 47.

108. *Mukteshwari,* p. 39 (verses 115–16).

109. There are many resources to which the interested reader may turn to explain the mantra as deity. See for example *Understanding Mantras,* edited by Harvey P. Alper (Albany: State University of New York Press, 1989), or the long chapter on mantra in Brooks's *Auspicious Wisdom.*

110. *Play of Consciousness,* p. 52.

111. *Play of Consciousness,* pp. 52–53.

112. *Kundalini,* p. 13.

113. Barbara Hamilton, Siddha Yoga Experience Archives.

114. *Kundalini,* p. 11.

115. Swami Muktananda, *The Perfect Relationship* (South Fallsburg, New York: SYDA Foundation, 1985), p. 40.

116. *The Perfect Relationship,* p. 39.

117. *The Perfect Relationship,* pp. 40–41.

118. *Resonate with Stillness,* June 4.

119. *The Perfect Relationship,* p. 39.

120. *The Perfect Relationship,* p. 39.

121. For further discussion, see the article on shaktipat in this volume.

122. Janet L. Dobrovolny, "Just Keep Thinking You're a Great Meditator," *Darshan* No. 77–78 (August–September 1993), p. 107.

123. See *Śiva Saṃhitā*.

124. *Jñāneśvarī* 6.211–16, 219–21, 224. This and all subsequent passages from *Jñāneśvarī* are from Swami Kripananda's *Jnaneshwar's Gita: A Rendering of the Jnaneshwari* (Albany: State University of New York Press, 1989).

125. *Kundalini*, p. 19.

126. Peggy Bendet, Siddha Yoga Experience Archives.

127. Śaivism generally holds the view that Śiva the Yogi is the author or the guru of the Vedas and all related forms of scripture.

128. On the different degrees and types of shaktipat see the article on that subject included in this volume.

129. *Kindle My Heart* (1996 edition), pp. 215–16.

130. *Jñāneśvarī* 6.239–44. In the maze of metaphors Jñāneśvar offers here, it seems clear that his goal is to describe the process by which multiple forms regain their ultimate unity. Thus, dispersed elements reunite into a single elemental form, breaths unite into the breath, and the process of Self-awakening is understood as the transformation of worldly poison into immortal nectar. Another element of this passage is a reference to bodily mastery so common to esoteric yoga. The point is that an internal awakening allows subtle awareness to direct the course of physical forms.

131. *Jñāneśvarī* 6.250, 253–54.

132. Swami Muktananda clearly affirms the traditional view of Kuṇḍalinī's culmination in the *sahasrāra*: "When the *sushumnā* fully unfolds, the seeker becomes one with Lord Shiva. As a result of the union of Shiva and Shakti in the *sahasrāra*, one who has finally established himself in that ever-blissful Shiva is recognized as a Siddha; such an attainment is called the state of Siddhahood. The *Shiva Sūtras* say, *siddhaḥ svatantra bhāvaḥ*, 'Such a one enjoys perfect freedom.'" This passage is from Swami Muktananda's *Light on the Path* (South Fallsburg, New York: SYDA Foundation, 1994), pp. 60–61.

133. *Jñāneśvarī* 6.269–77, 281, 287, 290–91.

134. *Play of Consciousness*, p. 147.

135. *Play of Consciousness*, pp. 204–205, 207.

136. *Jñāneśvarī* 6.372, 387–88.

Chapter 8. Siddha Yoga as Mahāyoga

1. Swami Muktananda, *Kundalini: The Secret of Life* (South Fallsburg, New York: SYDA Foundation, 1994), p. 18.

2. For more on Kuṇḍalinī and how this inner power is viewed in Siddha Yoga, see the chapter on this subject by Douglas Renfrew Brooks and Constantina Rhodes Bailly.

3. See "The Canons of Siddha Yoga: The Body of Scripture and the Form of the Guru" by Douglas Renfrew Brooks for a more complete discussion of Siddha Yoga's relationship to the texts of these traditions.

4. Swami Muktananda, *Play of Consciousness* (South Fallsburg, New York: SYDA Foundation, 1994), p. 26.

5. *Swami Muktananda Paramahamsa in Australia* (Ganeshpuri, India: Gurudev Siddha Peeth, 1973), p. 47.

6. Swami Muktananda, *Where Are You Going? A Guide to the Spiritual Journey* (South Fallsburg, New York: SYDA Foundation, 1994), p. 63.

7. For more about Swami Muktananda's understanding of *mahāyoga* as the distinctive experiential realization of the siddha's teachings and practices, see the articles in this book on the siddha, Kuṇḍalinī, shaktipat, and the guru-disciple relationship.

8. See *Play of Consciousness*, p. 98, for description of this experience.

9. *Yogaśikhā Upaniṣad* 1.69.

10. *Yogaśikhā Upaniṣad* 1.68–69a.

11. *Kūrma Purāṇa Uttarārdha* 11.1–44.

12. *Vāyavīya Saṃhitā* 29.27.

13. *Yogaśikhā Upaniṣad* 1.29.

14. *Kāmika Āgama* 26.12–19.

15. Quoted in *Play of Consciousness*, p. 25.

16. *Yogaśikhā Upaniṣad* 1.134.

17. *Niśvāsa Kārikā Āgama* 6.14.

18. *Yogaśikhā Upaniṣad* 1.133. See also Sir John Woodroffe (Arthur Avalon), *The Serpent Power* (New York: Dover Publication, Inc., 1974), p. 198.

19. This technical term of *haṭhayoga* is not to be confused with the usage of the word in Siddha Yoga, where *kriyā* refers to spontaneous movements of the awakened *śakti*.

20. See *Darśana Upaniṣad* 6.21–32; *Dhyānabindu Upaniṣad* 65–68; and *Nādabindu Upaniṣad* 31–41.

21. *Yogatattva Upaniṣad* 24b–25. See also Woodroffe, *The Serpent Power*, pp. 185, 189.

22. *Yogatattva Upaniṣad* 26–27.

23. Śrī Aurobindo, *The Synthesis of Yoga* (Pondicherry: Śrī Aurobindo Ashram Trust, 1976), p. 508.

24. *Gheraṇḍa Saṃhitā*, as quoted in the *Mahāyoga Vijñāna*, p. 430.

25. The *Kiraṇa, yogapāda* section; *Mataṅga Pārameśvara*, yogapāda section; and *Sārdha Triśati Kālottara Āgamas*.

26. *Yogasaṅgraha* 3.126.

27. "The *śakti* is awakened through *prāṇāyāma* or through the grace of a powerful Guru. Motivated by the *ātma-śakti* when the *prāṇa* becomes roused and lodged in the *adharacakra* [*mūlādhāra cakra*, the energy center at the base of the spine], the seeker's body starts to shiver and out of joy he starts to dance." *Yogaśikhā Upaniṣad* 6.28.

28. The *Kulārṇava Tantra* (14–63) says, "After a disciple receives shaktipat he has six experiences, one after the other: joy, tremors, levitation and hopping like a frog, swaying, sleeping, and fainting."

29. *Play of Consciousness*, p. 96.

30. *Play of Consciousness*, p. 34.

31. *Play of Consciousness*, p. 101.

32. *Jñāneśvarī* 6.211–21, from Swami Kripananda's *Jnaneshwar's Gita: A Rendering of the Jnaneshwari* (Albany: State University of New York Press, 1989), p. 75.

33. Swami Vishnu Tirtha Maharaj, *Devatma Shakti* (Delhi, India: Swami Shivom Tirth, 1974), p. 52.

34. Vishnu Tirtha, *Devatma Shakti*, p. 53.

35. *Play of Consciousness*, pp. 116–17.

36. Yogendrajnani, *Mahā Yoga Vijñāna* (Rishikesh, India: Srimati Annapurna Devi, 1990), p. 339.

37. Swami Chidvilasananda, *The Yoga of Discipline* (South Fallsburg, New York: SYDA Foundation, 1996), p. 164.

38. Vishnu Tirtha, *Devatma Shakti*, pp. 60–61.

39. *Play of Consciousness*, p. 132.

40. *Yogasaṅgraha*, as quoted by Sri Jñanaprakasa Sivacarya, *Śiva Yoga Saram* (from a handwritten manuscript prepared by the author's *dīkṣāguru*, Sri Rajaganesa Diksitar, p. 54). See also *Varāha Upaniṣad* 5.10 and commentary.

41. *Haṭhayogapradīpikā*, as quoted by Sri Jñanaprakasa Śivacarya, in the *Śiva Yoga Ratna* (from a handwritten manuscript, p. 54).

42. Woodroffe, *The Serpent Power*, p. 225.

43. See *Mahānirvāṇa Tantra*: "Just as the body has no power to function where there is no *prāṇa*, so even millions of repetitions of mantra will not bear fruit unless the *prāṇa-śakti* of the mantra is activated." (3.30.31)

44. Quoted in Kṣemarāja, *Śiva Sūtra Vimarśinī* 2.1.

45. *Kulārṇava Tantra* 17.54.

46. *Play of Consciousness*, p. 35.

47. *Sarvajñānottara* 6.15–17.

48. See Swami Muktananda, *Secret of the Siddhas* (South Fallsburg, New York: SYDA Foundation, 1994), p. 82.

49. Swami Muktananda, *In the Company of a Siddha* (South Fallsburg, New York: SYDA Foundation, 1985), p. 144.

50. *Yogaśikhā Upaniṣad* 1.130–31.

51. *Makuṭa Āgama* 11.39.43.

52. The verse says, "The supreme Śakti, whose nature is to create, constantly expresses herself upward in the form of exhalation and downward in the form of inhalation. By steadily fixing the mind on either of the two spaces between the breath, one experiences the state of fullness of Bhairava."

53. Swami Muktananda, *I Am That* (South Fallsburg, New York: SYDA Foundation, 1992), p. 39.

54. *Play of Consciousness*, pp. 73, 75.

55. *Where Are You Going?* pp. 82–83.

56. *Sarvajñānottara* 6.15–17.

57. *Mataṅga Pārameśvara Āgama*, chapters 4 and 5.

58. *Haṭhayogapradīpikā* 4.3–4.

59. *Jñāneśvarī*, 6.320, from Swami Kripananda's *Jnaneshwar's Gita*, p. 78.

60. *Yogaśikhā Upaniṣad* 2.20.

61. See *Play of Consciousness*, pp. 185–86.

62. *Haṃsa Upaniṣad* 18.20.

63. *Secret of the Siddhas*, p. 196 (verse 405).

64. *Play of Consciousness*, pp. 185–86.

65. *Play of Consciousness*, p. 184.

66. Yogendrajnani, *Mahāyoga Vijñāna*, pp. 301–12.
67. *Mṛgendra Āgama, yogapāda* 51–53; *Mataṅga Pārameśvara, yogapāda,* chapters 3 and 4.
68. Yogendrajnani, *Mahāyoga Vijñāna*, pp. 301–12.
69. *Play of Consciousness,* pp. 146–47.
70. Quoted in *Play of Consciousness,* p. 167.
71. *Play of Consciousness,* pp. 205–206.
72. *Raurava Āgama, vidyāpāda* 7.5; *Mataṅga Pārameśvara Āgama, yogapāda* 1.6; *Amṛtanāda Upaniṣad* 6.
73. *Kiraṇa Āgama, yogapāda* 1.3; *Dhyānabindu Upaniṣad* 41.
74. *Maṇḍala Brāhmaṇa Upaniṣad* 2–11; *Tejobindu Upaniṣad* 1.14–37.
75. *Haṭhayogapradīpikā* 4.3–4.
76. Woodroffe, *The Serpent Power,* pp. 185–86.
77. *Play of Consciousness,* p. 202.
78. *Jñāneśvarī* 3.78.
79. *Kundalini,* pp. 19–20.
80. Vishnu Tirtha, *Devatma Shakti,* pp. 81–82.

Chapter 9. The Ashram

1. Paul Zweig, "The Master of Ganeshpuri," *Harper's* (May 1977), p. 85.
2. Linda Johnsen, *Daughters of the Goddess: The Woman Saints of India* (St. Paul, Minnesota: Yes International Publishing, 1994), p. 78.
3. Virendra Kumar Jain, "An Ambrosial Experience of Baba's Grace," *Shree Gurudev-Vani* (1968), p. 31.
4. The language here is reminiscent of Mircea Eliade's influential but now somewhat dated *The Sacred and the Profane: The Nature of Religion,* translated by Willard R. Trask (New York: Harcourt Brace & World, 1959).
5. Eliade, *The Sacred and the Profane,* pp. 10–11.
6. For a phenomenological discussion of such an emergence of the sacred into the profane, see Mircea Eliade, (ibid.) passim, but especially Chapter One: "Sacred Space and Making the World Sacred," pp. 20–65.
7. Zweig, "The Master of Ganeshpuri," *Harper's,* p. 87.
8. Zweig, "The Master of Ganeshpuri," *Harper's,* p. 87.
9. Swami Muktananda, *Ashram Dharma* (South Fallsburg, New York: SYDA Foundation, 1995), pp. 11–12.
10. Swami Muktananda, from an unpublished transcript, December 16, 1978.
11. Interview with Venkappanna Shriyan, "How to Hold What the Guru Gives," *Darshan* No. 81 (December 1993), p. 28.
12. *Ashram Dharma,* pp. 3–4.
13. Here Swami Muktananda is consistent with his view of this power as the universal Goddess. For more on this topic, see Douglas Renfrew Brooks and Constantina Rhodes Bailly, "Kuṇḍalinī: Awakening the Goddess Within," elsewhere in this collection.
14. *Ashram Dharma,* pp. 19–20.
15. *Ashram Dharma,* p. 4.
16. Jane Ferrar, "Ashram Thesis," Siddha Yoga Experience Archives.

17. Devotees have experienced everything in Gurudev Siddha Peeth as "love in a physical form" and as "the Guru personified." See the collection of devotees' testimonies in "Even the Dust Gives Blessings," *Darshan* No. 30–31 (September–October 1989), pp. 9–32.

18. Interview with Swami Vasudevananda, 1995.

19. Interview with Swami Vasudevananda, 1995.

20. *Ashram Dharma*, p. 4.

21. "Report from Ganeshpuri," *Siddha Path* (December 1977), p. 5.

22. Swami Muktananda, *Satsang with Baba*, Vol. 1 (Ganeshpuri, India: SYDA Foundation, 1974), p. 326.

23. See Patañjali's *Yoga Sūtra*, e.g., 1.18, 1.50, 3.9, 3.10, 3.18, 4.9, 4.27.

24. Swami Muktananda, *Satsang with Baba*, Vol. 2 (Ganeshpuri, India: SYDA Foundation, 1976), p. 254.

25. *Ashram Dharma*, p. 21.

26. Swami Chidvilasananda, *Kindle My Heart* (South Fallsburg, New York: SYDA Foundation, 1996), p. 178.

27. *Satsang with Baba*, Vol. 2, pp. 101–102.

28. Interview with Venkappanna Shriyan, "How to Hold What the Guru Gives," *Darshan* No. 81, pp. 28–29.

29. Swami Muktananda, *Satsang with Baba*, Vol. 3 (Ganeshpuri, India: SYDA Foundation, 1977), p. 169.

30. *Ashram Dharma*, pp. 20–21.

31. *Ashram Dharma*, pp. 20–21.

32. From Swami Shantananda's "Introduction" to *Ashram Dharma*, pp. ix–x.

33. Swami Shantananda's "Introduction," *Ashram Dharma*, p. x.

34. *The Nectar of Chanting*, (South Fallsburg, New York: SYDA Foundation, 1983), p. xiii.

35. Swami Shantananda's "Introduction," *Ashram Dharma*, pp. x–xi.

36. Swami Shantananda's "Introduction," *Ashram Dharma*, p. xi.

37. Swami Muktananda, *From the Finite to the Infinite* (South Fallsburg, New York: SYDA Foundation, 1994), p. 144.

38. Swami Chidvilasananda, "Understand What You Are," *Darshan* No. 80 (November 1993), p. 36.

39. Swami Muktananda, *What Is an Intensive?* (South Fallsburg, New York: SYDA Foundation, 1995), p. 1.

40. Peggy Bendet, *Shri Gauri-Shankara Yajna* (South Fallsburg, New York: SYDA Foundation, 1993), p. 6.

41. Swami Muktananda, *American Tour 1970* (Piedmont, California: Shree Gurudev Siddha Yoga Ashram, 1974), p. 94.

42. See *Dhātupāṭha* 4.95 and Bhānuji Dīkṣita on Amarasiṃha's *Amarakośa* 2.7.3. References here come from a similar discussion by Patrick Olivelle in his *The Āśrama System* (New York: Oxford University Press, 1993), pp. 9–17.

43. See for example *Ṛgveda* 1.72.2, which describes the gods as "weary" (*śrama*) after chasing Agni.

44. See for example *Ṛgveda* 10.114.10, which notes that horses win a prize for their hard work (*śrama*).

45. *Śramaṇāsana*. See *Rāmāyaṇa* 4.13.6.

46. *Āśramaṃ śramaśokavināśanam.* (*Mahābhārata* 3.82.423).

47. *Aṣṭādhyāyī* 3.3.19.

48. Olivelle refers to the commentator Bhānuji Dīkṣita's explanation of Amarasiṃha's *Amarakośa* (2.7.3-4) as *ā samantāc chramo 'tra*: "There is toil all around [or completely] here." See Olivelle, *The Āśrama System*, p. 17, n. 3.

49. See for example *Ṛgveda* 4.12.2, in which a person is said to exert himself strenuously to bring wood to burn in the ceremonial offertory fire, or *Taittirīya Saṃhitā* 1.7.13, in which the primordial ancestor of the human race, Manu, is said to toil at cooking the sacrificial oblation.

50. See *Kātyāyana Śrauta Sūtra* 25.

51. See *Baudhāyana Dharma Śāstra* 2.5.1.

52. See *Śatapatha Brāhmaṇa* 14.6.8.10.

53. Thus, we read in the *Śatapatha Brāhmaṇa* 6.1.1.1, for example, that "in the beginning, only Prajāpati existed, alone. He wished, 'May I exist. May I reproduce myself!' He toiled, and he practiced austerity. From him, tired and heated, the waters were created. From that heated Person the waters are born. From his mouth he produced Agni [the god of fire]." See also *Taittirīya Brāhmaṇa* 1.1.35.

54. *Śatapatha Brāhmaṇa* 6.1.1.1. See also *Taittirīya Brāhmaṇa* 1.1.35.

55. *Bṛhadāraṇyaka Upaniṣad* 1.2.2.1 and 1.2.2.6.

56. See *Śatapatha Brāhmaṇa* 6.1.1.1.

57. *Taittirīya Upaniṣad* 3.1–5.

58. *Śvetāśvatara Upaniṣad* 6.21.

59. *Maitrī Upaniṣad* 4.3.

60. See *Vaikhānasa Dharma Sūtra* 1.6.7 and 2.1.4.5, *Baudhāyana Dharma Sūtra* 2.11.15, *Gautama Dharma Sūtra* 3.27, *Vaikhānasa Gṛhya Sūtra* 1.8.

61. See *Vinaya Piṭaka* 1.71, *Dīgha Nikāya* 2.339, and *Majjima Nikāya* 1.501, which describe residents of a Buddhist *assama* as using fire in their worship; and *Baudhāyana Dharma Sūtra* 2.11.15, *Gautama Dharma Sūtra* 3.27, and *Vaikhānasa Dharma Sūtra* 9.10, which note that the *śrāmaṇaka* fire of a Hindu *āśrama* must be installed properly.

62. See *Anguttara-Nikāya* 1.67, *Dīgha-Nikāya* 3.16.95ff, *Saṃyutta-Nikāya* 1.45, and *Dhammapada* 184. References in T. W. Rhys Davids and William Stede, *The Pali Text Society's Pali-English Dictionary* (London: Pali Text Society, 1921–25, reprint edition 1979), *s.v.* "Samaṇa," p. 682.

63. Sukumar Dutt, *Buddhist Monks and Monasteries of India* (London: George Allen & Unwin, Ltd., 1962; New York: Humanities Press, 1962), pp. 35–44, 112–13.

64. See *Taittirīya Ārayaka* 2.7. Reference and text in Olivelle, *The Āśrama System*, p. 12.

65. See *Ṛgveda* 1.55.4.

66. See, for example, *Ṛgveda* 10.109.4.

67. Sāyaṇa, on *Ṛgveda* 10.136.2.

68. For a lively song regarding such *keśins*, see *Ṛgveda* 10.136.

69. *Ṛgveda* 8.3.9, 8.6.18, 10.72.7.

70. *Kaṭha Upaniṣad* 3.6.10–11.

71. *Śvetāśvatara Upaniṣad* 4.14.

72. The wording in the latter part of this paragraph is similar to that in Radha Kumud Mookerji, "Ancient Indian Education," in *The Cultural Heritage of India*,

Vol. II, Second Edition (Calcutta: The Ramakrishna Mission Institute of Culture, 1963, reprint edition 1982), p. 640.

73. See Patañjali's *Yoga Sūtra* 2.30.

74. See *Yoga Sūtra* 2.32.

75. *Kaṭha Upaniṣad* 2.8.

76. *Bṛhadārayaka Upaniṣad* 3.5.1.

77. On the *vihāra*, see *Cullavagga* 6.2 and 6.15. See *Cullavagga*, translated by I. B. Horner, Volume 20 of *Sacred Books of the East*, Series VII (London: Pali Text Society, 1952, reprint edition 1975), pp. 160–69 and 209.

78. For discussion, see Sukumar Dutt, *Early Buddhist Monachism*, revised edition (London: George Allen & Unwin, Ltd.; New York: Humanities Press, 1962), pp. 125–36, 146–63.

79. On the history and contributions to Indian culture of Buddhist monasteries, see Dutt, *Buddhist Monks and Monasteries of India.*

80. *Suttanipāta* 5.1.1–3.

81. See *Chāndogya Upaniṣad* 7.14 and *Bṛhadāraṇyaka Upaniṣad* 6.2.1–7.

82. See *Baudhāyana Dharma Sūtra* 1.1.5–6, translated here by P. V. Kane in *History of Dharmaśāstra*, Second Edition (Poona: Bhandarkar Oriental Research Institute, 1974), Vol. 2, p. 971. See also *Mānavadharmaśāstra* 12.109 and *Vāsiṣṭha Dharma Sūtra* 6.43.

83. See *Pañcatantra* 4.4. Reference for this and the following note from G. S. Ghurye, *Indian Sadhus*, Second Edition (Bombay: Popular Prakashan, 1964), pp. 41–42.

84. *Pañcatantra* 1.4 and 2.1.

85. Kane refers to *Rājataraṅgiṇī* 6.300, which notes that Queen Diddā (tenth century) constructed a *maṭha* as a residence for people from Madhyadesha, Lata, and Saurashtra. See Kane, *History of Dharmaśāstra*, Vol. 2, p. 910.

86. Sometimes the affairs of a *maṭha* were overseen by a small group of people rather than by one individual. *Pañcatantra* 4.4 mentions such an arrangement in a *maṭha* in the Kanauj region.

87. For a discussion of the legal implications and a review of decisions regarding such succession, see Kane, *History of Dharmaśāstra*, Vol. 2, p. 908.

88. The eleventh- and twelfth-century Visiṣṭādvaita theologian and teacher, Rāmānuja, also founded *maṭhas* at Shrirangam and at Melkote. The Dvaita teacher, Madhva, (twelfth to thirteenth century) and the Kṛṣṇa *bhakta*, Vallabha, also founded *maṭhas* based on their own traditions.

89. *Vālmīki Rāmāyaṇa* 1.28.2. Translation here by Robert P. Goldman, *The Rāmāyaṇa of Vālmīki: An Epic of Ancient India*, Vol. 1: *Bālakāṇḍa* (Princeton: Princeton University Press, 1984), p. 178.

90. *Vālmīki Rāmāyaṇa* 1.27.15–18, translated here by Goldman, p. 178.

91. *Vālmīki Rāmāyaṇa* 1.28.12, Goldman, p. 179.

92. *Vālmīki Rāmāyaṇa, Araṇyakāṇḍa* 1.1–8, translated here by Sheldon I. Pollack in *The Rāmāyaṇa of Vālmīki: An Epic of Ancient India*, Vol. III, *Araṇyakāṇḍa* (Princeton: Princeton University Press, 1991), p. 87.

93. For Sanskrit text and translation, with Sanskrit commentary by Rāghavabhaṭṭa, see M. K. Kale, *The Abhijñānaśākuntalam of Kālidāsa*, Tenth Edition (Delhi: Motilal Banarsidass, 1969; reprint edition, 1980).

94. All quotations from the *Mahābhārata* in this and the following two paragraphs come from *The Mahābhārata,* translated and edited by J. A. B. van Buitenen, Vol. 1: *The Book of the Beginning* (Chicago: University of Chicago Press, 1973, Phoenix Edition, 1980), pp. 157–60.

95. *Abhijñānaśākuntala,* Act I, verses 10–12. For text, with commentary by Rāghavabhaṭṭa, see Kale, *The Abhijñānaśākuntalam of Kālidāsa,* 1980.

96. *Abhijñānaśākuntala,* Act I, verses 13–15.

97. *Abhijñānaśākuntala,* Act I, verse 31.

98. *Abhijñānaśākuntala,* Act II, verse 7.

99. Lazlo Slomovits, "Ashram Thesis," Siddha Yoga Experience Archives.

100. The dates of the developments presented in this paragraph follow C. D. Ullal's "Shree Gurudev Ashram," *Guruvani* (1964), pp. 57–60.

101. Ullal reports that after this year's stay, Muktananda "decided to resume his roaming in the lone places for *tapasya.* He went first to Trimbakeshwar near Nasik, then to Kasara, next to Yeola and lastly in the lonely Nagad hills situated near Chalisgaon. Here, he was doing intense *sadhana* and as usual no one knew where he was." See C. D. Ullal's "Shree Gurudev Ashram," *Guruvani* (1964), pp. 57–60.

102. "Editorial: The Unfolding of a Siddha Pitha," *Shree Gurudev-Vani* (1972), p. 1.

103. "Editorial: The Unfolding of a Siddha Pitha," *Shree Gurudev-Vani* (1972), p. 1.

104. Swami Muktananda, *Satsang with Baba,* Vol. 5 (South Fallsburg, New York: SYDA Foundation, 1978), p. 209.

105. "Editorial: The Unfolding of a Siddha Pitha," *Shree Gurudev-Vani* (1972), pp. 1–2.

106. Interview with Alberto Ferrario, 1994.

107. C. D. Ullal, "Shree Gurudev Ashram," *Guruvani* (1964), p. 58.

108. Interview with Janet Dobrovolny, June 23, 1992.

109. Jane Ferrar "Ashram Thesis," Siddha Yoga Experience Archives.

110. Interview with Swami Durgananda, 1995.

111. *Abhijñānaśākuntala,* Act I, verse 31.

112. Zweig, "The Master of Ganeshpuri," *Harper's,* p. 91.

113. Swami Muktananda, *Satsang with Baba,* Vol. 4 (Ganeshpuri, India: SYDA Foundation, 1978), pp. 117–118.

114. *Ashram Dharma,* p. 49.

115. *Kindle My Heart,* Vol. II (1989 edition) p. 118.

116. Gurumayi Chidvilasananda, "The Fire of Love," *Darshan* No. 2 (May 1987), p. 71.

117. Swami Muktananda, "The Embodiment of Grace," *Darshan* No. 30–31 (September–October 1989), p. 55.

Bibliography

PRIMARY TEXTS

Abhijñānaśākuntala, with commentary by Rāghavabhaṭṭa. Edited by M. R. Kale as *The Abhijñānaśākuntalam.* Tenth Edition. Delhi: Motilal Banarsidass, 1969, reprint edition, 1980.

Aitareya Āraṇyaka. Edited and translated by Arthur Berridale Keith. Oxford: Clarendon Press, 1909; reprint edition, Oxford: Oxford University Press, 1969.

Aitareya Brāhmaṇa. 2 volumes. Ānandāśrama-saṃskṛta-granthāvaliḥ, granthāṅkha 32. Pune: Ānandāśrama, 1931.

Aitareya Upaniṣad. In *Daśopaniṣads, with the Commentary of Śrī Upaniṣadbrahmayogin.* Revised Edition. Edited by the Pandits of the Adyar Library under the supervision of C. Kunhan Raja, revised by A. A. Ramanathan. 2 volumes. Madras: The Adyar Library and Research Centre, 1984. Volume 1.

Aitareya Upaniṣad Bhāṣya, by Śaṅkarācārya. Edited by Swami Gambhirananda. Calcutta: Advaita Ashrama, 1978.

Amarakośa of Amarasiṃha. Edited by A. A. Ramanathan. Madras: Adyar Library and Research Centre, 1983.

Aparokṣānubhūti, by Śaṅkarācārya. Edited by Swami Vimuktananda. Calcutta: Ramakrishna Math, 1973.

Āpastamba Dharma Sūtra. Edited by U. C. Pandey. Kashi Sanskrit Series, Number 59. Varanasi: Chowkhamba Sanskrit Series Office, 1971.

Āpastamba Śrauta Sūtra. 3 volumes. Edited by Richard Garbe. Calcutta: Royal Asiatic Society of Bengal, 1882–1902.

Aṣṭādhyāyī of Pāṇini. Edited by Sumitra M. Katre. Austin: University of Texas, 1987.

Āśvalāyana Gṛhya Sūtra. Edited and translated by N. N. Sharma. Delhi: Eastern Book Linkers, 1976.

Atharvaveda Saṃhitā. (Śaunaka rescension) 4 volumes. Edited by V. Bandhu. Hoshiarpur: Vishveshvaranand Vedic Research Institute, 1960–62.

Bahvṛcā Upaniṣad. In *The Śākta Upaniṣads, with the Commentary of Śrī Upaniṣadbrahmayogin.* Second Edition. Edited by Pandit A. Mahadeva Sastri. Madras: The Adyar Library and Research Centre, 1986.

Baudhāyana Dharma Sūtra. Edited by U. C. Pandeya. Kashi Sanskrit Series, Number 104. Varanasi: Chowkhamba Sanskrit Series Office, 1972.

Bhakti Sūtra. [See *Nārada Bhakti Sūtra.*]

Bhaktivijaya of Mahapati. Pune: Yasavana Prakāsana, 1974. Translated by Justin E. Abbott and Pandit N. R. Godbole as *Stories of Indian Saints.* Reprint Edition. Delhi: Motilal Banarsidass, 1982.

Brahma Sūtra, by Bādarāyaṇa. Edited and translated by Swami Gambhirananda. Third Edition. Calcutta: Advaita Ashrama, 1977.

Brahma Upaniṣad. In *The Sāmānya Vedānta Upanishads, with the Commentary of Śrī Upaniṣadbrahmayogin.* Edited by Pandit A. Mahadeva Sastri. Madras: Adyar Library, 1921.

Brahmabindu Upaniṣad. In *Upaniṣat-Saṃgraha.* Edited with Sanskrit Introduction by J. L. Shastri. Delhi: Motilal Banarsidass, 1970; reprint edition, 1984.

Bṛhadāraṇyaka Upaniṣad. In *Daśopaniṣads,* with the commentary of Śrī Upaniṣadbrahmayogin. Revised Edition. Edited by the Pandits of the Adyar Library under the supervision of C. Kunhan Raja, revised by A. A. Ramanathan. 2 volumes. Madras: The Adyar Library and Research Centre, 1984. Volume 2.

Chāndogya Upaniṣad. In *Daśopaniṣads,* with the commentary of Śrī Upaniṣadbrahmayogin. Revised Edition. Edited by the Pandits of the Adyar Library under the supervision of C. Kunhan Raja, revised by A. A. Ramanathan. 2 volumes. Madras: The Adyar Library and Research Centre, 1984. Volume 2.

Cūllavagga. [See *Vinaya Piṭaka.*]

Dhātupāṭha of Pāṇini. [See *Pāṇinīyadhātupāṭhasamīkṣa.*]

Dīgha Nikāya. Edited by T. W. Rhys Davids and J. Estlin Carpenter. London: H. Frowde for the Pali Text Society, 1890.

Gautama Dharma Sūtra. Edited by Manmatha Nath Dutt. In *The Dharma Śāstra Texts.* Calcutta: M. N. Dutt, 1908.

Īśā Upaniṣad. In *Daśopaniṣads, with the Commentary of Śrī Upaniṣadbrahmayogin.* Revised Edition. Edited by the Pandits of the Adyar Library under the supervision of C. Kunhan Raja, revised by A. A. Ramanathan. 2 volumes. Madras: The Adyar Library and Research Centre, 1984. Volume 1.

Īśvarapratyabhijñākārikā of Utpaladeva with his *vṛtti.* Edited by Madhusudan Kaul Sastri. Srinagar: Govt. Press, 1921 (Kashmir Series of Texts and Studies, no. 34).

Īśvara-pratyabhijñā-vimarśinī of Abhinavagupta. Edited by Mukunda Rāma. Kashmir Series of Texts and Studies, nos. 22 and 33. Srinagar: Research Department, Jammu and Kashmir Government, 1918 and 1921.

Īśvarapratyabhijñā Vivṛti Vimarśinī of Abhinavagupta with the *Bhāskarī.* Edited Madhusudan Kaul Sastri. Srinagar: Govt. Press, 1938-43 (Kashmir Series of Texts and Studies, nos. 60, 62, 65).

Jaiminīya Brāhmaṇa. Edited by R. Vira and L. Chandra. Nagpur: Sarasvati Vihara Series, 1954.

Jaiminīya Upaniṣad Brāhmaṇa. Edited and translated by Hanns Oertel. *Journal of the American Oriental Society* 16 (1896), pp. 79-260.

Jñāneśvarī, by Jñāneśvara (also known as Jñānadev). Rendered into English by Swami Kripananda. Albany, NY: State University of New York Press, 1989.

Kāmakalāvilāsa by Punyānanda. Edited and translated by Arthur Avalon (Sir John Woodroffe). Second edition. Madras: Ganesh and Co., 1953.

Kaṭha [*Kaṭhavallī*] *Upaniṣad.* In *Daśopaniṣads, with the Commentary of Śrī Upaniṣadbrahmayogin.* Revised Edition. Edited by the Pandits of the Adyar Library under the supervision of C. Kunhan Raja, revised by A. A. Ramanathan. 2 volumes. Madras: The Adyar Library and Research Centre, 1984. Volume 1.

Kaulavijñānanirṇaya. Edited by P. Ch. Bagchi. In *Kaulajñānanirnaya and Some Minor Texts of the Schools of Matsyendranātha.* Calcutta: University Press, 1934.

Kauṣītaki Brāhmaṇa. Edited by H. Bhattacharya. Calcutta Sanskrit College Research Series, 73. Calcutta: Sanskrit College, 1970.

Kauṣītaki [*Kauṣītakibrāhmaṇa*] *Upaniṣad.* In *The Sāmānya Vedānta Upanishads, with the Commentary of Śrī Upaniṣadbrahmayogin.* Edited by Pandit A. Mahadeva Sastri. Madras: Adyar Library, 1921.

Kena Upaniṣad. In *Daśopaniṣads, with the Commentary of Śrī Upaniṣadbrahmayogin.* Revised Edition. Edited by the Pandits of the Adyar Library under the supervision of C. Kunhan Raja, revised by A. A. Ramanathan. 2 volumes. Madras: The Adyar Library and Research Centre, 1984. Volume 1.

Kṣurikā Upaniṣad. In *The Yoga Upaniṣads, with the Commentary of Śrī Upaniṣadbrahmayogin.* Edited by Pandit A. Mahadeva Sastri. Reprint edition. Madras: The Adyar Library and Research Centre, 1968.

Kulārṇava Tantra. Edited by T. Vidyāratna, Calcutta: University Press, 1917 (Tantrik Texts, V); second edition, Madras: Ganesh and Co., 1956.

Mahābhārata. Edited by Vishnu S. Sukthankar. 19 volumes. Pune: Bhandarkar Oriental Research Institute, 1927–66.

Mahānirvāṇa Tantra. Edited and translated by Arthur Avalon as *The Great Liberation.* Calcutta: University Press, 1913 (Tantrik Texts, XIII); fifth edition 1952, reprinted Madras: Ganesh and Co., 1963.

Mahārthamañjarī. By Maheśvarānanda, edited by Madhusudan Kaul Sastri. Srinagar: Govt. Press, 1918 (Kashmir Series of Texts and Studies, no. 11); translated into French by L. Silburn. Paris: Institut de Civilisation Indienne, 1968.

Mahāvagga. [See *Vinaya Piṭaka.*]

Maitrī [*Maitrāyaṇīya*] *Upaniṣad.* Edited and translated by S. Radhakrishnan, *The Principal Upaniṣads.* Reprint edition. London: George Allen & Unwin, Ltd.; New York: Humanities Press, Inc., 1978.

Mālinīvijaya Tantra. Edited by Madhusudan Kaul Sastri. Srinagar: Govt. Press, 1922 (Kashmir Series of Texts and Studies, no. 37).

Māṇḍūkya Upaniṣad. In *Daśopaniṣads, with the Commentary of Śrī Upaniṣadbrahmayogin.* Revised Edition. Edited by the Pandits of the Adyar Library under the supervision of C. Kunhan Raja, revised by A. A. Ramanathan. 2 volumes. Madras: The Adyar Library and Research Centre, 1984. Volume 1.

Mantramahodadhi, by Mahīdhara. Edited by K. Śrīkṛṣṇadās. Bombay: Śrī Sat Guru Publications, 1962; recently reedited and translated in two separate volumes by "a panel of scholars." Delhi: Śrī Sat Guru Publications, 1984.

Manu Smṛti. 5 volumes. Edited by J. H. Dave. Bhāratīya Vidyā Series. Bombay: Bhāratīya Vidyā Bhavan, 1972–82.

Mṛgendra Tantra (*Vidyāpāda* and *Yogapāda*). Edited by Madhusudan Kaul Sastri. Srinagar: Govt. Press, 1930 (Kashmir Series of Texts and Studies, no. 50).

Muṇḍaka Upaniṣad. In *Daśopaniṣads, with the Commentary of Śrī Upaniṣadbrahmayogin.* Revised Edition. Edited by the Pandits of the Adyar Library under the supervision of C. Kunhan Raja, revised by A. A. Ramanathan. 2 volumes. Madras: The Adyar Library and Research Centre, 1984. Volume 1.

Nārada Bhakti Sūtras. Edited and translated by Swami Prabhavananda. Madras: Ramakrishna Math, 1972.

Nārada Sūtra. (See *Nārada Bhakti Sūtra*).

Netra Tantra with the *Uddyota* of Kṣemarāja. Edited by Madhusudan Kaul Sastri. 2 vols. Bombay: Nirnaya Sagar Press, 1926-39 (Kashmir Series of Texts and Studies nos. 46 and 61). See Brunner, *Netra Tantra.*

Nityāṣoḍaśikārṇava [Tantra]. Edited by V. V. Dwiveda. Varanāsī: Sampurṇānand Sanskrit Viśvavidyālaya, 1968.

Nityotsava, by Umānandanātha. Edited by A. M. Sastri. Baroda: Oriental Institute, 1923 (GOS, 23), revised edition by Swami Trivikrama Tirtha. Baroda: Oriental Institute, 1948.

Nṛsiṃhottaratāpanī Upaniṣad. In *The Vaiṣṇava Upaniṣads, with the Commentary of Śrī Upaniṣadbrahmayogin.* Edited by Pandit A. Mahadeva Sastri. Second edition. Adyar: The Adyar Library and Research Centre, 1979.

Pāṇinīyadhātupāṭhasamīkṣa. Edited by Bhagirathaprasada Tripathi. Varanasi: Sampūrānand Sanskrit Viśvavidyālaya, 1984.

Paramārthasāra, by Abhinavagupta. Edited (with a French translation) by L. Silburn. Paris: Institut de Civilisation Indienne, 1957.

Paraśurāmakalpa Sūtra with the commentary by Rāmeśvara Sūri entitled *Saubhāgyodaya.* Edited By A. M. Sastri and S. Y. Dave. Baroda: Oriental Institute, 1950, second edition (GOS 22).

Paratriṃśikā with the *Vivaraṇa* of Abhinavagupta. Edited by Madhusudan Kaul Sastri. Bombay: Nirnaya Sagar Press, 1918 (Kashmir Series of Texts and Studies, no. 18).

Parimala, by Maheśvarānanda. The auto-commentary on the *Mahārthamañjarī.* See above.

Parātrīśikā-laghuvṛtti of Abhinavagupta. Edited by Jagaddhara Zādoo. Kashmir Series of Texts and Studies, no. 68. Srinagar: Research Department, Jammu and Kashmir Government, 1947.

Prapañcasārasaṃgraha. Edited at Varanāsī, V.S. 1935 (C.E. 1878) (IOL-SB, III, p.1946); also recently as part of the Tanjore Sanskrit Library Series in 2 volumes, 1983.

Prapañcasāratantra, attributed to Śaṅkarācārya. Edited by T. Vidyāratna. Calcutta: University Press, 1914; with the Sanskrit commentary *Vivarana,* attributed to Padmapāda, edited in Calcutta: University Press, 1935 (Tantrik Texts, XVIII-XIX).

Pratyabhijñāhṛdayam of Kṣemarāja. Translated under the title *The Secret of Recognition.* With notes by E. Baer and Kurt F. Leidecker. Adyar, Madras: Adyar Library, 1938; Hindi translation by Jaideva Singh. Delhi: Motilal Banarsidass, 1973; English translation by Jaideva Singh. Delhi: Motilal Banarsidass, 1963; English translation and commentary named *The Secret of Realization.* By I. K. Taimni. Adyar, Madras, 1974.

Rāmāyaṇa. (See *Vālmīki Rāmāyaṇa*).

Ṛgveda Saṃhitā. Edited by Theodor Aufrecht. Published as *Die Hymnen des Rigveda.* 2 volumes. Reprint edition. Vienna: Otto Harrassowitz, 1988.

———. Edited by F. Max Muller. 4 volumes. Chowkhamba Sanskrit Series, Volume 99. Reprint Edition Varanasi: Chowkhamba Sanskrit Series Office, 1966.

Śaktisaṃgama Tantra. Edited (in 4 volumes) by Bhattacharyya. Baroda: Oriental Institute, 1932-47 (Vols. I-III) (GOS, nos. 61, 91, 104). Vol. I: Kālikhaṇḍa;

Vol. II: Tārākhaṇḍa; Vol. III: Sundarīkhaṇḍa; Vol. IV: Chinnamastākhaṇḍa, Edited by V. V. Dwiveda. Baroda: Oriental Institute, 1979 (GOS, no. 166).

Śatapatha Brāhmaṇa. (Mādhyandina rescension) 5 volumes. Bombay: Laxmi Venkateshwar Steam Press, 1940.

Śiva Saṃhitā. Edited and translated by Rai Bahadur Srisa Chandra Vasu. Delhi: Sadguru Publications, 1984.

Śiva Sūtra with Kṣemarāja's commentary, *Vimarśinī.* Edited by Jaideva Singh as *Śiva Sūtras: The Yoga of Supreme Identity.* Delhi: Motilal Banarsidass, 1979.

The Spanda Kārikās. With the *Vivṛtti* of Rāmakaṇṭa. Kashmir Series of Texts and Studies, no. 6. Srinagar: Research Department, Jammu and Kashmir Government, 1913.

Suttanipāta. Edited by Dines Anderson and Helmer Smith. Reprint Edition. London: Pali Text Society, 1966.

Svacchanda Tantra with the *Uddyota* of Kṣemarāja. Edited by Madhusudan Kaul Sastri, 7 vols. Srinagar: Govt. Press, 1921-35 (Kashmir Series of Texts and Studies, nos. 31, 38, 44, 48, 51, 53, 56).

Śvetāśvatara Upaniṣad. In *The Śaiva Upaniṣads, with the Commentary of Śrī Upaniṣadbrahmayogin.* Edited by Pandit A. Mahadeva Sastri. Madras: The Adyar Libary and Research Centre, 1950.

Taittirīya Āraṇyaka. 2 volumes. Ānandāśrama-saṃskṛta-granthāvaliḥ, granthāṅkha 38. Pune: Ānandāśrama, 1978.

Taittirīya-Brāhmaṇa. 3 volumes. Ānandāśrama-saṃskṛta-granthāvaliḥ, granthāṅkha 37. Pune: Ānandāśrama, 1979.

Taittirīya Upaniṣad. In *Daśopaniṣads, with the Commentary of Śrī Upaniṣadbrahmayogin.* Revised Edition. Edited by the Pandits of the Adyar Library under the supervision of C. Kunhan Raja, revised by A. A. Ramanathan. 2 volumes. Madras: The Adyar Library and Research Centre, 1984. Volume 1.

Tantrāloka by Abhinavagupta with the *Vivaraṇa* of Jayaratha. Edited by Madhusudan Kaul Sastri and Mukunda Rama Sastri. Srinagar: Govt. Press 1921-38 (Kashmir Series of Texts and Studies, vols. 27-39); reedited by R. C. Dwivedi and N. Rastogi, Delhi: Motilal Banarsidass, 1985; translated into Italian by R. Gnoli as *La Luce delle Sacre Scritture.* Torino: Classici Utet, 1972.

Tantrarāja Tantra. Part I (Chapters 1-18). Edited by Laksmana Sastri. Calcutta: University Press, 1918 (Tantrik Texts, VIII); Part II (Chapters 19-36), edited by Sadashiva Misra, Calcutta: University Press, 1926 (Tantrik Texts, XII); reprinted Delhi: Motilal Banarsidass, 1981 in one volume.

Tantrasāra by Abhinavagupta, Edited by Mukunda Rama Sastri. Srinagar: Govt. Press, 1918 (Kashmir Series of Texts and Studies, no. 17); translation into Italian by R. Gnoli *Essenza dei Tantra.* Torino: Boringhieri, 1960.

Tripurā Upaniṣad. In the *Śākta Upaniṣads,* with the Commentary of Śrī Upaniṣadbrahmayogin. Second Edition. Edited by Pandit A. Mahadeva Sastri. Reprint edition. Madras: The Adyar Libary and Research Centre, 1986.

Tripurātāpinī Upaniṣad. In *The Śākta Upaniṣads, with the Commentary of Śrī Upaniṣadbrahmayogin.* Second Edition. Edited by Pandit A. Mahadeva Sastri. Reprint edition. Madras: The Adyar Libary and Research Centre, 1986.

Upadeśasāhasrī, attributed to Śankarācārya. Edited and translated by Sengaku

Mayeda as *A Thousand Teachings*. Albany: State University of New York Press, 1992.

Upaniṣat-Saṃgraha. Edited with Sanskrit Introduction by J. L. Shastri. Delhi: Motilal Banarsidass, 1970; reprint edition, 1984.

Vaikhānasa Smārta Sūtra. Edited by W. Caland. Bibliotheca Indica, no. 242. Calcutta: Royal Asiatic Society of Bengal. 1927. Translated by W. Caland. Bibliotheca Indica, no. 251. Calcutta: Royal Asiatic Society of Bengal, 1929.

Vaikhānasa Śrauta Sūtra. Edited by W. Caland. Bibliotheca Indica. no. 265. Calcutta: Royal Asiatic Society of Bengal, 1941.

Vālmīki Rāmāyaṇa: Critical Edition (1960-75). 7 volumes. General editors: G. H. Bhatt and U. P. Shah. Baroda: Oriental Institute, 1960–75.

Varāha Upaniṣad. In *The Yoga Upaniṣads, with the Commentary of Śrī Upaniṣadbrahmayogin*. Edited by Pandit A. Mahadeva Sastri. Reprint edition. Madras: The Adyar Library and Research Centre, 1968.

Vāsiṣṭha Dharma Sūtra. Edited by Manmatha Nath Dutt. In *The Dharma Śāstra Texts*. Calcutta: M. N. Dutt, 1908.

The Vijñāna-Bhairava. With commentaries by Kṣemarāja and Shivopadhyāya. Edited by Mukunda Rāma Sastri. Kashmir Series of Texts and Studies, no. 8. Srinagar: Research Department, Jammu and Kashmir Government, 1918.

Vijñānabhairava Tantra. Edited and translated into French by L. Silburn. Paris: Institut de Civilisation Indienne, 1961 (Publications de l'Inst. de Civilisation Indienne, serie in-8, fasc. 15).

Vinaya Piṭaka. Edited by Hermann Oldenburg. Volume I: *Mahāvagga*. London: Pali Text Society, 1879, reprint edition 1969. Volume II: *Cūlavagga*. London: Pali Text Society, 1880, reprint edition 1977.

Vivekacūḍāmaṇi, attributed to Śaṅkarācārya. Edited and translated by Swami Madhavananda as *Vivekacudamani of Shri Shankaracarya*. Ninth Edition. Calcutta: Advaita Ashrama, 1974.

Yogatattva Upaniṣad. In *Upaniṣat-Saṃgraha*. Edited with Sanskrit Introduction by J. L. Shastri. Delhi: Motilal Banarsidass, 1970; reprint edition, 1984.

Yoga Sūtra of Patañjali. Edited and translated by Swami Hariharananda in *The Yoga Philosophy of Patañjali*. Albany: State University of New York Press, 1983.

Yoginī Tantra. In Arthur Avalon, *Tantra of the Great Liberation [Mahānirvāṇa Tantra]* London: Luzac and Co., 1913; reprint edition, New York: Dover Publications, 1972.

Yoginīhṛdaya [Tantra]. Edited G. Kaviraj. Varanāsī: Sampurānand Sanskrit Viśvavidyālaya, 1963, second edition (Sarasvati Bhavana Granthamala, 7), with the Sanskrit commentaries *Dīpikā* by Amṛtānanda and *Setubandha* by Bhāskararāya.

SECONDARY TEXTS AND REFERENCES

Abbott, Justin E. and N. R. Godbole. *Stories of Indian Saints*. 2 volumes. Poona, 1933; two volumes bound as one, Delhi: Motilal Banarsidass, 1982. Includes translation of the *Bhaktivijaya*.

Agrawala, V. S. *India as Known to Pāṇini*. Second edition. Varanasi: Prithivi Prakashan, 1963.

———. *The Thousand-Syllabled Speech.* Part 1: *Vision in Long Darkness.* Varanasi: Vedāraṇyaka Ashram (Distributed by Prithivi Prakashan, Varanasi), 1963.

Alper, Harvey P., editor. *Understanding Mantras.* Albany: State University of New York, 1989.

Aurobindo, Śrī. *The Synthesis of Yoga.* Pondicherry: Śrī Aurobindo Ashram Trust, 1976.

Babb, Lawrence A. *Redemptive Encounters: Three Modern Styles in the Hindu Tradition.* Berkeley: University of California Press, 1986.

Bailly, Constantina Rhodes. *Shaiva Devotional Songs of Kashmir: A Translation and Study of Utpaladeva's Shivastotravali.* Albany: State University of New York Press, 1987.

Bagchi, Prabodh Chandra. *Studies in the Tantras.* Calcutta: University of Calcutta, 1975.

Banerji, S. C. *Tantra in Bengal.* New Delhi: Manohar, 1992.

Basham, A. L. *The Wonder That Was India.* New York: Grove Press, Twenty-first printing, 1977.

Bharati, A. *The Tantric Tradition.* London: Rider and Co., 1965; Revised American Paperback Edition, New York: Samuel Weiser, 1975.

Bhattacharyya, N. N. *History of the Tantric Religion.* Delhi: Manohar, 1982.

Bhattacharyya, Narendra Nath. *History of the Śākta Religion.* New Delhi: Munshiram Manorharlal, 1973.

Biardeau, Madeleine. *Théorie de la connaissance et philosophie de la parole dans le brahmanisme classique.* Paris: Mouton, 1964.

Brooks, Douglas Renfrew. *Auspicious Wisdom: The Texts and Traditions of Śrīvidyā Śākta Tantrism in South India.* Albany: State University of New York Press, 1992.

———. "Encountering the Hindu 'Other': Tantrism and the Brahmans of South India," *Journal of the American Academy of Religion,* LX/3, 1993.

———. *The Secret of the Three Cities: An Introduction to Hindu Śākta Tantrism.* Chicago: University of Chicago Press, 1990.

Brown, C. Mackenzie. *The Triumph of the Goddess.* Albany: State University of New York Press, 1990.

Bühler, Georg. *The Laws of Manu.* Oxford: Oxford University Press, 1886; reprint edition, New Delhi: Motilal Banarsidass, 1979.

Burns, Edward McNall, Robert E. Lerner, and Standish Meacham. *Western Civilizations: Their History and Their Culture.* London, 10th Edition, 1984.

Chakravarti, Chintaharan. *The Tantras: Studies on their Religion and Literature.* Calcutta: Punthi Pustak, 1963.

Chatterji, J. C. *Kashmir Shaivism.* Albany: State University of New York Press, 1986.

Clifford, James and George E. Marcus, editors. *Writing Culture: The Poetics and Politics of Ethography.* Berkeley: University of California Press, 1986.

Coburn, Thomas B. *Devī Māhātmya: The Crystallization of the Goddess Tradition.* Delhi: Motilal Banarsidass, 1984.

———. *Encountering the Goddess.* Albany: State University of New York Press, 1991.

Chaudhary, Radhakrishna. *Vrātyas in Ancient India.* Chowkhamba Sanskrit Studies, Volume 38. Benares: Chowkhamba Sanskrit Series Office, 1964.

Conze, Edward. *Buddhist Thought in India.* London: George Allen & Unwin, 1983.

Dandekar, R. N. *Der Vedische Mensch: Studien zu Selbstauffassung des Inders in Ṛg- und Atharvaveda.* Heidelberg: C. Winter, 1938.

Das, H. C., assisted by D. Panda. *Tāntricism: a Study of the Yoginī Cult.* New Delhi: Sterling Publishers, 1981.

Dasgupta, S. *Obscure Religious Cults.* Calcutta: Firma KLM private, 1976.

Davis, Richard. *Ritual in an Oscillating Universe.* Princeton, New Jersey: Princeton University Press, 1991.

Deussen, Paul. *The Philosophy of the Upanishads,* translated by A. S. Geden. Reprint edition. NewYork: Dover Publication, 1966.

Dimmitt, Cornelia and van Buitenen, J. A. B., editors and translators. *Classical Hindu Mythology: A Reader in the Sanskrit Purāṇas.* Philadelphia: Temple University Press, 1978.

Dimock, E. C. *The Place of the Hidden Moon. Erotic Mysticism in the Vaiṣṇava Sahajiyā Cult of Bengal.* Chicago: University of Chicago Press, 1966.

Dowman, Keith, translator. *Masters of Enchantment: The Lives and Legends of the Mahāsiddhas.* Rochester, Vermont: Inner Traditions International, Ltd., 1988.

———. *Masters of Mahāmudrā.* Albany: State University of New York Press, 1985.

Dumont, Louis. "World Renunciation in Indian Religions." *Contributions to Indian Sociology* 4 (1960), pp. 33-62. Reprinted in *Religion, Politics and History in India: Collected Papers in Indian Sociology.* The Hague: Mouton Publishers, 1970, pp. 33-60.

Dumoulin, Heinrich. *A History of Zen Buddhism.* Translated by Paul Peachy. Boston Beacon Press, 1963.

Dutt, Sukumar. *Buddhist Monks and Monasteries of India: Their History and Their Contribution to Indian Culture.* Delhi: Motilal Banarsidass, 1989.

———. *Early Buddhist Monachism.* London: George Allen & Unwin, Ltd. New York: Humanities Press, 1962.

Dwiveda, V. V. "Alaṃkārasaṃgrahakāra Amṛtānanda Kī Yoginīhṛdayadīpikākāra Se Abhinnatā," in: *Ṛtandharā,* January-March 1972, pp. 55–62.

———. *Tantra-Yatra, Essays on Tantra-Āgama Thoughts and Philosophy, Literature, Culture and Travel.* Varanāsī: Ratna Publications, 1982 (in Sanskrit).

———. "Tripurādaśanasya parcitā ācāryah krtayaś ca." In *Sarasvatī Susamā* (Journal of the Sanskrit Visvavidyālaya). Varanāsī, Samvat 2022 (1971, C.E.), pp. 13-26.

———. *Upodghāta.* Introduction to the edition of the *Nityāṣoḍaśikārṇava* (in Sanskrit). See *Nityāṣoḍaśikārṇava* in this Bibliography under Primary Texts.

Dyczkowski, Mark S. G. *The Aphorisms of Śiva: The Śiva Sūtra with Bhāskara's Commentary, the Varttika.* Albany: State University of New York Press, 1992.

———. *The Canon of the Śaivāgama and the Kubjikā Tantras of the Western Kaula Tradition.* Albany: State University of New York Press, 1988.

———. *The Doctrine of Vibration. An Analysis of the Doctrines and Practices of Kashmir Śaivism.* Albany: State University of New York Press, 1987.

———. *The Stanzas on Vibration.* Albany: State University of New York Press, 1992.

Eggeling, Julius, translator. *The Śatapatha Brāhmaṇa.* 5 volumes. Sacred Books of the East, Volumes 12, 26, 41, 43 and 44. Oxford: The Clarendon Press, 1882-1900; reprint edition, Delhi: Motilal Banarsidass, 1963.

Eliade, Mircea, et al., editors. *The Encyclopedia of Religion,* 16 volumes. New York: Macmillan and Free Press, 1987.

———. *The Sacred and the Profane: The Nature of Religion.* Translated by Willard R. Trask. New York: Harcourt, Brace & World, 1959.

———. *Yoga: Immortality and Freedom.* Second Edition. Translated by Willard R. Trask. New York: Bollinger Foundation, Inc., 1975.

Falk, Maryla. *Nāma-rūpa and Dharma-rūpa: Origin and Aspects of an Ancient Indian Conception.* Calcutta: University of Calcutta, 1943.

Filliozat, Jean. "La Force organique et la force cosmique dans la philosophie médicale de l'Inde et dans le Véda." *Revue philosophique* 116 (1933), pp. 410-29.

Findly, Ellison Banks. "*Mántra kaviśastá*: Speech as Performative in the Ṛgveda" in Harvey P. Alper, editor, *Understanding Mantras* (Albany: State University of New York, 1989), pp. 15-47.

Fort, Andrew and Patricia Mumme. *Living Liberation in Indian Thought.* Albany: State University of New York Press, 1996.

Geertz, Clifford. *Works and Lives, The Anthropologist as Author.* Stanford, California Stanford University Press, 1988.

Ghurye, G. S. *Indian Sadhus.* Second edition. Bombay: Popular Prakashan, 1964.

Gonda, Jan. *Four Studies in the Language of the Veda.* Gravenhage: Mouton, 1959.

———. "The Indian Mantra." *Oriens* Volume 16 (1953), pp. 244-97. Reprinted in Jan Gonda, *Selected Studies, Presented to the Author by the Staff of the Oriental Institute, Utrecht University, on the Occasion of his Seventieth Birthday.* 4 volumes. Leiden: E. J. Brill, 1975.

———. *Notes on Brahman.* Utrecht: J. L. Beyers, 1950.

Green, William Scott. "The Otherness Within." In E. Frerichs and J. Neusner, editors, *To See Ourselves as Others See Us: Christians, Jews, and "Others" in Late Antiquity.* Atlanta, Georgia: Scholars Press, 1985.

———. "Something Strange, Yet Nothing New: Religion in the Secular Curriculum." In *Liberal Education* 73, Nov/Dec 1987, pp. 21-25.

———. "Storytelling and Holy Man: The Case of Ancient Judaism." In *Take Judaism, for Example.* Edited by Jacob Neusner. Chicago: University of Chicago Press, 1983.

Griffith, Ralph T. H. *Hymns of the Ṛgveda.* edited by P. L. Shastri. Reprint edition. Delhi: Motilal Banarsidass, 1973.

Goldman, Robert P. *The Rāmāyaṇa of Vālmīki: An Epic of Ancient India.* Volume I: *Bālakāṇḍa.* Princeton: Princeton University Press, 1984.

Goudriaan, Teun. *Māyā Divine and Human. A Study of Magic and Its Religious Foundations in Sanskrit Texts.* Delhi: Motilal Banarsidass, 1978.

———. editor. *Ritual and Speculation in Early Tantrism: Studies in Honor of André Padoux.* Albany: State University of New York Press, 1992.

———. editor and translator. *The Vināśikhatantra. A Śaiva Tantra of the Left Current.* Delhi: Motilal Banarsidass, 1985.

Goudriaan, Teun and Sanjukta Gupta. *Hindu Tantric and Śākta Literature.* (*A History of Indian Literature,* edited by Jan Gonda, Volume II, fasc. 2). Wiesbaden: Otto Harrossowitz, 1981.

Gupta, Sanjukta; Dirk Jan Hoens; and Teun Goudriaan. *Hindu Tantrism.* Leiden: E. J. Brill, 1979.

Gupta, Sanjukta. *Lakṣmī Tantra: A Pāñcarātra Text.* Leiden: E. J. Brill, 1972.

Haberman, David. *Acting As a Way of Salvation.* New York: Oxford University Press, 1988.

Hayes, Peter. *The Supreme Adventure.* New York: Dell Publishing Group, Inc., 1988.

Heesterman, J. C. *The Broken World of Sacrifice.* Chicago: University of Chicago Press, 1993.

———. *The Inner Conflict of Tradition.* Chicago: University of Chicago Press, 1985.

Hoover, Thomas. *The Zen Experience.* New York and Scarborough, Ontario: New American Library, 1980.

Hume, Robert Earnest. *The Thirteen Principal Upanishads.* New Delhi: Oxford University Press, 1995.

Huxley, Aldous. *The Perennial Philosophy.* New York: Harper & Row, Publishers, Inc., 1970.

Isherwood, Christopher. *Ramakrishna and His Disciples.* New York: Simon and Schuster, 1970.

Jagadananda, Swami, translator. *Upadeśasāhasri.* Seventh edition. Mylapore: Ramakrishna Math, 1984.

Jaini, Padmanabh. *The Jaina Path of Purification.* Berkeley: University of California Press, 1979.

Johnsen, Linda. *Daughters of the Goddess.* St. Paul, Minnesota: Yes International Publishing, 1994.

Kakar, Sudhir. *Ascetics, Mystics, and Shamans.* Chicago: University of Chicago Press, 1993.

Kale, M. R. *The Abhijñānaśākuntalam of Kālidāsa,* with the commenary of Rāghavabhaṭṭa. Tenth Edition. Delhi: Motilal Banarsidass, 1969; reprint edition, 1980.

Kane, P. V. *History of the Dharmaśāstra.* 5 volumes., Pune: Bhandarkar Oriental Research Institute 1930-62, Reprinted 1968-77.

Kaviraj, Gopinath. *Tantra o Āgama-Śāstrer Digdarśan.* Calcutta: 1963 (Calcutta Skt. College Research Series, No. XXV, Studies, no. 12, in Bengali).

———. *Tantrik Vānmaya me Śaktidṛṣṭi.* Patna: Bihar Rastrabhasa Parisad, 1963 (in Hindi).

———. *Tāntrika Sādhana aur Siddhānta.* Patna: Bihar Rastrabhasa Parisad, 1979 (in Hindi)

———. *Tāntrika Sāhitya.* Lucknow: Rajarsi Purusottam Das Dandan Hindi Bhavan, 1972 (in Hindi).

Keith, Arthur Berriedale. *Religion and Philosophy of the Veda and Upanishads.* Harvard Oriental Series 31. Cambridge: Harvard University Press, 1925. Reprint edition Delhi: Motilal Banarsidass, 1976.

Kinsley, David. *Hindu Goddesses: Visions of the Divine Feminine in the Hindu Religious Tradition.* Berkeley: University of California Press, 1988.

Klostermaier, Klaus. "The Creative Function of the Word." In Harold G. Coward, editor, *"Language" in Indian Philosophy and Religion.* SR Supplements 5. Corporation Canadienne des Sciences Religieuses/Canadian Corporation for Studies in Religion, 1978. pp. 5-18.

Kramrisch, Stella. *The Presence of Śiva.* Princeton, New Jersey: Princeton University Press, 1981.

Kripananda, Swami. *Jnaneshwar's Gita: A Rendering of the Jnaneshwari.* Albany: State University of New York Press, 1989.

Laksman Joo, Swami. *Kashmir Shaivism: The Supreme Secret.* Albany: The Universal Shaiva Trust, 1988.

Larson, Gerald J. *Classical Sāṃkhya: An Interpretation of Its History and Meaning.* Delhi: Motilal Banarsidass, 1979.

Lorenzen, D. N. *The Kāpālikas and Kālāmukhas, Two Lost Śaivite Sects.* Reprint edition, New Delhi: Motilal Banarsidass, 1972.

Mahony, William K. "Dharma: Hindu Dharma." In *Encyclopedia of Religion.* Edited by Mircea Eliade, et al. 16 volumes. New York: Macmillan Co. and The Free Press, 1987. Volume 4, pp. 329–32.

———. "Soul: Indian Concepts," In *Encyclopedia of Religion.* Edited by Mircea Eliade, et al. 16 volumes. New York: Macmillan Co. and The Free Press, 1987. Vol. 13, pp. 438–43.

———. "Spiritual Discipline" in *The Encyclopedia of Religion.* Edited by Mircea Eliade, et al. 16 volumes. New York: Macmillan and The Free Press, 1987. Volume 14, pp. 19–29.

———. "Upaniṣads." In *The Encyclopedia of Religion.* Edited by Mircea Eliade, *et al.* 16 Volumes. New York: Macmillan Co. and The Free Press, 1987. Volume 15, pp. 147–52.

McDaniel, June. *The Madness of the Saints: Ecstatic Religion in Bengal.* Chicago: The University of Chicago Press, 1989.

Monier-Williams, Monier. *A Sanskrit-English Dictionary.* Oxford: Clarendon Press, 1899; Reprint edition 1974; also first Indian edition, 1970.

Mookerji, Radha Kumud and U. N. Goshal, "Ancient Indian Education." In *The Cultural History of India,* Volume II. Second Edition. Calcutta: The Ramakrishna Mission Institute of Culture, 1963, reprint edition 1982: pp. 640–54.

Muller-Ortega, Paul Eduardo. *The Triadic Heart of Śiva, Kaula Tantricism of Abhinavagupta in the Non-Dual Śaivism of Kashmir.* Albany: State University of New York Press, 1989.

———. The Power of the Secret Ritual: Theoretical Formulations from the Tantra," *Journal of Ritual Studies,* 4:2 (Summer 1990): 41–59.

———. "Tantric Meditation: Vocalic Beginnings" in *Ritual and Speculation in Early Tantrism: Studies in Honor of André Padoux.* Teun Goudriaan, ed. Albany: State University of New York Press, 1992.

Natarajan, B. *Thirumandiram, A Classic of Yoga and Tantra by Siddhar Thirumoolar.* Edited by M. Govindan. Montreal: Babaji's Kriya Yoga Publications, Inc., 1993.

Neusner, Jacob. *Midrash in Context, Exegesis in Formative Judaism.* Atlanta, Georgia: Scholars Press, 1988.

———. *Judaism in the American Humanities.* Brown Judaic Studies 28. Chico, California: Scholars Press, 1981.

———. editor. *Take Judaism, for Example.* Chicago and London: University of Chicago Press, 1983.

O'Flaherty, Wendy Doniger. *The Rig Veda.* Harmondsworth: Penguin Books, 1981.

Olivelle, Patrick. *The Āśrama System.* New York: Oxford University Press, 1993.

———. translator. *Upaniṣads.* Oxford: Oxford University Press, 1996.

Padoux, André. "Contributions à l'étude du Mantraśāstra. I: La selection des mantras *(mantroddhara)*." In *BEFEO,* 65, 1978, pp. 65–85.

———. *Vāc: The Concept of the Word in Selected Hindu Tantras.* Albany: State University of New York Press, 1990.

———. *Recherches sur la symbolique et l'énergie de la parole dans certains textes tantriques.* Paris: Institut de Civilisation Indienne, 1964.

Pal, Pratapaditya. "The Fifty-One Śākta Pīṭhas," *Orientalia Iosephi Tucci Memoriae Dicata, Serie Orientale Roma LVI, 3.* Roma: Instituto Italiano Per Il Medio Ed Estremo Oriente, 1988.

———. *Hindu Religion and Iconology.* Los Angeles: Vichitra Press, 1981.

Pandey, K. C. *Abhinavagupta, An Historical and Philosophical Study.* Varanāsī: Chaukhamba Publication, reprint 1963, second edition.

Panikkar, Raimundo. *Mantramañjarī: The Vedic Experience.* Berkeley and Los Angeles: University of California Press, 1977.

Pandit, B. N. *History of Kashmir Shaivism.* Srinagar: Utpal Publications, 1990.

Pennington, Kenneth. *Popes and Bishops: The Papal Monarchy in the Twelfth and Thirteenth Centuries.* Philadelphia: University of Pennsylvania Press, 1984.

Peterson, Indira. *Poems to Śiva: The Hymns of the Tamil Saints.* Princeton: Princeton University Press, 1989.

Pollack, Sheldon I. *The Rāmāyaṇa of Vālmīki: An Epic of Ancient India,* Volume III, *Araṇyakāṇḍa.* Princeton: Princeton University Press, 1991.

Potter, Karl. *Presuppositions of India's Philosophies.* New Delhi: Prentice-Hall of India, 1965.

Proudfoot, Wayne. *Religious Experience.* Berkeley: University of California Press, 1985.

Rabinow, Paul. *Reflections on Fieldwork in Morocco.* Berkeley: University of California Press, 1977.

Radhakrishanan, Sarvepalli. *The Principal Upaniṣads.* London: George Allen & Unwin, Ltd.; New York: Humanities Press, 1978.

Ramana Sastri, V. V. "The Doctrinal Culture and Tradition of the Siddhas." In *The Cultural Heritage of India.* Calcutta: The Ramakrishna Mission Institute of Culture, 1978.

Ramanujan, A. K. *Speaking of Śiva.* London: Penguin Books, 1973.

Ranade, R. D. *Mysticism in India: The Poet-Saints of Maharashtra.* Albany: State University of New York Press, 1983.

Rastogi, Navjivan. *Introduction to the Tantrāloka.* Delhi: Motilal Banarsidass, 1987.

———. *The Krama Tantricism of Kashmir.* Delhi: Motilal Banarsidass, 1979.

Rigopoulos, Antonio. *The Life and Teachings of Sai Baba of Shirdi.* Albany: State University of New York Press, 1993.

Robinson, Richard and Willard L. Johnson. *The Buddhist Religion, A Historical Introduction.* Third Edition. Belmont, California, Wadsworth Publishing, 1982.

Sanderson, Alexis. "Mandala and Āgamic Identity in the Trika of Kashmir." In *Mantras et diagrammes rituels dans l'Hindouisme.* Edited by André Padoux. Paris, 1986.

———. "Purity and Power Among the Brahmins of Kashmir." In *The Category of the Person: Anthropological and Philosophical Perspectives.* Edited by Michael Carrither, et al. Cambridge: Cambridge University Press, 1985.

———. "Saivism and the Tantric Traditions." In *The World's Religions*. Edited by Stewart Sutherland, et al. London: Routledge, 1988.

———. "The Visualization of the Deities of the Trika" in *L'Image Divine: Culte et Méditation dans l'Hindouisme*. André Padoux, ed. Paris: Éditions du Centre National del la Recherche Scientifique, 1990.

Sax, William S. *Mountain Goddess: Gender and Politics in a Himalayan Pilgrimage*. New York: Oxford University Press, 1991.

Schimmelpfennig, Bernhard. *The Papacy*. Translated into English by James Sievert. New York: Columbia University Press, 1992.

SenSharma, Deba Brata. *The Philosophy of Sadhana*. Albany: State University of New York Press, 1990.

Sethi, V. K. *Kabir, The Weaver of God's Name*. New Delhi: Radha Swami Satsang Beas, 1984.

Silburn, Lilian, translator. *Śivasūtra et Vimarśinī de Kṣemarāja*, Institut de Civilisation Indienne, fasc. 47. Paris: Diffusion E. de Boccard, 1980.

———. *Kuṇḍalinī, the Energy of the Depths*. Albany: State University of New York Press, 1988.

Singh, Jaideva, translator. *The Doctrine of Recognition: A Translation of Pratyabhijñā-hṛdayam*. Albany: State University of New York Press, 1990.

———, translator. *Śiva Sūtras: The Yoga of Supreme Identity*. Delhi: Motilal Banarsidass, 1979.

———, translator. *A Trident of Wisdom*. Albany: State University of New York Press, 1989. (*Parātriṃśikā-vivaraṇa* of Abhinavagupta.)

———, translator. *The Yoga of Delight, Wonder, and Astonishment: A Translation of the Vijñānabhairava*. Albany: State University of New York Press, 1991.

———, translator. *The Yoga of Vibration and Divine Pulsation: A Translation of the Spanda Kārikās with Kṣemarāja's Commentary, the Spanda Nirṇaya*. Albany: State University of New York Press, 1992.

Singh, Huzur Maharaj Sawan. *Tales of the Mystic East*. Punjab, India: Radha Soami Satsang Beas, 1983

Smart, Ninian. *Doctrine and Argument in Indian Philosophy*. London: George Allen and Unwin, Ltd., 1969.

Smith, Brian K. *Classifying the Universe: The Ancient Indian Varṇa System and the Origins of Caste*. New York: Oxford University Press, 1994.

———. *Reflections on Resemblence, Ritual and Religion*. New York: Oxford University Press, 1989.

Tagore, Rabindranath. *Songs of Kabir*. A rendering of the poems of Kabīr. New York: Samuel Weiser, 1974.

Thursby, Gene R. "Swami Muktananda and the Seat of Power." In *When Prophets Die: The Post-Charismatic Fate of New Religious Movements,* edited by Timothy Miller. Albany: State University of New York Press, 1991.

Tirtha, Swami Shankar Purushottam. *Yoga Vani*. Varanasi, India: Ayurvedic Holistic Center Press, 1992.

Vail, Lise. "Renunciation, Love, and Power in Hindu Monastic Life," Ph.D. Dissertation, University of Pennsylvania, 1987.

van Buitenen, J. A. B. *The Bhagavadgītā in the Mahābhārata*. Chicago and London: University of Chicago Press, 1981.

———, translator. *The Mahābhārata.* Volumes I-III (Books 1-5). Chicago: University of Chicago Press, 1973–78.

Varenne, Jean. *Yoga and the Hindu Tradition.* Chicago: University of Chicago Press, 1976.

Venkatesananda, Swami. *Sivananda Yoga: A Series of Talks by Swami Venkatesananda to the Students of the Yoga-Vedanta Forest Academy.* Sivanandanagar, India: Divine Life Society, 1980.

Vishnu Tirtha Maharaj, Swami. *Devatma Shakti.* Delhi: Swami Shivom Tirth, 1974.

Washington, Peter. *Madame Blavatsky's Baboon.* New York: Schocken Books, 1984.

Wheelock, Wade T. "The Mantra in Vedic and Tantric Ritual." In *Mantra.* Edited by Harvey P. Alper, Albany: State University of New York, 1989, pp. 96-122.

White, David Gordon. *The Alchemical Body.* Chicago: University of Chicago Press, 1996.

Whitney, William Dwight, translator. *Atharva Veda Saṃhitā.* 2 volumes. Harvard Oriental Series, 7 and 8. Cambridge: Harvard University Press, 1905; reprint edition Delhi: Motilal Banarsidass, 1962.

Woodroffe, Sir John (Arthur Avalon). *The Serpent Power.* New York: Dover Publications, Inc., 1974.

Yogendrajnani. *Mahā Yoga Vijñāna.* Rishikesh, India: Srimati Annarpurna Devi, 1990.

Zweig, Paul. "The Master of Ganeshpuri." *Harper's.* May 1977, pp. 85-91.

———. "Shaktipat," *Three Journeys.* New York: Basic Books, Inc., 1976.

SIDDHA YOGA PUBLICATIONS

Bendet, Peggy. *Shri Gauri-Shankara Yajna.* South Fallsburg, New York: SYDA Foundation, 1993.

Butler, Ram. "No One Else Can Do It." *Darshan* No. 44, November 1990, pp. 60-68.

Chidvilasananda, Swami. *Ashes at My Guru's Feet.* South Fallsburg, New York: SYDA Foundation, 1990.

———. "Creating a Body of Light." *Darshan* No. 41-42, September 1990, pp. 159–73.

———. "The Fire of Love." *Darshan* No. 2, May 1987, pp. 68–81.

———. "Four Means of Recognizing the Self." *Darshan* No. 79, October 1993, pp. 26–31.

———. "Give Your Blessings to Others." *Darshan* No. 21, December 1988, pp. 73–84.

———. "Go Deep Within Yourself." *Darshan* No. 57, December 1991, pp. 41–53.

———. "God in His Creation." *Darshan* No. 53, August 1991, p. 42.

———. *Inner Treasures.* South Fallsburg, New York: SYDA Foundation, 1995.

———. "Live in the Realm of Great Experiences." *Darshan* No. 62–63, May–June 1992, pp. 82–97.

———. "Love and Nothing Else." *Darshan* No. 24, March 1989, pp. 77–88.

———. *Kindle My Heart,* Volumes I & II. South Fallsburg, New York: Prentice Hall Press, 1989.

———. *Kindle My Heart* Revised Edition. South Fallsburg, New York: SYDA Foundation, 1996.
———. "Knowledge Has to Be Practiced." *Darshan* No. 92, November 1994, pp. 40–45.
———. "More Power than the Atom Bomb." *Siddha Path,* June 1984, p. 19.
———. *My Lord Loves a Pure Heart: The Yoga of Divine Virtues.* South Fallsburg, New York: SYDA Foundation, 1994.
———. "One Day It Will Just Happen." *Darshan* No. 61, April 1992, pp. 42–51.
———. "Polish the Mind Again and Again." *Darshan* No. 28, July 1989, pp. 49–56.
———. "Shaktipat: Like a Ring of Lightning." *Darshan* No. 59, February 1992, pp. 41–45.
———. "See the Same Self in All." *Darshan* No. 106, January 1996, pp. 40–45.
———. "Siddha Gita: Song of the Siddhas." (Part I) *Siddha Path,* July 1984, pp. 29–34.
———. "The Supreme Self Is Changeless, Unborn, Ancient." *Darshan* No. 56, November 1991, pp. 51–59.
———. "This Precious Gift." *Darshan* No. 23, February 1989, pp. 89–95.
———. (An interview with) "To Experience the Inner Love." *Shree Gurudev-Vani,* 1982, pp. 18-22.
———. "A Torch on the Path to the Highest Attainment." *Darshan* No. 3, June 1987, pp. 67–77.
———. "Transform Your Vision Into One of Wisdom." *Darshan* No.82, January 1994, pp. 37–42.
———. "The Truth Is I Am." *Darshan* No. 20, November 1988, pp. 61–68.
———. "Understand What You Are." *Darshan* No. 80, November 1993, pp. 36–41.
———. *The Yoga of Discipline.* South Fallsburg, New York: SYDA Foundation, 1996.
———. "You Must Trust Yourself." *Darshan* No. 52, July 1991, pp. 40–54.
Chidvilasananda, Swami (Malti). "Devotion to You." *Siddha Path,* April 1980, pp. 4–5.
———. "Growing up with Baba." (Part One) *Siddha Path,* February 1982, pp. 12–14.
———. "Growing up with Baba." (Part Two) *Siddha Path,* March 1982, pp. 14–18.
———. "The Guru Is the Means." *Siddha Path,* March 1980, pp. 10–11, 17.
———. "Interviews." *Siddha Path,* June-July 1982, pp. 12–14.
Chidvilasananda, Swami; Muktananda, Swami. *Resonate with Stillness: Daily Contemplations from the Words of Swami Muktananda, Swami Chidvilasananda.* South Fallsburg, New York: SYDA Foundation, 1995.
Dalal, B. P. "Experience at Ganeshpuri." *Guruvani,* 1964, pp. 25–29.
Dobrovolny, Janet L. "Just Keep Thinking You're a Great Meditator." *Darshan* No. 77–78, August-September 1993, pp. 104–09.
Durgananda, Ma (Swami). "Letter from Melbourne." *Siddha Path,* November 1978, pp. 4–17.
———. "Letter from Miami." *Siddha Path,* May 1980, pp. 3, 18.
———. "Letter from South Fallsburg." *Siddha Path,* June–July 1981, pp. 9–17.
———. "Pattabhishek." *Siddha Path,* June-July 1982, pp. 32–35.
———. "Report from Ganeshpuri." *Siddha Path,* December 1977, pp. 5–23.
———. "Report from Ganeshpuri." *Siddha Path,* March 1978, pp. 5–15.
———. "Report from Ganeshpuri." *Siddha Path,* September 1978, pp. 9–24.

———. "Silence Is a Sadhana: Letter from South Fallsburg." *Siddha Path,* August 1981, pp. 5–7.

———. "The Whole World Is Home." *Siddha Path,* October-November 1981, pp. 5–17.

Ferrar, Harold. "The Cosmic Key." *Shree Gurudev-Vani,* 1980, pp. 77–81.

Franklin, George. "A Harvest of Grace." *Darshan* No. 30–31, October 1989, pp. 67–97.

Greco, Tony. "More than You Remember Being." *Darshan* No. 35, February 1990, pp. 68–69.

Jain, Virendra Kumar. "An Ambrosial Experience of Baba's Grace." *Shree Gurudev-Vani,* July 1968, pp. 29–33.

Kemter, Robert. "The Quickening Force." *Darshan* No. 52, July 1991, pp. 6–12.

Kripananda, Swami. *The Sacred Power: A Seeker's Guide to Kundalini.* South Fallsburg, New York: SYDA Foundation, 1995.

Marwah, R. N. "My Second Birth." *Swami Muktananda Paramahamsa: 60th Birthday Commemoration Volume,* 1968, pp. 74–77.

Muktananda, Swami. *American Tour 1970.* Piedmont, California: Shree Gurudev Siddha Yoga Ashram, 1974.

———. *Ashram Dharma.* South Fallsburg, New York: SYDA Foundation, 1995.

———. *Bhagawan Nityananda of Ganeshpuri.* South Fallsburg, New York: SYDA Foundation, 1996.

———. "Dhyana Chakra Pravartana." *Dhyana Chakra,* 1976, pp. 8–9.

———. "The Embodiment of Grace." *Darshan* No. 30-31, October 1989, pp. 49–55.

———. *From the Finite to the Infinite.* South Fallsburg, New York: SYDA Foundation, 1994.

———. *Getting Rid of What You Haven't Got.* South Fallsburg, New York: SYDA Foundation, 1974.

———. "The Guru Principle." *Darshan* No. 75, June 1993, pp. 20–27.

———. *I Am That.* South Fallsburg, New York: SYDA Foundation, 1982.

———. *I Have Become Alive.* South Fallsburg, New York: SYDA Foundation, 1995.

———. *In the Company of a Siddha.* South Fallsburg, New York: SYDA Foundation, 1985.

———. "Intensive Talk." *Siddha Path,* December 1980, pp. 4–20.

———. *Kundalini: The Secret of Life.* South Fallsburg, New York: SYDA Foundation, 1994.

———. *Kundalini Stavah.* Ganeshpuri, India: Gurudev Siddha Peeth, 1980.

———. *Light on the Path.* South Fallsburg, New York: SYDA Foundation, 1994.

———. *Meditate.* Albany: State University of New York Press, 1991.

———. *Muktananda Thanks You.* Oakland, California: SYDA Foundation, 1976.

———. *Mukteshwari.* South Fallsburg, New York: SYDA Foundation, 1995.

———. "The Nature of the Guru." *Baba Company,* Midsummer 1980, p. 5–9.

———. *Paramartha Katha Prasang: Spiritual Conversations with Swami Muktananda.* Ganeshpuri, India: Shree Gurudev Siddha Peeth, 1981.

———. *The Perfect Relationship: The Guru and the Disciple.* South Fallsburg, New York: SYDA Foundation, 1985.

———. *Play of Consciousness.* South Fallsburg, New York: SYDA Foundation, 1994.

———. *Reflections of the Self.* South Fallsburg: SYDA Foundation, 1993.

———. *Sadgurunath Maharaj ki Jay.* New York: SYDA Foundation, 1975.
———. *Satsang with Baba,* Volumes 1–5. Oakland, California: SYDA Foundation, 1974–78.
———. *Secret of the Siddhas.* South Fallsburg, New York: SYDA Foundation, 1994.
———. *Selected Essays.* South Fallsburg, New York: SYDA Foundation, 1995.
———. "Shakti—The Universal Energy." *Siddha Path,* August 1980, pp. 4–6, 14–16, 20.
———. *Siddha Meditation.* Ganeshpuri, India: Gurudev Siddha Peeth, 1982.
———. *Swami Muktananda Paramahamsa in Australia.* Ganeshpuri India: Shree Gurudev Ashram, 1973.
———. "To Know the Knower." *Siddha Path,* March 1981, pp. 4–16.
———. "Truly Know Others." *Darshan* No. 56, November 1991, pp. 43–47.
———. *What Is an Intensive?* South Fallsburg, New York: SYDA Foundation, 1995.
———. "What Is Greater Than the Self?" *Siddha Path,* September 1980, pp. 4–20.
———. *Where Are You Going? A Guide to the Spiritual Journey.* South Fallsburg, New York: SYDA Foundation, 1994.
Nirmalananda, Swami. "The Guru Makes You Full of Life." *Siddha Yoga,* May 1982, pp. 23–28.
Obel, Gita. "Muktananda's Joy." *Swami Muktananda Paramahamsa: 60th Birthday Commemoration Volume,* 1968, pp. 62–63.
Pahelvan, Babu Rao (An interview with). "The Early Days." *Darshan* No. 18–19, September–October 1988, pp. 9–16.
Prajnananda, Swami (Amma). "Discovering the Guru." *Shree Gurudev-Vani,* 1981, pp. 9–13.
———. "Editorial: An Ashram Discipline." *Shree Gurudev-Vani,* 1969, pp. xi–ix.
———. "Editorial: The Unfolding of a Siddha Pitha." *Shree Gurudev-Vani,* 1972, pp. 1–5.
———. *A Search for the Self: The Story of Swami Muktananda.* India: Gurudev Siddha Peeth, 1979.
Ram Dass (Richard Alpert). "Meeting Babaji." *Shree Gurudev-Vani,* July 1971, pp. 29–33.
Shantananda, Swami. "A Monk's Dharma." *Darshan* No. 15, July 1988, pp. 43–47.
Shriyan, Venkappanna. "How to Hold What the Guru Gives." *Darshan* No. 81, December 1993, pp. 26–29.
Speeth, Kathleen Riordan. "The Guru in the Context of Western Psychotherapy." *Shree Gurudev-Vani,* 1975, pp. 33–36.
SYDA Foundation. *The Nectar of Chanting.* South Fallsburg, New York: SYDA Foundation, 1983.
———. *The Nectar of Self-Awareness.* A translation of *Amritanubhav* by Jnaneshwar Maharaj. South Fallsburg, New York: SYDA Foundation, 1979.
———. *Transformation: On Tour with Gurumayi Chidvilasananda,* Volumes 1–3. South Fallsburg, New York: SYDA Foundation, 1985–87.
———. *We Have Met Before: On Tour with Gurumayi Chidvilasananda.* South Fallsburg, New York: SYDA Foundation, 1996.

Index

Transliterated Sanskrit words have been alphabetized according to spelling, not pronunciation. For example, Śakti *appears under "Sa" while the related Westernized word Shaktipat appears under "Sh." References to endnotes in the index are expressed as, for example, 598n90 (page 598, note 90). References to footnotes are expressed as, for example, 125fn* (footnote * on page 125).*

A

Abhijñānaśākuntala 551–56
Abhinavagupta 38, 181, 214, 283, 294, 296, 319, 623n25
  on shaktipat 417, 430–32
  on Śiva's will 440
  See also Kashmir Śaivism
Absolute
  names for 372
  triadic form and function of 634n151
  as Vedāntic Brahman 370–73
  See also Brahman; Consciousness; God
Absorption
  of disciple in guru 267–68
  See also *Layayoga*
Ācārya, as spiritual teacher 239–41
Accessibility, of Siddha Yoga to public 151, 152
Action in inaction 456
Action, yoga of (*karmayoga*) 518
  See also Seva
Addictions, Swami Muktananda on 89–90
Ādivāsīs 7
  and Bhagawan Nityananda 8–9, 14–15, 152
  and Swami Muktananda 95, 152–53
Advaita (nondual) Vedānta 364–66, 375–77, 383–84
  primary texts of 294
  in Siddha Yoga canon 284, 286, 293–94
  See also Nondualism; Vedānta
Āgamas, Śaiva 497, 499–500, 519–20
  in relation to Tantras 289
  as support for spiritual experiences 519–20
Ahaṃkāra 253
Akalkot, Swami 23, 197
Akkamahādevī 121, 295, 598n90
Alchemical traditions 466–68
  view of liberation in 210–11
Allamaprabhu 121, 295, 598n90
Alpert, Richard. *See* Ram Dass
Ānanda. See Bliss
Anandamayi Ma 29
Āṇavamala 38
  destruction of 437–39
  nature of 433–34
  See also *Malas*
Animiṣayya 598n90
Āratī
  devotional elements in 262
  as Siddha Yoga chant 367
  See also Chanting
Āsana(s) 501–3, 516
  See also *Haṭhayoga*
Ascetics 543
  in Indian epics 550–51
Ashram(s) 521–68

Ashram(s) (*continued*)
 in *Abhijñānaśākuntala* 551–56
 accessibility of 556
 atmosphere of 554–55
 beauty of 526, 550
 as bridge between sacred and profane 524, 555–56, 565–68
 as center for spiritual discipline 531–40
 definitions of 540–44
 effects of, on residents 528, 529, 532, 555–56
 etymologies of 540–43
 as form of guru 528
 highest authority in 555
 in Indian literature 549–56
 need for discipline in 534
 need for reverence in 529
 paradoxical aspects of 523–25, 531, 540–44
 as physical embodiment of divine Śakti (energy) 524–29
 as place of inner peace 524
 as place of spiritual intensity 523, 533
 qualities of 554–55
 and related Indian religious institutions 544–49
 remembrance of 554, 555, 565–67
 seen as refuge 551
 sense of unity in 555
 taken into the world 565–68
 tapasya in 531–33
 for teaching personal dharma 554–55
 See also Ashram dharma; Ashram life; Ashram schedule; Ashrams, Siddha Yoga
Ashram dharma 80, 102–3, 533–34, 554–55, 564–65
 See also Ashram(s); Ashram life; Ashram schedule; Ashrams, Siddha Yoga
Ashram life
 discipline in 59–62
 reverence for 529, 556–57
 schedule for 59–60
 See also Ashram(s); Ashram dharma; Ashram schedule; Ashrams, Siddha Yoga
Ashram schedule 534
 generating intense *tapasya* 532
 origins of, at Gurudev Siddha Peeth 534
 as support for spiritual discipline 534
 See also Ashram(s); Ashram dharma; Ashram life; Ashrams, Siddha Yoga
Ashrams, Siddha Yoga 556–65
 activities in 537–39
 chanting in 534–37
 cleanliness in 564
 culture of 564–65
 established by Swami Muktananda 562
 as *gurukula* 564, 565
 guru's example in 539
 in Oakland 94–95
 scriptural study in 537–38
 taking leave of 565–68
 worldwide development of 109
 worship ceremonies (*pūjā*) in 538–39
 See also Ashram(s); Ashram dharma; Ashram life; Ashram schedule; Gurudev Siddha Peeth; Oakland, Siddha Yoga ashram of; Shree Muktananda Ashram
Ātman (Self) 377–83
 in contrast to Brahman 378
 etymology of 377–78
 five layers of 381
 as identical to Brahman 383–87
 nature of 378, 379–82
 in relation to individual soul 378, 381–83
 as Self within microcosm 378
 See also Brahman; Self
Austerity
 as source of endurance xl
 of Swami Muktananda's earliest ashram 44–45
 See also *Tapasya*

Australia, Swami Muktananda in 78–79, 81, 83
Authority, spiritual
and canons 306–9
as proof of experiences 519
scriptures as 519
of siddha gurus 307–9, 311–19
three sources of 317–19
See also Guru; *Guruvāda*; Scripture(s); Siddha(s)
Avadhūta 177
Bhagawan Nityananda as 177
etymology of 177
Avidyā. *See* Ignorance
Awareness, pre- and post-revelatory 339–41, 343

B

Babu Rao Pahelvan 32
Balbhojan Center (Ganeshpuri) 14
Banārsi 338–39
Bandha(s) (locks) 502–5
See also *Haṭhayoga*
Being 357–59
as indivisible 354
as nature of Self 354
as seen in Upaniṣads 363
in Vedānta 370–75
Bhagavadgītā
on dharma 392–94
on equality consciousness 392–94
on guru-disciple relationship 257–59
on immanent Lord 392–93
on moral responsibilities 392–94, 403–4
as part of Vedāntic canon 364
on serving God 404
on seva 249–50
in Siddha Yoga canon 283
taught by Siddha Yoga gurus 283, 295–96
on worldly responsibilities 392–94, 403–4
See also *Jñāneśvarī*; Vedāntic traditions
Bhagawan, meaning of term 8fn*
Bhagawan Nityananda. *See* Nityananda, Bhagawan
Bhakti, Nārada's uses of term 259
See also Bhakti traditions; Devotion; *Nārada Bhakti Sūtras*
Bhakti traditions
on seva 250–51
in Siddha Yoga 365–66
See also *Bhaktiyoga*; Devotion; *Nārada Bhakti Sūtras*
Bhaktivedanta, Swami 73
Bhaktiyoga 517
See also *Bhakti*; Bhakti traditions; Devotion
Bhartṛhari 365
Bhopi, Gangubai 8–9
Bhūtātman. *See* Self, individual
Bible 279, 621n2
Bindu, symbolism of 192–93
See also Blue Pearl
Bliss (*ānanda*) 357
as Brahman 373–74
as fifth layer of Self 380–81
as goal of meditation 436–37
as nature of Self 357–59
Swami Chidvilasananda on 357
See also Joy
Blue Pearl (*nīlabindu*) 494
Jñāneśvar Mahārāj on 597n80
in *layayoga* 514
Swami Muktananda on 514–15
Swami Muktananda's experiences of 40, 494
Tukārām on 597–98n80
Body, physical
as abode of Self 384, 386–7
disciplining, through *haṭhayoga* 502–3
ego's effects on 506
purified by Kuṇḍalinī 469
in relation to subtle body 448
respect for 400–1
and Self within it 378, 380–81
of a siddha 176, 177–79
Swami Muktananda on 400–1
as temple of God 400–1

Body, physical (*continued*)
  transmutation of, in Nātha tradition 466
  See also *Haṭhayoga*; Heart; Senses
Body, subtle
  and ascent of Kuṇḍalinī 492–94
  in *haṭhayoga* 502
  Kuṇḍalinī within 447–48, 449–50, 459–60, 469
  and Nātha tradition 466, 468
  physiology of 475–76
  in relation to physical body 448
  in Siddha Yoga 466–67
  Swami Muktananda on 475–76
  See also Chakras; *Suṣumṇānāḍī*
Bombay, Swami Muktananda in 54
Boulder (Colorado) 93–94
Brahmācārya 545–46
Brahman 363
  as the absolute 370–72
  aphorisms on 364
  as "breath of life" (*prāṇa*) 373
  earliest senses of word 368–70
  etymology of 368–69
  forms of 373–75
  as identical to Ātman 383–87
  ignorance of 376–77
  nature of 373–75, 383–86
  as Self within macrocosm 378
  Upaniṣadic descriptions of 373–74
  Vedic hymn on 370–72
  See also Absolute; Consciousness; God; Self
Brahma Sūtra 364, 366
Brahmins 538–39
Brazil, Siddha Yoga in 151
Breath 373, 377
  and Kuṇḍalinī 473–77
  middle space of 474
  See also *Prāṇa*
Buddha 306
  See also Buddhism
Buddhism 297
  ashrams of 542–43
  canons of 306–7
  concept of *nirvāṇa* in 209
  and concept of Self 350
  enlightenment in 209–10
  mendicants in 547
  monasteries (*vihāras*) of 547–48
  passing of lineage in 598–99n90
  siddhas in 182, 189
  South Asian 349, 350
  Zen 350–51, 598–99n90
  See also Buddha
Butler, Ram 91fn*, 93
  See also Correspondence Course

C

Caitanya 366
California, Swami Muktananda in 83
  See also Oakland
Canon(s)
  in Buddhism 306–7
  in Christianity 306–7
  confirmed by guru 313–17
  different meanings of 277–78
  dynamic quality of 303
  embodied in guru xlvii–xlviii, 278, 305–9, 312–17, 345–46
  enduring quality of 303
  functions of 302–4
  inclusive 283–85
  as independent authority 306–7
  in Islam 306
  as lineage traditions 277–80, 284
  as more than words 303
  mutability of 278, 284
  nature of xlvii–xlviii
  role of guru in creating 278–80, 281, 283–89, 298
  and role of sages 305
  sacredness of 303
  in spiritual traditions 277–78
  three textual types in 278–79
  value of 302–4
  of Vedānta 362–64
  See also Canon, Siddha Yoga; Teachings, Siddha Yoga
Canon, Siddha Yoga 277–346
  absence of hidden elements in 300–1
  and Advaita (nondual) Vedānta 284, 286, 293–94

aphorisms in 292–95
and Bhagawan Nityananda 299
breadth of 297
chants in 290–1, 298
dynamic nature of 300, 301–2
essential qualities of 339
ethical values of 282, 290, 327–39
guru principle in 301–2, 310–21
guru's words in 299–300, 301
and Kashmir Śaivism 284, 286, 293–94
and multiple levels of truth 344
nondogmatic nature of 388–89
nonhierarchical quality of 300–1
nonsectarian nature of 288–89, 291
potential 301–2
preconditions for scriptural choices in 323–45
and saints 295–97
Śāstra texts in 292–95
scriptural sources of 280–301
and Swami Muktananda 299–300
Tantric traditions in 289–91
traditional Hindu texts in 282–89
treatises in 292–95
and use of technology 301
See also Canon(s); Teachings, Siddha Yoga
Celibacy 338, 627nn. 123, 124
Center Leaders
training for 95–96
Swami Muktananda to 113
See also Centers, Siddha Yoga
Centers, Siddha Yoga
1974–76 expansion of 82–83, 93–94, 102
role of, in 1990s 143–44
seva in 143–45
and SYDA Foundation 95
See also Center Leaders
Chaitanya Mahāprabhu 82fn*
Chakras 449, 450
See also Body, subtle; *Mūlādhāra cakra*
Chalisgaon 41
Change, seen as illusion 471
Chanting
at core of ashram life 59–60
developed by Swami Chidvilasananda 155–56
purifying effects of 59–60
in Siddha Yoga ashrams 534–35, 537
as spiritual discipline 537
Swami Muktananda's love for 31–32
See also Chants, of Siddha Yoga; Practices, spiritual
Chants, of Siddha Yoga:
Āratī 262, 367
Āratī Karūn 298, 299
Gurugītā 262–63, 290–91, 299 (see also *Gurugītā*)
Hymn Praising the Avadhūt 595n12
Jyota se Jyota 298, 299
as part of canon 290–91, 298
Śivamānasapūjā 291
Śrī Guru Pādukā-Pañcakam 270–71
Viṣṇu Sahasranāma 299
See also Chanting
Charitable works, of Siddha Yoga gurus 14–15, 152–55, 561
See also *Ādivāsīs*; Prison Project
Chidvilasananda, Swami 135–61
accessibility of 151
and chanting 155–56
charitable activities of 153–55, 561
and children 155
communication modes of 5–6
culture around 5–6
darshan of 158–61, 275–76
early tours of 127–30
ecumenical approach of 145fn*
and emphasis on love 129–30, 138–40
as eternal disciple xxxv–xxxvi, 135–36, 308
as example for her students xxxv, 128, 135–36
and global Siddha Yoga movement 3, 5–6
initiation of 118–22
installed as co-successor 126
installed as sole head of lineage 131
and Intensives 415
later tours of 140–41, 145

Chidvilasananda, Swami (*continued*)
message(s) of 136, 138
mission of 135–61
morning programs with 155–61
personalized concern for students, of 128, 129, 138–40, 145, 158–59
poetry of 326–27
programs with 155–61
and role of scriptures 319
shaktipat experience of 64–65
as siddha guru xx, 128–30, 135–40, 148–50, 159–61, 237
tested during transitional period 133–34
yajñas held by 135–36
See also Chidvilasananda, Swami, quoted on; Malti
Chidvilasananda, Swami, quoted on:
attaining purity 330
bliss 357
compassion 401–2
contemplation 400
gentleness 156–58
guru-disciple relationship 232–33
her experience of divine light 491–92
her experience with Swami Muktananda 491–92
her initiation 118–22
impurity 329, 330
initation 4, 237, 418, 428, 444, 458, 480–81
joy 357, 359
Kuṇḍalinī 398, 447, 459–60, 470, 472
nature of God 213
relationship with her guru 326–27
sadhana 399
Second world tour 410–11
shaktipat initiation 4, 237, 418, 428, 444, 458, 480–81
Siddha Yoga courses 292
spiritual practices 486
steadfastness in yoga 339
yoga xxii, xxiii
See also Chidvilasananda, Swami; Malti
Children 19, 155
Christianity 297, 306–7, 604n227
Cit. See *Citi*; Consciousness
Citi (consciousness), knowledge of 216, 218–19
See also Citi Śakti; Consciousness
Citi Śakti 526
embodied as ashrams 526
in form of Kuṇḍalinī 459–65
in form of mantra 481–82
nature of 460–61
permeating ashrams 526
Swami Muktananda on 460–61, 463, 473
See also Consciousness; Goddess; Kuṇḍalinī
Clinic, mobile 152–53
Cloud Messenger 556
Command, of guru
following of 231
forms of, in Siddha Yoga 256
in guru-disciple relationship 252–53, 255–56
and seva 250
Compassion
of guru for disciple 241–42
as nature of Self 401–3
Swami Chidvilasananda on 401–2
Concentration, in *haṭhayoga* 502
Consciousness
as breath (*prāṇa*) 473–75
forms of 469
four states of 379–80
as identical to Self 351–52
light of 214–16
in Śaivite philosophy 425–28
within subtle body 475–76
turīya state of 380
See also Citi; Citi Śakti; Equality consciousness
Consciousness movement 72–73, 85
Constitution, of Siddha Yoga 591n16
Contemplation 400
See also Self–inquiry
Correspondence Course, Siddha Yoga 91fn*, 145, 154
See also Butler, Ram

Cosmogony, of Kashmir Śaivism 468–73
Courage 403
Courses, Siddha Yoga
 beginning of 97–98
 purpose of 292
 scripture-based 150
 Swami Chidvilasananda on 292
 on video 109
 See also Teacher(s); Teachings; Trainings; Appendix 3, 581–88
Creation, in Kashmir Śaivism 456
Cults, Western fears of 109–10

D

Daily life, for Siddha Yoga students 98–99, 138–40
Dandaka Forest 550
Darshan 275–76
 etymology of 275
 forms of 275, 276
 with Swami Chidvilasananda 158–61, 275–76
Dattātreya 60
 and Swami Muktananda 187, 611n47
Dayananda, Swami (Shaligram Swami) 44
Delusion. See *Māyā*
Devotion (*bhakti*)
 as awakened by shaktipat 443–44
 to awakened Kuṇḍalinī 448–49
 different types of 259–60, 260–61
 as essential for disciple 247
 as expressed by meditation 461–62
 for guru 266–67
 of Muktananda for his guru 175-81, 226–28, 234
 in *Nārada Bhakti Sūtras* 259–61
 through selfless service 392–94
 and story of Eklavya 267
 as supreme path to liberation 247, 257, 258–62
 yoga of (*bhaktiyoga*) 517
 See also *Bhakti*; Bhakti traditions; *Bhaktiyoga*
Dharma
 of ashram life (*see* Ashram dharma)
 Bhagavadgītā on 392–94
 as expression of universal love 404
 as learned in ashram living 554–55
Dhoot, Murlidhar 107
Diachronic truth 320–21
Dialogues, scriptural
 and guru-disciple relationship 223–24
 from Upaniṣads 372, 374, 378–79, 380
Dīkṣā
 etymologies of 407–8, 437
 See also Initiation; Shaktipat
Disciple
 and darshan 275–76
 and different aspects of guru 266–75
 following guru's command 231
 and goal of becoming guru 450–51
 grace of 243
 as identical to guru 252–53, 255
 imperfect understandings of 339–40
 and inner guru 272–73
 and learning of truth 233
 and love for guru 226–28
 as merged into guru 231–32, 264–66
 as needing guru 224–26
 qualifications of 243–49
 responsibilities of xxxix, xl
 role of devotion for 247
 Sanskrit terms for 235
 in Siddha Yoga 249
 Swami Muktananda on 271
 in Tantric tradition 248
 trust in guru of 241–43
 when away from guru 266
 See also Discipleship; Guru-disciple relationship; Student
Discipleship
 as best path to liberation 234–35
 Bhakti tradition on 249
 of guru 307–8
 role of discipline in 235
 Śaṅkarācārya on 244–48
 seva in 249–56

Discipleship (*continued*)
Swami Chidvilasananda on 256
Swami Muktananda on 231, 235
Tantric tradition on 248
Vedāntic view of 243–48
Yogic tradition on 248–49
See also Disciple; Guru-disciple relationship; Surrender
Discipline, spiritual
in ashram life 59–62, 80, 533
in discipleship 235–36
in *haṭhayoga* 502–3
purpose of xxxix
in Siddha Yoga 506
in Yogic tradition 545
See also Practices, spiritual; Sadhana
Discrimination (*viveka*) 245, 531
developed through ashram life 531
Dispassion (*vairāgya*) 245, 246–47
Dissolution, as goal of *kuṇḍalinīyoga* 456–57
Diversity, seen as forms of the Self 354–55
Doctrine of the guru. See *Guruvāda*
Doership 255
Dreams, initiation in 192, 197
Dualism. *See* Duality
Duality 446–47
assumed by the One 470
as cause of delusion 330, 331
dissolution of 456–57
as root of suffering xxviii
See also Māyīyamala; Nondualism
Duḥṣanta, King 550–51. *See also* Duṣyanta
Durgananda, Swami, as historian of Siddha Yoga xliv–xlv
Duṣyanta 565–67
in *Abhijñānaśākuntala* 551–56
See also Duḥṣanta, King

E

Effort. *See* Self–effort
Egalitarianism, of Siddha Yoga 318–19
Ego
becoming free of 253–54, 340
of disciple 253
in Indian philosophy 253
and individual self 381
as worst enemy 340
See also Egolessness; Self, individual; Selfishness
Egolessness
fruits of 255
of guru 253–54
and knowledge of Self 253–54, 255
of siddha gurus 230
as spiritual goal 230
See also Ego
Ekaguru xxii–xxiii
Ekagurūpāsti 324–27
Ekalavya (Eklavya) 267
Eknāth 186
Emptiness, in Indian Buddhism 350
Enemies, inner 139
Enlightenment 208–21
best attained through discipleship 234–35
in Buddhism 209–10
devotion on path to 247
in Hindu traditions 208–9, 210
in Jainism 209–10
longing for 246–47
nature of 210–11, 212–13
in siddha traditions 210–11, 213–19
Vivekacūḍāmaṇi on 257
See also Freedom; Liberation; Self–realization; Siddha(s)
Equality consciousness
Bhagavadgītā on 392–94
in Siddha Yoga xxxii, xxxiii
Swami Muktananda on 395, 395–96
Erhard Seminars Training (*est*) 81
Erhard, Werner 81
est (Erhard Seminars Training) 81
Ethics, of Siddha Yoga 282, 290, 308–9, 327–39, 359–60
and effect on scriptural choices 334
with guru as exemplar 333–35
and nondiscrimination 328
as reflection of inner Self 329, 330
and respect for God in all 329
and Self-knowledge 347–48

See also Guru-disciple relationship; Purity; Renunciation; Responsibilities; Virtues
Etymologies of:
ashram 540–43
ātman 377–78
avadhūta 177, 594n12
Bhārata 554
brahmacarya 545
brahman 368–69
darshan (*darśana*) 275
dīkṣā 407–8, 437
disciple 235, 615n44
discipline 235, 615n44
guru 239, 262–63
haṭha 501
Hinduism 628n4
kriyā 411
mantra 508
mūlādhāra 474
sādhana 235
sādhu 235
śaktipāta 407
samādhi 456
saptah 537
siddha 308
siddha guru 408
Siddha Peeth 557
veda 368
Vedānta 362
yoga xxii
Europe, Siddha Yoga students in 140
Experience, as primary in Siddha Yoga 464–65
Experiences, spiritual
at core of Siddha Yoga 519–20
of the Goddess 452
in Gurudev Siddha Peeth 524–25, 528–29, 556–57, 559–60
of Kuṇḍalinī 467, 470
in meditation 486–87, 561–62
of physical *kriyās* 489–90
of *samādhi* 455
of shaktipat (initiation) 412–13, 414–15, 415, 479–80, 483–84
of Siddha Yoga students 534, 561–62, 567
of Swami Muktananda 36–38
Eye camps (Netraprakash) 153–54

F

Fallsburg, South. *See* Shree Muktananda Ashram
Family life, in Siddha Yoga 361–62
Feet, of guru 269, 270–71
See also Sandals, of guru
Field, knower of 351–52, 355
Fire
inner and outer 542–43
ritual (*yajña*) 135–36
See also Fire, yogic
Fire, yogic 136
in Swami Chidvilasananda's initiation 118–19
in Swami Muktananda's meditation 36
of yogic masters 19
See also Fire
Fivefold cosmic actions, of Śiva 432
Food, as viewed by Swami Muktananda 535
Forgetfulness, of Self 395
See also Remembrance
Foundation, SYDA. *See* SYDA Foundation
Freedom
of guru xxxiv–xxxvii
of siddhas 335
Functions, of Śiva 432

G

Gandhi, Mohandas (Mahātma) 297
Ganeshpuri (India)
Bhagawan Nityananda in 8–10, 14–15, 22
early development of 22
source of name of 557
See also Gurudev Siddha Peeth
Gavdevi 41–42
Germany, Swami Muktananda in 410–11
Global Siddha Yoga community 139–40

Goals, of Siddha Yoga 347, 354
God
absorption in 230
aspects of 388
as guru 256–57, 257–58, 260, 263–65, 274–75, 397–98
as identical to Self 229–32, 263–65, 274–75, 355–57
as immanent 392–93
as indweller xxviii
in Islam 349, 350
on knowing, as *śiva* 388
as love 260–61, 360
revealed through guru-disciple relationship 231, 232–33
as seen in others 392–93, 404
as understood in Siddha Yoga xxxviii–xxxix
See also Brahman; Consciousness; Goddess; Grace; Self; Śiva
Goddess
forms of 426
in Śākta Tantric tradition 388–89
vision(s) of 452
See also Citi Śakti; Kuṇḍalinī; *Śakti*
"God dwells within you as you" xxxvii, 15, 138, 397, 447
Gorakṣanātha 466
Gosavi, Rajgiri 41
Grace
bestowal of 432
of disciple 243
drawn by seva 144–45
guru as power of 272–73
need for 432–33
and self-effort 337, 399, 485–87
See also Grace, of guru; Self-effort
Grace, of guru 229, 229–30, 232
beneficial effects of 398
in continuing lineage 234
as divine grace 238, 397–98
drawn by disciple's longing 238
as essential to Kuṇḍalinī awakening 465–66
in Kashmir Śaivism 477
as means to Self-knowledge 397
and meditation 391, 485–87
in *Nārada Bhakti Sūtras* 260
and self-effort 399, 485–87 (*see also* Self-effort)
Self-knowledge through 391
in Siddha Yoga 480–81, 485, 495
in Vedānta 477
See also Grace; Guru, as grace-bestowing power
Guru 226–31, 266–75
absorbing disciples' karmas 106
absorption in 267–68
as canon xlvii–xlviii, 298, 312–17
command of 231, 250, 252–53, 255–56
compassion of, for disciple 241–45
as confirmer of canon 313–17
contemplation on 99, 267–68
darshan of 275–76
definition of xx
as determiner of canon 278–80, 281, 283–89, 298, 312–17
disciple merging into 264–66
as divine power 238, 272–73
effect of, on disciple 238
as ego-destroyer 253–54
egolessness of 230, 253–54
as embodiment of Self 229–32, 274–75
as eternal disciple xxxv–xxxvi, 308
etymologies of 239, 262–63
false 109–10, 251–52, 623–24n38
feet of 270–71
as grace-bestowing power xxii, 229, 238, 272–73, 432–33
as guide of awakened Kuṇḍalinī 450
as guru principle (*gurutattva*) 271–72
how to choose 251–52
as identical to God 257–58, 260
as identical to his ashram 528
as identical to Kuṇḍalinī 450, 452–53
as identical to Self 263–65, 274–75
identifying oneself with 451–52
identity of 397–98
as incarnation of God 257–58
inner 141, 228, 268–71, 272–73, 275–76, 450–53

intention (*saṅkalpa*) of xxiv–xxv, 98, 409
as Kṛṣṇa for Arjuna 255, 257–59
in Left-Current (Tantric) paths xxxiv–xxxv
as living canon 278, 312–17
and love for disciple 226–28
as mantra 270–71
as means to liberation 238, 272, 313–14
as means to Self-knowledge xxii–xxiii, 224–26
meditation on 267–68
mental worship of 267–68
nature of 34–35, 397–98
nondualism of 253
as one with disciple 231–32
outer 226, 450–51, 453
as perfect disciple 248
perfect freedom of xxxiv–xxxvii, 290
perfect love of 333–34
as pervading his ashram 528
physical form of 226, 229–30
qualifications of 180–81
qualified only when a siddha 236
qualities of 230, 247, 451
in Śaiva yoga 311–12
as Śakti 311
sandals of 35, 270–71
seeker's need for 224–26, 545
as seen in West xx–xxi, xxiii–xxiv
selection of xxiii
as Śiva 202–3, 229–30, 272, 311, 312, 314, 318
six types of 228
soteriological functions of 256–63
as supreme reality 273–74
Swami Muktananda on 314, 325, 330–31, 332, 334, 335, 336–37
in Tantric tradition 248
tests given by 254
as transformative power 241–42
true 251–52, 270
as truth 320–21
as ultimate reality 273–74
unity of forms of 274–75
when *ekaguru* xxii–xxiii
See also Grace, of guru; Guru-disciple relationship; Guru principle; Siddha(s); Siddha guru; Teacher
Gurubhāva 267–68
Gurudev Siddha Peeth
appearance of 525, 528
ashram schedule in 534–37
chanting in 534–37
as charitable trust 49
democratic qualities of 31, 51
early development of 557–60
early discipline in 80
entryway sign in 540
expansion of 54–56, 61, 560
experiences of Siddha Yoga students in 412–14, 524–25, 528–29, 534, 556–57, 559–60, 567
founding of 49–51
gardens of 51, 525–26
geographical setting of 521, 557
historical traditions about 557
legal title for 560
meditation spaces in 534–35
names of 557
scriptural study in 150
subtle initiations in 412–14
Swami Muktananda's stewardship of 560
as traditional *gurukula* 151–52
See also Ashrams, Siddha Yoga; Ganeshpuri
Guru-disciple relationship 223–76
as basis for scriptural canon 324
becoming the guru through 252–53
Bhagavadgītā on 223–24, 257–59
Bhakti tradition on 249
darshan in 275–76
and different aspects of guru 266–75
earliest scriptural references to 223–24
ethical boundaries in xxxvi
grace and self-effort in 337
and guru as disciple xxxv–xxxvi
and guru as ethical exemplar 333–34

Guru-disciple relationship (*continued*)
Gurugītā on 60
guru's role in 336–37
in Hindu tradition 239–41
Jñāneśvar Mahārāj on 265–66
Kabīr on 19
in Left-Current (Tantric) paths xxxiv–xxxv
mutual responsibility in 336
nature of 237–38, 450–51
nonduality within 264–66
redemptive function of 261
role of love in 226–28
role of mantras in 508
Śaṅkarācārya on 244–48
seva in 249–56
in Siddha Yoga 5, 141–50, 230–32
soteriological aspects of 256–63
surrender in 140, 335
Swami Chidvilasananda on 232–33, 243
Swami Muktananda on 45–47, 252–53
Tantric tradition on xxxiv–xxxv, 248
transforming power of 260–61
ultimate merger within 264–66
Upaniṣads on 258
Vedāntic view of 243–48, 305
virtues in 243–49
Yogic tradition on 248–49
See also Command, of guru; Disciple; Discipleship; Guru
Gurugītā (chant) 535, 619n164
in ashram life 60
as chanted with Swami Muktananda 535
on the guru 262–63, 273–74
in Siddha Yoga canon 290–91
See also Chanting
Guru, inner 228, 268–71, 272–73, 275–76, 450–53
experiences of 145–48
need to find 141
Self as 268–69, 272–73
See also Guru; Guru principle
Gurukula (school of the guru)
in ancient times 546
in Oakland ashram 96
reasons for studying in 546
in Siddha Yoga ashrams 564
and similar Indian institutions 548–49
in Swami Muktananda's ashrams 59
Guru Nānak 296
Guru principle (*gurutattva*) 310–21
and canonical authority 301
experienced in transitional period (1981–85) 126–27
in form of physical guru 263, 271
as inner Self 271
nature of 262
in Siddha Yoga 311
Swami Muktananda on 271
as yogic goal 311
See also Guru
Gurusevā. *See* Seva
Gurus, false 623–24n38
dangers of 251–52
Swami Muktananda on 109–10, 251–52
Western fears of 109–10
Gurus, true, Swami Muktananda on 308–9, 451, 483, 484–85
Gurutattva. *See* Guru principle
Guruvāda (doctrine of the guru) 306–9
Guruvani (magazine) 57

H

Haṃsa (mantra) 509–10
See also Mantra(s)
Hare Krishna movement 73
Hari Giri Baba 39, 52, 172
Harmony, in Vedic worldview 368
Haṭhayoga 501–7
etymology of 501
and Kuṇḍalinī 465–66, 469
progressive steps in 502
role of, in Siddha Yoga 503
samādhi state in 517
in Siddha Yoga ashrams 537
spontaneous, in Siddha Yoga 498, 502–3, 507
See also *Mahāyoga*

Havanas (fire rituals) 538
Heart
as abode of Self 386–87, 402
as Kuṇḍalinī's destination 493
nature of 386
opened by awakened Kuṇḍalinī 476
See also Compassion; Love
Hinduism
canonical authority of 621n1
as colonialist misnomer 628n4
etymology of 628n4
guruvāda tradition in 306–9
primacy of oral tradition in 305
as similar to Islam 350
six philosophical schools (*darśanas*) of 292
traditional texts of, in Siddha Yoga canon 282–89
See also Bhakti traditions; Nātha traditions; Śaiva traditions; Smārta traditions; Tantric traditions; Vaiṣṇavite traditions; Vedāntic traditions; Vedas; Yogic traditions
Hospital, mobile 152–53
Hubli 27–29, 367
Human development movement(s) 81

I

Identification, false 382–83
Idols and images xl–xli
Ignorance (*avidyā*)
of Brahman 376–77
as cause of suffering 394–95
ended by shaktipat 434–35, 437–38
as illusion 395
in nondual Vedānta 364
of reality 376–77
due to three *malas* 433–34, 438–39
See also *Malas*
Impurities. *See* Impurity; *Malas*
Impurity 328–30
arising from dualism 329
Swami Chidvilasananda on 329, 330
See also *Malas*; Purity
Inclusive canon 283–89
Inclusivism, of Siddha Yoga theology xxix–xxxiii
Individuality. *See* Ego; Self, individual
Individual self. *See* Self, individual
Initiation
in dreams 192, 197
early ritual forms of 408–9, 416–17
and mantras 507, 511
shaktipat as essence of 407–8
by siddha guru 408
Swami Chidvilasananda on 237
See also Shaktipat
Inner enemies 139
Inner guru 228, 268–71, 272–73, 275–76, 450–53
experiences of 145–48
need to find 141
See also Guru; Guru principle
Inner Self. *See* Self
Integral Yoga Institute 73
Intensive(s) 150–51, 538
development of 92–93
early experience of 414–15
given by Siddha Yoga teachers 98
under Swami Chidvilasananda 5–6, 143, 150–51, 415
as vehicle for Siddha Yoga initiation 412, 538
Intention, of guru. *See* Will, of guru
International Society for Krishna Consciousness 73
Inversion, in symbolism around Kuṇḍalinī 454–57
Islam 297, 306, 349, 350
Iyer, Ishwara 10–11, 595n15

J

Jainism, path to enlightenment in 209–10
Jain, Jinendra 82, 97, 99
Janananda, Swami 44
Janmasiddha 196–97
Japa. *See* Mantra repetition
Jīva. *See* Self, individual

Jīvanmukta 211
as a siddha 191
See also Enlightenment
Jñāna Sindhu (text) 268
Jñānayoga 517
Jñāneśvarī 295–96, 318, 322
See also *Bhagavadgītā*; Jñāneśvar Mahārāj
Jñāneśvar Mahārāj 185–86
admired by Swami Muktananda 185–86
on ascent of Kuṇḍalinī 492–93
on guru-disciple relationship 265–66
on his guru 256
on his lineage 185
honored in Siddha Yoga 295–96
on *kriyās* 488, 504
on mental worship of guru 269
nonsectarian views of, on Kuṇḍalinī 463
on seva 250, 251
in Siddha Yoga teaching 283
See also Jñāneśvarī
Jñānī (knower of truth), perspective of 201–4
Joy, Swami Chidvilasananda on 221, 257, 359
See also Bliss
Judaism 593n49, 621n1

K

Kabīr 19, 121, 186, 242–43
Kabirdas (of Hubli) 28
Kālidāsa 551–56
Kanhangad 13, 44
Kaṇva Kāśyapa 551–55
Karma
absorbed by shaktipat guru 106
dissolution of 18
purified through *kriyās* 487–92
and receiving shaktipat 440–42
at time of initiation 18
Kārmamala 433, 434, 438–39
See also *Malas*
Karmayoga 518
Kashmir Śaivism
canonical choices in 345
and classical yoga 446
on creation 456, 468
and forms in Siddha Yoga xl–xli
and Kuṇḍalinī in Siddha Yoga 446
Left-Current teachings in 327–28
levels of reality in 341–45
and the One in many 345
primary texts of 294
on shaktipat 430–33
in Siddha Yoga canon 284, 286, 293–94
and Siddha Yoga gurus 463
and Siddha Yoga worldview 361–62
as taught by Swami Muktananda 96–97
and the three *malas* 236, 615n45
translated by Jaideva Singh 97
on valid knowledge 319
See also Abhinavagupta; Śaiva traditions
Knowledge
levels of 201
ultimate 342–44
valid 319
yoga of (*jñānayoga*) 517
Krishna (Kṛṣṇa), as guru to Arjuna 257–59
Krishna Consciousness, International Society for 73
Kriyā(s) 19, 439, 487–92, 498, 503
beneficial nature of 488–90
etymology of 411
experienced by Malti 66
experienced by Swami Muktananda 36–37, 491, 504–5
experiences of 489–90
as forms of yoga 488–90
great diversity of 488
and *haṭhayoga* 503, 507
during initiation 411
Jñāneśvar Mahārāj on 488, 504
as movements of Kuṇḍalinī 487–92
as reaction to initiation 411, 428–29, 439–40
rooted in Indian traditions 490–91

scriptural basis for 488
Swami Muktananda on 439
visual 429
See also Initiation; Kuṇḍalinī; Shaktipat
Kṛpāsiddha 197
Kṛṣṇa, as guru to Arjuna 257–59
Kulārṇava Tantra 334
Kuṇḍalinī
apparent dual nature of 470–71, 473, 494
ascent of 38, 449–50, 459–60, 470, 492–93
ascent of, Swami Muktananda on 459, 470, 476, 480
awakened during shaktipat 421
awakened when pleased 398
awakening of 4, 413–14, 448–50
becoming Śiva 457
beneficence of 449–50, 478–79
best awakened by siddha guru 465
channeled by shaktipat guru 485
as Citi Śakti 459–65
cosmogonic 459–65
descent of 454, 469
directed by guru's grace 476–77
divine manifestations of 460–61
as Divine Mother 458
earliest texts on 447–48
effects of 498, 500
embodied in mantra 481–82
experiences of 467 (*see also* Shaktipat, experiences of)
explained by Swami Muktananda (1974–76) 91–92
as form of Goddess 448
forms of 447, 449, 452–55, 462, 473–75
free movement of 486–87
as guided by guru 450
identifying oneself with 451–52, 452–53
ignorance of 454
individualized effects of 478, 486–87, 491
as inner guru 450–51, 452–53
intelligence of 449–50
as Light's reflection 472
mahāyoga as result of awakening 500, 518
and *māyā* 469–72
and meditation 461, 485–87
as microcosm and macrocosm 453–55, 462, 464
as name for God 448
names for 460
need for devotion to 449
omniscience of 478
playfulness of 451
as principal deity of Siddha Yoga 446
qualities of 447
reuniting with Śiva 456–57, 492–94
as revealer of truth 453
and role in Siddha Yoga xxxviii, 446
and shaktipat 478–85
as Śiva's sacrificial offering 468–69
and sound(s) 472
special locations of 474–75, 476
Swami Chidvilasananda on 398, 447, 459–60, 470, 472
Swami Muktananda on 461, 462, 470, 473
in Swami Muktananda's sadhana 36–40
and Tantric traditions 289, 641n2
universal need to awaken 462
when "asleep" 454–56, 469–70, 471, 494
See also Citi Śakti; Goddess; *Kriyās*; *Kuṇḍalinīyoga*; Shaktipat
Kuṇḍalinī Śakti. *See* Citi Śakti; Kuṇḍalinī
Kuṇḍalinīyoga
basic model of 447–48
dissolution as goal of 456–57
nature of 461
and relation to *haṭhayoga* 465–66
in Siddha Yoga teaching 448–49
traditions' consistency on 448
and yogic traditions 463–64
See also *Mahāyoga*

L

Laukika (worldly) perspective 201

Layayoga 456, 512–15, 517
See also *Mahāyoga*
Learning, in ancient India 544
Left-Current (Tantric) paths xxxiv–xxxv, 290, 327–28, 457
See also Tantric traditions
Liberation
from bondage of three *malas* 236
as goal of Śaivism 425
as goal of Siddha Yoga 5
and shaktipat 438
Swami Muktananda on 40, 168, 169
See also Enlightenment; Freedom; Self-realization
Lifestyle, of Siddha Yoga students xxx–xxxi, 98–99
Light
primordial 373
reflected by *Citi* 472
See also Light(s), divine
Light on the Path (Swami Muktananda) 67–69
Light(s), divine 401
Swami Chidvilasananda's experiences of 491–92
Swami Muktananda's experiences of 494–95
See also Blue Pearl; Light
Lineage
as essential for siddha guru 190–91
mystical understanding of 192–93, 194–96
as part of ecumenical meta-lineage 194–95
passing of, in different traditions 48, 598–99n90
passing of, in Siddha Yoga 47–48, 121–22
of Siddha Yoga xxiv–xxvi, xxxvi
of teachers of truth 233
See also Siddha lineage(s), Siddha traditions
Lineage canon 283–84, 284–89
Lingananda Swami 29
Literature, Indian, on ashrams 549–56
Love
as awakened by shaktipat 443–44
as central to Siddha Yoga theology 359–60
as core of human life 443–44
as expressed through dharma 404
as foundation for sadhana 401–2
for God 568
in guru-disciple relationship 226–28, 232–33
in *Nārada Bhakti Sūtras* 259–61
as nature of God 260, 360
as nature of Self 359–60, 402, 405
for one's body 400–1
perfect, of guru 333–34
secondary, as path to supreme love 259
and Self 378–79
Swami Muktananda on 400–1, 405
as taught by Swami Chidvilasananda 129–30, 138–40
See also Devotion; Heart

M

Macrocosm, as identical to microcosm 453–55, 462, 463, 464
Madhva 365–66
Magical powers (*siddhis*) 187–89
Mahābhārata
ashrams in 550–51
in Siddha Yoga canon 282–83
Maharashtra
Bhagawan Nityananda settles in 14
history of 31
poet-saints of 361, 368
siddhas in 186
spirituality in 31
See also Jñāneśvar Mahārāj; Tukārām Mahārāj
Maharishi Mahesh Yogi 73
Mahāvākyas 361
Mahāyoga 477–78, 497–520
different names for 501
meaning of 481
as result of Kuṇḍalinī awakening 477–79, 500, 518, 520
Siddha Yoga as 197–98, 497–99, 518
Swami Muktananda on 497–99, 518

visions in 514–15
See also Yoga
Maitreyī, in Upaniṣadic dialogue 378–79
Malas (impurities) 236, 438–39, 440, 615n45
as cause of impurities 330
overcome only by shaktipat 432–35, 437
removed by awakened Kuṇḍalinī 470
self-imposed by Śiva 437, 440
weakening of 441–42
See also *Āṇavamala*; Impurity; *Kārmamala*; *Māyīyamala*
Mallikarjuna Swami 28
Malti
awakened Kuṇḍalinī in 65–67
childhood of 62
early sadhana of 62–67
as example to others 100
meeting Swami Muktananda 62
named as successor 115
physical *kriyās* of 66
sannyāsa initiation of 115, 118–22
scriptural talks by 111–12
in service to Swami Muktananda 100–1, 112, 113
shaktipat initiation of 64–65
spiritual training of 99–101, 111–13
Swami Muktananda's plans for 106–7
and SYDA Foundation 113
as translator 99
See also Chidvilasananda, Swami
Manana (reflection) 546
Mandagni Mountain 7–8
Mangalore 11–13, 25
Mantra(s)
bestowal of, in Siddha Yoga 482
Bhagawan Nityananda on 35
enlivened (*caitanya*) 482, 507
as essential to meditation 270
etymology of 508
as form of Citi Śakti 481–82
as form of guru 270–71
as form of Kuṇḍalinī 481–82
given by Bhagawan Nityananda 35, 510–11
in guru-disciple relationship 508
Haṃsa (mantra) 509–10
in initiation 417–18, 431–32, 511
and inner guru 270–71
as manifestation of Kuṇḍalinī 507
nature of 508
Oṃ Namaḥ Śivāya (mantra) 35, 58, 509–11
seen as divine forms 481–82
siddha's words as 220
of Siddha Yoga 482, 509–11
So'ham (mantra) xxxix, 271, 474, 509–10
Swami Muktananda on 482
types of 508
as used in meditation 58fn*, 509
See also Mantra repetition; *Mantrayoga*; *Oṃ Namaḥ Śivāya*
Mantra repetition (*japa*)
as *ajapajapa* 482
as key practice 481–82
as means to awaken Kuṇḍalinī 481–82
and role of grace in 482
See also Mantra(s); *Mantrayoga*
Mantravīrya 417
Mantrayoga 507–11
goal of 508
and Kuṇḍalinī 507
and levels of speech 511
samādhi state in 517
See also *Mahāyoga*; Mantra(s)
Manu the Law-Giver 627n133
Matsyendranātha 466
Māyā (illusion) 434
as gift of Creator 454
and Kuṇḍalinī 470–72
limitation of (see *Māyīyamala*)
See also Ignorance; *Malas*
Māyīyamala 433, 434, 438–39
See also *Malas*
"Meditate on your own Self" 15, 138, 397
Meditation 485–87
as concentration turned inward 58fn*, 400
by "contagion" 58–59

Meditation (*continued*)
as core of Siddha Yoga sadhana 399–401, 403
as expression of devotion 461–62
experiences in 486–87, 561–62
goal of 58fn*, 486
as key spiritual practice 485
as key to Self-realization 461–62
and Kuṇḍalinī 485–87
on one's guru 267–68
as path to Self-knowledge 389–91
purpose of 568
to quiet the mind 390–91
in relation to grace 391
Revolution 81–83, 151, 409–10, 412
and role in forming siddhas 169
self-effort and grace in 486
and Self-knowledge 347
as Self-remembrance 485–86
as spontaneous form of yoga 485
as state 58fn*
Swami Muktananda's experiences in 36–39, 40
as teacher of meditation 58fn*, 485
Upaniṣadic instructions for 389–91
See also Practices, spiritual
Meghadūta (Cloud Messenger) 556
Melbourne 78, 79, 82
Memorization, of sacred texts 304–5
Merging, of guru and disciple 264–66
Message
of siddhas xxxvii
of Swami Chidvilasananda 136, 138
of Swami Muktananda xxxvii, 15, 138, 397
Microcosm, as identical to macrocosm 453–55, 462, 463, 464
Mind
in Indian thought 544–45
light of God in 401
respect for 401
steadied by meditation 391
Mokṣa. *See* Enlightenment
Monasteries
in Buddhist traditions 547–48
in Indian traditions 547, 548–49
Monks, Siddha Yoga 103–5
of both genders 103
initiations of, by Swami Muktananda 103–5, 118
leaving Siddha Yoga 127
vows of 104
Moral conduct. *See* Ethics; Moral responsibility; Purity; Virtues
Moral responsibility
Bhagavadgītā on 392–94
in Siddha Yoga teachings 402–4
in Vedānta 391–94, 403–4
See also Ethics
Mudrā(s) 503–5
of the siddhas 219–21
See also *Haṭhayoga*
Muktananda, meaning of name 28–29
Muktananda, Swami
absorbed in his guru 33–35
and abundance 52–53
and attitude to food 535
autobiography of 69, 491–92
Āyurvedic studies of 29
becoming a monk 28–29
birth of 26
books of 300; Appendix 1, 569–71
and chanting as spiritual discipline 535
charitable activities of 561
as contributor to yogic understanding 455
core teachings of 219, 403–4
daily schedule of 60–61
death of 122–25
and descriptions of higher states 455
as disciple xxxv–xxxvi, 32–36, 45–47, 324–26
and earliest seva 28
early devotees' memories of 54–56
early initiations by 57–59, 78–79, 82, 85
early life of 25–35
and early stays in ashrams 27–28, 367
early teaching by 56, 61–62
early writings of 67–69

ecumenical approach of 145fn*
egalitarianism of 318–19
ethical standards of 334–35
and ethical teachings 359–60
as explainer of shaktipat 420–21, 422
fiery aspects of 61–62
and first meeting with his guru 26–27
First world tour of 73–80
heart attack of 106
and his ashrams 44–45, 48–49, 53, 54, 60–62, 524–29
and his gardens 558
and his global mission 48–69
and his guru's commands 48–49, 54, 69
at his guru's death 47–48
and his love for his guru 175–81, 226–28, 234
during his sadhana 32–41, 499, 558–59
and his study of shaktipat 421–44
and his use of term "siddha" 167, 184–87, 190–91
and Indian poet-saints 368
and informal shaktipat 412–14
and initiation by touch 414
initiation of 34–36
inner sounds heard by 513
itinerant years of 29–31
and Jñāneśvar Mahārāj 185
and Kashmir Śaivism 56, 96–97
kriyās experienced by 36–37, 504–5
last will and testament of 106–7
leaving home 27
liberation of 40–41
as lineage guru xxiv–xxvi, xxxvi
as "lion of Ganeshpuri" 54–56, 61–62
and love for chanting 31–32
in Maharashtra 31–32
mahāsamādhi of 122–25
meditation experiences of 36–39, 40, 422–23
and meditation revolution 81–83, 409–10, 412
meeting his guru 26–27, 32–35
1974 departure speech of 81–82
nondualist teachings of 367–68
and *Oṃ Namaḥ Śivāya* 25–26
and other Indian saints 27–29, 170–74, 224
and overcoming addictions 89–90
passes lineage to co-successors 122
philanthropy of 152–55
and plans for succession 106–7, 117–18
power of initiation on 206–7
practical advice from 89–90, 95
receiving his name 28–29
as re-establisher of shaktipat 420–21, 422
revival of ancient traditions by 165–66
sadhana of 36–40
Second world tour of 80–99
as shaktipat guru 4–5
as siddha guru 237
with Siddharudha Swami 27–29
simple living of 52–53
spiritual generosity of 116–17
as spiritual scholar 48, 367–68, 421–22
as student of Vedānta 48, 367
subtle initiations by 412–14
and suffering 88–89
as teacher 58fn*, 96–97
and term "Siddha Yoga" 208
tested by his guru 33–34
and texts used in his sadhana 297–98
Third world tour of 107–13
and training of disciples 101
and training of Malti 99–101, 111–13
and transmission of Siddha Yoga 3
and use of scriptures 519–20
and view of Śiva 169
See also Muktananda, Swami, quoted on
Muktananda, Swami, quoted on:
ascent of Kuṇḍalinī 459, 470, 476, 480
Bhagawan Nityananda 9, 16, 33, 175, 176, 179, 180, 219, 254

Muktananda, Swami, quoted on:
(*continued*)
Blue Pearl 494–95, 514–15
body as temple 400–1
Citi Śakti 460–61, 463, 473
daily life 89–90
dharmic life 404
discipleship 231, 234–35
equality consciousness 395, 395–96
false gurus 109–10, 251–52
guru-disciple relationship 45–47, 252–53, 336, 450–51
guru principle (*gurutattva*) 271
Hari Giri Baba 172
his final realization 494–95
his initiation 418, 419–20
honoring the Self 397
Kuṇḍalinī 461, 462, 470, 473
liberation 40
living as a siddha 404
love 400–1
mahāyoga 497–99, 518–20
mantra 482
nature of guru 325, 331, 332, 334, 335, 336–37
nature of true siddha 190–91
qualifications of a guru 180–81
renunciation 337–39
role of scriptures 318–19, 321–22, 323
selfless service 404
siddha's state 168, 169, 202–4, 207, 208, 210, 214
Siddha Yoga as religion xxvii, xxix, xxxi–xxxii
siddhis 10fn*
subtle body 475–76
surrender to guru 335
true disciples 271
true gurus 251–53, 308–9, 314, 451, 484–85
Zipruanna 170–72
See also Muktananda, Swami
Mūlādhāra cakra, as abode of Kuṇḍalinī 474–75, 476
See also Chakras; Body, subtle
Mumukṣutva 246–47
Muppinarya Swami 28
Music. *See* Chanting

N

Nāḍīs. *See* Body, subtle
Nagad 39
Nāmdev 186
Nārada, in Upaniṣadic dialogue 374
Nārada Bhakti Sūtras 259–61
Nātha siddhas 183–84, 185–86
Jñāneśvar Mahārāj among 185
lineage of 185
and Swami Muktananda 186–87
See also Nātha traditions
Nātha traditions 466–68
Native Americans 145fn*
Nectar of Chanting 298–99
Neem Karoli Baba 76
Netraprakash (eye camps) 153–54, 608n306
New Delhi, Swami Muktananda in 54
New York, Swami Muktananda in 71
Nididhyāsana 546
Nirvāṇa 209–10
Nityananda, meaning of name 8
Nityananda, Bhagawan 7–24
and *ādivāsīs* 8–9, 14–15
apparent lack of guru of 193
as archetypical siddha xxvii
arriving in Tansa Valley 8
asceticism of 9
and attitude to *siddhis* 205
as *avadhūta* 9–10, 22, 177
bliss of 175–76
body of 176, 177–79
as born siddha (*janmasiddha*) 10–11, 196–97
as canonical "text" 324–26
and children 19
cryptic language of 9, 16, 35
culture around 22–24
darshan of 16–19, 23, 179–80, 275
death of 47–48
early life of 10–15
equality consciousness of 354–55
ethics of 327

as exemplary siddha 175–81
feasts given by 8–9
fierce demeanor of 19–22
and first meeting with Swami Muktananda 26–27
followers of 6
and Gavdevi temple 41–42
guru of 10–11, 616–17n50
as head of siddha lineage 193
initiating Swami Muktananda 35–36, 418, 419–20
initiatory methods of 18–19, 22, 35–36, 413–14
inner state of 9, 11, 23
installing Swami Muktananda in temple 41–42
life of 7–24
mahāsāmadhi of 47–48
on mantra repetition 35
monastic disciples of 44
naming of 11
as siddha guru 18fn*, 237
and Siddha Yoga canon 299
special powers (*siddhis*) of 8–10, 11–14
and start of Siddha Yoga 3, 5–6
stories about 8–9, 9–10, 11–13, 14–15, 16, 23, 26–27
Swami Muktananda on 9, 16, 175, 176, 179, 180, 219, 326
as Swami Muktananda's guru 32–36, 41–45, 47–48, 254, 418, 419–20, 557–58
on Swami Muktananda's liberation 41
and Swami Muktananda's love for 175–81, 226–28, 234
as teacher 15–24, 33, 324, 325–26
testing Swami Muktananda 33–35, 254
and Tulsi Amma 13
words of 180
"yogic fire" of 19–22

Nityananda, Swami 115–33
as co-successor to Swami Muktananda 115–33
initiation of 107
installed as co-successor 126
personal qualities of 117, 128, 131
questions about actions of 117–18, 130–33
relinquishment of vows by 131
resignation of 115–16, 131–33
tours of 127–28

Niyama (yogic self-control) 545

Nondualism xxxiv
of egoless guru 204
guru principle in 310
in Siddha Yoga xxviii, 367
in Siddha Yoga canon 288, 294–95
as taught by Bhagawan Nityananda 15
as taught by siddhas 202
as taught in Siddha Yoga 5
theism of 310
in Vedānta 364–65
See also Advaita Vedānta; Unity of being

O

Oakland (California) 94–95, 96, 145
Siddha Yoga ashram of 525, 561–62

Offering 529

Oṃ 447

Oṃ Namaḥ Śivāya (mantra)
as nonsectarian mantra 481
at Siddharudha Swami's ashram 27
as Siddha Yoga mantra 481–82, 509–11
in Swami Muktananda's initiation 35
and Swami Muktananda's mother 25–26
See also Mantra(s)

Oral traditions 304–5

P

Pādukā-Pañcakam, Śrī Guru 270–71

Pahelvan, Babu Rao 32

Pañcavidha-kṛtyas 432

Pāṇini 240–41, 541

Paramahaṃsa, meaning of term 41fn**

Paramārtha Katha Prasang (Swami Muktananda) 56

Patañjali 233–34, 463–64, 643–44n52
Peacock wand 86, 93
Perennialism
of Siddha Yoga theology xxix–xxx, xxxi–xxxii, xxxviii–xxxix
and Swami Muktananda 195–96
Perfectibility, human 329–30
See also Perfection
Perfection xl
as attainable goal xxxix
attained through discipleship 237
in different forms xl, xli
as quality of siddhas 167–68, 203–4
See also Perfectibility; Siddha(s)
Perspectives, epistemological 201
of siddhas 201–4
Philanthropy, Siddha Yoga 14–15, 152–55, 561
See also Ādivāsīs; PRASAD Project; Prison Project
Play of Consciousness (Swami Muktananda) 40, 69
effects of, on Swami Chidvilasananda 491–92
Poet-saints
of Maharashtra 361, 368
quoted in Siddha Yoga 295
See also Saints
Poland, Siddha Yoga in 151
Pope 306–7
Practices, spiritual 568
absorption in guru 267–68
benefits of 401
as body of God 486
contemplation 400 (*see also* Self-inquiry)
darshan 275–76
love as basis for 401–2
necessity for 399
in relation to Kuṇḍalinī 460
sharing experiences as 491
Swami Chidvilasananda on 486
See also Chanting; Meditation; Sadhana; Scriptural study; Seva
Prajāpati 542
Prajnananda, Swami 67
Prakṛti 208–9
Prāṇa 501–2, 507
five functions of 477
as form of Brahman 373
and *Haṃsa* mantra 510
and Kuṇḍalinī 473–77
nature of 473–74
as universal consciousness 473–75
See also Breath; *Haṭhayoga*; *Prāṇāyāma*(s)
Prāṇāyāma(s) 501, 503
in *rājayoga* 516
See also *Haṭhayoga*; *Prāṇa*
PRASAD Chikitsa 561
PRASAD Project 153–54, 561, 608n306
Prison Project, Siddha Yoga 109, 145, 154–55
Profane
in contrast to "sacred" 523, 531, 556
made sacred through ashram life 567–68
meaning of 523
and saṃskāras 531
Pūjā. *See* Worship
Purification
by awakened Kuṇḍalinī 37–40, 119, 459–60
begun through shaktipat xxxviii
through chanting 59–60
in *haṭhayoga* 502–3
through *kriyās* 411, 428–29, 439–40, 487–92
as means to liberation xxxix
after shaktipat 411, 428–29, 439–40, 469, 470
See also Body, subtle; *Kriyā*(s); Kuṇḍalinī, ascent of; Purity
Purity
attainment of 330, 331
in Siddha Yoga ethics 327–39
Swami Chidvilasananda on 330
See also Impurity; Purification
Puruṣa 208–9

Q

Qualandi (Kerala) 10–11

R

Rājayoga 515–17
eight "limbs" of 515–16
samādhi state in 517
See also *Mahāyoga*
Ramakrishna Paramahamsa 23, 48, 72, 168–69, 297, 609n8
Ramana Maharshi 29, 286
Rāmānuja 366
Rama Tirtha, Swami 72
Rāmāyaṇa 7, 549–50
Ram Dass (Richard Alpert) 75, 76, 81
Reality
as seen in classical yoga 208–9
as seen in Sāṃkhya traditions 208–9
as seen in Siddha Yoga xxviii
See also Reality, ultimate
Reality, ultimate
guru as form of 273–74
in Hinduism 349
in nondual Vedānta 375–76, 383–84
as seen in Upaniṣads 363
See also Reality; Truth
Recollection (*smṛti*) 305
in Siddha Yoga canon 282–89
Reincarnation, liberation from 437
Relationship, of guru and disciple. *See* Guru-disciple relationship
Religion, Siddha Yoga's status as xxvii–xxxiv, 288
Remembrance
of ashram 554, 555, 565–67
through forms and images xl–xli
of God 259, 540
See also Forgetfulness
Renunciation 245
and effect on Siddha Yoga canon 338–39
of sexual activity 337, 338
in Siddha traditions 216–18
in Siddha Yoga 337–40
as spiritual necessity 337–40
in Upaniṣads 209
Repetition, of mantra. *See* Mantra repetition
Respect
in compassion 402
for oneself 359
for others 359, 392–94
Responsibilities
moral, in Siddha Yoga teachings 402–4
moral, in Vedānta 391–94, 403–4
worldly 401–4
See also Ethics
Restraints (*yamas*) 515, 545
Retreats, spiritual
during Second world tour 85–86
in South Fallsburg 111
with Swami Muktananda 80
trainings during 95–96
See also Intensive(s)
Revelation (*śruti*) 305
in Siddha Yoga canon 282–89
Revolution, meditation 81–83, 151, 409–10, 412
See also Meditation
Right-Current (Tantric) paths xxxiv–xxxvii, 290, 327–28, 458
See also Left-current paths; Tantric traditions
Rudi (Albert Rudolph) 71
Rudolph, Albert (Rudi) 71
Russia, Siddha Yoga in 150–51

S

Sacred
in contrast to "profane" 523, 531, 556, 565–68
experience of, in ashrams 528–29, 565–67
meaning of 523, 531
as way of seeing 531
See also Profane; Sacredness
Sacrifice 529
inner and outer 542–43
of Kuṇḍalinī by Śiva 468–69
as seen in Siddha Yoga 136
Sadhana
compassion as practice in 402
confusion in 39–40
as destroyer of *malas* 438

Sadhana (*continued*)
emphasized in Second world tour 90–91
etymology of 235
grace and self-effort in 399
love as basis for 401–2
necessity for 399
rate of progress in 449
Swami Chidvilasananda on 399
See also Discipline, spiritual; Practices, spiritual
Sādhanasiddha 197
Sahasrāra
as Creator's entrance 633n136
and inner guru 269–70, 271
reunion of Śiva and Śakti 456–57
Sai Baba of Shirdi 125fn*, 168–69, 186, 196–97, 297
Śaiva Āgamas 289, 497, 499–500, 519–20
Śaiva traditions
on divine power 544–45
on five functions of Śiva 432
identity of Śiva in 229
kriyās in 490–91
on *malas* (impurities) 433–35
on shaktipat 416–18, 424–42
and the siddha 181–82
Śiva as original guru in 229
soteriology in 416
supreme deity of 388
Upaniṣads of 634n145
and views of Śiva 425
See also Abhinavagupta; Kashmir Śaivism; Śaiva Āgamas; Śiva
Śaiva yoga
goal of 310–11
guru principle in 310–12, 320–21
Śaivite traditions. *See* Kashmir Śaivism; Śaiva traditions
Śakti 426–27
concealing aspect of 427
concretized as world 427
cosmic nature of 427, 429–30
creative aspect of 426, 429–30
dynamic nature of 470–71
intelligence of 427–28
in nondualist yoga traditions 310–11
as one with Śiva 426
as power of consciousness 426–27
in relation to Śiva 310–11, 345, 426, 468–69
reunion of, with Śiva 456–57
revelatory aspect of 426, 427, 429
true nature of 451
See also Citi Śakti; Goddess; Kuṇḍalinī; Shaktipat
Śaktipāta. See Shaktipat
Śakuntalā, in *Abhijñānaśākuntala* 551–56
Samādhi
in different yogas 516
etymology of 456
sahajasamādhi 215–17, 218–19, 221
states of 214–16, 221
Swami Chidvilasananda on 274
Sāṃkhya traditions
ego in 381
and enlightenment 208–9
view of reality in 208–9
Saṃsāra, in nondual Vedānta 377
Sanatkumāra 374
Sandals, of guru 35, 270–71
Saṅkalpa (will, intention), of guru 98, 409
in Siddha Yoga xxiv–xxvii
as Śiva's will 409
Śaṅkara. *See* Śaṅkarācārya
Śaṅkarācārya 291, 364, 366–67
on Brahman 383–84
as founder of monasteries and monastic orders 548–49
on great beings 242
on guru-disciple relationship 244–48
on ignorance of reality 376
in Siddha Yoga teaching 283
Sannyāsa
and inner renunciation 337–38
as one path to enlightenment 337–38, 340
of Siddha Yoga gurus 338
See also Monks, Siddha Yoga

Sanskrit
etymologies (*see* Etymologies)
German study of 71–72
and powers of its letters 508
Saptah (long chant) 528–29
Sārasvatī Order (of monks) 28fn**, 366, 549
Śāstras 301
in Siddha Yoga canon 292–94
Satchidananda, Swami 73
Sat-cit-ānanda (truth, consciousness, and bliss)
as Brahman 375
Self as 357–59
Satellite broadcasts, of Intensives 5–6, 143, 150–51
Scholarship, about Siddha Yoga xli–xliii, xliv
Scriptural study
purpose of 293, 499
in Siddha Yoga 150, 321–23, 537–38
See also Scripture(s)
Scripture(s)
as corroborative of experience 317, 323, 499
defined in relation to guru 278–80
on guru's authority 312–14
limitations of 315–16, 321, 322–23
in Siddha Yoga 318–19, 321–23, 463
Swami Muktananda on 318–19, 321–23
See also Canon(s); Scriptural study
"See God in each other" 15, 138, 139, 360
Seeker. *See* Disciple; Discipleship; Student
Self 347–405
as abiding in heart 386–87
as absolute existence 357–59
as actor on own stage 454
in all love 379
as awareness 379–80
as being 354
as bliss (*ānanda*) 357–59, 380–81
Brahma Upaniṣad on 225
in Buddhism 349, 350–51
at center of Siddha Yoga ethic 347–48
as compassionate 402
as consciousness (*cit*) 351–52, 357–59
as defined by siddha gurus 351–60
as different gods 387–88
as distinct from body 348, 351
as distinct from "small" self 348, 351–52
as distinctively Hindu concept 349
as embodied in guru 229–32
experienced as love 401–2, 405
as expressed in selfless service 402–4
fruits of knowing 227
as God 229–32, 274–75, 349, 355–57
guru needed to find 224–26
in Hinduism 349
as inner guru 268–69, 272–73
as inner witness 384
and Islam 349
as "knower of the field" 351–52, 355
as love 359–60
names for 460
as one in many 310
as only reality 349
qualities of 356–57
as *sat-cit-ānanda* 357–59
as sense objects 392
as supreme reality 349, 354–55
Swami Muktananda's message about 15, 138, 397
as universal Lord 387–89
as universal subject 349–54, 384–85
as universal truth 358
as unknowable by mind 384–86
as without qualities 379
as witness 351–52
See also Ātman; Self, individual; Self, inner; Self-knowledge
Self-effort xxxix, xl, 148
and grace 337, 399, 485–87
in Kuṇḍalinī awakening 480
need for, after shaktipat 429
in practices 485–86
on spiritual path 399

Self, individual (*jīva*)
as Brahman 383–87
as outer form of Kuṇḍalinī 453–54
in relation to Ātman 381–83
in Vedānta 381–83
Self-inquiry 139, 149–50
See also Contemplation
Selfishness, compassion as antidote for 402
See also Ego
Self-knowledge
benefits of 227, 354
cultivated by practices 347
to end suffering 395–96
as goal of Siddha Yoga 347
through grace 391, 397–98
through grace of Self 398
guru needed for 224–26
liberating effects of 353, 368, 389, 396
through meditation 389–91
only through sadhana 399
strengthened by scriptural study 347
Selfless service. *See* Seva
Self-realization
Jñāneśvar Mahārāj on 493
nature of 493, 495
Swami Muktananda on 40
See also Enlightenment; Liberation
Self-Realization Fellowship 72
Sense objects, seen as Self 392
See also Senses
Senses, as seen in Siddha Yoga 362
See also Sense objects
Separation
freedom from 500
from God 253, 254
Service
to one master (*ekagurūpāsti*) 324–27
to others 393–94, 404
selfless (*see* Seva)
Seva (*gurusevā*, selfless service) 249–56
in ancient India 250–51
in ashrams 59, 532
Bhagavadgītā on 249–50, 261
as central Siddha Yoga teaching 136, 143–45
fruits of 532–33
in Gurudev Siddha Peeth 535–37
as one's *dharma* 393–94, 404
performed for disciple's sake 254
in Siddha Yoga 143–44, 250
with Swami Muktananda 83–84, 101–2
Swami Muktananda on 404
in Swami Muktananda's early life 28
during world tours 83–84
as worship 394
Sevananda, Swami 57
Shaivism. *See* Kashmir Shaivism; Śaivism
Shaktipat 407–44
Abhinavagupta on 430–32
around a siddha 59
as awakening of Kuṇḍalinī energy 421, 426–27
and awakening of love 443–44
as beginning of spiritual journey 399, 415
bestowed by Śiva's will 440–42
bestowed during Intensives 5–6, 150–51, 538
bestowed only by *sadguru* 436
in *Bhagavadgītā* 397
by Bhagawan Nityananda 18–19, 22, 413–14
as central to Siddha Yoga xxxvii–xxxviii
conceptual structure for 424–28
differences in experiences of 431, 438–39
earliest texts on 407, 408–9
in early days of Gurudev Siddha Peeth 57–59
effects of 4, 443–44
etymology of 407
experiences of 57–59, 64–65, 75, 78–79, 86–88, 412–13, 414–15, 428, 479–80, 483–84
experience vs. theory of 422
experiential evidence for 442–44
by guru's will 98
heart-opening effect of 443–44
as highest form of initiation 428
historical rarity of 408, 410, 428

as indispensable for liberation 425–26, 438
informal transmissions of 412–14, 483–84
as initiating *mahāyoga* 477–78
and karma 18, 440–42
in Kashmir Śaivism 430–33
and Kuṇḍalinī 478–85
levels of intensity of 431, 438–39
Malti's experience of 64–65
mass bestowal of 92–93
means of bestowing 409
as means to Self-knowledge 398, 399
necessity of 433
as new birth 444
as planting seed of liberation 436
prerequisites to receiving 408
in relation to initiation 407–8, 409
responses to 428–29 (*See also Kriyās*)
as revelatory act 426, 427–28
as safest through guru's grace 480
in Śaiva Siddhānta tradition 18
in Śaivite philosophy 424–42
seen as birthright, in Siddha Yoga 458
by self-effort 480
as sole means to overcome *malas* 433, 434–35
Swami Chidvilasananda on 4, 418, 428, 458, 480–81
Swami Muktananda's experience of 35–36
textual sources on 416, 423–24
and timing of bestowal 440–42
by touch 93, 414
transforming power of 410–11, 442–44
as transmission of spiritual power 409
universality of 420
in Vedāntic narratives 397
See also Initiation; Intensive(s); *Kriyās*; Kuṇḍalinī; Shaktipat guru
Shaktipat guru 48
Shaligram Swami (Swami Dayananda) 44
Sharing, in Siddha Yoga 57, 152, 491
Shetty, Subhash 107, 115
See also Nityananda, Swami
Shirdi, Sai Baba of 125fn*, 168–69, 186, 196–97, 297
Shivananda Swami 29
Shree Gurudev Ashram Trust 560
Shree Muktananda Ashram 110–11
accessibility of 152
appearance of 523
development of 562
founding of 110–11
geographical setting of 521–23
renaming of 110fn*
See also Ashram(s); Ashrams, Siddha Yoga
Shriyan, Venkappanna 44–45, 51, 65, 107, 525–26, 532–33
Siddha(s) 165–221
associated with mountains 183
as *avadhūta* 177
Bhagawan Nityananda as example of 175–81
from birth (*janmasiddhas*) 10–11
bliss of 175–76, 210
complete freedom of 189
defined as a state 297
definitions of term, in Sanskrit 187, 609n3
as dwelling in *siddhaloka* 187, 193, 212
earliest uses of term 182–83
as enlightened in this world 217–18
as enlightened teacher 220–21
equality consciousness of 214–15
equivalent terms for 191
essential role of lineage for 190–91
etymology of 280
examples of 169–172, 175–81
gesture (*mudrā*) of 219–21
Hari Giri Baba as example of 172
hidden qualities of 170
in Indian spirituality 165–221
as *jīvanmukta* 174–75
as knower of the truth 203
as link in a meta-lineage 194–95
meanings of term 187–88, 190–91, 194–96, 609n3

Siddha(s) (*continued*)
meanings of term, typology of 190–200
omniscience of 219–20
from other religions 191, 194–96
as pan-Indian category 181–82
paradoxical nature of 168–75, 203, 210, 214–15
perfection of 203–4, 219–20
as philosopher's stone 202–3
popular Indian notions of 187–89, 206
and relationship to *siddhi*s 204–7
retroactive identifications of 181
revolutionary nature of 220–21
in Śaivite traditions 181–82
as sectarian term 183–84
significance of body of 176, 177–79
speech of 220
state of 167–69, 200–4, 230, 297
Swami Muktananda's typology of 196–97
Swami Muktananda's understandings of 167, 184–87, 190–91
as teacher of nonduality 202
as term connecting all enlightened beings 191, 194–96
as term marking initiatory connection 190
as term marking institutional affiliation 190
as transhistorical category 194–96
words of 220
Zipruanna as example of 169–72
See also Enlightenment; Guru; Shaktipat guru; Siddha guru; Siddha lineage(s); *Siddhaloka*; Siddha traditions
Siddha guru
as bestower of shaktipat 408, 409
and disciple's karmas 18
as ethical exemplar 333–34
etymology of 408
as grace-bestower 313, 314, 315, 325
for guiding Kuṇḍalinī 480–81
throughout history 236–37
as identical with Kuṇḍalinī 447
as the means 238
as perfect disciple 237
primary function of 462
purity in freedom of 331
qualifications of 236–37
as shaktipat guru 408
in Siddha Yoga 237
as Śiva 435–36
and source of power of 238
teaching methods of 19
will (*saṅkalpa*) of xxiv–xxv, 98, 409
See also Enlightenment; Guru; Siddha
Siddha lineage(s)
according to Swami Muktananda 187, 615n38
blessings from 211
as ecumenical concept 193–96
as lineage of Bhagawan Nityananda 193
as linked to Śiva 192–93, 196
Śaivite orientations of 169, 181–82
Swami Muktananda on 615n38
typology of 191–96
See also Lineage; Nātha siddhas; Siddha; Siddha traditions
Siddhaloka 106, 187, 193, 195, 196, 211–12
Siddharudha Swami 27–28, 59, 116fn*
Siddha traditions
created from other traditions 281
enlightenment in 210–11, 213–19
historical background of 181–89
in Maharashtra 186
Jñāneśvar Mahārāj in 186
recent scholarship on 609n2
renunciation in 216–18
and Śaivite traditions 181–82
and their canons 278–80, 285–86
See also Siddha; Siddha lineage(s)
Siddha Yoga
accessibility of 151, 152
apolitical nature of xxxiii
basic teachings of xxxvii, 397
canon of 277–346
celebrations in 135
as collective path 144

Constitution of 591n16
as contemporary term xxv–xxvi
core concepts of 49, 447
culture of 95–96, 98–99, 105
definition of 447
as different from Vedānta 361–62
discipleship in 141 (*see also* Discipleship; Guru-disciple relationship)
ethical values of 281–82 (*see also* Ethics)
first use of term 67–69
goal of 49–51, 208, 449, 462
and guru principle 311
and guru's intent (*saṅkalpa*) xxiv–xxvi
haṭhayoga in 503
inclusivist theology of xxix, xxx–xxxiii
and Kashmir Śaivite worldview 361–62
as *mahāyoga* 197–98, 497, 518
mainstream nature of 151
mantras in 482
meanings of Sanskrit term 167, 208
meditation in 485–87
mission of 4, 81–83, 409–10
on moral responsibility 402–4 (*see also* Ethics)
mystical basis for xxix–xxx, xxxii–xxxiii
as mystical Hinduism xxxiii
as named by Swami Muktananda xxiv–xxvi
nondogmatic nature of 288–89, 297
nondualism of xxviii, 5
nonsectarian nature of 288–89, 291
as path of devotion 198
as path of guru's grace 198
as path of love 198
perennialist theology of xxix–xxx, xxxi–xxxii, xxxviii–xxxix
renunciation in 337–39
as Right-Current (Tantric) path xxxiv–xxxvii, 290, 327–28
role of guru in 447
sacrifice in 136
scriptural sources of 280–301
scriptures in 318–19, 321–23
sharing in 491
spiritual continuity within 6
and status as religion xxvii–xxxiv, 288
and its students' lifestyle xxx–xxxi, 98–99
subtle body in 447–50
and Tantric traditions 289–91
and term's significance 208
Vedāntic values in 403–4
and view of reality xxviii
as world religion xxvii–xxxiv
See also Canon, Siddha Yoga; Chidvilasananda, Swami; Muktananda, Swami; Nityananda, Bhagawan; Siddha guru; Siddha Yoga gurus; Siddha Yoga (history of); SYDA Foundation; Teachings, Siddha Yoga
Siddha Yoga (history of) 3–161
broadening of base of 80–83
expansion of 80–83, 136–38, 140–43
first Western students of 71
as global community 5–6, 139, 140
organizational development of 80–83, 92–95, 140–43
post-Muktananda transitional period in 126–34
as story of three masters 3, 6
See also Chidvilasananda, Swami; Muktananda, Swami; Nityananda, Bhagawan; Siddha Yoga; Succession, in Siddha Yoga
Siddha Yoga gurus
experiential primacy for 463, 464–65
and interest in *haṭhayoga* 465
nonsectarian teachings of 463
source of authority of 308, 311–19
and teachings of Patañjali 463–64
See also Guru; Siddha Yoga
Siddha Yoga lineage, transmission of
by Bhagawan Nityananda 47–48
by Swami Muktananda 106–7, 115–18, 121–22

Siddhi(s) (supernatural powers)
of Bhagawan Nityananda 8–10, 11–14
Bhagawan Nityananda's attitude to 205
secondary 204–5
siddha's relationship to 204–7
supreme 204–7
Swami Muktananda on 10fn*
Sikh gurus 296–97
Silence 322–23, 344
Sin xxxix
Singh, Jaideva 97
Śiṣya (disciple) 235
See also Disciple; Discipleship; Student
Śiva
as all reality 321, 344–45
in apparent bondage 430–31, 433–35
as cause of grace 430–31
concealing play of 430–31, 433–35
divine sport of 430–31
embodied to bestow grace 435–36
fivefold cosmic actions of 432
free will of 440–42
grace-bestowing power of 432–33, 434–35
as guru 311, 312, 314, 318
guru's identity with 202–3, 208
as head of all siddha lineages 192
as name for consciousness 425
in nondualist yoga traditions 310–11, 312
nonpersonal forms of 425
as one with *śakti* 426
personified forms of 425
in physical form of guru 174, 272, 435–36
as primordial guru 192, 199, 229
in relation to Śakti 310–11, 345, 456–57, 468–69
returning to himself 425–26, 434–35
reunion of, with Śakti 456–57
as seen by Śaivism 229–30
as seen by Swami Muktananda 169
as source of Siddha Yoga 199
viewpoint of 201–4
See also Śaiva traditions; *Śivo'ham*
Śivamānasapūjā (chant) 291
Sivananda, Swami (of Rishikesh) 23, 73
Śiva Sūtras 313
Śivo'ham ("I am Śiva"), experiencing truth of 425, 438
Sleep, of Kuṇḍalinī 454–56, 469–70, 471, 494
Smārta traditions 286–87, 292
See also Recollection
Smṛti. *See* Recollection
Social service. *See* Philanthropy; PRASAD Chikitsa; PRASAD Project; Prison Project
So'ham mantra xxxix, 271, 474, 509–10
See also Mantra(s)
Sound(s)
associated with Kuṇḍalinī 472
inner (unstruck) 512–13
and *layayoga* 512–13
in Śabda Advaita Vedānta 365
South Fallsburg. *See* Shree Muktananda Ashram
South India, and Siddha Yoga canon 295
Spanda, as pulsation of consciousness (Citi) 468–69
Speech
of a siddha 220
three levels of 511
Spiritual experiences. *See* Experiences, spiritual
Śravaṇa 546
Śruti. *See* Revelation
Stories
crow king and owl king 202
Eklavya's devotion 267
Kabīr and the millstone 242–43
Student
as *adhikārin* 546
as *antevāsin* 546
in Indian traditions 240–41, 545–46
See also Disciple; Discipleship
Students, of Siddha Yoga 143–48
ashram stays of 145

daily life for 138–40
diversity of 145fn*, 148, 151
in Europe 140
as a global community 139–40
lifestyle of xxx–xxxi, 98–99
self-effort of 148
social service by 152–55
Swami Chidvilasananda as example for 128, 135–36
See also Disciple; Guru-disciple relationship; Sadhana; Seva; Yoga
Study, scriptural. *See* Scriptural study
Subhash Shetty 107, 115
See also Nityananda, Swami
Succession, in Siddha Yoga
after Bhagawan Nityananda 47–48
controversy around, in 1980's 115–18, 130–33
manifestation of guru principle in 126–27
after Swami Muktananda 115–34
Swami Muktananda's plans for 106–7, 115–16
transitional period in (1981–86) 126–34
See also Chidvilasananda, Swami; Lineage; Malti; Nityananda, Swami; Subhash Shetty
Suffering
as result of ignorance 394–95
due to separation from God 242–43
Swami Chidvilasananda on 128
See also Ignorance; Separation
Sufi stories 297
Suki 39
Superimposition, in nondual Vedānta 376–77
Surrender 140
to one's guru 335
in Siddha Yoga teachings 140
of Swami Muktananda to his guru 34–35
See also Guru-disciple relationship; Renunciation
Suṣumṇānāḍī 474–76
ascent of Kuṇḍalinī through 449, 459, 475–76
representing path of Siddha Yoga 476
See also Body, subtle
Śvetaketu, in Upaniṣadic dialogue 380
Swamis, Siddha Yoga. *See* Monks, Siddha Yoga
SYDA Foundation
establishment of 94–95, 562
first president of 95
Malti's service to 113
Symbolism
erotic, around Kuṇḍalinī 457
through inversion 454–57
Synchronic truth 320–21

T

Tamil Sittars 186
Tansa River Valley 7–8
Tantra
of the Left-Current xxxiv–xxxv, 290, 327–28, 457
of the Right-Current xxxiv–xxxvi, 290, 327–28, 458
See also Tantric traditions
Tantric traditions
in Buddhism 189
esoteric claims of 289
Goddess in 388–89
on guru-disciple relationship 248
and *Gurugītā* chant 290–91
on guru's transforming power 262
Kuṇḍalinī energy in 231
and *kuṇḍalinīyoga* 641n2
Śākta Upaniṣads of 634n147
on shaktipat 416–18
and Siddha Yoga canon 289–91, 292
and *smārta* traditions 286–87
See also Tantra
Taoism 297
Tapas (heat). See *Tapasya*
Tapasya (austerity) 531–33, 541–42, 543
as destroyer of *saṃskāras* 531
fruits of 531–32, 533, 568
in Indian scriptures 541–42
meanings of 541–42

Tattvas 228–29
See also Guru principle (*gurutattva*)
Teacher(s)
in Hindu tradition 239–41
lineages of 233–34
need for, to transmit truth 233–34
Sanskrit terms for 239
Siddha Yoga monks as 103
training of 95–96, 97–98
types of 239
See also Guru; Student
Teachings, Siddha Yoga
ecumenical aspects of 145fn*
through formal study 96, 97–98
through Intensives 150–51
new forms for 148–50
practical emphasis of 138–40
preservation of 95–96
through questions and answers 79–80, 85, 96
through scriptural study 150, 321–23, 537–38
self-inquiry in 139, 149–50
on selflessness 136, 143–44
surrender in 140
See also Canon, Siddha Yoga; Courses; Teachers; Trainings; Appendix 3, 581–88
Technology
and Siddha Yoga canon 301
and transmission of traditions 305
Theism, in Upaniṣads 257
Tirtha, Swami Rama 72
Tours, of Swami Chidvilasananda 127–30, 140–41, 145
Tours, of Swami Muktananda 71–113
in Australia 79, 83
in California 83
challenging conditions in 84–85, 101
and development of centers 82–83, 102
emphasis on sadhana during 90–91, 101
First world tour 73–80
Indian traditions preserved in 83–84
instruction on Kuṇḍalinī in 91–92
Intensives during (1974–76) 92–93
itineraries for, *see* Appendix 2, 575–79
on-the-job learning in 84–85
organizational development during 92–95
retreats during 85–86
role of swamis (monks) in 105
Second world tour 80–99
seva during 83–84
Third world tour 107–13
as traveling ashram 83–84
Tours, of Swami Nityananda 127–28
Traditions
oral 304–5
transmitted by canons 302–5
transmitted by different means 304–5
See also Buddhism; Canon(s); Traditions, Hindu
Traditions, Hindu. *See* Bhakti traditions; Nātha traditions; Śaiva traditions; Smārta traditions; Tantric traditions; Vaiṣṇavite traditions; Vedāntic traditions; Vedas; Yogic traditions
Trainings, Siddha Yoga 95–98
See also Courses; Teacher(s); Teachings
Transcendental Meditation (TM) 73
Triadic form, of absolute 634n149
Trivedi, Pratibha. *See* Prajnananda, Swami
Trust, of disciple in guru 241–43
Trust, Shree Gurudev Ashram 560
Truth
aparā (ordinary) level of 342
embodied in guru 320–21
multiple levels of 340–45
as nature of Self 358
nature of 233
parā ("beyond") level of 344
parāparā (mixed) level of 343
and relation to scriptures 321–23
revealed by Kuṇḍalinī 453
synchronic and diachronic 320–21

timelessness of 320–21
See also Knowledge; Reality, ultimate
Tukārām Mahārāj 186, 192
Tulsi Amma 13
Turīya state 380

U

Uddālaka, in Upaniṣadic dialogue 380
Unity. See *Layayoga*
Unity of being 310–11
See also Nondualism
Universalism 195
and Swami Muktananda 195–96
Universe
created by divine playfulness 456
as pulsation (*spanda*) of Citi 468–69
Upaniṣads 362–64
core teaching of 363
dialogues in 372, 374–75, 378–79, 380
guru-disciple relationship in 223–24
on meditation 389–91
on nature of Brahman 373–74
path to liberation in 209
renunciation in 209
in Siddha Yoga canon 282
Usgaon 608n306

V

Vaiṣṇavite traditions 366
and Siddha Yoga 287
supreme deity of 388
Upaniṣads of 634n146
Vajreshwari (village) 7, 95, 558
Vajreśvarī 7
Vallabha. *See* Vallabhācārya
Vallabhācārya 364–65, 395
Vālmīki. *See Rāmāyaṇa*
*Vārkarī*s (in Maharashtra) 31, 295
Vedānta (the)
canon of 362–64
defined 362
etymology of 362
and experience of siddha gurus 405
forms of 364–66
forms of, in Siddha Yoga 364–66
and identity of Brahman with Ātman 383–87
and Kuṇḍalinī 464–65
on moral responsibilities 391–94
nondual (Advaita) 364–66, 375–77, 383–84 (*see* Vedānta, Advaita)
Self in 347–405
and Siddha Yoga 347–405
significance of 363–64
as source for other Hindu traditions 361
as source for Siddha Yoga teachings on Self 361
and Swami Muktananda's teachings 403–4
See also *Bhagavadgītā*; Brahman; Śaṅkarācārya; Upaniṣads; Vedānta, Advaita; Vedāntic traditions; Vedas
Vedānta, Advaita (nondual) 364–66, 375–77, 383–84
primary texts of 294
in Siddha Yoga canon 284, 286, 293–94
See also Nondualism; Vedānta
Vedāntic traditions
on guru-disciple relationship 243–48
on the Self 263
on seva 250–51
See also Vedānta; Vedānta, Advaita; Vedas
Vedas
attributed to sages 305
authority of 319
etymology of 368
great teachings of 361
oral transmission of 305
origins of 311, 312
when taught by guru 311–12
worldview of 368
See also Upaniṣads; Vedānta; Vedāntic traditions
Venkappanna Shriyan 44–45, 51, 65, 107, 525–26, 532–33
Venkatesananda, Swami 23, 73

Venkateshwar Rao 131–33
See also Nityananda, Swami; Shetty, Subhash
Vihāras (Buddhist monasteries) 547–48
Vīraśaivism 295, 598n90, 622n24
and Swami Muktananda 186
view of liberation in 211
Virtues
developed through discipleship 237
emphasized in Siddha Yoga 327
needed by disciple 243–49
need to protect 540
as reflection of human perfection 329
Swami Chidvilasananda on 249, 617n102
See also Ethics
Vishnudevananda, Swami 73
Visions
after shaktipat 429
See also Light(s), divine
Viṣṇu Sahasranāma 298–99
Vivekacūḍāmaṇi 234
on guru-disciple relationship 244–48
on paths to liberation 257
Vivekananda, Swami 72, 286

W

Waste, avoided by Swami Muktananda 53
Western seekers 71–73
in Siddha Yoga 79–80
See also Tours, of Swami Chidvilasananda; Tours, of Swami Muktananda
Will, of guru xxiv–xxv, 98, 409
Witness
as identical to Self 351–52
within individual self 384
See also *Puruṣa*
Worship
through ashram activities 529, 538–39
ashram's formal ceremonies of (*pūjā*) 538–39
mental, of guru 269

Y

Yajña (fire ritual) 135–36, 538–39
Yājñavalkya, in Upaniṣadic dialogue 372–73, 378–79
Yama (yogic restraint) 515, 545
Yande, Pratap (Dada) 51
Yeola 31, 32, 36
Yoga
commitment to 500
definitions of xxii–xxiii
etymology of xxii
goals of 500
kinds of 464, 477, 497–501, 517–18
need for teacher in xxii
in Śaiva Āgamas 497, 500–1
steadfastness in 339
Swami Chidvilasananda on xxii–xxiii
See also *Mahāyoga*; Siddha Yoga; Yoga traditions
Yoga Sūtras 292
Yoga traditions
in *Bhagavadgītā* 166
and enlightenment 208–9
and *kuṇḍalinīyoga* 463–64
self-discipline in 545
on seva 250–51
view of reality in 208–9
See also Yoga
Yogananda, Paramahamsa 72

Z

Zen Buddhism 350–51, 598–99n90
See also Buddhism
Zipruanna 32, 169–72, 332–33
Zweig, Paul 86–88

Author Index

Citations to works by Swami Chidvilasananda, Swami Muktananda, and other primary sources (or their translations) have been omitted from this index. References to endnotes in the index are expressed as, for example, 598n90 (page 598, note 90). References to footnotes are expressed as, for example, 125fn (footnote * on page 125).*

A

Agrawala, V. S. 616n63
Alper, Harvey 646n109
Aurobindo, Śrī 648n23

B

Babb, Lawrence 606n262
Bailly, Constantina Rhodes 625n70
Basham, A. L. 589n1
Bendet, Peggy 651n40
Bharati, Agehananda 622n13
Brooks, Douglas Renfrew 592n34, 593n47, 621n1, 622n13, 625n67, 634n149, 641n2, 643nn. 30, 31; 646n99
Burns, Edward McNall 604–5n227

C

Clifford, James 593n47
Conze, Edward 613n85

D

Dalal, B. P. 600n109
Dasgupta, S. 610n33
Davis, Richard H. 637n1, 638n17
Deussen, Paul 632n101, 635n158
Dimmitt, Cornelia 642n27
Dobrovolny, Janet L. 647n122
Dowman, Keith 187–89
Dumoulin, Heinrich SJ 599n90, 604n227
Durgananda, Swami 620n180
Durkheim, Emil 592n31
Dutt, Sukumar 652n63, 653nn. 78, 79
Dvivedi, V. V. 622n13
Dyczkowski, Mark 610n31

E

Eliade, Mircea 184, 609n1, 610n41, 613n94, 650nn. 4, 5, 6

F

Ferrar, Harold 642n25
Ferrar, Jane 650n16, 654n109
Fort, Andrew 613n88
Franklin, George 602n188, 603n192

G

Geertz, Clifford xlv, 593n48
Ghurye, G. S. 653n83
Goldin, Marilyn 609n315
Gompers, Alan 608n309
Goudriaan, Teun 622nn. 12, 13
Greco, Tony 607n290
Green, William Scott 593n49, 621n1
Gupta, Sanjukta 622nn. 12, 13

H
Haberman, David 612n84
Hatengdi, M. U. 623n28
Hess, Linda 611n45
Hoover, Thomas 598n90, 604n227
Huxley, Aldous 591n21, 611n57

I
Isherwood, Christopher 609n8

J
Jain, Virenda Kumar 650n3
Jaini, Padmanabh 613n86
Johnsen, Linda 607n268, 608n311, 650n2
Johnson, Willard L. 605n227
Joshi, Keshav Ramchandra 590n10

K
Kakar, Sudhir 642n28
Kane, P. V. 653nn. 85, 87
Kemter, Robert 641n63
Kripananda, Swami 641n61, 645n63

L
Larson, Gerald J. 612n82
Lerner, Robert E. 605n227

M
Mahony, William K. 615n44
Marwah, R. N. 600n103
McDaniel, June 610n15
Meacham, Standish 605n227
Mookerji, Radha Kumud 652n72
Muller–Ortega, Paul 592n34, 610n25, 646n93
Mumme, Patricia 613n88

N
Nanda, B. N. 600n102
Neusner, Jacob 593n49, 621n1
Nirmalananda, Swami 600n111

O
Obel, Gita 600n104
Olivelle, Patrick 651n42, 652n48

P
Padoux, André 622n13
Pennington, Kenneth 604n227
Potter, Karl 612n68
Prajnananda, Swami 596nn. 44, 53; 600n123, 639n31
Proudfoot, Wayne 589n3

R
Rabinow, Paul 593n47
Ram Dass 76, 299, 601nn. 144, 147, 148, 153
Ramanujan, A. K. 598n90, 610n28, 611n46
Ranade, R. D. 610n32
Rigopoulos, Antonio 609n9
Robinson, Richard H. 605n227

S
Sanderson, Alexis 638nn. 17, 18
Sastri, V. V. 610n27
Sax, William S. 593n47
Schimmelpfennig, Bernhard 604n227
SenSharma, Debabrata 640n53
Sethi, V. K. 41fn*, 596n36
Shantananda, Swami 651nn. 32, 33, 35, 36
Sharma, Baldev Raj 632n101
Sharpe, Don 79
Shāstrī, Mukund Rām 637n3
Silburn, Lillian 642n14
Singh, Huzur Maharaj Sawan 599n90
Singh, Shukdev 611n45
Smart, Ninian 612n68
Speeth, Kathleen 602nn. 164, 169
Spiro, Melford 592n31

Staal, Fritz 645n66

T

Tagore, Rabindranath 611n45
Thursby, Gene 604n226, 605nn. 244, 245; 606n262
Tirtha, Swami Shankar Purushottam 646n91
Toomey, Tom 608n310

U

Uchiyama, Kōshō 629nn. 8, 9
Ullal, C. D. 654nn. 100, 101, 107

V

Vail, Lise 604n227
van Buitenen, J. A. B. 11, 589nn. 4, 6; 620n178, 642n27
Varenne, Jean 642nn. 10, 12
Vaudeville, Charlotte 611n45
Venkatesananda, Swami 22, 596n40
Vishnu Tirtha, Maharaj, Swami 39fn*, 593n4, 646n91, 649nn. 33, 34, 38

W

Washington, Peter 601n138
White, David Gordon 183–84, 591n14, 609n2, 610nn. 24, 29, 30, 34, 37, 43; 642n9, 644n59
Woodroffe, Sir John 648n18, 649n42, 650n76

Y

Yogananda 601n140
Yogananda, Paramahamsa 72
Yogendrajnani 649n36

Z

Zenji, Dōgen 629n8
Zweig, Paul 602n165, 650nn. 1, 7, 8; 654n112

The Muktabodha Indological Research Institute

The Muktabodha Indological Research Institute is a not-for-profit educational center dedicated to Indological research and to the publication of studies, historical research, and interpretations and translations of South Asian texts. Agama Press is one of the imprints of the Muktabodha Institute. The Institute recognizes and honors different approaches and forms of scholarship that make significant contributions to our understanding of South Asian studies and seeks in every effort to sustain standards of excellence and academic integrity. In addition to research and publications, the Muktabodha Institute also supports such archival work as the microfilming of texts and the video documentation of traditional *yajñas*, and periodically sponsors international gatherings for scholars of Indology.

MEDITATION REVOLUTION

A History and Theology of the Siddha Yoga Lineage

This groundbreaking collection of essays explores the origin, development, teachings, and practices of a contemporary spiritual movement. The subject is Siddha Yoga, a path of meditation rooted in the Indian philosophical tradition that has had tremendous impact on contemporary students of spirituality since the 1970s. This book centers around the work of two teachers: Swami Muktananda, who introduced Siddha Yoga and its teachings to the West, inspiring what he termed a "meditation revolution," and Gurumayi Chidvilasananda, who has brought Siddha Yoga to maturity as a global spiritual movement. *Meditation Revolution* examines one particular tradition in its historical and theological context, illumining issues that will be of interest to serious students of religion and spirituality.

From the Foreword:

Paul Muller-Ortega, Douglas Renfrew Brooks, William K. Mahony, Swami Durgananda, et al., offer herein a rich feast of historical and theological reflection that is sympathetic to Siddha Yoga but at the same time is fully faithful to the canons of critical inquiry characteristic of serious history of religions work. . . . One very much hopes that this collection may be the first of many other collections that dare to move away from purely descriptive scholarship in order to address some of the great spiritual issues of our time.

GERALD J. LARSON

Rabindranath Tagore Professor of Indian Cultures and Civilizations
and Director, India Studies Program, Indiana University, Bloomington

ISBN 0-9654096-0-0
90000>
9 780965 409605

AGAMA PRESS